Donald Brode M.D.

WITHDRAWN

D1270951

MEDICINE *throughout* ANTIQUITY

MEDICINE
throughout
ANTIQUITY

by

Benjamin Lee Gordon, M.D.

Member American Association of the History of
Medicine and American Academy of Ophthalmology
and Otolaryngology. Certified by American Board of
Ophthalmology. Attending Ophthalmologist to Shore
Memorial Hospital, Somers Point, New Jersey, and to
Atlantic County Hospital for Tuberculous Diseases
and Atlantic County Hospital for Mental Diseases,
Northfield, N. J. Authorized Medical Examiner for
Civil Aeronautics Administration, Dept. of Com-
merce, Washington, D. C. Author of "The Romance
of Medicine."

Foreword by

Dr. Max Neuburger

157 Illustrations

PHILADELPHIA
F. A. Davis Company • Publishers
1949

PRINTED IN THE UNITED STATES OF AMERICA

To my wife DOROTHY,
the following pages are
affectionately dedicated

Foreword

THE AUTHOR of this volume is one of the few practitioners who combines a lively interest in the history of medicine with sound and solid method in historical research. For quite some time now, he has been proving his capacity along these lines. Each of his technical articles in the *Archives of Ophthalmology* shows historical background in keeping with the standard set by Hirschberg. The author's publications dealing with medicine among the Hebrews rest on deep and critical scholarship, reminiscent of Preuss. Gordon's book *Romance of Medicine* combines enjoyable readability with richness of content. It has been widely acclaimed, gone through two editions, and is being translated into Spanish. Its virtues characterize, but to a still greater extent, this distinguished and comprehensive work: *Medicine throughout Antiquity*.

This book, in many ways, is distinctive in the literature on medical history. Hitherto, writers have provided only the briefest account of prehistoric medicine and, after a more or less sketchy description of medicine in the Orient, give us the main chapters of ancient medicine: those on Greece and Rome. In Gordon's work, however, pre-Greek medicine fills Part I, comprising 429 pages. In Part II, he admirably describes Greek, Alexandrian, and Roman medicine from the sources and with reference to general cultural environment; to this he adds an account of Talmudic medicine.

Gordon distinguishes three periods in ancient medicine: (1) the prehistoric, starting from the earliest times; (2) the protohistoric; and (3) the age that began with Ionic philosophy and ended with the fall of Rome. He has worked through a vast body of material, with reference to the results of the latest research on the subject. His work is critical, and in some ways organized and synthesized along completely new lines. Time and again, Gordon throws light on modern medicine, and at every turn the reader feels that the book hails from the pen of a practicing physician.

DR. MAX NEUBURGER

vii

Preface

THE PURPOSE of this book is to present an historical résumé of medicine as it was conceived, developed, and practiced by the various peoples of antiquity. A determined effort has been made throughout this work to emphasize outstanding historical facts. With so large a field and with such a vast and varied mass of material, many subjects could not be discussed as fully as their importance might seem to warrant.

In pursuing his investigations, the writer was careful to confine himself to widely recognized sources and to discoveries in the fields of archeology, anthropology, and paleopathology, which in recent years have thrown a flood of light on prehistoric medicine. He has endeavored, as far as is feasible, to permit the ancient records and the ancient doctors to speak for themselves.

No effort has been spared in collecting and critically sifting the material used and the pictures employed to illustrate the text. The author has sought to supplement rather than to parallel other texts. In a work of this kind, one must anticipate considerable divergence of opinion among the various authorities. Every author needs must view the subject through his own spectacles, notwithstanding how objective he strives to be.

The purpose of the present writer was not to promulgate obtuse speculations but to collect and systematize facts. He trusts that he has succeeded in bringing within the covers of a single volume a comprehensive account of the essential aspects of ancient medicine.

The writer has deemed it advisable to divide the present work into two parts: the first dealing with the prehistoric and protohistoric periods, upon which the science of archeology has thrown much light; and the second part dealing with the Greco-Roman period (which terminated with the fall of Rome in 476 A.D.,), upon which considerable historical data are available.

When writing on any subject pertaining to art, science, or literature, one, of course, becomes deeply indebted to the efforts of all one's predecessors. This is particularly true when writing on an historical subject. The writer humbly expresses his gratitude to the multitude of authors whom he has consulted in the preparation of this work.

The author has avidly strived to refer in the text or in the footnotes to the sources from which the following chapters have been derived;

but owing to the fact that one's personal thoughts are so inextricably interwoven with the thoughts of others, which have been integrated throughout the years, he may have expressed unwittingly as his own an occasional idea that was previously uttered by others. For such unintentional infringements, the author asks forgiveness.

The writer wishes to thank his colleagues and others from whom he received ideas that are incorporated in this book.

To Professor Max Neuburger, the renowned medical historian, who so kindly read the page proofs of this work and gave such sincere encouragement, the author tenders his deepest appreciation.

To his oldest son, Dr. Cyrus H. Gordon, Professor of Assyriology and Egyptology at Dropsie College, Philadelphia, he is grateful for reading much of the manuscript and proffering his valuable critical observations and corrections.

To his youngest son, Maurice B. Gordon, M.D., he is indebted for the great interest he has manifested in both the literary and mechanical aspects of this work. He watched over the publication from its inception to its completion and made an important contribution to this work. The chapter "Ancient Hebrew Medicine" is largely the work of his pen.

The author's secretary, Mrs. Elizabeth Shrope, also rendered invaluable assistance. She copied and recopied the manuscript with thoroughness, good will, and understanding and made numerous valuable suggestions with regard to the arrangement of the material. For her unceasing help, the author expresses his sincere thanks.

Any expression of appreciation would be incomplete without mentioning the generous assistance received from various libraries: especially the New York Academy of Medicine, the New York Public Library, the Library of the College of Physicians of Philadelphia, the Library of the Jefferson Medical College, the Library of the Smithsonian Institute, and above all the public and medical libraries of Atlantic City, New Jersey.

The author expresses his thanks to the many friends who so kindly supplied interesting photographs, drawings, or restorations, and to the editors of medical journals for permission to use certain parts of his own articles, previously printed in their publications.

Last, but not least, it is a great pleasure to acknowledge gratefully the cooperation and unfailing helpfulness of the publishers, the F. A. Davis Company.

BENJAMIN LEE GORDON, M.D.

Table of Contents

Part I

PREHISTORIC AND PROTOHISTORIC MEDICINE

Part II

THE GRECO-ROMAN PERIOD

Part I

PREHISTORIC AND PROTOHISTORIC MEDICINE

1

Introduction

Remember the days of old,
   Consider the years of many generations;
Ask thy father, and he will declare unto thee,
   Thine elders, and they will tell thee. [1]

THE TERM "historia" was used by the Ionian philosophers (sixth century B.C.) to connote the search for knowledge in the wider sense of the word. It included the results of inquiry and investigation but not narratives. Two centuries later, the *historicos*, or the reciters of stories, superseded the *historeans*, the seekers of knowledge.

History, in the early stages of human life, existed purely as oral tradition of folklore, practices, customs, and religious beliefs transmitted from one generation to another. The art of healing goes far beyond the confines of written history. It extends back into the dimly distant recesses of a period before man completely evolved from a lower species of anthropoid life, from a time when instinct and intelligence were first combined in the search of measures to allay the individual's own pain and cure his own sickness.

Later, as intelligence came more to the fore and animal instinct slipped more into the background, efforts to allay pain and combat disease extended to one's family and friends. Thus, medicine originated at a period when man's intelligence began to work on his primal sympathy to help those of his kindred who were in sorrow, need, and sickness.

Three Periods of Ancient Medicine: Medicine of antiquity may be divided into three unequal periods. The first, or long period, began with the very birth of man and terminated when history began to be recorded. The second, or protohistoric period, began when history was first recorded and persisted until the rise of the philosophical

3

school of Ionia (about 600 B.C.). The third period began with the Ionian philosophers and terminated with the decline and fall of Rome.

First Period: Information concerning the first period has been derived by paleopathologists, from evidence of disease discovered in fossilized human remains, from rude paintings and carvings on walls of caves and stones, and from stone instruments which may have been used for surgical operations. Such evidences are often more trustworthy than inscriptions and books.

Second Period: The records of the second period, of course, are not confined to medicine or surgery. They are more often of a general nature. For example, the code of Hammurabi deals with legal matters, and surgery is merely brought in from a legal point of view. The same is true of the Old Testament, which is the chronicle and anthology of the Hebrew people and which refers to medicine only incidentally.

In the Iliad, while describing the heroes at the battlefield, Homer tells of surgical operations performed upon them. Antiquity has occasionally afforded direct evidence dealing with physicians and remedies, such as, for example, the Egyptian papyri and the Babylonian medical tablets.

Third Period: The third, or rational, period begins with Thales of Miletus and the Greek school of philosophers. The last is the best known period of ancient medical history. From the start of this period, medical history has been committed to writing. Greece and Rome have supplied most of the scientific medical information of the third period. The philosophical speculations of Pythagoras, Empedocles, Alcameon, and others of the Ionian school culminated in the "natural" investigations of Hippocrates and his school, which in turn transmitted its heritage to the students of the school of Alexandria and their Roman successors.

Importance of History: Hippocrates, in his Corpus, strongly advocates the importance of studying the views of ancient healers:

> I do not say that the old art of healing should be abandoned as of no account as though its investigations were wrongly conducted; on the contrary I maintain that its way of thinking came so near the truth that one should take it more into consideration and wonder at the discoveries made in spite of so great a lack of knowledge.

Hippocrates insisted that his followers be grounded in the history of their predecessors.

An old Chinese proverb declares: "To understand the present, one should examine antiquity." But for antiquity, things would not be as they are now.

The importance of history to any given branch of human knowledge was emphasized by Cicero who stated:

Not to know what has been transacted in former times is to continue always a child; if no use is made of the labors of the first ages, the world must remain always in the infancy of knowledge.

Herodotus: The greatest historian of all time, Herodotus (484–425 B.C.), was not an idle tourist. He was a critcial observer of all that he saw and was told, and he tested his evidence whenever possible. His work remains a scientific achievement, remarkable for its careful observation. He also added to the scientific spirit an artistic sense which enabled him to cast his material into the best literary form.

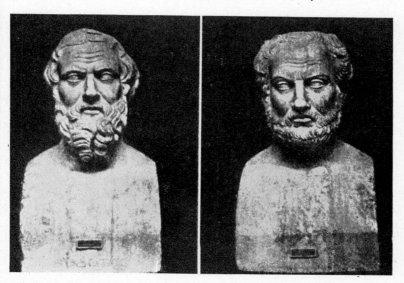

Fig. 1: *Left:* Herodotus was called the "Father of History"; he was above all a born narrator. *Right:* Thucydides looked at events more critically and sought causes and effects. He was the first pragmatic historian. (Both faces are on one marble sculpture in Naples.)

Thucydides: The next great Greek historian was Thucydides (c. 460–339 B.C.) who also combined artistic skill with higher science. He scorned the storyteller "who seeks to please the ear rather than speak the truth." He withdrew from vulgar applause, conscious that his narrative would be considered "disappointing to the ear"; he recast the materials out of which he constructed his history so as to lift his narrative into the realm of pure literature. He reworded his speeches, letters, and documents to be in tone with the rest of the story. Both historians record medical fact with great accuracy. In Roman times history still attained the great purpose laid down by the Ionians as may be seen from the works of Ovid, Livy, Tacitus, Strabo, and others.

Medical History: Medicine did not have a Herodotus nor a Thucydides to record its progress, but the scope of medical history differs from that of general history. "History," said Gibbon, "is little more than the register of crimes, follies, and misfortunes." This cannot be said of medical history. It deals with compassion, mercy, pity, and kindness. It does not deal with kings and warriors; the only war it recognizes is that which is against diseases, and the only chieftain it admires is the physician who knows best how to combat pestilence.

A branch of knowledge, so conducive to human welfare and so essential to the preservation of the human race, like the healing art should naturally have its history imbued with a kind of religious veneration on the part of medical students and physicians. This, however, more often than not, is not the case. Few doctors appear to have heeded the remarks of the historian, Thomas Fuller (1608–1661):

History maketh a young man to be old without either wrinkles or gray hair, privileging him with the experience of age, without the infirmities or inconvenience thereof. Yea, it not only maketh things past present, but enables one to make a rational conjecture of things to come.

The reason for this lack of interest lies not so much with students and physicians as with the schools which appear to find little or no room in their curriculum for the history of the subject with which they endeavor to interest the student and leave upon him a lasting impression.

The history of medicine, as has been pointed out, antedates the Egyptian papyri and Babylonian inscriptions. Paleontologists read its history in fossilized human remains. Archaeologists unravel historical medical data from paintings on the walls of prehistoric caves, from certain figures on stones, and from artifices used by prehistoric man. Antiquity can no longer be measured by the short rod of tradition, just as distance cannot be estimated by means of the "horse and buggy." Historians gather more reliable information from the dust heaps of Mesopotamia and fragments of papyri found in the hot sand of the Egyptian desert, than from the writing of the greatest travelers of antiquity who supposedly gathered their data from the priests of "On" and "Sais" and from the magi of the valleys of the Euphrates and Tigris. The term "prehistoric" has lost its original significance in the presence of new discoveries. So-called "prehistoric accounts" become historic as new discoveries throw back the curtain of history.

SOURCES OF INFORMATION: The meager sources of information derived from the records left by the peoples occupying the valleys of the rivers Euphrates, Tigris, Indus, and Nile (originally known from the references found in the writing of Greek historians) have been augmented during the past century by discoveries of inscriptions on sculptures, tablets, papyri, and other articles. These new discoveries, which are still largely fragmentary, have already, pieced together, furnished valuable medical information.

Egyptian: The several Egyptian papyri reveal that the people of the Nile, as far back as 3500 B.C., already possessed a well-grounded knowledge of the art of medicine. They believed that some internal driving force was responsible for the faculties of motion, sensation, and thought; but not being aware of the anatomy and the mechanism of the cerebral centers, they placed these phenomena under the direct supervision of the gods. They bestowed upon the heart, which is the organ that makes itself most readily manifest to the primitive mind, being always in action during life and checked at once by death, the central properties of life.

Babylonian: Babylonian medicine perhaps never reached the standard of proficiency of Egyptian; but as will be shown, it reached a progressive state of development. A medical compendium discovered in the library of Ashurbanipal,[2] comprising three cuneiform tablets, reveals that the Babylonians, regardless of their strong belief in magic and occult cures, had a comprehensive knowledge of medicine. Some of these tablets show that they attributed disease to living creatures which acted as carriers.

Babylonian mythology frequently exhibits symbolical significance. Nergal, the god of pestilence and destruction, for example, appears in the form of an insect. The fly-god of Ecron, *Baal-zebub*,[3] was perhaps a Philistine name for Nergal.

Hindu: It is not known how early the Hindus began to cultivate the science of medicine. It will be shown that at the beginning of the third millennium B.C., medicine was already well developed in the valley of the Indus, at Mohenjo-daro, Harappa, and elsewhere.[4] The Hindus were perhaps the first to practice scientific healing. They cultivated those sciences which helped them in their worship; it will be shown in the chapter dealing with India that a knowledge of medicine was most essential to their religious practices.

According to tradition, Atreya, the famous physician, taught medicine at Kasi and Benares and that Susruta taught surgery at Taxilla.[5] The work of the latter seems to be verified by a Sanskrit text which is still extant. There is considerable evidence that Indian medical ideas influenced the schools of Asia Minor and, through them, those of Greece.

Chinese: The Chinese were the only ancient people who were little influenced by outside sources. They isolated themselves, as it were, within the "Chinese wall" where they remained until comparatively recent times. They consequently developed their own theories and practices.

Greek: In the state of society portrayed by Homer, it is clear that as early at 1000 B.C. medicine in Greece was already a distinct and organized profession; surgery especially had been based on long experience. The Homeric nomenclature for the various parts of the body is substantially the same (according to Daremberg) as that employed long afterwards in the writings of Hippocrates. However imperfect medicine might have been in Homer's time as compared with later times, it was far from being in its infancy. The Homeric heroes themselves are represented as having considerable skill in surgery and being able to attend to ordinary wounds and injuries. There were also a professional class, represented by Machaon and Podalirius, the two sons of Aesculapius, who are treated with great respect. It would appear, too, that the duties of these two were not precisely the same. Machaon's task was more specifically to heal injuries, while Podalirius had received from his father the gift of "recognizing that which was not visible to the eye, and tending to what could not be healed." In other words, a rough indication is seen of the separation of medicine and surgery.

Aesculapius appears in Homer as a Thessalian king, not as a god, although in later times, divine honors were extended to him. There is no sign in the Homeric poems of the subordination of medicine to religion, such as is the case in the writings of ancient Egypt, Babylonia, and India, nor were priests charged in Greece as they were in other countries, with medical functions.

Homer, writing probably in the ninth century B.C., credits the origin of the arts of medicine and surgery to the Egyptians.

> From Paeon sprung their patron-god imparts,
> To all the Pharian race his healing arts.
>   Odyssey IV, 231 (Pope)

It is difficult to ascertain to what extent Homeric surgery was introduced from Egypt. There is no question, however, that Egypt had a great influence on Greek scientific thinking. The intercourse of the Greeks with the Egyptians was made possible by the "open door" policy of King Psamtichus (c. 660 B.C.). This contact proved to be a great stimulant to Greek thought and intellectual activity. Perhaps the vein of mysticism which overgrew the primitive simplicity of Homeric religion was also of Egyptian origin.

The first attempts made in Greece to separate science from the religion and mysticism imported from the land of the Nile were made by Thales of Miletus, Xenophanes of Colophon, and Pythagoras of Samos. They advanced philosophical and scientific methods to create the "know how" to solve natural problems. The Greeks word "physis" denoting nature, its derivatives "physics" and "physiology," and the term, "cosmos," denoting the mundane system, were unknown to Homer and Hesiod, the early Greek writers and poets. They first appeared with the Ionian philosophers. In the words of the historian, Grote:

> The elemental analysis of Thales of Miletus, the one unchangeable cosmic substance varying only in appearance but not in reality as suggested by Xenophanes, and the geometrical and arithmetical combinations of Pythagoras, all these were different ways of approaching the explanation of physical phenomena and each gave rise to a distinct school of philosophers where they all agreed in the parting from the primitive method and in recognizing determinate properties, invariable sequence and objective truth in nature.

Xenophanes disclaimed all knowledge concerning the gods, and pronounced that no man can have any means of ascertaining when he is right and when he is wrong with respect to them.

The first result of such concepts was the conversion of the empirical rules derived from Egypt to deductive sciences. The Ionian philosophers sought reality in matter and slowly developed a theory of primary elements which culminated in the atomism of Leucippus and Democritus. Medicine to them was a part of philosophic speculation.

The importance of the Ionian school of philosophy lies in the fact that for the first time in history the processes of the whole universe were conceived as natural and potentially explicable by ordinary knowledge and rational inquiry. The idea that matter is composed of indestructible primordial elements tended to encourage skepticism in the minds of these people who took their gods seriously.

Despite the fact that Anaxagoras was driven from Athens as an atheist and the same charges were maliciously trumped up against Socrates, science came out of the conflict victorious. The Greek religion, characterized by its dynamic flexibility, its myths, and adaptability to the needs of poetic and artistic beauty, as well as its readiness to accept new ideas, led to a liberal outlook on universal phenomena.

At the beginning of the fifth century B.C., the Ionian philosophy became a highly controversial subject. The chief opponent of the philosophical system of Ionia was Hippocrates, who believed in natural observation (*vis medicatrix naturae*).

Celsus states that Hippocrates was the first to separate medicine, not from priestcraft, but from philosophy.[6] Hippocrates treated all human phenomena as scientifically determinable. He was not against religion; he merely believed that divine and scientific reasoning are one and the same. In discussing some physical diseases found among the Scythians he observed:

The Scythians themselves ascribe the cause of disease to the gods and revere and bow down to such sufferers, each man fearing that he may suffer the like, and I myself, think that these affections as well as all others are divine. . .nevertheless, each of them has its own physical condition and not one occurs without such physical condition.

Greek medicine culminated in the school of Hippocrates (c. 420 B.C.), the father of scientific medicine, whose methods, if not altogether modern in the present sense, are at least modern in principle. They were far in advance, not only of his own generation, but also of succeeding ages.

The conquests of Alexander the Great carried Hellenic civilization to the east. The intellectual center he founded in Alexandria was particularly noted for its medical erudition. A new method of investigation was applied to science, in the capital of the Ptolemies, which was separated from philosophic theories. The methods of Aristarchus, Archimedes, and Hippachus who solved great natural problems for the first time, were adopted by Herophilus and Erasistratus with regard to medicine. Nothing was taken on trust. Each medical problem had to be solved on natural principles. The idea that animal dissection was as reliable as human dissection was discarded. With the aid of the liberal Ptolemies, human dissection was openly pursued; the knowledge thereby gained, proved a boon to the science of physiology.

Auxiliary Sciences: Gradually, with the passing of centuries, a group of auxiliary sciences, including chemistry, physics, physiology, biology, botany, anthropology, and archaeology became associated with medicine, each of which served either as a basis for testing results or as a tool for investigating facts. The knowledge of medicohistorical events that occurred between the teaching of Hippocrates and the writing of Galen formed a long chain in the evolution of medicine. It makes interesting reading and must not be lost sight of by the followers of Hippocrates.

Oliver Wendell Holmes, in one of his addresses, urged his students not to look with contempt on ancient and outmoded medical books:

That debris of broken systems and exploded dogmas forms a great mound, a mountain Testaccio of the shards and remnants of all vessels which once held human beliefs. If you take the trouble to climb to the top of it you will widen the horizon and in these days of specialized knowledge your horizon is not likely to be too wide.

The greatest enemy of medicine in all ages was superstition. The healer of diseases was generally looked upon as a miracle worker. Medicine was the only profession which elevated its practitioners to the lofty position of godhood. Egypt had its Imhotep, Greece its Aesculapius, Persia its Thrita, and India its Dhanwantari. Until this unwarranted exaltation of doctors gave way to the pressure of reason, scientific medicine was not possible. Under the pressure of scientific reasoning, each old and erroneous theory gave way to a more modern and rational one.

The atomic doctrine of Democritus and the doctrine of the four elements of the Ionian philosophers were the forerunners of modern chemistry. The concept of invisible malignant demons entering the body to cause disease was a premonition of bacteriology. The doctrine of humoral pathology has evolved into the science of endocrinology. The science of anatomy did not begin with Herophilus nor even with Galen. It commenced even before the Egyptian priest looked over the viscera of animals to determine their eligibility for sacrifice. Physiology did not begin with Dalton and his associates. It commenced before the doctrine of pneuma, *spiritus animalis,* and certainly before the human faculties of sensation, perception, and coordination were localized in the brain. History constantly repeats itself, making only such changes of progress as the growth of the centuries requires. The sage of old lives again in us. "The water is fresh but the fountain is old."

Early Medicine: The practice of medicine in early times may have been extremely simple. There are those who claim that when man first appeared on the earth, human disease had not yet attained that complexity of character which at the present time calls for the utmost skill in diagnosis and treatment and had not yet acquired that virulence which has so often wreaked havoc with the lives of men and the efforts of the physician. At any rate, in the early days of human history, man's food and habits were infinitely simpler and more in harmony with nature than at present. The desire for luxury and artifacts had not yet overwhelmed him and vice had not insidiously eaten away into his constitution. A few simples of the vegetable kingdom appeared ample to cure most of the diseases of the Egyptian. Civilization not only advanced new ideas which benefited humanity, but brought with it new diseases and complexities. The art of medicine has grown in proportion to the growth of the complexity of disease.

Modern Medicine: The vast structure of modern medicine represents one of the greatest triumphs of the human mind, but the story of its development and its achievements is one of the least known parts of history. Medical history is not merely an account of books and authors; it is the history of human suffering and human errors. To quote Voltaire:

It is the history of one who having studied nature from his youth knows the properties of the human body; the disease which assails it; the remedies which will benefit it; exercises his art with caution and pays equal attention to the rich and poor alike.

AUTHOR'S AIMS

An attempt will be made in the following chapters to survey the medical history of antiquity. It has been the writer's aim to bring together facts scattered in large and varied fields of literature which are not ordinarily accessible to the average busy practitioner, and certainly not to the circle of lay readers whose interest in medical history is purely objective.

The present author has chosen to close his work with the fall of the western empire (476 A.D.)—the date where many histories of medicine begin. No attempt has been made to discuss medieval medicine from the fifth to the fifteenth century, nor modern medicine from the fifteenth century on. Those who desire to read the history of modern medicine may find at their disposal a number of excellent works.

The chapters on evolution and paleontology were presented because of their close association with the evolution of medicine. This holds true also with the chapters dealing with the Ionian and Athenian schools of philosophy. Chapters 5 and 6, dealing with primitive concepts of disease and death, and early concepts of nature, have been included as a kind of introduction to the succeeding chapters. Chapters on Talmudic medicine cover a subject that is little known to the English reader. The Talmud was written at a period in world history when medicine was at a very low ebb; the reader will find there, not only the current medical tenets of the period, but also the ingenious medical doctrines of the ancient Hebrews, as well as those of the Greeks, Romans, and eastern nations.

In order to understand the development of medicine properly, a knowledge of its growth is essential. Such a knowledge is as important to medicine as the doctrine of evolution is to biology or as knowledge of embryology is to an understanding of histology and anatomy. No physician would expect to establish a diagnosis without ascertaining the clinical history of a given case. Racial factors must often be taken into consideration when diagnosing certain diseases. Schottky, in a work entitled "Rasse und Krankheit," demonstrated how the principles of susceptibility and immunity depend on racial factors. He believes that heredity and racial factors are historic and phylogenic. The term "ethnic pathology" has been applied to diseases of certain groups of people possessing the same physical characteristics and maintaining a common susceptibility and immunity from ages back. In other words, one must focus upon the ills of bygone time in order to analyze adequately the manifestations of disease of the present times.

No one can comprehend correctly and look intelligently into the future if he does not follow the road of his knowledge along historical lines. Every current that makes up the large stream of our present sum total of knowledge goes back to distant sources and is tied up with other streams. History follows the current of ancient medical thought:

> That which hath been is that which shall be
> And that which hath been done is that which shall be done,
> And there is nothing new under the sun.'

It is of course true that modern science has provided man with better knowledge and more accurate methods of investigating natural phenomena. Yet science has not changed the natural order of things one iota. The discovery of the growth of grain and edible plants from seeds buried in the ground by early man was certainly a greater boon to mankind, than, let us say, the modern discovery of vitamin C. The first man to spin wool for clothing purposes was certainly a greater inventor than the discoverers of rayon and nylon. Ancient man's discovery of fire without a doubt surpasses modern man's discovery of electricity. The world got along for millenniums without electricity, but one cannot conceive how man's life would be without the use of fire. Without fire many foods would not be suitable to eat and metals would remain useless in the ores. The passage of civilization from the Stone Age to the Iron and Bronze Ages was effected to a large extent by fire, and without fire the area of the world suitable for human habitation would be confined to the tropical and subtropical climates, and man would not have been able to migrate to the temperate and frigid parts of the world.

The genius of man is by no means strictly a product of the scientific age. Ancient men made fundamental discoveries with regard to medicine, and many surgical and pharmacological principles may be traced to remote antiquity. Even the recent discovery of penicillin, which is derived from a mold, may find a counterpart in the ancient use of the mold found on human skulls which had been exposed to the air. This was employed in antiquity as a hemostatic and to hasten the recovery of the injured. As late as 1644, Schröder, the author of the "Pharmacopeia Chymica," pointed to the value of a "down-like excrement" growing on the skulls of those killed on the battlefield as being excellent for bleeding. He states that the moss growing on other bones is not as effective. At present, scientists distinguish between the therapeutic advantages and strengths of various molds. The mold of rye was used by midwives long before the modern doctor prescribed ergot.

For ages the Chinese and Hindus have used dried pulverized sponges, which contain iodine, for many diseases. The use of ephedrine originated with the Chinese in bygone years. The Ebers Papyrus, 1600 B.C., recommends ox liver as a therapeutic agent in diseases of the eye. Hippocrates prescribed it mixed with honey, in cases of nightblindness, not knowing that nightblindness is due to vitamin A deficiency. Digitalis was originally a witch's brew. In our pharmacopoeia are found many other drugs which may be traced to the ancient healer.

Modern medicine, therefore, cannot be considered independent of the practices of the ancient doctors. It is merley a link, to be sure a strong link, in the long medical chain that stretches throughout the ages past and the ages to come.

References and Notes

1. Deuteronomy 32:7.
2. Assyrian Medical Text: Proc. Roy. Soc. Med., Sec. History of Medicine, 17, 1924.
3. II Kings 1:3, 16.
4. Sarton, G.: Isis, 70:223, 1936 (quoting Sir John Martial, London, 1931).
5. Ibid., p. 76.
6. Preface to "De Medicina."
7. Ecclesiastes 1:9.

2

The Antiquity of Medicine

THE EARLY MAN

BEFORE discussing prehistoric medicine, it may be proper to give a short review of what is known of the early man: his origin, geography, morphology, mentality, and environment.

Origin

The exact time when the accident or the series of events took place which led man to separate from his original species to become a biological entity is not known. As a matter of fact, man has no more knowledge of his racial origin than a child has of its individual birth. A child, however, as it grows, gradually derives some knowledge of its relationship to its parents, and observing generations, going and coming, becomes familiar with the circumstances of birth and death. But man, in the long years of his existence, has had no such experience that might cast light on the origin of his race, for he has not personally witnessed the birth of any new species, nor has he had recourse to anyone who has.

Theories of Evolution: Not quite a century ago the prevailing belief was that man, as other forms of life, had been created in his present form only a few thousand years ago. The teaching of geology and biology that the earth and all living creatures upon it were evolved by a process of gradual development extending back many millions of years was denounced as heresy. The narrative of the first chapters of the Book of Genesis[1] had firmly established, among people at large, the belief that man, in his present form, was an object of Divine creation; opposition was not only unpopular but was even considered dangerous. The doctrine of evolution caused consternation, particularly in the minds of churchmen. They bitterly resented any implica-

15

tion of relationship between man and any other species. They saw in the theory of evolution a sinister attempt to upset the long established Biblical tenet regarding man's origin. The violent tempest aroused by Darwin's "Origin of Species" (1853) has continued up to the present day. The polemic between Huxley, Gladstone, and the Duke of Argyll of two or three generations ago is well known to students of the history of evolution. In recent times one may recall with amusement the controversy between William Jennings Bryan and a young instructor over the teaching of the descent of man. The young teacher was discharged from the school because of his views concerning the genesis of man.

Naturally, so long as it was believed that the earth was a creation of only a few thousand years, no theory of evolution could gain any headway. But since geology revealed the continuous changes of the earth extending throughout its many millions of years of existence, the theory of the origin of species has gained ground gradually.

Theories of Greek Philosophers: The doctrine that the human being, as well as all other living species, came about in a natural way, was really not new. Natural ideas of the origin of living organisms were suggested millenniums ago by the Greek philosophers: Anaximenes, Heraclitus, Empedocles, Democritus, Diogenes of Apollonia, and others. Of course their views were far from the modern theory of evolution. They believed that all kinds of living beings had a natural independent origin from the material of the earth. Aristotle was the first biologist of antiquity to maintain that there was a gradual succession of living beings from the very simplest to the most perfect form. Life itself, according to Aristotle, arose through direct metamorphosis of organic matter:

. . . plants came early in the succession for although endowed with power of nourishment and reproduction, they have neither feeling nor sensibility. Later came the plant animals or zoophytes; and still later animals properly gifted with sensibility and even to some extent with powers of thought. Highest of all came man, the one form capable of abstract thought. The process of nature is a struggle towards perfection. The expression of a perfecting principle is inherent in the universe. The result is a gradual evolution from the lower to the higher. At the back of the perfect principle is the efficient cause. [2]

Aristotle does not indicate whether the original cause that gave the first impulse remained outside the operation of nature or whether it is all the time constantly at work. Aristotle is not exact in detail; the idea of progressive changes in the organic world, however, stands out clearly enough. He did not point out the particular natural agency through which changes might be brought about. He reflects the idea of survival of the fittest, anticipated in a crude form by Empedocles, who perhaps did not have sufficient facts at his disposal to observe the phenomena of variation normally found among living things.

Theory of European Scholars: The Greek idea of evolution made no impression upon the learned world. The idea remained dormant until the seventeenth and eighteenth centuries when a free independent spirit began to prevail among many European scholars; the theory of

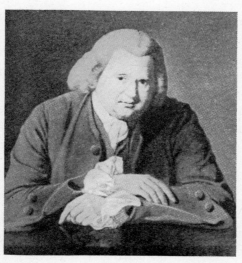

Fig. 2: Dr. Erasmus Darwin (1731-1802). Erasmus Darwin was born at Elton in Nottinghamshire on Dec. 12, 1731. He studied medicine and the sciences at St. John's, Cambridge, and Edinburgh. He began his medical practice in Nottingham (1750), but he soon moved to Lichfield, which city offered him greater opportunities. He was interested greatly in the treatment of alcoholic patients. His fame, however, he derived as a scientist. His "Zoonomia" (1794-1796) contained a system of pathology and a treatise on generation, in which (according to his famous grandson Charles R. Darwin) he anticipated the views of Lamarck. The essence of his views was contained in the following conclusions, "One and the same kind of living filaments is and has been the cause of all organic life." He was also known as a botanist and poet. The merit of his "Botanical Garden" (1791) lay in its scientific enthusiasm and interest in nature, which pervaded it. In 1781, he moved to Derby, where he died suddenly on April 18, 1802. (After a painting by Joseph Wright [1734-1797]. Original in the National Portrait Gallery, London.)

succession was discussed sympathetically by Bacon, Leibnitz, Spinoza, Hume, Linnaeus, Buffon, and Kant.

Many more scientists of note probably held similar views about the mutability of species on the ground that variation in animal and plant form could have been brought about directly by environmental changes, and that these changes could remain fixed by heredity. Out of deference to Biblical teaching, however, they remained silent.

Buffon (1753–1778) verbally questioned the orthodox idea that the human has no relation to other species, although in his writings, out

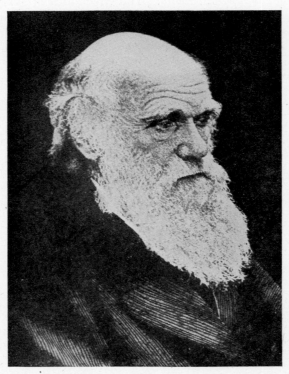

Fig. 3: Charles Robert Darwin (1809-1882). Charles Robert Darwin, the son of Dr. Robert Waring Darwin, was born in Shrewsbury, England, on February 12, 1809. He studied at the Universities of Edinburgh and Cambridge. His interest in the natural sciences was probably derived from his grandfather Erasmus Darwin, who was a great naturalist. At the age of thirty-one, he set out on a five-year voyage to many lands, where he studied animals, plants, and rocks. His main interest was the origin of species. His great work "The Origin of Species" (1859) stirred the intellectual world and is considered the most important work of the 19th century. He was a cautious student, devoted to truth. His kindliness of character and honesty of purpose made him beloved to all who knew him. He died April 9, 1882.

of respect to religious doctrine, he expressed himself at times in favor of the Biblical conception of creation.

The idea of evolution was greatly enhanced by the writings of Erasmus Darwin (1731–1802) (grandfather of the famous author of "Origin of Species") and the famous scientist Lamarck (1744–1829) of France.

Both accepted the doctrine of mutability of species, and each advanced a theory of evolution of his own and adopted an hypothesis to explain how the transformation of species might be brought about. They both believed that a variation of environment was at the bottom of the specific changes.

Morphology

Basis of Modern Doctrine of Evolution: While the idea that man may have come into existence by modification of lower vertebrates is as old as speculative thought, evidence to this effect was vague until the middle of the nineteenth century when the modern doctrine based on certain scientific observations was promulgated by Darwin and his collaborators. They based their opinions on the following facts:

1. There are few ideas more ingrained in ancient and low civilizations than that of the relationship by descent between lower animals and man. Savage and barbaric religions recognize this, and few beliefs in the mythology of ancient peoples all over the world are more universal than that man is in some way related to animals.

2. Man presents the same fundamental plan of structure as the lower vertebrates.

3. Rudimentary and apparently useless structures exist in one species which are fully developed and have definite function in another species.

4. There is evidence that organisms are homologous in their intrauterine development.

5. Human remains in the fossilized state show that the present inhabitants of the globe are a product of a long process of evolution.

6. Diseases among fossilized animals show a similarity to those of early man.

7. Handicraft has successively developed.

Darwin[3] has said:

It is notorious that man is constructed on the same general type or model as other mammals. All the bones in his skeleton can be compared with corresponding bones in a monkey, bat, or seal. So it is with his muscles, nerves, blood-vessels, and internal viscera.

The brain, the most important of all the organs, follows the same law, as shown by Huxley and other anatomists.

The Darwinian theory was strongly seconded by A. R. Wallace, who stated:

By universal consent, we see in the monkey tribe a caricature of humanity. Their faces, their hands, their actions, and expressions present ludicrous resemblances to our own. If the skeletons of the higher anthropoids are compared with those of man, we find all of the bones with very few exceptions, correspond, the differences being of degree and not of kind.

This resemblance is so pronounced that Professor Owen says:

I cannot shut my eyes to the significance of that all pervading similitude of structure—every tooth, every bone, strictly homologous—which makes the determination of the difference between Homo and Pithecus the anatomist's difficulty.

This is also emphasized by Huxley[4] in his work "Man's Place in Nature":

Whatever system of organs be studied, the comparison of their modifications in the ape series leads to one and the same result—that the structural differences which separate man from the gorilla and the chimpanzee are not so great as those which separate the gorilla from the lower apes.

Elie Metchnikoff, the famous scientist of the Pasteur Institute, expressed himself on the subject of descent of man as follows:

Close examination of the structure of man has proved in a most definite fashion the existence of a near kinship with the higher monkeys or anthropoids. Now that all the details of the human organism have been studied and the anatomical structure of man and large monkeys without tails has been compared bone with bone and muscle with muscle, a truly astonishing analogy between their organisms is made manifest; an analogy apparent in every detail.

David Starr Jordan maintained:

Man is connected with the lower animals by the most perfect homologies. These are traceable in every bone and muscle and every blood vessel and gland in every phase of structure even including those of the brain and nervous system. The common heredity of man with other vertebral animals, is as well established as any fact can be.

Ernst Haekel finds it very difficult to show why man should not be classed with the large apes in the same zoological family: "We all know a man from an ape but it is quite another thing to find differences which are absolute and not of degree only."

Mentality

Mentality of the Ape: The (highest) anthropoids among mammals designated as manlike apes are the four types known as the gorilla, chimpanzee, orangutan, and gibbon. They are designated as "manlike apes" because of their similarity to the human form and the relatively large size of their brains. They are provided with hands and that highly specialized digit called the "thumb." It has been asserted that man ascended to the peak of the evolutionary scale with the development of his thumb, producing a hand of great dexterity for the fashioning of weapons and implements. That assertion seems weakened when

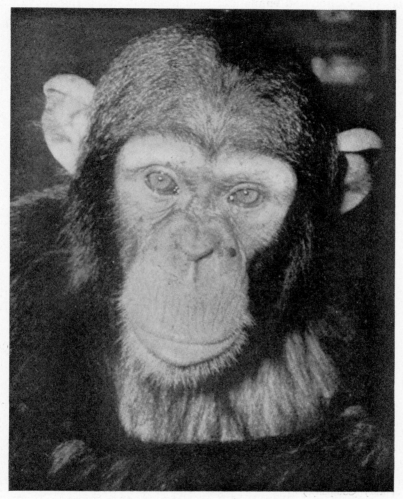

Fig. 4: Young Chimpanzee. (Courtesy of Zoological Society of Philadelphia. Photograph by Mark Mooney, Jr.)

one looks at the hands of an anthropoid ape, for here are dexterous thumbs and hands of great strength. In facial appearance, the chimpanzee is nearest in resemblance to man. Its skull architecture, eyes, and hands are almost human.

The orang has learned to drive nails, remove tight nuts with a wrench, and select a key from several on a ring and then open a lock. Such actions which were not only acquired by training, but also by mere observation and emulation, tend to elevate the orang above the mental plane of mere animals.

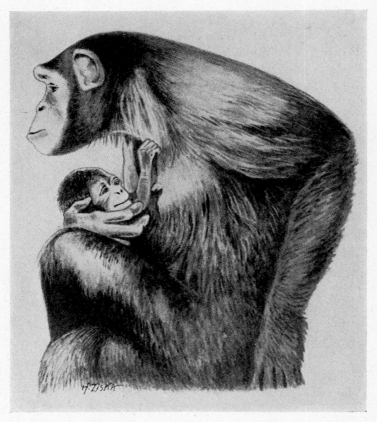

Fig. 5: One of our nearest living relatives: Female chimpanzee and young. (From Yerkes, R. M.: Almost Human. Courtesy of the author and The Century Company.)

Darwin observed that monkeys are susceptible to all human tastes and vices. They develop a strong liking for coffee, tea, and alcoholic beverages. He observed monkeys smoking tobacco with pleasure; he cites Bohem to the effect that natives of Africa catch wild baboons by exposing vessels filled with beer as bait.[5] The average wild gorilla,

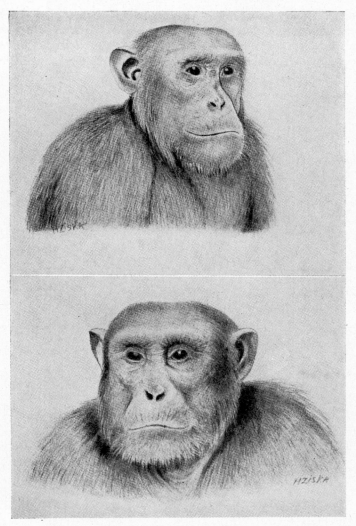

Fig 6: Male and female chimpanzees. (After Allen, J. A. From photographs by Herbert Land.)

chimpanzee, and orangutan are tremendously strong for their weight, possessing twice the strength of the human—pound for pound.

Limitations: Owing to the mentality of these animals, which is at a considerably lower level than a half-witted human's, they have not developed their hands to their full potential capacity. The apes build no shelters, store no food, and are wasteful and destructive in their feeding. The only time they even approach using their powerful hands for delicate manipulation is in making flat nests of branches in the trees, where they may sleep; but these crude gatherings are as nothing when compared with the skillfully prepared nests, shelters, and burrowed

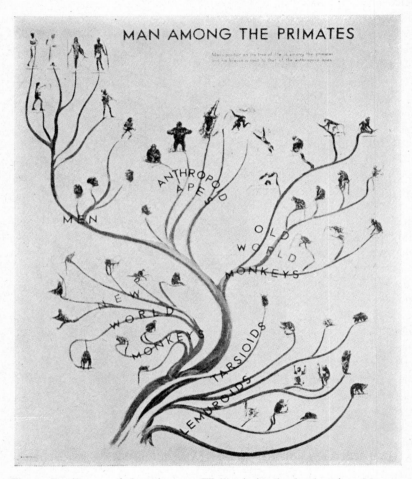

Fig. 7: Family tree of the primates. (Wall painting in the American Museum of Natural History, New York.)

homes of the smaller animals well down the scale of classification— where hands are absent.

The limited use of the hands by apes is probably due to the fact that in the struggle for existence against inimical beasts and the adverse elements of nature, they were best adapted to walk on all fours. They made use of their hands only by choice and not by habit. For similar reasons man has not learned to grasp things with his feet. He did not develop the faculty of pedal prehension, not because he does not possess the muscles and tendons which afford the faculty of grasping, but because he did not need this faculty. He never had any occasion to use his legs for prehension. It is known that in cases where both arms are amputated in man he has learned to pick up objects with his toes.[6]

Physiological Differences of Man and Ape: The apparent physiological differences between man and the manlike ape, such as, for example, the faculty of erect walking, the use of the hands, and above all the faculty of speech, cannot be held against the theory of the descent of man from anthropoid ancestry. Several of the anthropoid species assume an erect posture at will if not by habit.[7] "There is good testimony that various species of the gibbon readily take to erect posture." George Bennett is quoted to the effect that the Hylobates Syndactylus walks rather rapidly in the erect posture. Doctor Burroughs declares that the horlook or hoolock walks erect, and when placed in an open field balances himself very dexterously by raising its hands over the head and slightly bending the arms at the wrist or elbow.

Articulate Language: The absence of articulate language in the anthropoids is not inconsistent with the theory of evolution; it should be observed that language owes its origin to the imitation and modification of various natural sounds. The parrot, for example, will imitate man's sound and speech. Monkeys understand much that is said to them by man, and when wild, utter signal cries of danger to their fellows. Fowls are also commonly observed to give audible warning sounds of impending danger from hawks.

Anthropoid apes are potentially developed for articulate speech.[8] All anthropoids possess vocal organs constructed on the same general plan as those of the human. The vocal organs are used by many of them to express emotions such as joy and anger, and to issue warning to their young when danger is imminent.

In fact monkeys possess a vocabulary of their own. They produce sounds which mean definite things, and in speech, they rank higher than anthropoid apes. It is thus strange that anthropoid apes, standing at the head of the class zoologically, must be given second place in production of meaningful sounds. Monkeys are most vociferous, and the Old-World kinds excel in their vocabularies. To say that monkeys talk, would be stretching the point, but they utter sounds as definitely invariable as human words in expressing pleasure, condolence, assurance, relieving fear, calling to congregate, "conference" sounds when groups are assembled, sounds of caution, and sounds of imperative warning. Besides these sounds, many kinds of monkeys have developed facial grimaces, movements of the eyelids, wrinkling of the forehead—even wiggling of ears—and all having definite meaning. Monkeys beckon, point, make deprecating gestures, and extend their arms in supplication or begging (as they do when seen on the streets accompanying organ grinders).

Intelligence: The chief reason for lack of development of articulate speech may be ascribed to lack of intelligence. This brings up the questions as to why apes do not possess more intelligence than they do, and by what means man has so far outdistanced all other beings in his mental capacity and consequently in his struggle for life. The attempt to minimize this remarkable disparity between man and the anthropoid has not met with equal support from all investigators. The ultraevolutionists solve this problem by asserting that, since all evidence based upon careful experiments points to the cortex of the cerebrum as the seat of the intelligence, consciousness, sensation, volition, and memory associations, the increasing development of the cortex increases also the mental function, so that in higher vertebrates there is unquestionable evidence of what in ourselves we call psychic phenomena. Intelligence is thus not something that is the exclusive possession of man but apparently something which appears in the animal kingdom whenever the nervous system attains a certain type of development. Since it comes more and more into evidence with the increasing complexity and perfection of the nervous mechanism, it is to be regarded as an extension of those other organic functions of adjustment and regulation which render animal life possible. An animal is intelligent largely in the degree to which it consciously adopts means to an end. Man can direct his action towards certain ends by deliberately choosing the means to be employed in attaining those ends.

Cranial Sizes: The evidence is that, ordinarily, whenever an adult man has a skull less than 19 inches in circumference or less than 65 cubic inches of brain, he is idiotic. Those celebrated personalities who combined acute perception with great reflective power have had heads above the average size.[9]

Cranial Capacities: The difference of the cranial capacity of the lowest savage is said to be not less than five-sixths of the highest civilized races. The brain of the highest ape scarcely has the capacity of one-third that of man. The ratio runs as follows: anthropoid, ten;

savage, twenty-six; and civilized European, thirty-two. The differences are primarily in degree. There is no visible variation in the basic structure of the respective brains.

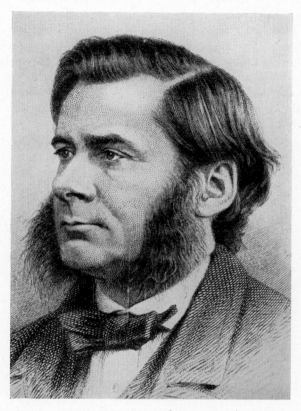

Fig. 8: Thomas Henry Huxley (1825-1895). Thomas Henry Huxley was born at Ealing, Middlesex, England. He studied at the Medical School of Charing Cross. After receiving his degree in 1846, he entered the Medical Service of the Royal Navy. In 1854, he was made Professor of Natural History in the Royal School of Mines and held that position until 1885. He was the first great teacher of biology by the laboratory method. He was a man of commanding intellectual power. He defended and explained Darwin's hypothesis on evolution with telling effect. Perhaps his greatest service was in promoting the advance toward intellectual honesty. His scientific researches filled four large octavo volumes, and his collected essays and books were published in 1892, in nine volumes.

The brain capacity of the average modern European skull is 1450 cc.; the cranial capacity of the largest male gorilla is not over 580 cc. The physical line of demarcation between the Bushman and the gorilla is no more sharply defined than between the gorilla and the orang, or between the orang and the gibbon. At birth and early infancy the human is no wiser—indeed often less wise—than the beast of that period. Man's mental make-up does not develop markedly until about two years of age.

Psychologists' Opinions: Psychologists, however, are not in accord with the doctrine that there is only a difference of degree in the mental manifestations of man and other mammals. Some are of the opinion that the principles of evolution are inadequate to account for the origin and workings of the higher faculties in man. Even Huxley, one of the greatest exponents of evolution, has expressed a different view on this phase of the subject:

I have endeavoured to show that no absolute structural line of demarcation, wider than that between the animals which immediately succeed us in the scale, can be drawn between the animal world and ourselves; and I may add the expression of my belief that the attempt to draw a psychical distinction is equally futile, and that even the highest faculties of feeling and of intellect begin to germinate in lower forms of life. At the same time, no one is more strongly convinced than I am of the vastness of the gulf between civilized man and the brutes; or is more certain that whether from them or not, he is assuredly not of them. No one is less disposed to think lightly of the present dignity, or despairingly of the future hopes, of the only consciously intelligent denizen of this world.[10]

St. George Mivart has this to say with reference to the mental evolution of man:

I have no wish to ignore the marvellous powers of animals, or the resemblance of their actions to those of men. No one can reasonably deny that many of them have feelings, emotions, and sense perceptions similar to our own; that they exercise voluntary motion, and perform actions grouped in complex ways for definite ends; that they to a certain extent learn by experience, and combine perceptions and reminiscences so as to draw practical inferences, directly apprehending objects standing in different relations one to another, so that in a sense, they may be said to apprehend relations. They will show hesitation, ending apparently, after a conflict of desires, with what looks like choice or volition: and such animals as the dog will not only exhibit the most marvellous fidelity and affection, but will also manifest evident signs of shame, which may seem the outcome of incipient moral perceptions. It is no great wonder, then, that so many persons little given to patient and careful introspection, should fail to perceive any radical distinction between a nature thus gifted and the intellectual nature of man. [11]

Dr. Daniel Giraud Elliot, discussing the brain development of anthropoid apes in his monograph "The Primates," states:

The brain of the chimpanzee corresponds in all its physical details very closely to that of man. The fissures and convolutions are identical; even "Broca's convolution," which is the seat of articulate speech, is also present. Why, then, if these apes are provided with a brain so like that possessed by man, do they not talk and accomplish many of those things which man, the greatest of all primates, is able to achieve? The only explanation that seems reasonable is, that the indescribable, mysterious, and powerful influence which is called the Ego or Will, is lacking in the ape, and the possession of which raises man alone above all created beings and makes him the responsible creature that he is.

Physiology

Genetics: The theory of evolution is supported on genetic grounds. Anthropoids, like man, are developed from a fertilized ovum of about the same size. In the early stages of gestation, the anthropoid embryo can hardly be distinguished from that of the human embryo, and at birth anthropoids are as helpless as are human infants at that period. Even with respect to maturity, there is a great similarity between man and the orangutan. Living under similar climatic conditions, both reach their maturity at the age of from ten to fifteen years.

Vestigial Organs: There is probably no more striking evidence as to the kinship of man to the anthropoid ape than the presence in both of them of useless organs, which are present and useful in lower animals. The semilunar fold, found in the human and anthropoid eyes, is a vestige of the third eyelid or nictitating membrane functioning in birds and reptiles. But in man and anthropoid it is vestigial and does not function.[12] Human and anthropoid ears also possess homologies, being considerably smaller in size and with less functional efficiency than in the lower animals. The muscles which extend from the cartilage of the ear to the bones of the skull, have, in most human individuals and higher anthropoids, no functions, whereas in the lower animals they are useful. The so-called "Darwin's tubercle" is absent or very inconspicuous in man and in the anthropoids. A number of vestigial organs are normally met with, or are occasionally present in the human body, such as, for example, the canine teeth, the coccyx, the cecum, the intercondyloid and supracondyloid foramens of the humerus, the vermiform appendix, and the fibrous traces of various muscles. The gluteus quadrus, levator claviculae, and several other muscles that occur occasionally in man are regularly present in the apes. Wiedersheim, in his "The Structure of Man: An Index of His Past History," has pointed out more than one hundred atavistic structures and peculiarities which occur constantly or occasionally in various parts of the human body. Haeckel has designated these structures as "useless primitive heirlooms," but some of them, such as the vermiform appendix, are considerably worse than useless.

Hair: The scanty growth of hair on man's body cannot be used as a valid argument against the evolutionary theory, because man's body is really covered with very fine short hair, and the arrangement of the hair is analogous to that of the anthropoid ape. Furthermore, in intrauterine life, the face and body of the human embryo are covered with short, fine wooly hair (lanugo), which usually disappears before birth. Human hair tends to reappear after maturity. Occasionally the embryonic hair continues to grow, forming, in the adult, a long fleecy covering of the face and body.[13]

Blood: There is also an hematological homology of man to certain simians. G. H. F. Nuttall found that, when the serum of the blood of a rabbit which has been immunized against human blood serum is mixed with moderate strength sera of higher apes and monkeys respectively, it reacts with all, although in a varying degree. When mixed with more highly diluted sera from such animals, it forms a precipitate only with man and higher apes, such as the chimpanzee, orang, and gorilla.

Gulliver has shown that the red blood cells increase progressively in diameter from the lemurs to man, but the difference is slight between the great apes and man. Landsteiner and Miller found that the blood of the higher apes contains the same four groups of agglutinins which serve to distinguish the four main types of human blood. It is also well known that the apes are especially susceptible to many diseases usually regarded as being peculiar to man. Induced syphilis takes a much more virulent form in the higher apes.

Bones: Sir Arthur Keith has pointed out that every bone of man's body is found in the ape and presents the same leading features, differing only in proportion, size, or other detail. The same may be said of the internal organs upon which the fundamental physiological reactions of the organism depend. According to Sontag, the vertebral column of the ape differs from that of man, mainly in its curvatures, and in the character of certain bones. Man has a typical anthropoid neck, except for the fact that it is somewhat longer and has less well developed musculature. A vestigial tail appears in the embryonic development of both ape and man, projecting outside the body to about the sixth week in the latter case, and then sinking into the body leaving only a depression on the outer skin.

Teeth: The young ape, like the human child, possesses a set of twenty milk teeth, and these are later replaced by thirty-two permanent teeth as in man. The dental formula for both ape and man is as follows: four incisors, two canines, four premolars, and six molars in upper and lower jaw. The basic pattern of the several kinds of teeth is much the same, the reduction in size of the canines in man offering the most outstanding difference. The organs of the mouth and throat of ape and man are homologous, and are highly similar for the most part. The larynx and accessory vocal organs follow the same general arrangement, although the vocal cords are soft and some of the other vocal structures are more or less rudimentary in the apes.

Sense Organs and Nervous System: The sense organs and nervous system of man represent another important heritage from the anthropoid level. The gradual recession of olfaction and the growing importance of vision and the other senses had reached an advanced stage long before the prehuman stock diverged. The correlative evolution of sense organs and nervous system is reflected in the elaboration of the neopallium, with special centers for vision, audition, skin sensitivity, motor control, and associative processes. The brain of the great apes is so well developed along these lines that the localization of cortical functions in man is determined largely by experimentation upon the ape brain.

Theories and Processes of Evolution

Variation: The underlying basis of evolution is variation. It is an unavoidable observation that children differ in many respects from their parents. While possessing traits of both parents, the offspring always differs from either of them. This fact is also true of the evolution of groups and races of people. A race which is made up of a succession of individuals (phylogeny) is subject to similar changes. Through heredity, animals maintain structural similarity but not identity. Through variation they tend to become different. Heredity and variation are the fundamental principles upon which the phenomena of evolution are based. Darwin designated the phenomena of variation in individuals as the start of potentially new species which might evolve into distinct species, and the variation of groups as the birth of families, genera, and races. That variation is the cause of evolution may be seen from the fact that man himself has been able to develop new varieties of plants and breeds of animals, which differ as much from the original ancestral forms as many wild species differ among themselves.[14]

Attitudes on Evolution: Darwin does not view the descent of man from lower beings as a blot on the human escutcheon. To the contrary, the fact that man has risen from a low beginning to his present height on the evolutionary scale should not be degrading any more than his formation from the "dust of the ground" or his embryologic development from an ovum which is not readily distinguished from that of a dog. In his psychic development, which he did not inherit from his earliest ancestors but developed gradually by evolution, lies the great difference between civilized man and the brute.

The origin of man may be distressing and revolting to those who count genealogy as the all-important factor in human life, and who delight in surrounding the cradle of man's birth with a brilliant halo; but those who consider mental superiority the great factor that distinguishes man from all other beings are not dismayed by learning the truth. Man's psychic faculties do not appear to have come to him as a heritage from his remote ancestry. He achieved them through the ages in a manner which even science finds difficult to explain.

Evolution is by no means the only discovery which forced ancient tradition to make way for scientific thought. When Galileo Galilei (1564–1642) demonstrated that the earth was not a fixed body in the center of the universe, and that the sun and all other celestial luminous bodies were not created as satellites to serve the earth as the property of man, society was violated, and Galilei was made to pay the supreme penalty for his revolutionary discovery. The general populace and even men of learning could not conceive that the sun and other "hosts of heaven" were created for other purposes than to serve man with light. Man is most unwilling to become disillusioned and submit to reality.

While the Darwinian doctrine has been generally accepted by science, there are many things with reference to the history of man which science thus far has not adequately explained. Science has not made clear the precise antiquity of man and his birthplace. Perhaps the strata which contain the secret of the antiquity of man and his place of birth are yet to be uncovered. For, after all, what has been discovered thus far has been largely by chance (i.e. during the digging of a road or a railway or by the violence of an earthquake). Africa, Asia, America, and even the greater part of Europe are still, paleontologically speaking, unexplored.

Three Principal Theories: Three principal theories were formerly advanced as to the progenitor of man. According to Lamarck, man's early ancestor was a chimpanzee, since this animal approaches man more than any other anthropoid ape in its physical characteristics. M. Vogt believes that man is only a cousin of the anthropoid, and that the ancestor common to both of them is still farther off. The third theory is that of Haeckel, who believes that man's remote ancestor was an ape of the old continent, a pithecian, which itself was derived from a lemur, in turn going back to a marsupial. He believes man's birthplace was in widely separated places such as in Madagascar, Ceylon, or the Sunda Islands. The difference of opinion arises from the

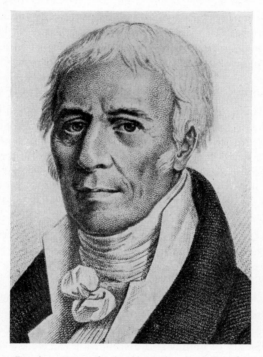

Fig. 9: Jean Baptiste Lamarck (1744-1829). Jean Baptiste Lamarck engaged in the study of medicine and botany after he resigned from the army on account of injury. In 1793, he was appointed to the *Jardin des Plantes* where he remained for 25 years as Professor of Invertebrate Zoology. Here he was joined later by Cuvier and St. Hilaire. In 1809, he published his famous "Zoologique," in which he supported the theory that all kinds of animals including man were derived from one species. This view was almost entirely superseded by Darwin's theory of natural selection. (Ambroise Tardieu.)

fact that each of the anthropoids, i.e. the chimpanzee, gorilla, orangutan, and gibbon, approaches man only in certain characteristics, but by no means in all. Even among the so-called "inferior races," no one race, not even the Bushman, is especially marked out as descending from an anthropoid. The precursor of man, then, is only analogous to the anthropoid apes. The human type is an improvement upon the general type of their family, but not of one of their known species in particular.

Peyrere's Doctrine: The controversy between the Monogenists and Polygenists is now only of academic interest. It is now recognized that all mankind originated from one stock and that racial difference is the result of natural selection, of crossing, and perhaps, to some extent, of external influences. The idea of polygenism was popular among religious philosophers of a bygone era. In 1655, Isaac de la Peyrere advanced the doctrine that there were pre-Adamite men and that Adam was the first man of the Semitic family only. To prove this assertion, he cited Genesis 4:15, "and the Lord set a sign for Cain lest any finding him should kill him." He claimed that this proved that there were in the days of Cain, other men who might attempt to kill him, for no other Adamites were left after Cain killed his brother Abel.

Peyrere goes on to remark that the expression in Genesis 6:2, "The sons of God saw the daughters of men," and then the term "nephilim" (giants) prove conclusively that Adamites were not referred to. Furthermore there is no record of Adam having any daughters. Thus, even according to Genesis, the creation of man goes back further than 5705 years.

Peyrere's Biblical "discovery" particularly appealed to Americans who favored slavery. They maintained that the pre-Adamites were ancestors of the modern Negro and that the whites are the only bonafide descendants of Adam.

Unity and Antiquity of Man: The unity of man is now upheld by religious thinkers; they attribute the traits of the different races of man to geographic distribution in accordance with the book of Genesis. The early antiquity of man is still disputed by the clergy. Science, however, has furnished ample evidence that man assuredly is of great antiquity. The exact time and place, however, when man separated from his forebearer is still a mystery. John Burroughs aptly remarked: "Man has climbed up from some animal form and he has, as it were, pulled the ladder with him."

Lamarck's Theory: While the evolution of man from a lower species of life has been generally accepted, biologists have not been in accord as to the process by which the change has taken place. Jean Baptiste Lamarck (1744–1829), in his "Philosophie Zoologique" (1809), presented a theory that environmental changes could lead to an alteration in the habits of an animal. This altered habit could consequently cause increased use of some organ, together with a compensatory decreased use of others, resulting in new acquired characteristics which could be transmitted from parents to offspring and cause the formation of a new species. Lamarck sums up his views in the following words:

All that nature has caused individuals to acquire or lose through the circumstances to which their race has found itself for a time exposed, and consequently, through the predominant exercise of certain organs, or through a failure to exercise certain parts, it preserves through heredity to the new individuals that are produced by them, provided the changes acquired are common to the two sexes, or to those that have produced these new individuals.

As an example, according to Lamarck, the remote ancestors of the present day long-necked giraffe originally had a short neck like other animals. The long neck was acquired by attempts to reach the foliage of the more lofty shrubs. With continued effort, the neck became elongated and this character was transmitted from one generation to another and finally became a fixed racial character. Lamarck's view was popular among biologists before the Darwinian doctrine was proposed. It was finally rejected when it was shown to be contrary to the facts.

If acquired characteristics would be transmitted to future generations by heredity, it was argued, then the practice of circumcision at the present time among certain races would not be necessary, for the male infants born certainly would have acquired from their parents the change in the character of the prepuce in the many thousands of years since the advent of this custom. Chinese women have compressed their feet from time immemorial without any change in the size of the feet of the newly born female infants. An Indian tribe which flattened the heads of their progeny in early life from remote ages, did not undergo any hereditary changes in skulls. Among the lower animals, dogs and sheep have been docked for many generations, and yet the young are still born with tails of the same length as their ancestors.

Darwin's Theory: Darwin (1809–1882) was inclined first to accept the Lamarck theory of transmutation but later he abandoned it. He writes:

If under changed condition of life, a structure before useful, becomes less useful, its demutation will be favorable for it will profit the individual not to have its nourishment wasted in building up useless structures...Thus I believe natural selection will tend in the long run to reduce any part of the organism as soon as it becomes through changed habits superfluous. [15]

Darwin explains his own theory of transmutation[16] as follows: No two offsprings of the same parents are quite similar to each other; indeed they often vary to a considerable extent. Under the conditions in which they live, some of these offsprings will have an advantage over the rest, dependent upon an inborn peculiarity. Since, therefore, more progeny are produced than can ever survive, those most fitted to these surroundings will have the better chance of living. These will, in larger numbers, perpetuate the race and transmit their unborn qualities to the race, thus gradually eliminating the less suitable ones.[17]

Getting back to the example of the giraffe, Darwin and Wallace would explain the length of the neck as follows: With Lamarck they believe that the ancestor was short-necked, but the subsequent elongation they explain in quite another way. During times when grass and foliage were scarce, the short-necked animals soon exhausted the herbage and shrubs. The taller shrubs and trees afforded subsistence to animals with a higher reach. Among the ancestral giraffes, those born with the longest necks would at such times have an advantage over the rest, who would in large numbers perish from starvation. The longer-necked ones, more suited to their environment, would perpetuate their inborn quality of long-neckedness. Again with the next generation, those with the longest necks would survive, and so on.[18]

In the "Origin of Species" (1859), Charles Darwin presented a new salient conception of evolution in the theory that man might have originated from a creature whose physical characteristics bore a very strong resemblance to those of the higher apes of the present day. He mentions specifically the gorilla, chimpanzee, and the orangutan as the most closely related to the human ancestral stock. Darwin proved his theories with a wealth of facts drawn from a variety of scientific fields, and he presented his subject so convincingly that it defied successful contradiction. The only opposition to his main thesis came from the pulpit and a part of the lay press who saw in this theory an effort to undermine the narrative of the Holy Writ.

"Natural Selection" Theory: In his doctrine of "Natural Selection," Darwin supplied a good working hypothesis as to how evolution might have been brought about. He immediately gained support of such contemporary scientists as Herbert Spencer, Alfred Russell Wallace, Henry Huxley, and the eminent geologist, Sir Charles Lyell. Lyell at first opposed the doctrine of transmutation of species, but he eventually became converted to Darwin's views.

Herbert Spencer (1820–1903), in an early essay "The Development of Hypothesis" (1852), opposed the theory of evolution, but in his "Principles of Psychology," he appears to treat his subjects from an evolutionary point of view.

Scientific men at present may differ as to the cause of evolution and may disagree with Darwin, particularly with regard to his "Natural Selection" theory, but they are unanimous in accepting the doctrine of some form of organic evolution.[19]

The doctrine of evolution, which is generally accepted at the present time, teaches that organic forms are not separate creations, but each bears a certain definite relationship to all other forms; that all organic forms undergo modifications; that all of our present plants and animals are the descendants of preexisting forms of organic life; and that the farther back we trace man, the more we find him approaching in bodily form those species of the anthropoid quadrumana which are most akin to him in structure. According to this theory, the first appearance of man on earth was followed by a vast period of human savagery which lasted until the ever-progressing development made the race capable of civilization.

SIX FUNDAMENTAL PROPOSITIONS: The principle of evolution, which is based by Darwin on the hypothesis of "Natural Selection," includes the following six fundamental propositions:

1. Living organisms are enormously fertile, yet the total number is approximately stationary, being kept down by the periodical deficiency of food and disease.

2. In the struggle for existence, a vast majority of the organisms which come into the world are doomed to early death.

3. As a consequence of the extensive variability in structures and activities, even among the very closely related individuals, some will fit better into the existing environment than others and so will carry an advantage.

4. Some of the huge number of individuals competing for a place in the world have advantageous variations and are consequently preserved, while those with unfavorable variations perish (natural selection or survival of the fittest).

5. Changing environment necessitates continued structural modifications.

6. If certain members of a given group meet the conditions of life through variation in one direction, and others in other directions, then divergence among the forms through the continued action of natural selection, generation after generation, must in time be sufficient to make them evolve into new species.[20]

The primary shortcoming in this process of natural selection as a causative principle lies in the fact that the mere act of sifting out the fit by exterminating forms which have undergone unfavorable variations cannot of itself initiate new variations.

Darwin applied his hypothesis of "Natural Selection" not only as a biologic factor in the "Origin of Species," but also as a sociologic factor in the preservation of most favored individuals, as well as the selection of the most efficient groups in the intertribal conquests. In his "Descent of Man," he states:

. . . the early progenitors of man must have tended, like all other animals, to have increased beyond their means of sustenance, and that they must, therefore, actually have been exposed to a struggle for existence and consequently to the rigid law of "Natural Selection." Beneficial variation tends to preserve; injurious variation tends to destroy. Man's favorable variation lies in his greater intelligence and development of social attitudes which lead to cooperation for mutual defense.[21]

It is often stated that "Natural Selection," in the social sense, has been done away with at the present time in view of our advanced civilization where there is no fear of wild beasts and other catastrophies. Weaklings who would perish under more primitive conditions are kept alive, and everything possible is done to prevent "Natural Selection" from eliminating the ill-favored members of the human race. But "Natural Selection" operates in other ways. While it is true that one form of "Natural Selection" has been done away with through modern civilization, other forms continue to operate.

Evolution against Disease: Dr. Reid points out in his "Present Evolution of Man" that man's advance is not mainly an evolution of physical or intellectual strength, as was the case with his remote ancestry, but also an evolution against disease. Reid is undoubtedly right in his contention that the course of human development has been greatly influenced by the selective action of various diseases, and that this will probably continue in the future. Races tend through the action of "Natural Selection" to become immunized to prevalent diseases. The white man's diseases have decimated the American Indian; the Negro is susceptible to tuberculosis and is relatively immune to malaria; and the Chinese resist typhoid.

The selective agency may act very differently upon different racial stocks. The complex of conditions presented by life in India weighs more heavily upon Europeans than upon the Hindus. In the United States, economic and climate factors are much more fatal to the Negroes than to the whites, and accordingly life expectancy among whites is much longer than among Negroes.

The effects of selective agencies upon different races unquestionably have had much to do with determining the present geographical distribution of the races of mankind. The Negro population could never invade the Arctic Circle, even if there were no other human competitors; and were it not for their relative immunity to malaria, they would probably long ago have been eliminated from Africa by invaders from other lands.

Dr. J. A. Lindsay has pointed out that the selective influence of disease cannot be treated in general terms. Some diseases, like the plague, cholera, and typhus, produce much greater ravages among the slum elements of the population than among the well-to-do, whereas influenza is much more apt to attack all classes and age groups, although not with equal virulence or mortality. The common diseases of childhood, such as whooping cough, measles, scarlet fever, and diphtheria, are very prevalent among all classes. The mortality of the first three is much greater among the children of the poor. Diphtheria, on the other hand, when allowed to run its natural course, has a high mortality among rich and poor alike. With measles, scarlet fever, and whooping cough, mortality is largely dependent upon general health, whereas with diphtheria this is not so. Any consideration of the role that "Natural Selection" plays in the destiny of man must also take into account the selective nature of disease.

Weismann,[22] a consistent follower of the Darwinian theory, has maintained that the so-called "inheritance of useful and unuseful organs or acquired instincts" may readily be explained by the law of selection:

The gradual increase for generations in the size of a useful limb or the perfection of a valuable organ of sense, may readily be explained by selection. The fact that the limb or organ is useful to the race in its struggle for existence will determine the survival of those born with these serviceable parts well formed and these in their turn will produce others as favorably or more favorably constituted from whom further selection can take place.

The study of the origin of disease shows that by far the greater number of severe constitutional derangements produce no effect upon the productive cells. They are incapable of producing a change that will be hereditarily transmitted. They can, however, produce racial changes by selection. In most diseases the blood composition tends to undergo changes, and many of the tissues suffer alteration in structure. These changes, however, are of a temporary character. When the attack is over, as in the case of smallpox for example, numerous diseases cannot be inflicted again upon the individual for a protracted period of time.

Metchnikoff explains the induced immunity as follows:

An army of the small cells called phagocytes which wander through the blood and tissues are able to attack the microbes of disease and after a struggle they are able in many cases to kill these voracious intruders.

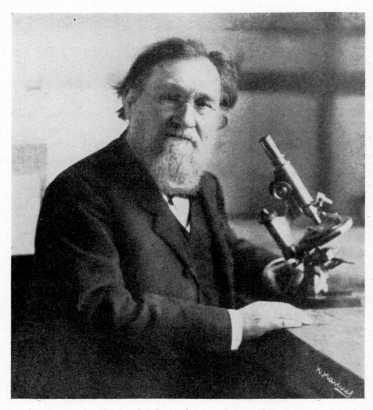

Fig. 10: Elie Metchnikoff (1845–1916). Elie Metchnikoff lived in Russia at a period when the academies of education were closely guarded by secret police against liberal thoughts. He attempted to commit suicide twice because of persecution. He finally managed to escape to Messina. One day, while watching moving cells of a transparent, star-fish larva through a microscope, he conceived the idea that mobilization of such cells might serve as a defence mechanism of the organism against the invaders of the body. This was the beginning of his theory of phagocytosis: the doctrine that, when microbes attack the body, multitudes of phagocytes rush to the injured part, hurl themselves against the bacterial enemies, and attempt to destroy them, He soon became known as a pathologist, although he had no medical training. Eventually, he joined the staff of the Pasteur Institute in Paris.

In so doing, however, numerous phagocytes succumb to the struggle while those which are left alive within the body of a convalescent patient possess the power of resisting and destroying the particular microbe which had undertaken the invasion. These resisting phagocytes selected from the rest, together with their descendants who share their resisting qualities, are able to prevent fresh inroads of the same enemy. This acquired immunity does not indicate any change in the ordinary muscle or brain cells of the body or that the reproductive cells are in anyway altered, for the immunity is due only to a change in the phagocyte army.

Just as children of the same parents are not exactly alike with respect to color of hair, shape of limbs, or temperament, so they differ in their capacity to combat the micro-organisms of disease. An epidemic disease will seek out for destruction those organically liable to fall prey to it. Those having greater resistance will not only survive but will produce progeny selected for survival.[23]

Since the rediscovery in 1900 of the Mendelian doctrine of heredity, the theory of "Natural Selection" has lost much of its former prestige. Biologists are not as ready to accept the "Natural Selection" as an adequate explanation of the origin of species, although their faith in the Darwinian theory of evolution remains intact.

There might have been more than one cause contributing to the evolution of man. From a medical point of view, however, the "survival of the fittest" was one of the most important causes. It is well known that bacterial organisms existed before man, that communities and entire districts were swept away by pestilence and famine, that only those favored with immunity in combating the ravages of the frequent epidemics survived, and that only those endowed with resourcefulness in the search for food remained alive.

References and Notes

1. Genesis 2:7.
2. Lewes, G. H.: Aristotle, p. 107.
3. Darwin, C.: Descent of Man. D. Appleton-Century Co., New York, 1871, p. 6.
4. Huxley, T. H.: Man's Place in Nature. D. Appleton-Century Co., New York, 1899, p. 143.
5. "Descent of Man." p. 7.
6. Ibid., pp. 50-53.
7. Ibid., pp. 52-53.
8. Ibid., pp. 88-89.
9. "Man's Place in Nature." p. 143.
10. Ibid., pp. 152-153.
11. Miyart, S.: Elementary Anatomy. 1873, p. 396.
12. The Anatomy of Expression. 1884, pp. 110-131 (cited by Darwin, p. 11).
13. "Descent of Man," pp. 18-32.
14. Wallace, A. R.: Natural Selection. The Macmillan Co., New York, 1871, pp. 34-35; see also Darwin: Descent of Man, p. 47.

15. Huxley, T. H.: Life and Letters. 2:14.
19. Osborn, H. F.: Biblical World. 4:67. Scott, W. F.: Theory of Evolution, 1917,
17. "Descent of Man," p. 47.
18. "Natural Selection," pp. 41 & 43.
19. Osborn, H. F.: Biblical World. 4: 67. Scott, W. F.: Theory of Evolution. 1917,
     p. 1. Park, G. H.: What Evolution Is. 1925, p. 62.
20. "Natural Selection," p. 302.
21. "Descent of Man." pp. 47-48.
22. Weismann, A.: Studies in the Theory of the Descent, translated by Raphael
     Meldola, p. 62. Essays upon Heredity, translated by Poluton. Schonland
     & Shiply, London, Vol. 1, published in 1889, Vol. 2 in 1892.
23. Haycraft, J. B.: Darwinism and Race Progress. London, 1895, pp. 3-27.

3

Paleolithic Evidence of the Antiquity
of Medicine

FOR AGES man paid little attention to his early history. The discoveries
of hieroglyphic writings in Egypt and cuneiform inscriptions in Babylonia during the last century forced the attention of the civilized world
to the fact that human history was vastly more ancient than had been
previously conceived. Archaeological investigations have brought to
view civilized peoples much further back in the past than history had
formerly supposed possible. Linguistic science has demonstrated that
man is much older than was generally supposed, and that many civilized
communities and family groups of languages did exist in remote antiquity. It was pointed out that many centuries, and perhaps millenniums, had elapsed before so complete a system as the hieroglyphic
and cuneiform scripts could have been evolved; and the development
of certain arts and sciences among the early Egyptians and Chaldeans
must also have required ages previous to the dawn of written history.
In consequence of these observations, the date of man's birth was pushed
further and further back beyond the 5705 years calculated according
to the book of Genesis.

No one even dared dream that the antiquity of man could be counted
into hundreds of thousands and perhaps millions of years. The doctrine of evolution changed the whole aspect of history. Instead of man's
being a strange creature made in the mold of his Creator by a supernatural hand and endowed at the dawn of his history with a high degree
of intellect and knowledge,[1] but who has undergone a progressive decline through the ages, it became clear that man was not created in
his present form; but like all other metazoans, he gradually developed

43

from forms of life physically and mentally inferior to himself. In other words, man during the ages of his existence has not fallen but risen.

FOSSILS

Paleontological records exhibit a progressive series of animal forms throughout the successive geologic strata. The more recent the strata, the higher the type, and the more nearly the approximation to the modern species. Whole groups of animals at times disappeared at the close of a geologic period to be replaced by other distinct groups of closely related species without the appearance of intermediate forms.

Early Interpretation of Fossils: For a long time fossilized human remains were looked upon by some as individuals of the nether world which cannot live when exposed to the air but are very much alive underground. Others assumed such remains to be the "fallen man"[2] transformed into stone as punishment for religious violations. Again there were crude notions that fossilized human remains were relics of the universal deluge which, according to the Hebrew tradition, destroyed all living beings[3] excepting those that were with Noah on the Ark. Still others opined that these relics were freaks of nature *(lusus naturae)*: the larger fossils the remnants of giants; the smaller ones the remains of pygmies.

In modern China "dragon bones," as fossils are called, have a highly commercial value. When powdered, dissolved in acid, and mixed with a liberal quantity of superstition they are considered highly efficacious remedies in almost every kind of disease, from malaria to compound fracture of the leg. The apothecary shops carry on a luxurious trade with fossils; and if a Chinese discovers a fossil-bearing locality, he guards it as if it were a gold mine.

Greek philosophers, such as the Pythagoreans, interpreted fossils as an effort of earthly matter to become living organisms. Aristotle and Xenophon, and Roman writers such as Strabo, knew of the existence of fossils and surmised in a crude way their relation to the history of the earth. When naturalists began to study the fossils buried in the rock of the earth's crust, they soon learned that the newer deposits contain forms akin to these now living on the earth and that the deeper strata hold remains that differ from present day animals.

Source of Prehistoric Events: Historic facts are gathered from written record in the form of inscriptions on clay tablets, stone, papyri, and other writing surfaces. Prehistoric events are deduced from unearthed flints, sherds, bones, horns, teeth, or houses. Fragments of fine art and good architecture indicate that the people of that period were advanced in culture. On the other hand, crude implements or weapons made of stone show that their owners were poorly advanced culturally. People, not capable of making even the most rudimentary works of art, leave evidence of their existence and their activities, which together with their bones, serve as records to those who are learned in examining them. The science of geology has provided a background upon which events long erased from human memory may be recovered. It supplies information as to the chronological sequence of changes of the earth's surface and elucidates the period of time when manlike apes or apelike men first appear on the scene. By subdividing the tertiary period, one may follow the history of the development of the modern type of life and may observe how the fauna of each period became gradually more and more like those of the present. The succeeding strata of the earth, and the remains encased within them, are like the pages of a book, each marked by different kinds of fossils. The lowest kind of fossils are imbedded in the deeper and older rocks and the highest in upper and newer rocks. Fossils commonly consist of shells, bones, teeth, and other hard parts of animals, since these are the remains most readily preserved in the sediment of streams.

In the Miocene strata of the tertiary period, anthropoid apes allied to the gibbon and chimpanzee appeared in Europe. Apelike men or manlike apes, such as the Pithecanthropus, of which certain bone fragments were found in Java in 1891, probably belong to a later tertiary period (Pliocene).

From towards the end of the tertiary period (Pleistocene), evidences of intelligent ape-men have been unearthed in the form of fossilized skeletons or bones, often intermingled with similar remains of extinct animals. These ape-men are characterized by overhanging brows, projecting jaws, and chin sloping back from the base of the lip. From their remains it is evident that they crouched as they walked, with head thrust forward and back bowed; their legs, of almost human proportions, were curved, and closely approximate those of modern man. The later tertiary period witnessed the appearance in Europe of man having the bodily characteristics of the present species. The ape-man, distinctly lower and less able to survive in his struggle for existence, had to yield to this higher form. The relations sustained in early times between various types of intelligent primates are a moot question. However, they all seem to have used various stone implements characteristic of the period during which they sojourned, and the handiwork of each succeeding period represented a great improvement over the eoliths of the early periods. Carved and furrowed bones, which have been

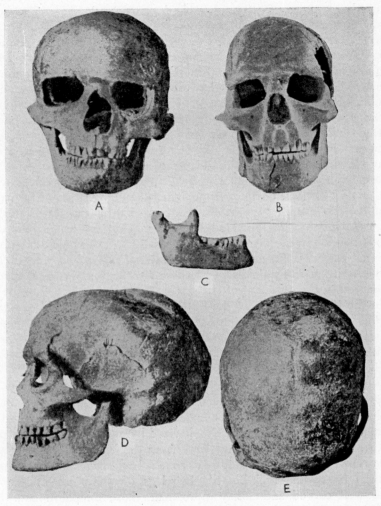

Fig. 11: Skulls of Aurignacian Age from Western Europe. *A, C, D, E:* Male skulls and lower jaw of Cro-Magnon type, from the *Grotte des Enfants* near Mentone (after R. Verneau). *B:* Male skull from Combe-Capelle, type of *Homo aurignacensis* (?) (after H. Klaatsch).

unearthed, indicate that they are not the product of the teeth or claws of carnivorous animals but unquestionably the handiwork of man.

Stone Age: The term "Stone Age," which is used to designate a certain prehistoric epoch, really does not refer to an exact time or place. There never has been a time nor a condition of life when man used nothing but stone tools and weapons. At all times he has had at his disposal other materials, such as wood, bone, ivory, horn, and shell. The term "Stone Age," excludes only metals. During this stage, man commonly made his implements, weapons, and tools largely of stone. The Stone Age therefore does not express a period of time which has passed, but rather any culture in which metals are not used in making implements.

Duration of Stone Age: While it is true that in western Europe the Stone Age ended when metal came into use, in North Africa there are still persons who use stone implements. Maspero relates that he saw a man who was still shaving his head with a flint blade; when he asked him why he didn't use a less painful instrument, his reply was, "This was good enough for my father and surely must be good enough for me." The man was well up in years. He stated that in his youth this was a common custom in Egypt. His head, which was bleeding after usage of the rough razor, he covered with leaves. He continued this manner of shaving to the end of his life.

In the Pacfic Islands, the Stone Age was in progress when the white man reached there; in North America, the Stone Age continued among Indians until the last century. In South America, there is no doubt that many tribes still live in the Stone Age.

Periods of Stone Age: The Stone Age is divided into two periods known as "paleolithic" and "neolithic." During the paleolithic period, rudely made tools were manufactured of stone by chipping; in the neolithic period man occasionally made tools of great beauty and delicacy, and in addition, he often polished his stone products.

Location of Implements: Stone implements have been found all over Europe, America, and parts of Asia. They are constructed from various flints and stones. Many of them are obviously intended for warlike purposes. To peoples long past the Stone Age, such mementos aroused a feeling of mystery and even awe. In the eleventh century, a "haven axe" was considered a suitable gift for a king. As late as the seventeenth century, a French ambassador brought a stone hatchet (which is still displayed in the museum of Nancy) as a present to the Prince Bishop of Verdun. This gift was believed to possess great healing virtues.

Folklores Regarding Implements: The peasants of western Europe revere the stone axes which are picked up occasionally in the fields or dug up in the course of excavations. Folklore has it that they are thunderbolts which have fallen from the sky and that they are efficacious in protecting their bearer from lightning. In Germany peasants call such a stone axe "Donnerkeile" (thunder chisel); these are kept in families as a protection from lightning. A common saying regarding the stone axe is the following: "He who chastely beareth this shall not be struck by lightning, nor the house, nor the town where this stone is." In Russia, when a peasant finds a stone axe, he guards it avidly. If he constructs a house, it is built into the house under the threshold, and is considered a positive protection against damage from tempest. If his house is already built, the stone is carefully guarded; and when the winds and clouds and roaring thunder announce a storm, it is brought out and placed upon the table. With it are also placed a candle blessed by a priest of the village and a holy crucifix; and surely with this triple guarding, combining charms of both ancient and modern times, objects connected with both paganism and Christianity, no ill can befall the peasant.

In Cornwall, water in which a celt is boiled is a cure for rheumatism; in Brittany, it is put in wells to purify the water and to keep up its supply; in Germany, it is considered good for diseases of man and beast—it increases the milk of cows, assists childbirth, and becomes most valuable as a remedy for children's diseases; in Saxony, rolled in the wool of sheep or the hair of goats, it brings good luck to the flock or herd, and prevents rot and putrid decay.

Arrowheads also were believed to possess magic power. In Scotland, Ireland, and other countries they are called "elf darts," and are believed to be weapons of the fairies. The superstition is entertained that arrowheads are never found when one is seeking them. They are often mounted in silver and worn as charms to ward off the attacks of occult agencies. When a peasant believes that the disease which ails his cattle is due to some evil mystic agency, he at times calls in a fairy doctor, who with much mystery proceeds to suck the part which is the seat of the disease, thus drawing out the fairy darts; then the occult physician places the invisible darts, together with a coin, into a vessel of water from which the animal is made to drink; this effects a cure. In southern Europe, also, curious notions regarding the stone arrowhead abound. A peasant, when finding such "a tongue of St. Paul," devoutly kneels before it, picks it up with his own tongue, and keeps it for a charm. In North Africa, Arabs wear necklaces of carnelian beads, which are imitations of old arrowheads, "because they are good for the blood."

When Europeans and Americans first visited Alaska, the Indian inhabitants were living in the Stone Age. They had stone axes, awls, adzes, knives, chisels, and the like. Now and then, when a native of Alaska wishes to undertake some enterprise of more than usual importance, he takes down the old stone adze to use in the day's work. In order that the full miraculous benefit may be reaped from the old tool, the wife at home is forbidden to speak a word during her husband's absence for fear of spoiling the charm. Notwithstanding the fact that the stone adze was perfectly well known to the natives, that it formerly was in common use, and that the nature of its manufacture and employment were well known, there was the tendency to look upon this aged tool, tried and true, with reverence.

The old stone tool superstition dies hard as the new and better implement comes into use. Many persist in their use of the old tool. The book of Joshua[4] distinctly states that Joshua used stone knives for circumcision. The Jews were certainly not in the Stone Age at this period. Unquestionably metallic tools and implements were used for ordinary purposes. But the old stone knife was continued in the religious ceremony harking back to the book of Exodus, "Then Zipporah took a sharp stone and cut off the foreskin of her son."[5]

The Egyptians used a knife of stone to cut open the body which was to be embalmed. This is seen from Herodotus:

The body being laid on the ground, he who is called a scribe first marks on its left side how far the incision is to be made, then the embalmer having an Ethiopian stone and cutting the flesh as far as the law allows, instantly runs off, the bystanders pursuing him and cursing him and pelting him with stones and, as it were, turning the horror of the dead upon him. [6]

Geological Study of Fossils

The study of fossils was retarded until the revival of learning in Italy. Scientists of the sixteenth and seventeenth centuries had some well-advanced ideas of fossilized man; but because of the rigid interpretation of the Biblical account of sudden creation, they did not openly express any opinion on the subject. The study of fossils was established as a branch of geology at the beginning of the nineteenth century and somewhat later became incorporated in the new science of paleontology.[7]

Lamarck and Cuvier: J. B. Lamarck (1744–1829) and Georges Leopold Cuvier (1769–1832) were the pioneers in this branch of geology; the first was the founder of invertebrate and the second of vertebrate paleontology. Their ideas on this subject prevailed from the close of the eighteenth century to the publication of Darwin's "Origin of Species" in 1859. To Lamarck, science is indebted for the hypothesis of "slow variation," both with regard to living forms and environment. To Cuvier, science owes a tribute for the first clear expression of the idea of "increasing organic perfection" in all forms of life from the lowest to the highest organisms.

Prehistoric Records in Rocky Strata: The study of geology has shown that the earth has undergone evolutionary changes through the millions of years of its existence. Upheavals occurring at different periods of the earth's history have exposed to view many of the rocky strata

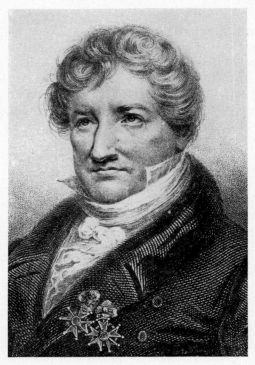

Fig. 12: Georges Leopold Cuvier (1769-1832). Georges Leopold Cuvier assumed a high position among French naturalists. He may be regarded as the first to classify animals in kingdoms. His first professorship of anatomy was held at the *Museum d' Histoire Naturalles.* In 1798, he became Professor of Natural History in the College of France. Among subjects taught was the study of fossils of mammals and reptiles, as well as the osteology of living forms belonging to these groups. The subject of paleontology may be said to have been one of his creations. He was a prolific writer. The results of his paleontological and geological investigations were published in a work of two volumes, "Recherches sur les Ossements Fossiles de Quadrupeds" (1812).

deposited in different geologic eras. By observing these strata in the different regions, geologists have been able to piece together a fairly well-connected history of the earth's crust. They were able to determine which deposits are very old and which are relatively recent, and to what particular chapter in the world's history a given stratum belongs. Scientists found in these rocky strata the records of prehistoric man. To quote Agassiz (1853): "The crust of our earth is a great cemetery where the rocks are the tombstones on which the buried dead have written their epitaphs."[8] The records disclose that man, as well as other living beings, existed in early geologic times.

Occasionally a cast of a living being is discovered. The organism itself, which was originally imbedded in mud or clay, has long since decayed with the space it occupied filled with infiltrations of foreign material, thereby forming a cast which assumed the outline of the organism replaced. Sometimes only an imprint is found as a result of an impression made in soft mud or clay by a living being.

But, most frequently, fossil remains are found which are formed as the result of petrifaction (i.e. the substance of the organic body is replaced by mineral matter). Human fossils throw much light upon the physical history of man and have made the greatest contribution to the doctrine of the origin of species and descent of man.

Fossils only occur in sedimentary strata such as sand, stone, shale, and limestone. Fossils are being formed at the present time just as they were a million years ago: when an animal dies, the body may be covered with sand or other sediments; then very slow changes ensue, cell by cell, until the animal substance is replaced by mineral matter; eventually petrifaction is completed, and the animal is changed to stone as it were. A region must have the proper age and geologic formation to exhibit fossil remains.

Three Periods of Prehistoric Archaeology: Prehistoric archaeology deals with three periods, known respectively as the "paleolithic," the "neolithic," and the "Bronze Age." Each is distinct from the other two, although the latter two show a certain amount of overlapping. However, there is no evidence that a neolithic race has ever gone back to paleolithic methods; there is no case of a people which has learned to use metal that has voluntarily gone back to limiting itself to stone.

Knowing the stratum in which a fossil is found, one may derive a fair idea as to the period in which the organism, that has been transformed into a fossil, existed. Taking the human skull as a starting point, one may observe the modification in the form and capacity of the skull between the Paleolithic, Neolithic, and Bronze Ages, and also of modern races. Geology, therefore, throws a bright light on the early history of man.

Knowledge Obtained from Fossils: Although, in the case of lower animals, one can form a definite idea of their habits and mode of life from the structure of their bones and teeth, as far as the present state of our knowledge of man is concerned, one cannot always distinguish between the skeleton of a savage and that of a philosopher. Man of past ages is to be studied principally by his works—by the houses he has built for the living, by the tombs he has constructed for the dead, by the fortifications he has erected for defense, by the implements he has fashioned to aid him in his tasks and by the ornaments he has manufactured for decorative purposes.

The data now available for the study of early man are thus manifold. Very interesting is the evidence to be derived from his handiwork. Stone implements give considerable knowledge concerning early man. The earliest products of the first human artisans consist of chippings made with implements of flint, probably the first material known to have been so used by man; these belong to the paleolithic period of the Stone Age.

Neolithic man was a different being. Although he continued to use flint implements, he greatly perfected them. He also adopted a permanent place of residence and became an agriculturist as well as hunter and fisherman. He buried his dead with the obvious expectation of life on the other side of the grave. He built houses and erected wonderful megalithic monuments. He at last discovered the art of smelting metals; and after an era of bronze weapons and ornaments, he eventually ushered in the Age of Iron.

Fossil remains of human bones have been found in numerous caves of England, France, Belgium, the Netherlands, and the Valley of the Rhine, intermingled with those of the rhinoceros, cave bear, and animals that have since disappeared from the earth, indicating that man has lived contemporaneously with animals that still persist and others that have been long extinct and swept away from the modern world. Such caves, which are mostly found in calcareous strata, are often closed with slabs of stone, evidently to protect the occupants from predatory animals.

In 1855, Lund, a Danish naturalist, discovered human fossils in eight different locations, all bearing signs of geological antiquity. In the province of Minas Geraes, Brazil, he found human skeletons in a fossilized state, among the remains of forty-four different species of now extinct animals, and under conditions which led him to the conclusion that all of them were contemporaneous inhabitants of the region where the vestiges were found.

Doctor Schmerling has examined a large number of localities in France and Liege where fossilized human bones and craniums, together with those of animals of extinct species, were found in caves. The human fossils were found in the same position as the animal remains; and near these relics, objects of human workmanship were discovered, such as fragments of vessels and flint implements imbedded in the clay.[9]

One of the first investigators in the field of paleontology was M. Boucher de Perthes. In 1838, he discovered, in the gravel-pits of Menchecourt in the valley of Somne, northern France, human bones associated with the remains of many extinct and nonextinct animals, such as the rhinoceros, the mammoth, the hippopotamus, the elephant, the cave bear, the hyena, the reindeer, the ox, and the urus. The human bones were mixed with scoriae, metals, pieces of pottery, and other vestiges of civilization of the period to which these buried men belong. A number of stone axes and other implements of human workmanship were also found. In his "Antiquities,"[10] he states:

My discoveries may appear trifling to some, for they comprise little save crumbling bones and rudely sculptured stones. Here are neither medals nor inscriptions, neither bas-reliefs nor statues—no vases, elegant in form, and precious in material—nothing but bones and rudely polished flints. But to the observer who values the demonstration of a truth more than the possession of a jewel, it is not in the finish of a work, nor in its market-price, that its value consists. The specimen most beautiful is that which affords the greatest help in proving a fact or realizing a provision; and the flint which a collector would throw aside with contempt, or the bone which has not even the value of a bone, rendered precious by the labor it has cost him, is prefered to a Murrine vase or to its weight in gold.

However great the number of ages which shroud the history of a people their intelligence may be ascertained by their works. If they have left no specimens of art, it is because they have merely appeared and vanished quickly. Experience proves that only races who have been cast upon an abnormal soil and under an unfriendly sky leave no mark behind them. They were a people who did not live a normal life; they only eked out a miserable existence and were always liable to extinction. But people who had a country and who were not brutalized by slavery and vice always leave traces behind them, a tradition of art, evanescent perhaps, but still sufficient to recall the physiognomy of the people, their social position, and the degree of civilization they had attained when that art was cultivated.

Among these specimens of primitive industry are arms and amulets which were intended to accompany their owners into the tomb, or even to follow them beyond the grave; for in all ages, men have longed for an existence after death. In these tokens from the tomb—these relics of departed ages—coarse and imperfect as they appear to an artistic eye, there is nothing that we should despise or reject; these are the last witnesses of the infancy of man and of his first footsteps upon earth; they present the only remains of nations who reared no columns nor monuments to record their existence. In these poor relics lie all their history, all their religion; and from these few rude hieroglyphics must one get an idea of their existence and the revelation of their customs.

If we were engaged with Egyptians, Greeks, or Romans, people who have furnished us with *chef-d'oeuvre* which still serve as our models, it would be irksome to examine the ancient oak to find whether it had fallen before the tempest or the axe, or to argue whether the angle of a stone had been smoothed by the hand of man or the action of running water. But when the soil we explore has no other signs of intelligent life, and the very existence of a people is in question, every vestige becomes history.

It is easy to conceive that, of all the works of man in those ancient deposits, instruments of stone would have the best chance to withstand the whips and scorns of time for they are best suited to resist the decomposing action of time. These stones bear marks of incessant friction which stone alone could have resisted.

The human remains discovered at the various excavations represent several varieties of the genus homo. Paleontologists can trace both physical and mental development from the older fossils up to the more recent forms. It is impossible to get away from the fact that very early man was a most primitive creature, not far removed from his animal ancestors, and far lower than present man. Indeed, all signs point to a time when he walked on all fours or at best in a semierect position; and his brain capacity, as appears from the skull cap of the Java man, was decidedly small. However, in spite of this apparent handicap, he did have, within his flat and poorly formed skull, something that was capable of continuous development, more capable of progress than the brain of any other animal.

Those whose minds are imbued with religious conviction detect in this apparent superiority the intervention and help of a supreme power— a certain purposeful entity, whose control has shaped the destiny of man and whose final goal is to the perfection of all his faculties to the end that he may be duly fitted for a future life when the earthly existence has come to an end. Others ascribe the same phenomena to a purely logical and physiological development and attribute such to man's superior cerebral equipment.

Henry F. Osborn is of the opinion that there is an impassable gap in the geological records between man and the anthropoid. After all, he argues, it is very uncertain as to just how he is related to the anthropoid ape, despite the fact that the physical homologies are close. He believes that the human ancestors and the anthropoid apes sprang from a common stock as far back as the Pliocene epoch.[11]

It is of interest to know at what particular stage of man's existence he became a thinking human animal. Naturally this development must have occurred long after his brain had attained a fairly high degree of impressionability.

The age of prehistoric man is calculated in terms of geologic deposits in which his remains are found. To quote Osborn again:

The antiquity of man is now reckoned not in the thousands but in the hundreds of thousands of years. And we will soon approach the period when it will be reckoned in millions of years.

The farther back we penetrate into the past, the more difficult it becomes to differentiate between a highly intellectual animal and the very rude human creature from whom man is said to have originated. Man slowly struggled up from a cultural phase where stones in their natural state were employed to serve his temporary purposes. This period, known as the "eolithic," was succeeded, after a vast interval, by a stage of human development where flint chipping was employed in the deliberate manufacture of tools.

MEN OF PALEOLITHIC PERIOD

There are four main groups of fossils of man or similar apelike creatures to be considered: (1) The Java man, or Pithecanthropus erectus; (2) the Dawn, or Piltdown, man; (3) The Neanderthal man; and (4) the Cro-Magnon man.

Java Man: Perhaps the most interesting and widely discussed fossilized human remains to be discovered is the Java man, or Pithecanthropus erectus, found in Trini, Java, by Dr. Eugene Dubois (1891–1892).[12] This discovery consisted of a calvarium, two molar teeth, and a left femur. Dr. Dubois made a comparative study of these bones with the human skeleton (both fossil and modern), and with the skeletal structure of the anthropoid apes. He concluded, in an exhaustive monograph (including photographs of each bone), published in 1891, that these bones came from an animal having an erect manlike attitude and a calvarium with characteristics partly human and partly animal— a missing link between the anthropoid ape and man.

Unfortunately, these bones, although found in the same Pliocene stratum, were not discovered close together. The skull cap was deposited 15 meters away from the femur, and some experts wondered if the bones were from the same individual. There was little difference of opinion among anatomists that the femur was human. It unmistakably belonged to a member of the genus homo who had assumed an erect attitude. Of the twenty experts who examined the teeth, some thought them to be human, some simian, and others insisted that they belonged to a transition form. The most significant feature of the Java calvarium is the small cranial capacity (1000 cc.). The distinctive features of the calvarium are the prominence of the supraorbital ridges and the occipital protuberance, and its remarkably low and receding forehead.

Piltdown Man: Another group of allegedly human remains, consisting of a shattered skull, a jawbone, and some teeth, apparently dating from

A   B

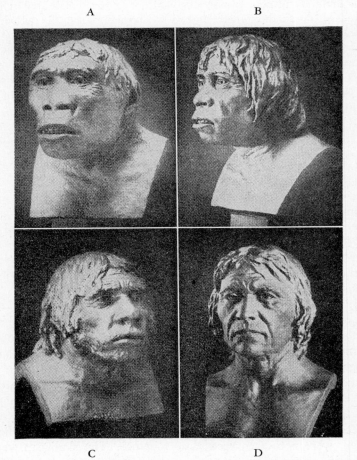

C   D

Fig. 13: Restoration of Prehistoric Men. *A: Pithecanthropus erectus,* the Java man. *B: Eoanthropus dawsoni,* the Piltdown man. *C: Homo neanderthalensis,* the Neanderthal man. *D: Homo sapiens,* the Cro-Magnon man. (From Lull, R. S.: Organic Evolution. The Macmillan Company, 1929.)

the Pliocene age, was discovered in Sussex, England, and is known as the "Piltdown man" or "Dawn man."[13] In this case the skull is very thick with a flat vertical forehead and a simianlike jaw. The general appearance of the skull suggests an intermediary form between chimpan-

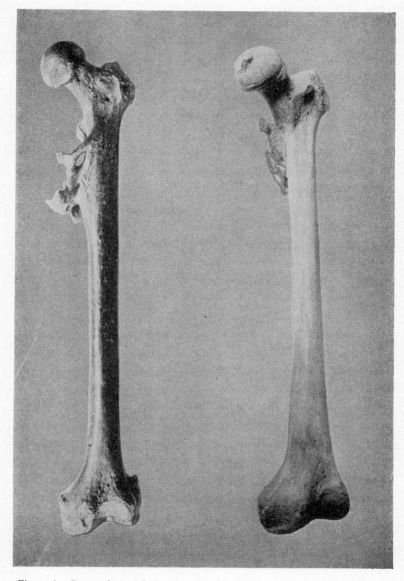

Fig. 14: Comparison of Femurs. *Left:* Femur of the *Pithecanthropus.* *Right:* Femur of a white American on the same scale. Both specimens show abnormal growth of bone near the upper end. The straightness of the bone shows that the *Pithecanthropus* had already acquired an erect posture. (Courtesy of the Smithsonian Institute, Washington, D. C.)

zee and Bushman. Owing to this extraordinary thickness of the skull and the simian character of the jaw, this man has sometimes been termed an "Eoanthropus." The brain capacity was estimated as 1070 cc. as compared with 1450 cc., the average capacity of modern man. The

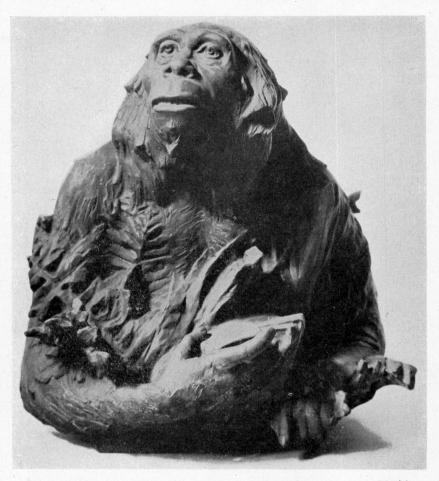

Fig. 15: Rutot's sculptor's conception of *Pithecanthropus erectus* (Smithsonian Institute photograph).

skull is remarkably large for these early times. It should be borne in mind that the cranial capacity of the largest male gorilla is not over 580 cc. Comparing this skull capacity with that of modern primitives, such as, for example, the Vedda tribes of East India, the Dawn man's

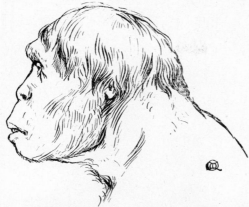

Fig. 16: *Pithecanthropus,* the subman of Java (restoration).

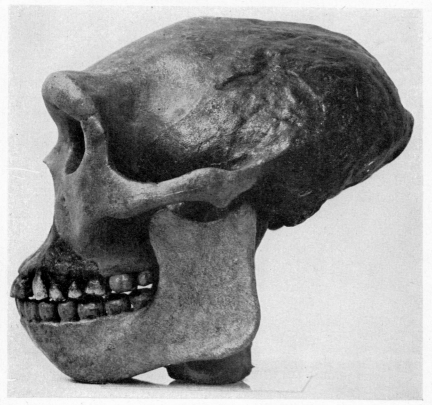

Fig. 17: Cast of Weidenreich's restoration of *Pithecanthropus'* cranium.
(Smithsonian Institute photograph.)

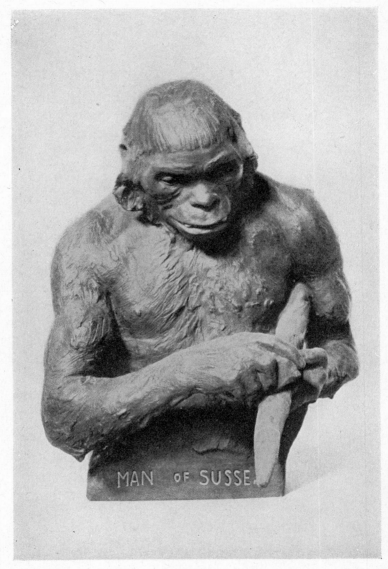

Fig. 18: Restoration of Piltdown man (Dawn man), shown using an eolith.
(Modeled by Mascre. Courtesy of the Smithsonian Institute.)

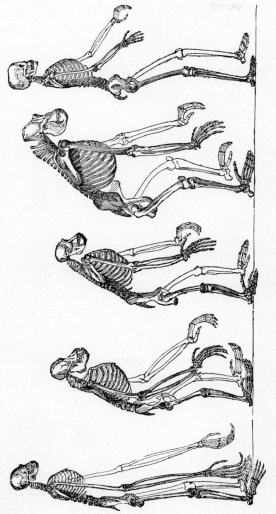

Fig. 19: Skeletons (from *left* to *right*) of the gibbon, orang, chimpanzee, gorilla, and man. (Photographically reduced from diagrams of the natural size [except that of the gibbon, which was twice as large as nature]. Drawn by Mr. Waterhouse Hawkins from specimens in the Museum of the Royal College of Surgeons.)

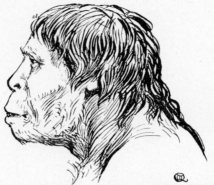

Fig. 20: *Eoanthropus Dawsoni,* the Piltdown man (restoration).

skull capacity was larger by 70 cc. The inner contour of the skull indicates that this Pliocene man had a developed speech area and a well convoluted forebrain. Two individuals of the same type have been found two miles apart. The caves where they were found were associated with flint and bone implements.

The Piltdown man, so far as our present knowledge goes, does not appear to be related to any other species of man found during the lower paleolithic period. Future discoveries of the Piltdown type may, however, raise him to generic rank.

Neanderthal Man: Another significant discovery was made in 1886 by workmen in a cave at the valley of Neander near Duesseldorf,[14] Germany, who found a human skull and some bones. Upon careful examination by Schaffhausen and other scientists, it was revealed that the form of the skull was that of a new type of man, something between

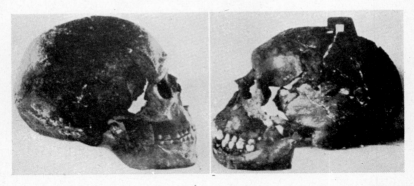

Fig. 21: Two prehistoric human skulls. *Right:* The skull of a Neanderthal man. *Left:* An Aurignacian skull.

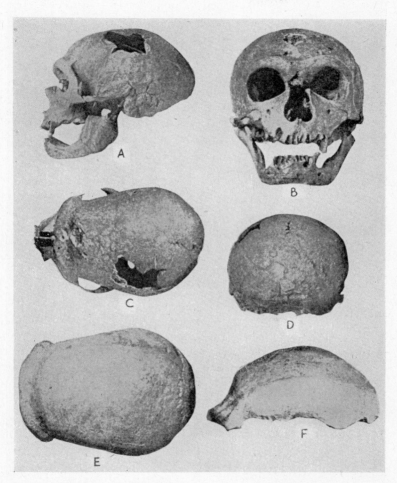

Fig. 22: Skulls of Neanderthal type. *A, B, C, D:* Skull from *La Chapelle-aux-Saints* (after M. Boule). *E, F:* Skull top of Neanderthal man (after H. Klaatsch).

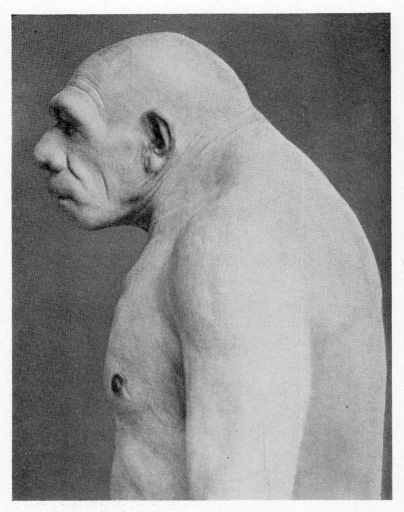

Fig. 23: Restoration of the Neanderthal man, showing especially the shape and carriage of the head. (Courtesy of the Museum of Natural History, New York.)

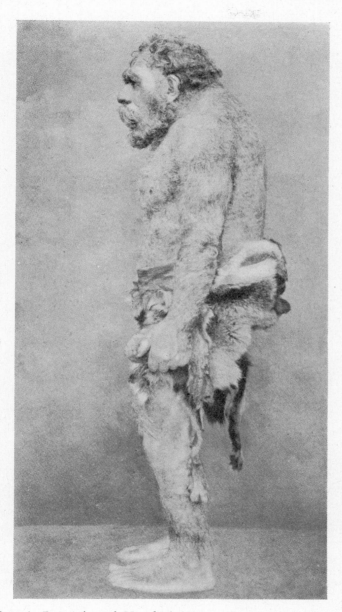

Fig. 24: Restoration of Neanderthal man. Note carriage of head; his skeleton shows that he could not quite straighten his knee joints. (Courtesy of the Field Museum of Natural History.)

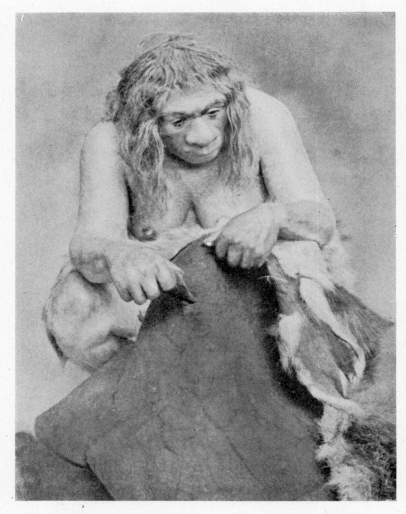

Fig. 25: Restoration of a Neanderthal woman scraping a hide. The large number of flint scrapers found indicates that the skins of animals were cured in Mousterian times. (Courtesy of the Field Museum of Natural History.)

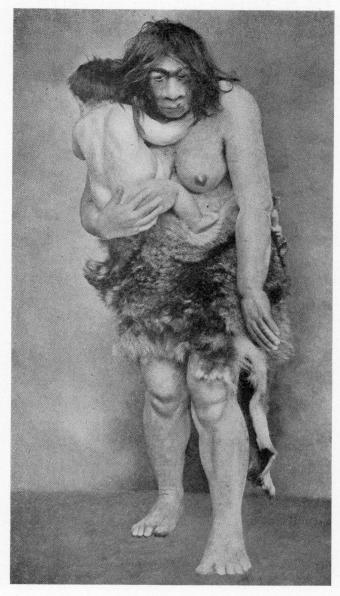

Fig. 26: Restoration of Neanderthal woman and child. (Courtesy of the Field Museum of Natural History.)

modern man and anthropoid apes. From the appearance of the skull and some of the bones, Schaffhausen reconstructed a picture of what is now known as the "Neanderthal man." Later, almost an entire skeleton of the Neanderthal man was discovered in a small grotto in France. This was examined by the noted French anthropologist, M. Marcellin Boule, who found it to be that of an old man. He described his frame-

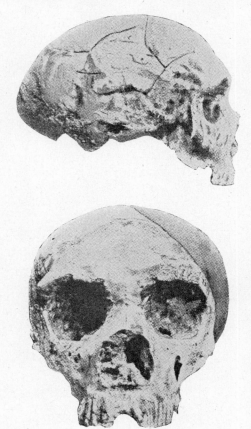

Fig. 27: The skulls of Gibraltar—Neanderthal type. (After A. Hrdlicka.)

work as follows: Large and flattened skull, prominent supraorbital ridges gradually sloping toward the back of the head, low retarding forehead, massive jaws, and a retarding chin. The head was long in proportion to its width (dolichocephalic).

Other characteristics of this Neanderthal man were short legs below the knee, a large perfectly formed hand, and well-formed grasping thumb and fingers. Judging from the evidences of his workmanship found in the same grotto, his hands were guided by a clever and designing mind. His stature as a whole was that of a stocky short man about 5 feet, 4 inches in height. His cranial capacity was 1530 cc., larger

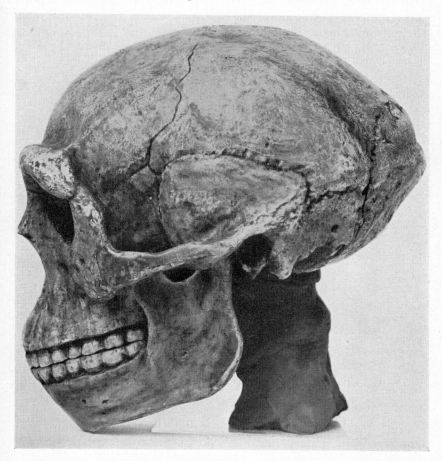

Fig. 28: Cast of Weidenreich's restoration of *Sinanthropus-hekinensis*-III cranium. (Smithsonian Institute photograph.)

than that of the average modern European skull, which is about 1450 to 1500 cc. On the basis of his observations, Schaffhausen gave as his opinion that this man was an intermediate between the simian and modern man. The skull became known as belonging to *Homo neanderthalensis*, and judging from the stratum and character of the earth in which it was discovered, the Neanderthal man probably existed 1,250,-000 years ago. The Neander valley type of man appears to have occupied parts of southern Europe and certain regions on the banks of the Mediterranean.

Some eighty-five years previous to this discovery, an English army officer stationed at Gibraltar found a human skull of great antiquity and unusual appearance. He forwarded the ancient relic to England where it was examined by Darwin and Huxley, but for some reason or other

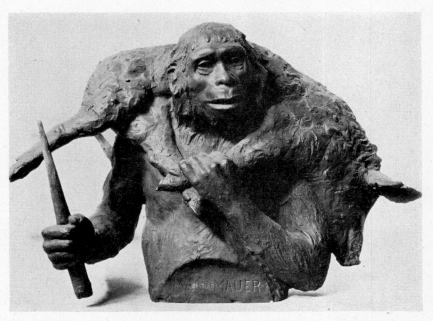

Fig. 29: Rutot's sculptor's conception of *Homo heidelbergensis.* (Smithsonian Institute photograph.)

they found little interest in it. This skull later proved to bear the same general character as that of the Neanderthal skull.

Related to the Neander valley race, but larger in stature, was the Heidelberg man, *Homo heidelbergensis.* He was discovered in 1807 amid lower Pleistocene deposits near Heidelberg. His lower jaw shows a close relationship to that of the Neanderthal man. He had projecting brow ridges. His brain appears to have been somewhat less developed.

Another type of great antiquity, which had a striking resemblance to the Neander valley race, is that of *Les Hommes de Spy,* discovered in

Belgium by M. M. Lohest and N. di Puydt in 1886. They found two women skeletons buried deeply in a mass of debris at the entrance of a cave at Spy. These skeletons were covered by a hardened layer composed of chippings of ivory and flint, pieces of charcoal, and some fragments of limerock. In the same cave, together with the allegedly human

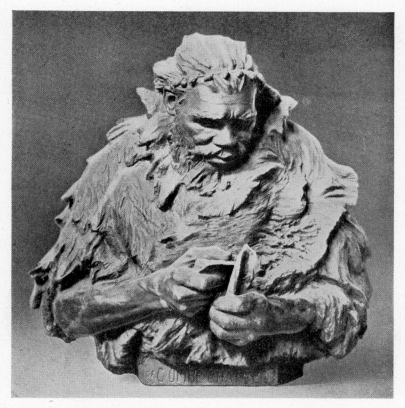

Fig. 30: Restoration of Cro-Magnon man, represented clad in furs and carving a piece of bone. (Modeled by Mascre under the direction of Rutot.)

skeletons, were found skeletons of the mammoth and other animals now extinct, and a variety of flint implements.

The Neanderthal man appears to have been somewhat skilled in fashioning instruments. In his cave were found crude and clumsy spears, clubs, and hand axes. He evidently made them primarily for the purpose of bagging game, for there were in these locations an abundance of reindeer, oxen, bison, and many other horned creatures

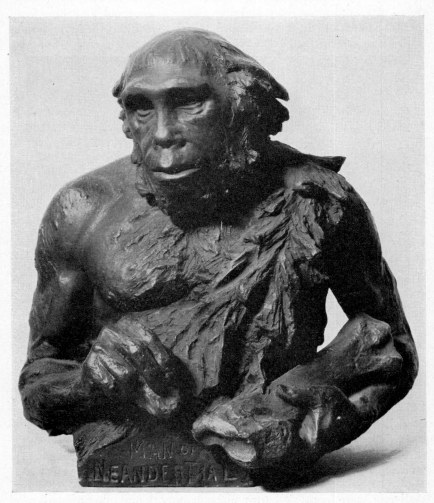

Fig. 31: Rutot's sculptor's conception of *Homo neanderthalensis*. (Smithsonian Institute photograph.)

whose capture was difficult without weapons. He needed also weapons for defense against ferocious lions, bears, hyenas, and wolves who were more than a match for the little Neanderthal man. What became of him is a mystery. Perhaps the struggle for survival was too much for him. At any rate he appears to have perished to make way for a more human race—the Cro-Magnon. While the Neanderthal man possessed definite animal characteristics, his successor, the Cro-Magnon, was certainly more human than beast.

Cro-Magnon Man: The Cro-Magnon[15] was a fine, tall person averaging 6 feet in height or even more. He was broad-shouldered and erect

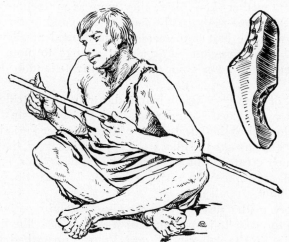

Fig. 32: The Spokeshave man (restoration).

in his standing attitude, bearing some resemblance to the American Indian. He was aggressive, thoughful, self-reliant, and ready to dominate all living things. From the walls and ceilings of his caves comes evidence that he possessed a surprising degree of artistic proficiency. Many most interesting relics made of bone, ivory, stone, or clay have been found in the various cave and rock shelters which he inhabited. These also show that he possessed a high degree of artistic and technical skill. The walls of his caves are thickly covered with colored drawings of animals, such as the mammoth, reindeer, horse, bison, ibex, and others; and in one cave, there is a picture of a remarkable rhinoceros with long-pointed horns and a coat of long thick hair. Many drawings represent female figures. These pictures are not all of equal artistic merit. Some are more accurate than others. Most of them show extraordinary artistic skill.

The ceiling of the cave at Altamira, Spain, depicts a veritable panorama of herds of animals in fairly natural color. This is probably the finest specimen of Cro-Magnon art so far brought to light. The Spanish government has taken over the grotto as a national monument to this artistic people. There are many more caves and rock shelters in Spain and France containing paintings of animal life. All of these are extremely interesting and instructive. The celebrated cavern of Font de Gaume, of Les Eyzies, France, is a veritable picture gallery.

The Cro-Magnons are said to have been the first manufacturers of needles. They made these needles from splinters of bone and employed them to sew together skins which they wore as protection against the cold. Their weapons were mostly made of bone and ivory. They were not as heavy as the flint implements of the Neander valley race who inhabited the same region. It is almost strange to note that these artists did not build houses, nor did they cultivate land or domesticate animals.

The skull of the Cro-Magnon man indicates a great stride in mental capacity over the Java, Neanderthal, and Piltdown man. The Cro-Magnon belonged to the latest phase of the Reindeer Period in France (about 25,000 years ago). It does not appear, however, that they possessed a much greater brain case than the Neanderthals, as would be expected of a people who displayed such fine artistic feeling and mechanical skill.

The history of the discovery of the Cro-Magnon race in brief is as follows: In the year 1858, workmen on a railway near the little village of Les Eyzies, in the valley of Vezere, France, unearthed three complete skeletons of men, two of women, and one of a child. This discovery was followed by numerous others during the next few years in the same neighborhood. The most perfect specimens were found in the Cro-Magnon cave; hence these prehistoric people became known as the Cro-Magnon race. In another cave at Baumes, Claudes, in the Vezere valley, thirty-five human craniums were found, with portions of skeletons attached. Evidences of the Cro-Magnon race have since been discovered all over Europe but nowhere else. The relics are most plentiful in Derdogne, in the Vezere valley, where eight sepulchral caves have been discovered.

The cranial capacity of the Cro-Magnon man is estimated to have been 1550 cc. The cephalic index varied from 70 to 73. The Cro-Magnon skull was narrow with prominent cheek bones, the jaw was thick and strong, the chin well developed, and the forehead high with reduced orbital ridges. In general appearance the skull suggests that of the present day Eskimo. The parts comprising the hardest and most durable part of the skeleton, and the least likely to be destroyed by the ravages of time, are the jaw, skull, teeth, and one or more of the long bones of the lower extremities. Even these structures are often found decayed and partly destroyed and have to be reconstructed. The reconstruction of fossils requires skill and a knowledge of comparative anatomy. The general outline and character of the skeleton can be determined by anatomists from only the examination of the skull and one or more of the long bones of the leg, such as the femur. Because of the fact that the human body presents a certain unity of structure, the relationship of one bone to the entire skeleton can be figured out by those who are skilled in the measurement of the skeleton.

The size and shape of the muscles and fleshy parts of the body can also be estimated by experts in this special work from certain landmarks appearing on the bones. Frequently even age and sex may be figured out if certain bones are intact. Diseases of primitive man, such as rickets and tuberculosis of the bones, may also be recognized.

The famous French anthropologist, de Quatriphages, has reconstructed, from observations made on many Cro-Magnon skeletons, the following picture:

Eyes depressed beneath the orbital vault; the nose straight rather than arched; the lips somewhat thick; the maxillary bones strongly developed; the complexion very brown; the hair dark and growing low on the forehead.

He states that the Cro-Magnon was tall, possessed firm limbs, and had a long head (dolichocephalic).

The nervous system tends to keep pace with the evolution of sensory-motor mechanisms in the organism. This is so true that the nervous system, and especially the brain, may be used as a rough index of sensory-motor evolution. The brain in the prehuman stock increased greatly in size, while the weight of the body remained approximately the same. The brain of the great apes ranges in weight from 300 to 500 gm., while the body weight is much greater than that of man. The average human brain weight is something like 1400 gm., being above 1000 gm. in the Australian pygmies, and reaching well over 2000 gm. in the more advanced races. The brain of Cromwell, for example, weighed 2231 gm., while that of Byron ran to 2294 gm. As Sir Arthur Keith has noted, the brain of ape and man at birth weighs 200 to 300 gm. and 300 to 500 gm. respectively, which shows that the enlarged adult brain is largely a postnatal development, and hence of relatively late evolutionary character.

Since the skull of the human fossil is nearly always recovered, the indices based upon skull measurements are of special interest and importance to the student of human evolution. The cranial capacity is measured in terms of cubic centimeters by filling the skull with liquid, millet seed, shot, or the like, and then emptying the contents into a graduated glass tube. The general shape of the head is expressed by the cranial index which corresponds to the cephalic index of living specimens, except that it is computed at two units less because of the absence of skin and other tissues. These and numerous other

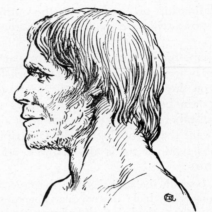

Fig. 33: The Cro-Magnon man (restoration).

head measurements enable the comparative anatomist or the physical anthropologist to interpret properly the evolutionary significance of skeletal remains with fair exactitude.

Our knowledge of the arts and customs of early man is based upon recovered implements and other evidences of human handiwork. Although such artifacts are somewhat rare from the earlier ages, cultural materials are much more plentiful than fossil remains when corresponding periods are considered.

The prehistoric antiquity of the Cro-Magnon race is attested by the fact that, during most of their sojourn on the earth, the members of this race had no knowledge of metals but used implements fashioned from stones and bones, that they were ignorant of agriculture, and that they had no knowledge of domesticating animals. In culture they were below the native tribes of present-day Africa and Australia. They lived primarily on hunting—particularly the reindeer—and hence they are often referred to as "the reindeer men."

At a later period they probably advanced beyond the stage of hunting, fishing, and nomadic life. It is probable that they reached the stage of agricultural development. Nevertheless they belonged essentially to the neolithic age.

From the time of the Cro-Magnon, down to historic times, the history of civilization has been classified on the basis of materials

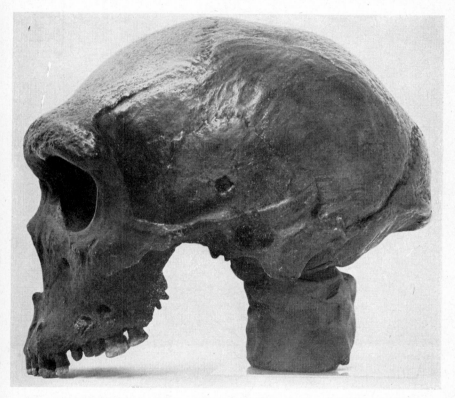

Fig. 34: Cast of *Homo rhodesiensis* skull. (Smithsonian Institute photograph.)

used for tools and implements. Thus following the neolithic period, came the Bronze and Iron Ages.

Another important paleontological discovery in relation to the descent of man was that of M. Lartet. In a cave near the French town of Aurignac, which had been used as a tomb by early Stone Age men, he found, in 1861, the remains of a number of human skeletons including men, women, and children, together with skeletons of a number of animals, including the cave-bear, the mammoth, the horse, the cave-hyena, the rhinoceros, and several other species now extinct which lived contemporaneously with man at that time. Many of these animal bones were found scraped and hollowed, evidently by the same stone implements found in the cave. Lartet estimated the antiquity of the contents of this cave as dating from 10,000 to 50,000 years ago.

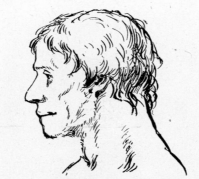

Fig. 35: *Combe-Capelle* man (restoration).

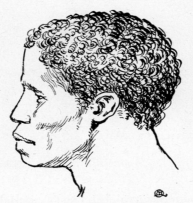

Fig. 36: *Grimaldi* man (restoration).

In Italy, at Monte Aperto, Capellini has discovered bones of a tertiary man and his manual instruments in clay deposits of the Pliocene age. He found ribs and scapulas marked by numerous deep incisions which could have been made only by sharp instruments.

Numerous craniums, supposed to be of great antiquity, the anatomical features of which do not apparently harmonize with those of the Piltdown, Neander, and Cro-Magnon specimens, have been recorded.

The two skeletons discovered by Dr. Verneau, in the grottos des Enfants near Mentone, appear not to fit in with any of these fossilized men. They are intermediate between the Neander valley man and the Cro-Magnon race. Both of these skeletons have prominent negroid jaws. The fact that near these skeletons was found a Cro-Magnon body need not cause too much dissension; this is probably due to the fact that, while a higher race had been developed, individuals of an older and lower race still survived in Europe.

The existence of man in a remote geological time cannot now be questioned despite the fact that the Pithecanthropus erectus is the only type which can be regarded thus far as definitely bridging the gulf between man and anthropoid apes. It is often difficult to recognize from very fragmentary remains the character of the man and the time of his existence.

Among the most clearly marked lines, whereby the lowest prehistoric culture has gradually risen to the highest modern level, are the succession of Stone, Bronze, and Iron Ages. The Stone Age represents the early condition of mankind in general and has remained in savage districts up to modern times. The introduction of metals did not always completely supersede the use of old stone hatchets and arrows. These often continued side by side with bronze and even iron implements.

With reference to the western hemisphere, no reliable evidence of any very great antiquity of man has come to light so far. Archaeological field parties in western Oklahoma, northeastern New Mexico, and southwestern Texas have come upon stone arrowheads of a peculiar type associated with the bones of an extinct species of bison. Some years ago Charles Abbott found a number of stone implements in Trenton, New Jersey. Dr. Hilborn T. Cresson found similar tools in Ohio. The antiquity of this human workmanship cannot be questioned. On the basis of this evidence, it is inferred that man inhabited the American continent for only from 10,000 to 25,000 years. Dr. W. H. Holmes, a prominent archaeologist, doubts even the extent of this period. There is no reason to believe that these early Americans were of any different stock than the American Indians. It is generally believed that the American Indian came here originally from Asia, probably by way of Bering Strait. Thus, human remains of a remote prehistoric age have not been positively identified in the Americas. Perhaps this is due to the fact that the anthropoid apes from whom man is descended are not known to have inhabited the western hemisphere.

MERGING OF PALEOLITHIC AND NEOLITHIC PERIODS

The passing of the Cro-Magnon man and the appearance of the neolithic man in Europe was a gradual process. Many of the Cro-Magnon men followed the reindeer into northern Eurasia, leaving their culture behind. Their descendants are said to have also found their way to Spain, Italy, and other parts of southern Europe. The age of the neolithic man is given as about 25,000 years ago. The neolithic stage ended with the Bronze Age which marked the dawn of civilization. Neolithic man was shorter in stature than the Cro-Magnon but both were dolichocephalic. Cro-Magnon skeletal remains have also been identified in the shell heap of Mugen, Portugal, and in a cave at Ofnet, Bavaria.

Neolithic man migrated into Scandinavia about 7000 B.C. The neolithic stage terminated in the Azilian and Tardnoisian stages.

The last period (of paleolithic times) lasted from about 10,000 to 7000 B.C. During this period the age of chipped flints definitely and finally ended in Europe. This period is known as the "Azilian." It takes its name from the *Mas d'Azil* or "House of Refuge," a large cavern in the eastern Pyrenees, named so because the Protestants took shelter there to escape persecution. The extensive deposits in this cave are typical of the Azilian epoch. The marked pebbles found there may be the earliest known traces of symbolic writing. It is well within the realm of possibility that the bow and arrow were developed by the people of this epoch. The Azilians are said to have been first to have round skulls, characteristic of the modern Mediterranean races. The Azilian age came to a close with the end of the neolithic period. The date of this era is put at 7000 to 8000 B.C. From that time on, the history of man has been recorded. The earliest organized governments, so far as our present knowledge goes, were Egypt and Sumer. Mystery still shrouds the origin of Chinese civilization.

The origin of nearly every essential thing of our present civilization is lost in the obscurity of passed ages, before the oldest historic period. The arts of writing, building, spinning, weaving, mining, and smelting metals came to us from prehistoric times. Neither history nor tradition has told us when or where these arts have originated, and our knowledge of Chaldea, Egypt, or China has not given a clear account of their beginnings.

References and Notes

1. Genesis 3:12.
2. Ibid., 6:4.
3. Ibid., 7:21.
4. Joshua 5:7.
5. Exodus 4:25.
6. Herodotus (Henry Cary's version, "Euterpe"). American Book Co., 2:86, 1847.
7. A name coined independently by de Blaindville, Fischer, and Von Waldheim, 1834.
8. The Lectures of Louis Agassiz, Mobile Daily Tribune, 1853.
9. Schmerling: Recherches, 1:59 and 66.
10. Boucher de Perthes, J.: Antiquites Celtiques et an ediluviennes. Paris, 1849.
11. Osborn, H. F.: Biblical World. 41:76.
12. The Java man, Pithecanthropus erectus, lived about 500,000 years B.C., was found near Trinil on the Island of Java, 1891, and was deposited in Tyler Museum, Haarlem.
13. The Piltdown man is dated about 100,000 years B.C., was found by Charles Dawson in a quarry 4 feet below the surface in Piltdown, Sussex, England, in 1911, and is found in the British Museum.
14. The Neanderthal man (Homo neanderthalensis) lived about 400,000 years B.C. He was found in the Neander valley between Eberfeld and Düsseldorf, Germany in 1857, in a cave 100 feet below the plateau and 60 feet above the Dussel River. It is deposited in Bonn, Germany.
15. The Cro-Magnon (Homo sapiens) is dated about 25,000 years B.C. He was discovered in 1867 in a rock shelter. Bones are deposited in the Jardin des Plantes Museum, Paris, France. He is supposed to be the first developed man.

4

Prehistoric Medicine

WILLIAM JAMES (1842–1910), in his "Human Immortality," states:

Bone of our bone, and flesh of our flesh, are these half brutish prehistoric brothers. Girdled about with the immense darkness of this mysterious universe even as we are, they were born and died, suffered and struggled. Given over to fearful crime and passion, plunged into the blackest ignorance, preyed upon by hideous and grotesque delusions, yet steadfastly serving the profoundest of ideals in their fixed faith that existence in any form is better than non-existence, they ever rescued triumphantly from the jaws of ever-imminent destruction the torch of life, which, thanks to them, now lights the world for us. [1]

Thanks to the painstaking investigations of the archaeologists and the paleopathologists, progress has been made in recent years in the study of prehistoric man in health and disease. Our knowledge of prehistoric man rests on documentary evidence which is just as trustworthy as written testimony. The medical evidence is derived first from the fossilized remains found in quarries, caves, gravel beds, mines, and graves of Europe and other continents, many of which have shown abundant evidence of disease; and secondly from primitive races which have not changed much from their paleolithic and neolithic ancestors and which are still living in Stone Age culture. Examples of such races may be found among the aborigines of Australia, Central Africa, Borneo, New Guinea, and New Zealand.

There is no hard and fast boundary to indicate where historic medicine begins and prehistoric ends. Prehistoric medicine is generally referred to a period antedating 4000 to 5000 B.C. Following this millenium human events are termed "historic" because of the availability of written documents. Archaeological discoveries tend to push the historic period further and further back toward deep antiquity.

The prevalence of disease in prehistoric times has been well summed up by a recent writer:

The pathological investigation of fossil remains is a new study. The work already done, however, justifies us in asserting that the commoner diseases of animals, plants, fish, and insects, originated shortly after the development of the genus or species, and are consequently almost as old as the genus or species subject to them. No matter how much living conditions varied in accordance with climatic changes, diseases, infections, epidemics and pests have followed the evolution of organic life, and carried on a constant warfare with them. [2]

K. Sudhoff, one of the most prominent investigators in the field of prehistoric medicine, states:

That disease abounded even in the imaginary Golden Age of early man, ten thousands of years ago, yes, even in the Palaeozoic Era, millions of years before, is demonstrated by the investigation of primordial and prehistoric times. [3]

ORIGIN OF MEDICINE

Animal Healing: The origin of medicine may be traced to an early biologic period, even before man completely evolved from a lower species of life.[4] Animals perform certain functions by intuition, or subordinated intellect. Birds and fish, for example, migrate from one climate to another at certain seasons of the year; the spider selects the corner in which to spin its web; the bees build their hive, the birds their nest; ants carry off their larvae to safety whenever their habitat becomes too damp and bring them back when it returns to proper humidity.

Naturalists have long observed that animals try to mitigate irritation and pain by resorting to various healing powers of nature. For example, animals refresh their heated bodies by submerging themselves in cold water. They rub, scratch, and change their position to alleviate irritated areas. They warm their stiffened limbs by exposing themselves to the sun. They lick their sores and wounds. They are known to suck or blow on injured parts. Monkeys are known to extract foreign bodies, such as thorns and burrs, from themselves and to help relieve their fellows of parasites. Monkeys have been seen to stem the flow of blood from a wound by placing their paws over the bleeding and applying pressure. A dog, when it fractures its leg, practically reflexly learns to run on three legs holding its injured leg immobilized in a position that allows proper healing with minimum damage. When sick, dogs commonly search for certain herbs or grass to produce emesis and purgation. Swallows heal their sore eyes with the juice of a certain plant known as "cetadine."

Pliny states that the hippopotamus, after having overeaten, presses its body over a sharp stump or reed to break a blood vessel and permit ready egress of blood from its body. Following this procedure, this animal assures hematosis by pressing the bleeding surface against limey soil. Man, according to Pliny, learned from the hippopotamus the art of bloodletting. He further states that a cat, when bitten by a snake, rolls itself on thorny grass in order to permit the poison to escape through the open skin. He mentions that a deer, when shot with an arrow, eats a certain grass which softens the tissue and loosens the arrow from her body, and that turtles use an antidote against snake bite.

The mongoose, when bitten by a snake, chews mimosa leaves; the toad, when stung by a spider, eats the leaves of Plantago major. According to Greek and Roman legends, man learned many therapeutic measures from animals.

There is a legend that Hippocrates came upon the idea of administering clysters to relieve constipation by observing an ibis taking water into its beak and injecting it into its own rectum. Another legend concerning Hippocrates is that he once saw a groundhog emerge from its hole for the first time in the spring and wipe its blinded eyes with a certain grass which restored sight.

Primitive Healing: Knowledge as to prehistoric medicine may be derived from present-day primitives who are still living in Stone Age culture. The aborigines of New Guinea, Borneo, Central Africa, New Zealand, and Australia have never advanced beyond the culture of their prehistoric forebears.

The common concepts and practices of widely scattered modern primitives must be assumed to have originated from a common source in deep antiquity before the descendants scattered across the face of the earth. They may hark back to the time when mankind occupied a small geographical section of the globe and had a common folklore and tradition. Unless this premise is postulated, it is difficult to conceive how Australian savages, aborigines of Africa, and prehistoric natives of America possess similar customs and practices. Surely there have been no direct communications between the aborigines of these diversified areas.

STUDY OF CAVES

The chief sources of information, leading to the conclusion that diseases prevailed in prehistoric times and that measures were taken by men to combat them, rests on observation of fossils found in caves, in lakes, under lake dwellings, in gravel beds, and in mines.

The search for fossils and the unicorn horn, which ranked so high in the therapeutic armamentarium of the sixteenth and seventeenth centuries, led to the discovery of many caverns containing human and

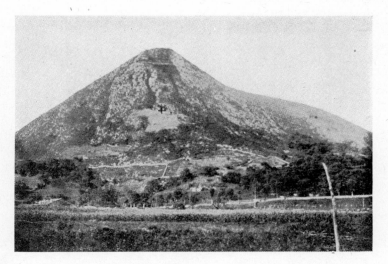

Fig. 37: The *Pico del Castillo,* showing the entrance to the Cave of *Castillo* (x) near Puente Viesgo, Santander.

animal remains. Caves and lake dwellings were employed by prehistoric men, not only for shelter and protection against the inclement weather, but also as safeguards against human enemies and ferocious beasts. Incidentally it may be interesting to note that in the second world war, caves were used by allied soldiers and civilians as dwelling places and air-raid shelters.

Classification According to Age: Caves may be classified, according to their age, as Pliocene or Pleistocene. The first, or older, caves contain the remains of animals only. The Pleistocene caves contain the remains of extinct animals and/or paleolithic man. In the latter caves, occasionally there are also implements of human workmanship. Caves of later prehistoric times contain the remains of domestic animals with or without man, and frequently more refined implements.

Contents of Caves: The French naturalist, Cuvier (1769–1832),[5] was among the first paleontologists to study the contents of caves. He identified the fossilized bones of the rhinoceros, hyena, lion, wolf, fox, and stag. Other observers[6] identified the reindeer, horse, bison, and cave-bear. From 1825 to 1841, McEnery discovered, in the famous "Kent's Hole" cave near Torquay, the first flint instrument near the bones of extinct animals, indicating that man existed in Devonshire contemporaneously with certain extinct animals. McEnery's conclusion has been verified by Pengelly, with the collaboration of the British Archaeological Association.

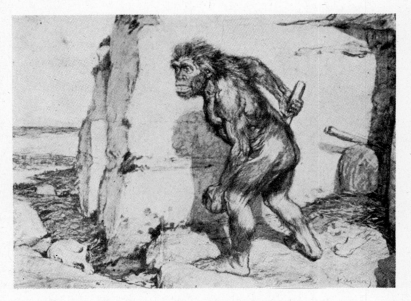

Fig. 38: The cave-man. (Found at Aix-la-Chapelle, France.)

In order to understand the circumstances that influenced the study of prehistoric pathology, a brief review of the subterranean habitations of man is here given.

KENT'S HOLE CAVE: The Kent's Hole cave was found to consist of four distinct strata. The upper stratum was composed of dark earth containing medieval remains. The stratum next to this contained Roman pottery and articles which proved that it was in use during the Iron, Bronze, and Neolithic Ages. The lowest stratum exhibited a stalagmite floor, varying in thickness from 1 to 3 feet, and covering a layer of red earth. This layer contained bones of the hyena, lion, mammoth, rhinoceros, and many other animals, extinct and nonextinct, in association with flint implements. The walls of the lowest stratum were found to be engraved with antlers, thus indicating that man inhabited the cavern during this earliest period. The exploration of the cave of Brixham near Torquay (1858) led to the identification of the bones of man with those of various extinct animals.

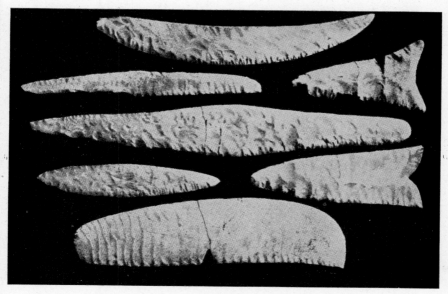

Fig. 39: Prehistoric flint knives and lances. (From Petrie, Sir F.: Seventy Years in Archaeology.)

FRENCH CAVES: The researches of Mortillet[7] (1821–1898) have shown that groups of men dwelt in the caves of France. The bones found fit in with the type of human remains found in the caverns of Spy and Neanderthal. The skull structure is intermediate between that of ape and human. The floors of the caves explored by Lartet[8] (1801–1871), in the valley of the Vezere and Dordogne, contain broken bones of animals killed for food mingled with rude implements and weapons made from bones and unpolished stone. Charcoal and burnt stones indicated the position of the fireplace. Axes, lance-heads, hammers, saws made of flint, bone needles, sculptured reindeer, bison, horse, ibex, antelope, and sheep were also found. These remarkable accumulations of debris represent the refuse cast aside and mark the places where the ancient hunters lived.

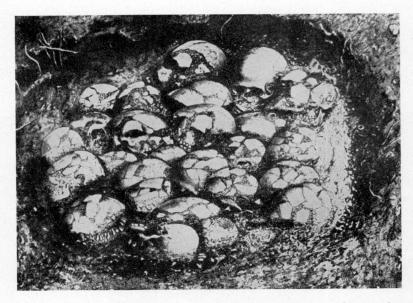

Fig. 40: In the *Ofnet* grotto in Bavaria, there has been discovered a collection of thirty-three human skulls from the Azilian and Tardenois periods. Most are dolichocephalic, but some are brachiocephalic. The last is rare in the olden Stone Age.

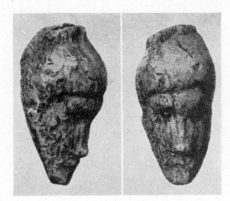

Fig. 41: One of Professor Absalo's finds in Moravia of Aurignacian date. Probably represents a woman, for men are hardly ever represented in this era.

Reindeer evidently supplied a good part of the food eaten by these primitive men. These animals appear to have roamed about central France in large herds. The most striking remains left behind in these refuse heaps are the sculptured reindeer antlers and figures engraved on fragments of rock and ivory. The most striking figure is that of

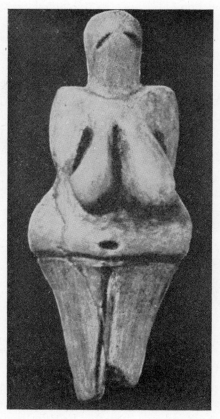

Fig. 42: Early Stone-Age, Bone Sculpture. In early sculptures from the Stone Age, women are usually represented with greatly developed breasts and hips. (Found in Moravia by the Czech archaeologist Absalon.)

the mammoth engraved on a fragment of its own tusk. The extreme curvature of the mammoth's tusks is not to be found at present in any living elephant, and the engraving proves that the artist was thoroughly familiar with this extinct animal. The drawings exhibit considerable artistic skill and are evidently drawn from life.

There has been much discussion as to what has become of the the cave-men of France. Some authors are of the opinion that they followed the reindeer who withdrew to the north, following the retreating ice of the glacial period, and are today the Eskimos. There are many features of the life of the Eskimo that remind one of the ancient Stone Age man of France. Both gained their livelihood by hunting; both used bone and horn to tip their lances; both employed spears and harpoons and had a passion for carving bone and ivory; both took delight in drawing animal forms from life; and both employed similar tools.

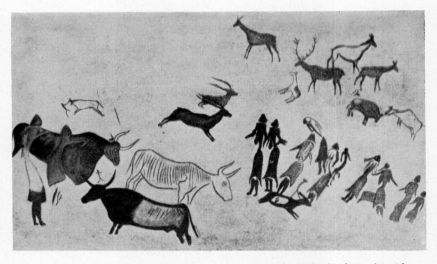

Fig. 43: Painting on a stone wall near Cogul, in eastern Spain, from the older Stone Age. The scene on the right shows nine women clad in short skirts dancing around a naked man. (Aquarelle by W. Tupy.)

Early cave-men ranged over middle Europe as far south as the Pyrenees and the Alps. They inhabited the caverns of Belgium, Germany, Hungary, Switzerland, and the British Isles. They lived by hunting and fishing and were clad in skins sewn together with the sinews of reindeer or strips of intestine. As intimated, they had a marvelous talent for drawing animal figures. They did not domesticate animals nor were they acquainted with the arts of spinning or pottery making. There is no evidence that they buried their dead. The interments, such as those at Aurignac, Les Eyzies, and Mentone, probably date from a later age. The later prehistoric caves can be distinguished from the Pleistocene caverns by the fact that they

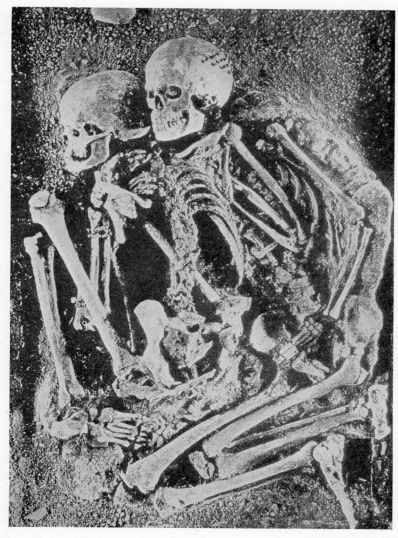

Fig. 44: The *Grimaldi* skeletons of a woman and a youth with negroid characteristics. (After Verneau. Courtesy of Smithsonian Institute, Washington, D.C.)

contain the remains of domestic animals and wild animals of a later date.

Classification According to Period: Caves may also be classified in accordance with the age during which man dwelt in them, i.e. Paleolithic, Neolithic, Bronze, and Iron Ages. The neolithic caves which are widely spread throughout Europe have been used also for burial purposes. Bodies were buried in these caves in a crouched posture. The skeletons are of short stature, the tallest being 5 feet, 6 inches, and the shortest, 4 feet, 10 inches.

Prehistoric caves have recently been explored in Palestine and in the Lebanons. Some years ago, Canon Tristram examined a cave in the Lebanons which contained flint implements along with charcoal and broken bones and teeth.

In North America, F. W. Putman explored a Kentucky cave in which he discovered rudely pleated clothes and other articles. Ornaments of various kinds and substances were found, ranging from small bones and teeth strung together to colored pebbles, gold, and precious stone ornaments.

Caves have excited the awe and wonder of mankind in all ages. They have been the center around which have clustered many legends and superstitions. In Persia they were connected with the obscure worship of Mithras. Their names frequently represent a survival of the superstitious ideas of antiquity, as for example, the "fairy," "dragon," or "devil's" caves of France and Germany. Long after the elves, goblins, and fairies had forsaken the forest and glens of Germany, they dwelt in their palaces deep in the Harz mountains in the dwarf holes, whence they came from time to time into the upper air.

STUDY OF LAKE DWELLINGS

Besides caves, man built, for his protection, dwellings in the midst of, or close to the shore of, bodies of water. The dwellings were built on lofty piles connected with each other by bridges or planks. They were reached from the shore by canoes. Among the first to describe dwellings built upon lakes was Hippocrates. Writing in the fifth century B.C., he concerns himself with the inhabitants of a lake named Phasis:

Their country is fenny, warm, humid, and wooded; copious and severe rains occur there at all seasons; and the life of the inhabitants is spent among the fens; for their dwellings are constructed of wood and reeds, and are erected amidst the waters; they seldom practice walking either to the city or the market, but sail about, up and down, in canoes constructed out of single trees, for there are many canals there. They drink the hot and stagnant waters, both when rendered putrid by the sun, and when swollen with rains. The Phasis itself is the most stagnant of all rivers, and runs the smoothest; all the fruits which spring there are unwholesome, of feeble and imperfect growth, owing to the redundance of water, and on this account they do not ripen, for much vapor from the waters overspreads the country. For these reasons the Phasians have shapes different from those of all other men; for

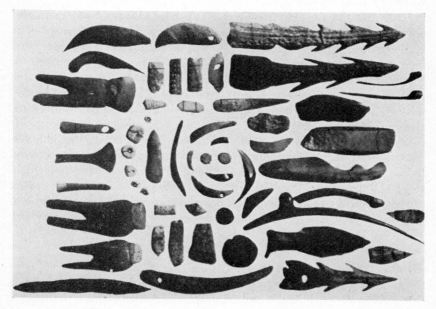

Fig. 45: Quantities of household utensils and tools of various kinds, like harpoons and needles, have been found in the lake dwellings. This collection comes from Vinelz, Switzerland.

they are large in stature, and of a very gross habit of body, so that not a joint nor vein is visible; in color they are sallow, as if affected with jaundice. Of all men they have the roughest voices, from their breathing an atmosphere which is not clear, but misty and humid; they are naturally rather languid in supporting bodily fatigue. [9]

Herodotus, writing also in the fifth century B.C., describes the people of Lake Phasis as living in houses constructed on platforms of planks fitted on lofty piles in the middle of the lake, which are approached from the land by a single narrow bridge.

They live in the following manner: every man has a hut on the planks, in which he dwells, with a trap door closely fitted in the planks, and leading down to the lake. They tie the young children with a cord round the foot, fearing lest they should fall into the lake beneath. [10]

Abulfeda, the Arabic geographer, writing in the twelfth century, notes that part of the Apamaen Lake was inhabited by Christian fishermen who lived on the lake in wooden huts built on piles. Sir John Lubbock (Lord Avebur) mentions that the Rumelian fisher-man on Lake Phasis "still inhabit wooden cottages built over the water, as in the time of Herodotus."

Since the days of Hippocrates, many lake villages have been dis-covered, chiefly in Switzerland, furnishing information on early man. Early man's artifacts which fell into the water have of late years been recovered and studied by archaeologists. The lake settlement at Moosedorf near Berne affords the most perfect example of such dwellings in the Stone Age. A large variety of stone implements and pottery, burnt wheat, barley and linseed, bones of stags, oxen, swine, sheep, and goats have been found in the water below.

In other lake villages, "kitchen middens," or dump heaps, contain-ing a variety of objects indicating human habitation have been found in the water. Stag horns used for medical purposes were present in most of the "kitchen middens." Lake dwellings, aside from affording protection from human foes and ferocious animals, were thought to exert a prophlyactic effect against disease.

PALEOPATHOLOGY

Ethnic Pathology: The story of medicine in prehistoric times is of interest, not only to students of anthropology and medical history, but also to the pathologist and clinician. The term "ethnic pathology" has been applied in recent years to include a group of diseases com-mon to a certain people who possess the same physical character-istics and who maintain a common susceptibility and immunity to certain ailments. From this viewpoint, primitive pathology is con-sidered in the light of transmissible factors and in terms of family line inheritance.

"Disease in general and infection in particular," stated Elie Metchni-koff, "were developed on the earth in a very remote epoch. Disease doubtlessly began with the inception of antagonism between two forms of life and this may be nearly as old as life itself. Phagocytosis unquestionably began very early in the history of animal life." Metchnikoff calls attention to the occurrence of epidemics of a severe nature among the protozoa and especially the amoeba. Henry Fair-field Osborn, the noted American paleontologist, thought that the extinction of certain groups of mammals of antiquity was influenced by widely spread disease epidemics. The same cause might have brought about the disappearance of many human groups from the face of the earth.

Importance of Paleopathology: The importance of paleopathology in the interpretation of modern medicine and medical history has been outlined by Klebs[11] (1834–1913):

We need only consider what definite influence diseases exert in our individual lives; what profound social upheavals were brought about through the influence of epidemics, less perceptible perhaps but none the less strongly, through widespread chronic ailments as through professional diseases; how whole districts and countries are forsaken because disease made them uninhabitable; how diseases affecting early childhood and others producing sterility led to gradual extinction of whole peoples.

For the grasp of such problems, the study of disease as it appears to us now, does not suffice. The traces left during immense periods of time have to be taken into account, and it is in just such questions not approachable by other methods that paleopathology in time to come may furnish important solutions.

Prevalence of Disease: The investigation of the history of disease and its manifestations in prehistoric times, known as "paleopathology," has shown that sickness prevailed since the first evidence of life on earth. Certain diseases were acquired by mammals from preceding forms. Some of these ancestral forms still persist from ages past; others became extinct. Bacteria, recognized at present as the principle cause of disease, were among the early biologic types. At a very early period simple forms of life became parasitical and pathogenic; they grew upon flesh long before there were men.

Fossilized remains of the dinosaurs reveal signs of disease and injuries, and there are signs of infection in other prehistoric fossilized animals. Inflammatory conditions due to bone infection, cavities, and impaction of molar teeth, have been noted in fossilized mammals. The studies of M. Bernard Renault have shown beyond any doubt that various forms of bacteria of the Micrococcus and Diplococcus types existed in fossilized fish and in the vertebral remains of the carboniferous period. In one skeleton of a dinosaur evidence of a leg abscess was found.

As has been intimated, there is strong evidence for the belief that diseases existed long before man made his appearance on the earth, and that many prevailing diseases are of great antiquity, extending back into geologic times for hundreds of thousands and perhaps millions of years. Disease organisms, one of the manifestations of life, have followed the same line of evolution and development as have plants and animals. Life processes in the past have been governed by the same laws as at present.

Scourges, such as malaria, syphilis, tuberculosis, rabies, glanders, encephalitis, amoebic dysentery, hookworm, elephantiasis, variola, herpes, spotted fever, and relapsing fever, have always been influenced by invading organisms; they have often been transmitted by animal carriers.

Transmission of Disease: Animals are liable to transmit disease to man and vice versa.[12] Bubonic plague, for example, has been transmitted through rats and flies. Yellow fever has been conveyed by one or more species of mosquito; typhus, by the body louse; and typhoid fever, by the common house fly.

Similarity of Diseases of Ape and Man: According to Rengger,[13] monkeys are susceptible to colds and manifest the same symptoms as man; they also readily acquire tuberculosis. They are subject to inflammatory disease of the eyes. Senile cataract is not uncommon among monkeys and dogs. The writer has observed various forms of cataract among dogs. Cataract extraction restores vision among canines as readily as among humans. Gastrointestinal diseases among animals are of frequent occurrence and respond to therapy such as is commonly employed on humans.

In the investigation of diseases of early man, therefore, one may be greatly assisted by observing pathological conditions common among primates and apes of the present time whose structure and physiology closely resemble those of man. A large number and variety of benign and pathological parasites are present in primates, and parasitic infection is recorded in many of the different species of monkeys and apes either wild or in captivity. Hegner (1928) thought that the protozoan parasites of primates, such as monkeys, apes, and man "belong for the most part to the same species or are so similar in their structure and life cycles, as to be practically indistinguishable."

Clark found among the wild monkeys of Panama, malaria of the tertian type. Malarial parasites have been discovered among the chimpanzees and gorillas of west Africa, corresponding to those present in man, with respect to the three species and the various stages. Small threadlike worms (filaria) are common alike among apes and men. They are found in unusually large numbers in the peritoneal cavity and in some cases also invade the thoracic cavity.

Schultz found the gibbons of northern Siam heavily infected with worms.[14] Schultz is of the opinion that, in view of the fact that parasitic infections are known to occur in wild apes, "it seems more reasonable to assume that early man suffered from parasitic infection rather than to assert that he differed radically in this respect from his evolutionary cousins."

Fox (1939) has described many cases of chronic arthritis in mammals. He found marked arthritic changes in the baboon, gorilla, and orangutan. Fifteen out of a total of eighty-nine gorillas and two of forty-nine orangutans were affected with arthritis. Among wild adult gibbons studied by Schultz, he found, in a few skeletons, arthritic changes in the phalanges and metacarpals. The joint surfaces of certain skeletons were hypertrophied, the bones rough and partially porous, which condition could have resulted either from an arthritic condition or some surface infection.

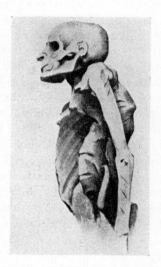

Fig. 46: Spinal curvature. (Ruffer.)

Evidence of Disease in Fossils: *Bacteria:* Additional evidence that many pathologic conditions existed in early prehistoric times may be derived from the presence of bacteria in fossils. In 1914, Charles D. Walcott discovered bacteria in the oldest fossils of North America. Renauld and Van Tegham have demonstrated viable bacteria of a later geologic age in decayed bones, and Moody found bacteria in prehistoric vertebrates.

Skeletal Changes: Schaffhausen (1858) observed pathologic lesions in the Neanderthal skeleton, the left humerus and the proximal end

of the left ulna of which were diseased. Virchow regarded the abnormality of the humerus and ulna as an indication of rickets. Bartel
states that the Heidelberg skeleton exhibits Pott's disease with
kyphosis. A case of Pott's disease was also reported by Smith and
Ruffer in the skeleton of an Egyptian priest of Amon of the twenty-
fifth dynasty (about 1000 B.C.). Virchow observed certain pathologic changes in the fossil bones of the Pithecanthropus erectus,
the Neanderthal man, and the cave-bear. Sir Auckland Geddes
thought that the Piltdown man's marked thickness of the skull was
pathological and indicative of tuberculosis.[15]

Fractures: One of the most frequent afflictions that confronted
prehistoric man was fracture of the limbs and, to a lesser extent,
the other bones of the body. Rigorous life and the daily struggle
against the elements and beasts of prey made such injuries prevalent.
Numerous healed fractures of the humerus, radius, ulna, femur, tibia,
and fibula have been found in graves of an age which extends far
beyond the oldest written records. A Neanderthal skeleton shows
the effect of an old and severe dislocation of the left elbow. A great
number of forearm fractures are present in the French neolithic skeletons. The large proportion of such lesions about the arms is probably
due to the fact that the upper extremities are extensively used for
offensive and defensive purposes. The Pithecanthropus erectus, the
oldest skeletal remains discovered by Dubois in 1891 near Trinil in
central Java, shows, according to Virchow and Duckworth, evidence
of fracture and marked exostosis of the left femur.

In some of the records collected by authorities on folklore, are
lines which suggest that the early medicine man knew the importance
of approximating the broken bones and tissues in case of fracture:

He put marrow to marrow; he put pith to pith; he put membrane to membrane; he put tendon to tendon; he put blood to blood; he put tallow to
tallow; he put flesh to flesh; he put fat to fat; he put skin to skin; he put
hair to hair; he put warm to warm; he put cool to cool. [16]

Such a statement shows a clear comprehension of the necessity of
correctly setting fractured bones.

Jager[17] attributed the perfectly healed fractures exhibited by the
skeletal remains of prehistoric and early historic man to the application of artificial aid. He grouped fractures into two categories: well-
healed and badly healed fractures. The efficient results in the former
group he ascribed primarily to the artificial help administered; the
poor results in the latter group he ascribed primarily to the fact
that the cases were left solely to nature. The many perfect recover-

ies among early man led Jager to the opinion that the art of setting and holding broken bones together is very old. Le Baron was also of the opinion that early man reduced fractures with great perfection. According to him, certain fractures, particularly those of the ribs and of the lower end of the radius, healed readily. Only six out of the eighteen cases he examined healed badly.

But good bony union was also found in fractures of anthropoid apes. In a series of 263 fractures in anthropoid apes, involving the humerus, radius, femur, tibia, and clavicle, nine were found perfectly healed and most of the remaining healed in varying degree. Only a few of the fractures exhibited bad union. Thus, the idea that early man received artificial manipulation in the care of his fractures is not a proven fact. It is more likely that nature attended to the healing processes of the fractured bones.

Nature of Early Lesions: Le Baron[18] divides the causes of lesions among early man into four categories: (1) mechanical, (2) accidental, (3) caused by trepanation, and (4) spontaneous. He gives a detailed account of surgical operations performed by early man and discusses the nature of the diseases to which he was subject. In one cave, Le Baron found many perforated metatarsal bones, arranged in the form of a necklace, a sculptured scapula in the form of a bird, and a fibula notched by a flint knife.

Bone Lesions: Among fossilized man, Le Baron found four cases of Colles' fracture. One fracture through the middle of the shaft of the ulna made good union. Another break at the lower third of the humerus and one fracture of the clavicle healed with good results. He noted a fracture of the body of the femur that was but poorly healed. A fracture of the tibia and fibula exhibited formation of callus. Five fractured ribs and two fractured clavicles showed good results. In one case there was erosion of eight teeth which he thought due to syphilitic influence. Certain tibias, allegedly syphilitic, showed hyperostosis. Le Baron observed thirty cases of arthritis and many cases of infected gums among the fossilized remains of early man. He is strongly of the opinion that violent and vicious plagues commonly raged at the expense of prehistoric man. He mentions scurvy as a ravaging disease in early times.

Head Lesions: It is notable, said Le Baron, that a large number of injuries were in the head and produced by blows from stones and arrows. Fractures of the skull were commonplace. Primitive man early came to the realization that the quickest method of subduing an enemy was to strike him over the head. Wounded skulls have been discovered in every part of the world. That these skull wounds were not always fatal is proven by the fact that many healed skull fractures have been recovered.

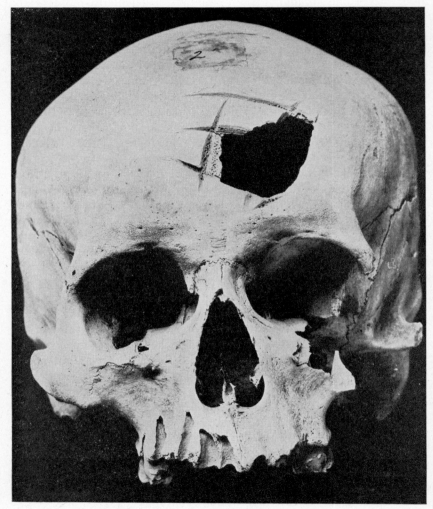

Fig. 47: Trephined Indian skull from Huarochiri, Peru. (Smithsonian Institute photograph.)

TREPHINING: Excavations conducted in various parts of the world, and particularly in Peru, reveal that as high as 2½ per cent of the prehistoric population exhibit evidences of skull trephining. The reasons for resorting to this procedure is not clear, since most of the victims with trephined skulls do not show head lesions. The famous anthropologist and cranial surgeon, Paul Broca[19] (whose fame is associated with the brain speech area and convolution bearing his name), is of the opinion that trephining was performed for

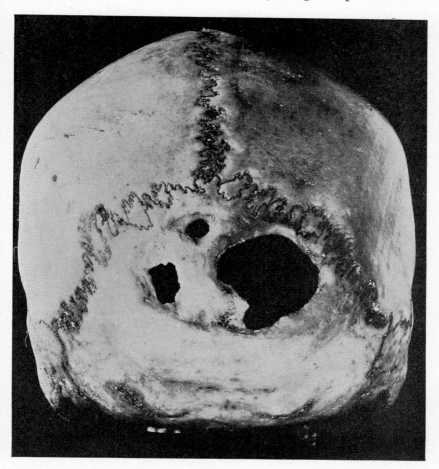

Fig. 48: Trephined Indian skull from near Cuzco, Peru. (Smithsonian Institute photograph.)

the relief of certain disorders such as epilepsy, insanity, and persistent headache. Perhaps the chief motive for this operation was to allow the demon causing the disease to escape and to render those who underwent the operation safe from further assault by evil spirits.

In the majority of cases, the operation was performed on the young, and Broca is of the opinion that whenever a neolithic child had fits, a perforation was made in its head to let out the incarcerated demon. If the operation was successful and the fits ceased, it was looked upon with great reverence; the excised fragments of bone were used

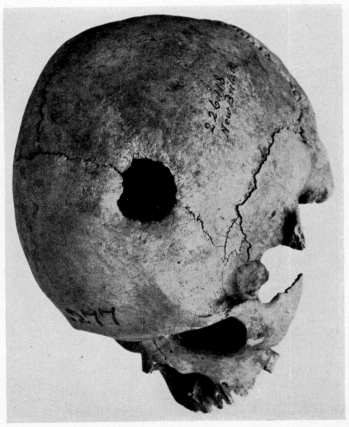

Fig. 49: Trephined Melanesian skull from New Britain. (Smithsonian Institute photograph.)

as amulets, as indicated by the number of them being perforated, and by the fact that many of them are found in the burial places. Opening the door for the evil spirit to escape brings back to mind an old custom in England which is not altogether extinct, i.e. of throwing open the windows of a room where death has recently occurred, with the idea of facilitating the exit of the departed spirit.[20]

Recent studies show that a large proportion of persons on whom trephining was performed in America had the operation performed in accordance with sound surgical principles, such as to aid depressed fractures of the skull. The operation among the American Indians appears to have been rarely fatal. In a number of cases there is evidence that the patient lived many years after the operation. There are, of course, some cases in which the skulls show no evidence of healing. These patients probably died before healing took place.

It is difficult to ascertain where the operation for trephining originated. The concensus is that it originated in one particular place in Europe or Asia during the Pleistocene period, before the human family was scattered to all parts of the globe, for it is hard to conceive how, otherwise, this operation could have spread from one continent to another, always performed with essentially the same technique.

The vault of the skull was the region most accessible to the operator at a time when beds or tables were not in use. Trephination was frequently performed several times on the same person. As many as three or four openings have been observed in some neolithic skulls. In a neolithic sepulchre at Vendrest, France, eight individuals out of 120, including both sexes, exhibited skulls that had been opened by trephining. Many of the patients appear to have survived the operation as is evident from the healing of the edges. The trephined skulls, found in France, mostly have single openings, although multiple openings are not rare. The openings, as a rule, are rather small, perhaps to avoid herniation of the meninges and cranial contents. Where the openings are large, plates, consisting of a part of a skull, another bone, a gourd, or a metal plaque, are employed to prevent such complications.

The method used for the operation included processes of drilling, scraping, cutting, and sawing. The surgical instruments employed were made of flint, stone, or fragments of shell.

The operation of trephining of the skull is still being attempted by present-day aborigines; and if a deduction is permitted from the present practice, the purpose of trephination (as intimated previously) was to afford relief from convulsions, epilepsy, headache, and mental disorders. This operation was not so much to affect the cranial contents or the skull but to afford an opening for the evil spirit to escape from the skull of the sufferer.

Primitive man still appears to have better resistance against infection than civilized man. While primitive man is more prone to succumb to disease once he acquires it, his wounds generally heal more quickly and recovery is more frequent.

Among the American Indians, trephination frequently resulted in uneventful recovery. There was usually no inflammatory reaction or suppuration; but when an Indian fell sick, he seldom recovered. There was an adage among Spanish American physicians, "When an Indian falls sick he dies."

Recently trephining has been reported among the Kabyles of New Algeria and the natives of the island of New Britain.

Fractures and other skull lesions were rather rare among early mammals. Their brain cases were solid and well protected by muscles. A very severe blow was needed to produce a fracture. Cuvier, however, observed a fracture of the skull of a hyena from the Pleistocene period in France.

In historic times the ancient Greeks practiced trephination in cases of skull injury. Heliodorus trephined the skull to prevent pus collection and other complications. Celsus regarded trephination as a last resort, to be employed when all other remedies, such as compresses, plasters, and the like, failed. Arab physicians sternly discouraged the operation. The famous founder of French surgery, Lanfranchi, confessed that he very seldom practiced trephination because "in such cases the surgeon is chiefly dependent upon the 'Holy Ghost.'" Guy de Chauliac (c. 1350), physician to three popes, was very cautious in recommending this operation. He practiced it only in very extensive skull fractures and for the excavation of dural exudates.

CAUTERIZATION: Primitive man did not limit his head surgery to trephination. He scarified or cauterized a "T"-shape figure on the vertex of the skull. The reason for such a practice is obscure. It was usually done on female heads. Perhaps this was a sign of disgrace similar to the sign put on Cain after he killed Abel,[21] or a form of mutilation which was practiced from a very early period as a religious rite, in deference to the dead. It might have been a measure to counteract the evil design of a demon which caused death in the family. The Hebrews prohibited such practices as is indicated in the Book of Leviticus, "ye shall not make any cutting in your flesh nor imprinting any marks upon you."[22] The very fact that the Hebrews felt obligated to promulgate this ban effectively demonstrates that the practice must have been in vogue at that period.

Herodotus states that the Lydians cauterized the scalp for many ailments. In the days of Avicenna, the Persians performed similar cauterization as a therapy against infantile convulsions.

Arthritis: The most common disease due to bone pathology is arthritis. No climate, no condition of life, and no diet has been able to obliterate it. It was found among all fossil vertebrates, and in some cases all the vertebrae were affected. Hoffschlager[23] is of the opinion that arthritis deformans was common not only in cave-men but also among cave-bears as well. The studies of Fox and Schultz have been discussed previously in this chapter.

Joint involvement was frequent. Joint surfaces of some skeletons were hypertrophied, rough, and spongy, a condition resulting either from an arthritic condition or other inflammatory process.

Pales[24] reported cases of ankylosis of the vertebrae, lipping, osteophytosis, and atrophic intervertebral discs in neolithic skeletons of France (c. 10,000 B.C.).

Six thousand prehistoric skeletons examined by Schultz and Jones exhibited no evidences of rickets, scurvy, or osteomalacia. Hrdlicka[25] is in accord with this observation as to the rarity of rickets among prehistoric men. On the other hand, Nielson of Copenhagen found, among 616 prehistoric skeletons, considerable evidence of this disease, as well as of arthritis deformans. Derry, Stricker, and Schmerling also found rickets to be common in prehistoric skeletons. Schmerling found it also common in fossil animals.[26] Rheumatism was a common illness among early cave-men.

Dental Lesions: Dental lesions have been observed in fossil mammals. Hrdlicka found an early Rhodesian skull with nine teeth badly destroyed and the remaining ones damaged. In a Neanderthal skull of LaChapelle, only two of the permanent teeth were found remaining, and one of these had an open pulp cavity with alveolar abscess.

Many dental diseases are known to occur among all major groups of primates. According to Sir Frank Colyer (1939), alveolar abscesses are common in all specimens with advanced attrition of the teeth. Schultz found alveolar abscesses among 59 to 62 per cent of chimpanzees and gorillas.

Alveolar abscesses occur in up to 62 per cent of anthropoid apes. Carious cavities in the permanent teeth of anthropoids have been observed to become more frequent as age advances. Among chimpanzees, whose homologies with the human are most striking, carious teeth are more common than among the orangutans.

Schultz[27] believes that the nutritional, social, and most other environmental factors of the recent anthropoid apes cannot be very far removed from the conditions which prevailed in the ages during and after which man separated from the common ancestral stock of all higher primates. Thus it is possible that the conditions for the acquisition of, and reaction to, diseases and injuries in early man were in all probability similar to those persisting among present-day apes.

Krogman,[28] summarizing the literature pertaining to dental pathology, concluded that in prehistoric times one out of four adults had one or more carious teeth. In ancient specimens of anthropoid apes, the prevalence of alveolar abscesses is still more pronounced; as for the chimpanzees, alveolar abscesses and dental cavities occur in 59 per cent of the specimens. This figure is increased to 62 per cent in the orangutan. Carious cavities in the permanent teeth grow more frequent with age among all anthropoids.

In one of the Assyrian medical texts, published by R. Campbell Thompson in the proceedings of the Royal Society of Medicine in London, from the Imperial Library of Ashurbanipal in Nineveh, there is an inscription:

If a man's mouth has mouth trouble, thou shalt bray lilium in well water, introduce salt, alum, and vinegar thereon; thou shalt leave it out under the stars in the morning; thou shalt wind a linen (strip) round his forefinger; without a meal thou shalt cleanse his mouth.

This method of cleansing the teeth and mouth reminds one of the modern pencil swab and was used as a hygienic measure to protect the teeth.

Syphilis: Some observers are of the opinion that lesions in neolithic craniums and tibias, and to a lesser degree in the other bones, are indicative of syphilis. Virchow was of the opinion that certain bony lesions found in prehistoric America were an indication that syphilis existed in America before Columbus. Syphilis of the skull frequently affects the nasal bones. Many skeletons showed erosion of the bones of the nose and hard palate. A thick and heavy skull commonly indicates a chronic syphilitic lesion. If the skull is marked also by vascular grooves and perforations, it indicates a more acute process. Bony changes, similar to those seen in syphilis, have been found in the graves of the mound builders of America; this helped convince some historians that syphilis was introduced into Europe by the sailors of Columbus returning from the New World. The evidence of syphilis among early men, however, is not conclusive. The skeletal changes mentioned above may also be the result of other affections.

Organic and Functional Disease: The evidence cited that prehistoric man was affected with diseases similar to those of the present time relates largely to ailments of the bones and teeth; the soft parts of the body are rarely preserved through petrifaction. It is obviously difficult to recognize organic and functional diseases from lesions found in fossilized skeletons of man or animals. There are, however, a few methods by which organic and even functional maladies of early man can be ascertained:

1. The observation of disease conditions among the present anthropoid apes whose mode of life has not materially changed from that of their remote ancestors.

2. Presence of disease in modern primitives who live under the same conditions and environment as their prehistoric progenitors.

3. The extinction of races of man and of entire species of animals, such as the trilobite, the mammoth, the dinosaur, and the cave-bear, can often best be explained on the basis that their disappearance was caused by pestilence. The disappearance of many racial groups of men through the ravages of epidemics is well within the memory of man. Cities and entire districts have been decimated or entirely wiped out through widespread epidemics. In Britain during the fifth century of our own era, the country was swept by what is referred to in the Welsh "Book of Alan Daf" as "the yellow plague" because "it made yellow and bloodless all whom it attacked." In 543 A.D., 10,000 persons died each day from the bubonic plague in Constantinople alone. In the fourteenth century, the plague in Europe is estimated to have wiped out over 25,000,000 persons. It destroyed at least 10,000,000 of the population of India. Asiatic cholera and maleria, endemic in Asia, have annihilated millions of peoples. Diseases in children have reaped a grim harvest throughout recorded history. Such calamities, in the absence of sanitary and healthful living conditions, undoubtedly struck man as well as other forms of life in early prehistoric times.

4. Hereditary evidence: Susceptibility and immunity to disease is transmissible from generation to generation. Practically everyone whose opinion is of any value concedes that heredity plays a certain role in the causation of disease. The few differences of opinion are due to the circumstance that the relative potency of the hereditary factor is often difficult to estimate. The study of pedigree has been the chief method of those whose aim it has been to show that physical and mental defects are transmitted according to the Mendelian law.

Bacteria, viruses, protozoa, fungi, and simple metazoa are now recognized to be the cause of all infectious diseases; and these more or less simple forms must have existed long before man evolved from the evolutionary ladder. Aside from diseases produced via the agency of these living organisms, man is subject to ailments produced by degenerations, endocrine unbalance, and dietary deficiencies. Diseases exemplifying the penetration of living organisms into the cells of man include tuberculosis, typhoid fever, cholera, anthrax, encephalitis, influenza, smallpox, measles, mumps, chicken pox, typhus, tetanus, scarlet fever, and yellow fever. Malaria and syphilis appear to have had their origin in deep antiquity. Degenerative diseases may follow bacterial invasion, as in certain diseases of the cardiovascular and renal apparatus. Living invaders of the cellular structure of man may effect degeneration by the production of toxic substances which are circulated throughout the blood stream. Endocrine diseases are commonly produced by either hyper or hypo activity of the hormones produced by the thyroid, pancreas, anterior pituitary, ovaries, testes, and parathyroids. The commonest dietary deficiencies include the avitaminoses. Worm infestations, blood dyscrasias, leukemia, malignancy, urinary and biliary concretions and obstructions, and pernicious (hyperchromic macrocytic) anemias are other disease classifications. All these maladies have apparently existed long before the dawn of recorded history.

Huxley came to the conclusion that the shaping or controlling forces which, in due season, were to give rise to both man and his pathologies lay latent in the germ plasm of that simian stock which ultimately blossomed into human and anthropoid shapes.

Immunity: A study of the causes of death in man, animals, and plants leaves no doubt that one of the principal characteristics possessing survival value is immunity to disease. Unfortunately, this is not a very permanent acquisition, because the agents of disease also evolve, and on the whole more rapidly than their victims. Immunity is often correlated with physical characteristics. In the United States the white and colored population die from very different types of infection.

It seems likely that, when a species is subjected to a series of attacks by an evolving parasite, it may be forced along a path of structural change by the temporary successful acquisition of immunity. But in the end it may be driven into a corner, so to speak, where further immunity involves structural changes which are disastrous to it in its everyday life. Disease may in this way have played a very important part in the decay of human civilizations.

From the number of diseased skeletons of antiquity discovered within the past century, one may form an idea as to the tremendous number of diseases that prevailed in prehistoric times. Since pathological changes affecting bones are relatively few when compared with diseases attacking the soft parts of the body, and since only a small fraction of human bones became fossilized and of these only a small fraction have as yet been discovered, one may get a quantitative idea of the ailments that prevailed in prehistoric times.

EARLY TREATMENT OF DISEASE

Cro-Magnon Humane Principle: Efforts to combat disease also date far back into antiquity. There is evidence to show that as early as 20,-000 years ago the Cro-Magnons made concerted efforts to take care of their diseased and injured. They appear to have been the first humans to join together in the struggle against disease by enlisting one of their tribesmen to occupy himself with the treatment of disease. They first introduced that humane principle, not to leave the sick and disabled alone but to aid them in their distress. Thus the Cro-Magnons were apparently the first recorded men to establish the profession, or vocation, of healer. They were the first to elevate themselves above the instinctive animal practice by which diseased or injured individuals hid themselves from their own kind and their enemies, took care of their own ills as best they could in solitude, and either perished or got well in a dark corner.

A picture discovered in one of their caverns in the French Pyrenees by the three sons of Count Begouen (since known as *Trois Freres* in honor of the three brothers) shows that as early as 20,000 years ago these men had a recognized chief to lead them in the battle against disease. It is, of course, idle to think that they had a doctor in the present sense of the word. They probably had no tribal organization but lived in scattered groups. They were not interested in agriculture or in domesticating animals. Each small Cro-Magnon group had a chief of its own. Life was hard, and a livelihood was obtained from hunting and fishing. The fight against animal brutes and savage tribes frequently resulted in bodily injuries and diseases. But the Cro-Magnons cultivated among themselves a feeling of sympathy toward each other in case of distress. Unlike the very early men who struggled against disease alone in dark caves and died neglected, the Cro-Magnons inspired a willingness among their tribesmen to aid the injured and the sick. The picture now under discussion depicts the figure of a medicineman of the early Stone

Age, wearing a deerskin about his body, antlers of a reindeer on his head, and mittens on his hands. His ears appear like those of a bear. A long flowing beard and a tail of a horse complete his costume. He is represented in a half crouching position, surrounded by his kinsmen and animals to whom he is administering magic

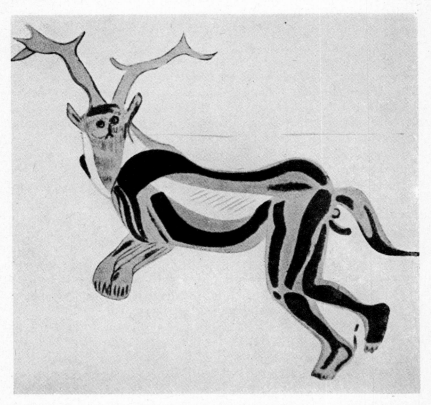

Fig. 50: The Sorcerer. The famous figure known as "the Sorcerer," partly engraved and partly painted in black, from the cavern of the *Trois Freres* in southwestern France. (From photograph by Count Begouen. Obermaier, H.: P. 223.)

cures. This picture recalls the present Australian or African savage medicineman who disguises himself in the skins of animals, and roars, shrieks, and dances, thus distracting his patient from his painful condition, and, by sorcery and magic, tries to cure him.

Evil-Spirit Theory: The term "medicineman," as used for primitive healers, has no connection with the knowledge of medicine, pharmacy, or even surgery. It is associated with appeasing the spirits. When the medicineman amputates a finger, trephines a skull, cauterizes a scalp, cuts the prepuce from a male child, sucks the blood or pus from a wound, or opens a vein for bloodletting, he does so without any intention of counteracting a pathological condition on a rational basis. His purpose is to permit the egress of an evil spirit from the body, and for this purpose alone he employs a surgical procedure. Both medicine and surgery appear to have had their beginning in shamanism, or magic. Early man tried to counteract his ills by intuition. The idea that disease is a punitive measure dispensed by the gods for violation of religious principles was a later conception. Man's concept of spirits antedated his belief in benevolent deities or gods. The idea of a god or gods was later conceived to intervene and protect him from the evil spirits.

Physical Measures of Paleolithic Man: The early paleolithic man evidently did not conceive of spirits being the cause of his ills. He resorted to physical measures practiced by his anthropoid ancestors instinctively. Gradually, as his mental faculties evolved, his medical practices also expanded. At first he resorted to measures, such as rubbing, scratching, soaking the swollen areas, pressing on painful parts, blowing over inflamed regions, moistening wounds with saliva, and applying cooling leaves on wounds. Later, when his knowledge and experience increased, he sought the help of his fellow being in the binding of his wounds and the setting of his broken bones. Still later, further benefiting from the experience gained by the march of time, he consulted one of his neighbors who made a practice of helping his fellow kinsmen in physical distress. The last development was the origin of the physician. The early healers were perhaps women (wise women) who attended to the sick and particularly to women in labor

Early Midwives: The profession of midwife has been the province of women since the dawn of civilization.

The great Mother was the head of the primitive family. She was the priestess and sorceress in one. She was considered able to put pain to flight; she was the originator of the healing god. From the darkness of her womb sprang new life, the first miracle of which man became aware. In her life-giving body, the primal forces of nature were at work and her maternal instinct made her better acquainted than the opposite sex, with charms and incantations necessary to protect the life she gave birth to, from malignant spirits.

Early Physical Therapy: Many practices employed by prehistoric peoples are continued not only by primitives but also by civilized people, but in the latter case the practices are regarded in quite another light. Modern massage and steam baths, for example, are lineal descendants of primitive rubbing and steaming. However, the object of the therapy to the prehistoric man was to drive out the evil demons from the diseased persons. The practice of kneading or pounding the body in a definite direction, usually toward the feet where it was believed the spirit escaped, or the cutting of the skin to allow the demon to depart with the sanguineous flow, led to the development of Swedish massage and bloodletting.

The results effected by massage, hydrotherapy, venesection, and for that matter diathermy, are frequently of a psychologic nature. Knowing the name of the evil spirit, using archaic and foreign words, or summoning medicinemen from other tribes as consultants were factors in producing a cure. In modern times a physician who can glibly give his patient a technical four-syllable diagnosis is also often held in great repute; and like as not, his fame is apt to be greater abroad than at home. Although the rational physical aspect of treatment has come more and more to the fore, there is no place in the world where the magical aspect has altogether disappeared.

Early Anatomical Knowledge: From drawings left on the walls of caves, it is evident that certain prehistoric men had a rude knowledge of visceral topography and an acquaintance with the vital organs of the body, such as the heart, lungs, and liver. The Pindal elephant is pierced with arrows imbedded in the heart. The Niaux bison is portrayed with weapons directed at the vital centers. One picture portrays the abdomen laid open by a slash, and another shows an exposed brain. Many such exhibits testify that prehistoric man had some knowledge of the gross anatomy and of the relationship of the organs to each other.

Amputations: On the walls of the caves of neolithic France and Spain (c. 7000 B.C.), drawings and silhouettes of amputated legs, arms, and fingers are seen. Amputation was performed with flint knives. In the Aurignacian period, several pictures depicting hands and feet shortened to the interphalangeal and metacarpal regions are observed. Fingers and toes were occasionally removed by tying a thread around them and exerting pressure until they dropped off. Hemorrhage was stopped by a compression bandage. When this was not available, the bleeding finger or hand was placed in hot sand. The need for amputation might have suggested itself to the prehistoric surgeon for the following conditions: (1) the realization that hopeless damage has been done to the parts; (2) the knowledge of the potentially fatal effects of snake bite; (3) for ceremonial and sacrificial reasons; and (4) the realization that a person with a badly injured organ might be better off when it is removed.

Decapitation: Certain Aurignacian skulls in Germany offer evidence of decapitation at or just before death. Chopping off a hand, forearm, or finger, gouging out an eye, castration, infibulation, and many other kinds of mutilation have been common and are still practiced among primitive men.

Puberty Ceremonies: An early practice, which is still widely employed, is the rite of knocking out teeth as a puberty ceremony in males. As a rule the incisors are removed, but canines often meet with the same fate. Wilke observed[29] such cases in the graves of neolithic Spain and England. Shukbas reports the same in Palestine. Valois and Cole have met with similar cases in early paleolithic sites in Africa. Ritualistic operations, commonly connected with sex, are circumcision and infibulation. Evidences of the former have been found in predynastic Egypt and Nubia.

Finger Mutilation: In the Cro-Magnon caves are imprints of human hands which had been laid on rock and then dusted around with colored earth.

The practice of finger mutilation among Australian Bushmen and American Indian tribes is associated with burial customs and disease therapy. A Bushman woman may cut off a joint of one of her fingers when a near relative is about to die.

American Indians have been known to cut off finger joints when burying their dead during a pestilence so as "to cut off death." They sacrifice a part of the body to save the whole.

Highland Gaelic mythology tells of heroes, who lie asleep to gather power which will enable them to combat monsters and fierce enemies. Heroines awake them by cutting off their fingers, a part of the ear, or a portion of the skin from the scalp.[30]

References and Notes

1. Williams, J.: Human Immortality. 1898, p. 33.
2. Brown, S.: Physician Throughout the Ages. 1928, Vol. 1, p. 4.
3. Sudhoff, K.: History of Medicine. 1926, p. 77.
4. "Physician Throughout the Ages." 1928, Vol. 1, p. 3.
5. Cuvier, G.: Recherches sur les ossemens fossiles de quadrupedes. Paris, 1812, 1821, 1825.

6. Busk, G.: Natural History. 1865.

7. Mortillet, L. L. G.: French anthropologist, who made a special study of the Swiss lake dwellings. His most important work is "Le Prehistorique," 1882.

8. Lartet, E.: French archaeologist, encouraged by Cuvier. He made excavations which led in 1835 to the discovery, in the vicinity of Auch, of a number of fossil remains which he described in a paper, "The Antiquity of Man in Western Europe," 1860.

9. Hippocrates: Air, Water and Places, Francis Adams, ed. William Wood and Co., New York, p. 172.

10. Herodotus: Terpsichore. V. Henry Cary, ed., New York, 1847.

11. Klebs, E.: Codiscoverer of the bacillus of diphtheria. Klebs was assistant to Virchow at the Pathological Institute of Berlin. Garrison places him next to Pasteur as the most important precurser in the bacterial theory of infection. He is the author of two books on pathology.

12. Lindsay, W. L.: J. Ment. Sc. (cited by Darwin) July, 1871, p. 7.

13. Cited by Charles Darwin: Descent of Man. D. Appleton-Century and Co., 1898, p. 7.

14. Schultz, A. H.: Diseases and Healed Fractures of the Wild Apes. Bul. Inst. Hist. Med., 71-81, July 19, 1939.

15. Geddes, Sir A.: Arch. Anthropol., 15, 1907.

16. Gilles, H. C.: Home Life of Modern Highlanders. 1911, p. 85.

17. Jager, K.: Beitrage zur Prohistorischen Chirurgie (Palachirurgis). Deutsche. Ztschr. F. Chir., 109-140, 1907-1909.

18. Le lesion osseuses de homme prehistorique du France. Juliet, 1881, pp. 1-118.

19. Broca, P.: Paleopathology, 360.

20. Broca, P.: Anthropol. Soc., Vols. 11 and 17.

21. Genesis 4:15.

22. Leviticus 19:28.

23. Hoffschlager, R.: Von der Heilkunst des Forgeschichtlichen Menschen Ciba Zeitsch. 6:19, 23, 24, 1937; 1939.

24. Pales, L.: Paleopathologie et pathologie comparative. Masson et Cie, 1930.

25. Hrdlicka, A.: Anthropological Work in Peru, 1913. Smith misc. collection 61, pub. n., 1918; 1914, pp. 22, 46, 69.

26. Ossements Fossiles. 2:180; Schmerling of Liege found, in the caves of Belgium, caries of the bones of the lower jaw and forelegs. He described a case of ankylosis of the cervical vertebrae and a lumbar vertebra which was nearly destroyed by disease before the animal died. The cave-bear seems to have been very liable to rickets and, in some cases, its joints present the characteristic deformities of rheumatoid arthritis.

27. Schultz, A. H.: Characters Common to Higher Primates and Characters Specific for Man. Quart. Rev. Biol., 11: 259-283.

28. Krogman, W. M.: The Pathology of Prehistoric and Protohistoric Man; The Skeletal and Dental Pathology of an Early Iranian Site. Bull. Inst. Hist. Med. 1:24-48, 1940.

29. Wilke, G.: Der Heilkunst in der Europaischen Forzeit. 1936.

30. Mackenzie, D. A.: Myths of Crete and Prehellenic Europe, pp. 30-31.

5

Primitive Concepts of Disease and Death

"MEN that look no further than their outside," said Sir Thomas Brown, "think health an appurtenance unto life, and quarrel with their constitution for being sick; but I that have examined the parts of men and know upon what tender filaments that fabric hangs, do wonder that we are not always so, and considering the thousand doors that lead to death do thank my God that we can die but once." The problem of disease and death has challenged the mind of men from time immemorial.

Early man could well understand disease and death brought about by violence but could not grasp the idea of disease or death coming without visible cause. For want of a rational explanation, he inferred that there had been an offended or jealous spirit, an evil force from without, that entered his body to afflict him with disease and possibly death.

PRIMITIVE THEORIES OF DISEASE

Spiritual Etiology: The spiritual etiology of disease may sound fantastic and superstitious to modern man, but considering the time, when man viewed disease without any idea of its causation, and when the treatment of disease was more or less folkloristic, a concept like demonology must be considered a progressive step in the evolution of medicine. It was a recognition of the fact that every natural occurrence must have a cause; but lacking positive knowledge, prehistoric man permitted his imagination to play a part in naming its origin. He visualized invisible disease-demons from the air as the cause of his ills, and left it to the modern bacteriologist with a microscope to isolate, describe, and cultivate these little demons which he has named "microbes."

115

The mere fact that, when medicine was in its infancy, external and invisible objects were thought to be the etiologic factors of disease was a great contribution to the future knowledge of medicine.

The animistic forces of evil, which primitive men believed were the agents that punished him with disease, were: (1) heavenly powers, such as gods and stars; (2) aerial powers, such as demons; (3) terrestrial forces, such as witchcraft and evil eye; and (4) subterranean powers, such as ghosts of the dead, worms, or serpents.

Millenniums have elapsed between the animistic and the bacterial theories of disease; concept after concept was proposed, only to be discarded by succeeding observers. Medical concepts based on non-scientific premises often last long. They may be retained in the minds of man long after they pass the primitive stage, and even after scientific data have disproved them. This ancient concept still prevails among primitive peoples in many countries. In upper Burma, cholera and smallpox are conceived as devils that lurk in the fog and filth.

To the Koreans, disease is personified; they have a notion that typhus devils, cholera devils, and smallpox devils roam the air; and in their attempt to scare them away, they beat gongs, drums, pots, and pans. This noisy ceremony is kept up incessantly for three days and nights after the funeral of one who has died of one of these diseases.

In China, the air still swarms with countless good and evil spirits. The good ones, they believe, move through the air in a curve, the bad ones in a straight line. This fantastic belief influenced the development of Chinese architecture. The roofs of houses, pagodas, gateways, and all other conspicuous structures are therefore curved. For the same reason, there are no straight highways in China, and the development of straight railways has been hindered.

In Oceania and Polynesia, it is believed that disease is due to an offended spirit which has to be propitiated by sacrifice. In Samoa, disease is considered a result of the wrath of some particular deity. The high priests of the village, who ascertain the causes of the malady, order sacrifices on behalf of the sick—a confession is obtained from every member of the patient's family as to the crimes each has committed or the curses uttered in anger against the sick person.

When a Polynesian takes sick, the priest-physician is sent for. As soon as he arrives, a young plantain tree procured by some member of the family is handed to him as an offering to the offended deity, together with a present of clothes furnished as a fee to the priest. The priest begins his rites by calling upon the god and beseeching him to abate his anger toward the sufferer. The priest propitiates the offended god and supplicates him for relief. The medicine administered is a mere vehicle by which the god would act and arrest the progress of the disease.[2]

Natives of Australia attribute disease and death to black magic perpetrated by persons who wish them harm. Any inimical native may act as a sorcerer. He goes away into the forest with his *irna* (a stick or a bone less than a foot long, sharpened at one end, the other being tipped with a certain kind of grass or resin) which he places in the ground while muttering some curse, such as "May your heart be rent asunder!" or "May your head and throat be split open!" Then he goes back to his camp, returning later to fetch the *irna* which he hides near his camp. He bides his time until a night when he can get near enough to distinguish his victim without being himself observed. He then stoops and, turning his back toward the camp, takes the *irna* in both hands and jerks it repeatedly over his shoulder muttering the same curse again. The pointing of the *irna* causes disease and death unless the evil magic which has emanated from the point of the *irna* can be removed. A string is usually attached to the end of the *irna,* and this the sorcerer often burns in the fire to insure the death of the victim. In place of a bone, a stone may be used, preferably of crystalline quartz, which is believed to be capable of directing the magic against the victim.[3]

There is a general agreement among observers of primitive communities that natives are extraordinarily open to suggestions, so far, at least, as the transmission of disease is concerned. One who believes that magic has been exercised upon him simply lies down, refuses food, and pines away. Among the Melanesians at New Guinea, diseases are thought to emanate from sorcerers; and after their death, such powers commonly pass to their daughters.[4]

In Celebes Island, ancestral spirits dwell to a great extent in the ethereal regions. The return of the departed spirits is dreaded; and at funerals, the relatives blacken each other's faces with charcoal (this custom is called "maha-wuwuringan"). The object is to prevent any recognition by the ghosts who may be hovering about the graves or returning to their former abodes. Black peoples, such as the Australians and Andamanese, try to disguise themselves by daubing their faces with white bands or patches. White is the mourning color in China.

The medicineman, or healer, employs various methods to counteract the animistic forces of disease. One of the methods still used is to cast out the evil spirit from the patient by the force of his own familiar spirit. Sometimes he appeals to his familiars to indicate the method of treatment.

When the sickness is thought to be caused by the soul's wandering away from the body of the patient, the medicineman, or *shaman*, endeavors to recapture it by sending his own soul in search of it. While in a trance, the *shaman* speaks of the hazardous chase connected with capturing the fugitive soul. Reviving from the trance, he exhibits a small object which he pretends to be the soul and which he returns to the patient.

The Minahassas have a novel notion that both sickness and death are caused by the soul's leaving the body to flutter about the air somewhere in the neighborhood. When one of their tribesmen is stricken with disease, the *walian* (priest, or *shaman*) is called to bring the soul back to the patient. While all his friends are around the patient, the *walian* goes out to the field or village to look for the fugitive soul. He builds a fire on which he cooks rice and chicken to entice the soul. He also whistles, or calls the soul by calling certain pet names such as are used in calling a favorite dog. Then he goes through the lists of the gods and performs a religious ceremony. At last the *walian* gives a start, as if he sees the soul moving in the grass. Having located the errant soul, the *walian* advances carefully and catches it in his clothes or hands, just as a school boy might catch a butterfly in his hat. The *walian* then returns to the patient, opens his clothes, and says, "Now here is your soul returned." If the patient does not get well promptly after such a stratagem, it is a good sign that his end is near.[5]

In Loango, for instance, the natives affirm:

Something takes the man by surprise, enters into him and ill-treats him. This something may be powers or malign influences or poisons—which emanate from natural objects, places, solid or liquid foods—but also from fetishes, men, and wizards. They may also be souls of any kind, which brush against the sick man and slip into him, or else definite souls which feed upon his vital forces, cause him pain, paralyze him, and trouble his mind, etc.[6]

To the Fijian mind, illness is like a wave, an outside influence which sweeps over the sick man and seems to possess him. This wave, this influence, generally proceeds from gods or devils or living beings, hardly ever from natural causes, such as cold or heat. There is no natural cause for sickness to the Fijians; they seek it *praeter naturum,* i.e. in an invisible world, existing side by side with this.

In Bombay, whatever the illness is which attacks man, woman, or child, or even cattle, the Kolies imagine that it arises from the action of an evil spirit or an offended deity; and at the end of a certain period, after having vainly endeavored to cure the malady by remedies known to them, they consult an exorcist able to expel evil spirits.[7] At Bahrel Ghazal, "even where disease is not directly attributed to the machinations of enemies, the idea of possession seems to hold."[8]

Practices of Diagnosis: The practices relating to diagnosis are the direct outcome of this mystic idea of illness. It is important to discover what malign power or influence has taken possession of the sick man, what witchcraft is being exercised upon him, and so on. This diagnosis, upon which everything else depends, can only be made by a man qualified to come in contact with mysterious forces and spirits, and powerful enough to fight them and expel them. The first step, therefore, is to appeal to the medicineman, *shaman,* wizard, doctor, exorcist, or whatever he may be called; and if this person consents to undertake the cure, his first care will be to put himself into the special state necessary to be able to communicate with forces and spirits, and effectively exercise upon them his potential influence. This necessitates a whole series of preliminary operations which may last for several hours, or even a whole night. There must be fasting or intoxication, and dances to the extent of complete exhaustion and excessive perspiration, until at last the "doctor" seems to lose consciousness and be "beside himself." It is at this moment that the diagnosis is accomplished, intuitively, and consequently without any possibility of error:

The most important among the paraphernalia of the *shaman* [when about to treat a sick man] is a head-dress made of a mat, which is worn in his incantations.....Before putting it on they blow upon it, and sprinkle it with water which has been poured over magic herbs. He puts himself into a trance by singing the song he had obtained from his guardian spirit at the time of his initiation. He dances until he perspires freely, and finally his spirit comes and speaks to him. [9]

Indifference to Physical Symptoms: Very little attention is paid to physical symptoms. "In West Africa," says Nassau, "this diagnosis is not made by an examination and comparison of the physical and mental symptoms, but by drum, dance, frenzied song, mirror, fumes of drugs, and conversation with the spirit itself."[10]

The indifference concerning physical symptoms also proceeds from the mystic idea of illness. The seat of the malady is not within the body or the visible organs; it is the mind or spirit which is attacked. Thus, in West Africa, "the dogma that rules [the doctor's] practice is that in all cases of disease in which no blood is showing, the patient is suffering from something wrong in the mind."[11] According to the Iroquois, "every illness is a desire of the mind, and one does not die unless the desire is unfulfilled." In Acadia, the sick man is refused nothing he asks, because in such a state his desires are orders from the guardian spirit; and when wizards are called in, it is because they can best learn from the spirits the cause of the trouble and the suitable remedy. It is the wizard's duty to discover the sorcery which has caused the illness.

Religious Factor in Early Medical Practice: The profession of doctor was, and still is, among many peoples, intimately connected with religion. The first doctor of whom records are available was a priest; and throughout Egyptian history, many of the functions of the priest were magical in character. The common methods of therapeutics were exorcisms by which demons were expelled. Frequently the expulsion was effected by words and gestures, and sometimes by the use of amulets or other substances which the magician charged with occult powers. Often the rite included a foul mixture to drink, accompanied by a recitation. The offensive mixture was intended, not to counteract the morbid condition of the patient, but so to disgust the demon who had taken possession of the patient that he would voluntarily leave the victim.

Secondary Place of Drug Therapy: The efficacy of the treatment depends entirely upon connections and participations of a spiritual or magic kind. As a consequence, the therapeutics of white people are valueless. Their remedies may possibly do harm (on account of the unknown mystic properties in them); it is certain they can do no good, and they are quite ineffectual in dealing with the maladies of primitives. The strong repugnance felt against European remedies, of whatever kind they may be, is very general. "He fears the white man, dreads his medicines, and shrinks from the outward applications which may, for aught he knows, be possessed of secret properties that will cause his destruction."[12] Certain observers have clearly penetrated the reason for this dislike. Of New Zealand, Elsdon Best writes:

A great distrust of European doctors is manifest in this district. It is probable that this is not due to any disbelief in the medical knowledge of the said profession, but that the natives have an instinctive fear that a doctor will interfere with the state of tabu, that the life principles will be endangered by the methods of Europeans.

Whatever may be the treatment prescribed for the sick man, the medicines he is to take, the regimen he must follow: whether he is to have steam baths. phlebotomy, or, in certain cases, trephining—it is the mystic forces which insure their efficacy. They don't set a value or trust on anything, unless it is connected in some measure with the supernatural.[13]

To the Negritos of the Philippines, "all disease is caused by spirits, which must be expelled from the body, before a cure can be effected."[14] It is plain that the component parts of any fetish are looked upon by them as we look upon the drugs of our materia medica. It is plain, also, that these drugs are operative, not as ours are, by certain inherent chemical qualities, but by the presence of a spirit to whom they are favorite media. And it is also clear that the spirit is induced to act by the pleasing enchantments of the magic doctor.[15]

The materia medica used by the medicinemen varies much. In some cases, their skill amazes explorers; in others, their resources are scanty.

Practice of Magic: It is astonishing to read of the many cures primative doctors effected despite their irrational concepts of disease. As an illustration, the New Testament story of the Gadarene swine may be mentioned.[16] The primitive practice of magic like the present practice of psychotherapy, was based on the power of suggestion. The old adage, "Nature cures the disease, while the remedy amuses the patient" has evidently more than an element of truth.

The ancient method of exorcism of spirits was based on a set of procedures which had a suggestive effect on the mind of the patient. The following passage, in "Life in Ancient Egypt and Assyria" by Maspero, gives a graphic picture of the methods ancient Egyptian healers employed to impress the sick whom they intended to heal. It tells of the famous exorcist, Nibamon of Thebes who was particularly known for his skill in curing the most violent headaches. He was summoned by a woman by the name of Khait to attend her husband. He arrived toward evening accompanied by two servants, one having in his hand a black book and the other a chest filled with the necessary materials for making all kinds of amulets, such as clay for modeling plants, assorted consecrated linens, red and black ink, and wax to make figures. As soon as he arrived and glanced at the sick man, Psarou, he knew that a dead man visited him every night and was devouring him. Thereupon he took out some clay from his casket, mixed it with a blade of grass, and kneaded it into a ball, over which he chanted an incantation from the black book.

The book states that the best way of driving away the rebellious spirits is to persuade them that their victim is placed under immediate protection of one of several divinities; in tormenting him, it is the gods themselves that they unconsciously provoke; and if they persevere in their evil designs, they risk annihilation from the person whom they expected to destroy with impunity. Nibamon's incantation commences by announcing that "The magic virtues of Psarou, son of the Lady Tentnoubit, are the virtues of Osiris-Atmu, the father of the gods"; and then, since this too general a proposition would not suffice to alarm the ghost, the magician enumerates the portions which compose the head of Psarou, and proves that they are all armed with divine charms, i.e. the magic virtues of his left temple are the virtues of the temple of Tmu; the virtues of his right eye are the virtues of that eye of Tmu which pierces the darkness with its rays. The virtues of his left eye are the virtues of that eye of Horus which destroys—in short, he is a god and one of the most formidable of the gods, that one to whom nothing in Heliopolis is closed. (This is an ingenious method of insinuating that Psarou is an incarnation of Ra, without, however, directly making the assertion.) Four times Nibamon repeats his formula and then slides the ball under the sick man's head; at night, when the dead man appears, he will not have sufficient strength to do any harm and will remain powerless as long as the ball remains in its place.

Some of the magical formulas were nothing more than meaningless gibberish with no mythological significance, but the procedure by the exorcist, or *shaman,* has always carried enough weight to impress the sick person.

The Brazilian Bororos do not as a rule use magical powers to cast out the demon of disease, but they carry the idea of suggestion to a ridiculous stage by having the father take the medicine in order to cure the sick child. "They almost invariably get well."

"Sympathetic" Therapeutics: But even supposing that for a certain disease they prescribe the same medicine as modern doctors would do, the chief consideration for them is to expel the influence of the spirit whose presence causes the trouble. "Sympathetic" therapeutics is practiced widely; European practitioners were still resorting thereto three centuries ago. To take but one example in British Columbia, "decoctions of wasps' nests or of flies are drunk by bar-

ren women, to make them bear children, as both bring forth many young."[17]

The healing virtues of the drug are, as a rule, governed by a good many conditions. If it is composed of plants, they must have been gathered by certain persons, at a given moment, with special incantations and instruments, the moon being in such and such a phase, etc.; if these conditions are not fulfilled, the remedy will not operate. The person must approach the plant from a certain direction, going around it from right to left one or four times, and reciting prayers all the time. Then he pulls up the plant by the roots and covers it with soil. Sometimes the *shaman* must leave the first three plants he sees, and take the fourth only, after which he may go back to the three others. The bark is always removed from the eastern side, because it will have received more healing power by being subjected to the sun's rays.[18]

If the sufferer is cured, all goes well, and the professional healer receives the gratitude of the relatives. But if, in spite of his efforts, the issue is unfavorable, he is held responsible. In more primitive societies, failure is as a rule attributed to "the malignant action of a superior magic on the part of some hostile spirit or individual."[19] In a general way, since the idea of illness and its causes and treatments remains a mystic one, the failure of the efforts made for the patient are accounted for as easily as their success. It is the more powerful "force" or "influence" or "spirit" upon which life and death depend.

The Shaman: The term "shaman" signifies magician or medicine-man. His functions consist chiefly in working cures by magic. Records from Egypt, Babylonia, and other ancient countries show that early medicine originated in magic. The doctor was a magician, and his methods of cure were magical.

The efficacy of a *shaman* depends on his ability of communicating with the invisible powers and departed spirits and receiving from them revelations as to the future. On these occasions the performer, in order to contact these forces, puts himself into a state of nervous excitement, in which his mouth foams and his limbs are convulsed.

The office of the *shaman* is often hereditary; both sexes are eligible. It may fall occasionally to those to whom spirits have revealed themselves or whom the spirits have supposedly chosen. *Shamanists* usually select, as their pupils, boys with epileptic or hysterical tendencies. Negro *shamans* prefer dwarfs or albinos as pupils. To prove their fitness for this important calling, they have to perform some unusual stunts, such as acting as though they themselves were possessed. Others are trained by an older member of the profession. If the budding Dyak *manang* has been cured by an older *shaman*, he is considered to have more aptitude for joining the profession. Among the Dyaks, the initiation of a *shaman* to his calling includes the committing to memory of traditional lore, such as charms, incantations, and symbolic practices.[20]

The similarity of the proceedings of the Siberian *shaman*, the North American medicinemen, and the African "doctor" constitutes important evidence that, at a remote prehistoric time, the ancestors of the present aborigines of the various parts of the world inhabited a common home where they cultivated a common tradition; and when separated by a series of migrations, they carried along with them their old customs and practices. It favors also the hypothesis that the new world was peopled by races once belonging to Northern Asia. Of course this implies the passing of periods which must be reckoned by millenniums, for the diversity of human races evolves as slowly as geologic change. There are many customs which have no meaning at present but which had a good reason in the far past, for every single thing man did was reasonable to him when he first began to do it. The continuation of such practices is expressed by the term "cultural survival."

The main difference in the performance between the Siberian *shaman* and the North American medicineman is that the former uses a magic drum, the latter a magic rattle. Both wear fantastically decorated cloaks.

That *shamanistic* practices have survived from the days of the Cro-Magnon to the present time, is due to the fact that human reasoning has been so weak that one success impressed upon the memory outweighs nine failures.

Other Animistic Concepts: Animistic concepts of disease are not confined to primitive peoples alone. In New England, in 1693, Cotton Mather wrote:

. . . this, the Destroyer, or the *"Divel"* that scatters Plagues about the World; Pestilential and Contagious Diseases; 'tis the Divel who do's oftimes invade us with them. 'Tis no uneasy thing for the Divel, to impregnate the Air about us, with such Malignant Salts as meeting with the Salt of our Microcosm, shall immediately cast us into that Fermentation and Putrifaction which shall utterly dissolve all the Vital Tyes within us. . . . And when the Divel has raised those Arsenical Fumes which become Venomous Quivers full of Terrible Arrows, how easily can he shoot the delecterious Miasma into those Juices or Bowels of Men's Bodies, which shall soon Enflame them with a Mortal Fire.

It is obvious that such concepts are not conducive to sanitation, for the "Divel" would probably pay scant respect to such things as hygiene, antisepsis, and quarantine. Epidemics, like cholera and the plague, which may be checked now before they have fairly started, formerly swept away thousands in their course.

One reason for the obscurity about disease was the ignorance of functional diseases of the body. If an arrow, for example, is shot into the eye causing blindness, the most determined opponent of natural laws will admit the connection between blindness and the lesion. But if blindness resulted from abuse of the eye, primitive man ascribed it to spiritual forces because he could not otherwise explain it. It is functional diseases that influence the uninitiated to resort to the supernatural. He cannot realize that changes in the structure produce functional derangement, although the changes cannot always be detected.

PRIMITIVE THEORIES OF DEATH

Spiritualistic Theory: Primitive theories of death, like those of disease, have been spiritualistic. Disease and death affect the utmost being of man. Even the most primitive savage holds that his inmost being is the spirit, not the body. How merely physical agencies can affect a spirit, and why a simple blow on the head should drive the soul from the body does not concern him. It is a question that puzzled Galen, who writes, "If Plato were alive, I should like to ask him why great losses of blood, a draught of hemlock or a severe fever should separate soul and body, for according to Plato, death takes place when the soul removes herself from the body."[21] If the primitive does not find this occurrence unnatural, it is because he has a supernatural solution to this problem. Sometimes this theory is carried out to its fullest extent. Thus, the Abipones hold that man is naturally immortal and that even those killed in battle die, not from their wounds, but from the enchantment of the hostile medicineman. If there were no medicinemen, there would be no death, despite the fact that an arrow or a branch of a tree can kill without the aid of sorcery. Faith in the spiritual origin of disease is too deeprooted to change the belief.

Death, like that of internal disease, has been attributed by primitives to violent or mystic sources. Neither was considered a natural occurrence. According to Spencer and Gillen,[22] the Australian aborigine, and in a smaller degree the American Indian and natives of Asia and Africa, are "quite unable to realize death from natural causes." There is no such thing as death from natural causes. Both disease and death are the direct outcome of the influence of some ghost, demon, or wizard.[23]

The native African cannot understand that one who was well two weeks ago should now be dead, unless some potent wizard had interfered and, by the art of magic, broken the thread of life. Natives of benighted countries will die after the infliction of even a most superficial wound if they believe that the weapon which inflicted the wound has been magically endowed. They simply lie down, refuse food, and pine away. The only possible cure for one wounded by a "charmed" spear is strong countermagic.[24]

Primitive man cannot conceive that death is brought about by disease; he believes that diseases are caused by the ghosts of the dead. He therefore endeavors to appease the dead.

Among certain Indians in Canada:

If fire should break out in a village where there are any dead bodies, they (the dead bodies) will be the first to be placed in safety. The people will despoil themselves of their most precious possessions to adorn the dead; from time to time they open their tombs to change their garments and they deprive themselves of food so that they may carry it to the graves and to the places where they imagine their souls of the dead to be wandering. . . . they are careful to cover their bodies in the grave in such a way that no soil will touch them.

How American Indians resort to ancient Egyptian practices can only be explained on the basis that both learned such customs in prehistoric ages from the same sources.

Communication with the Dead: There is no insuperable barrier separating the dead from the living. On the contrary, the living are constantly in touch with the dead and can do the dead good or harm, and can also be well or badly treated by them. To the primitive, there is nothing strange in communicating with the dead, and nothing unusual about being connected with "spirits," or with any occult force whose influence he feels, or which he fancies himself subduing. This is in a measure true to even cultural peoples, as in the case of the spiritualists in England and elsewhere.

The reality of the objects he perceives does not in the least depend upon his being able to verify that reality by what we call experience; indeed, as a rule, it is the intangible and invisible that are most real in his eyes. Moreover, the dead do not remain without revealing their presence even to the senses. Occasionally they are heard in the wind. They cannot be seen; they are like the wind; in fact the gentle rustling of the plantain leaves is said to be caused by the ghosts, and a whirlwind which carries up dust, leaves, and straws is said to be the ghosts at play.[25]

It is a positive conviction of the Chinese people that spirits of the dead exist, that they keep up with the living a most lively intercourse, as intimate almost as that among men. There exists, in fact, a line of separation between the dead and the living, but it is a very faint line, scarcely discernible. In every respect their intercourse bears an active character. It brings blessing and evil as well, the spirits thus ruling effectually man's fate.[26]

These concepts show that the dead are believed to be alive in their graves. Throughout the whole range of Chinese literature, coffins with a corpse inside are designated "animated encoffined corpses" or "animated coffins."[27] A young girl widowed as a bride, when she has acquired the consent of her own parents and those of her deceased bridegroom, may renounce conjugal life forever. She is, as a rule, allowed to settle for good in the mortuary house and is then formally united with the dead in marriage.[28] In ancient China, there existed the curious custom of placing deceased females in the tombs of lads who died before they were married.[29] Public opinion inclines favorably to the sacrifice of wives who follow their husbands to the tomb, and the act reflects so much honor on the families that widows often desire it, or at least resign themselves to it. Of course they may be constrained by their family circle.[30]

Theory of Disease Caused by the Dead: There is a strong belief among some primitives that the dead may cause disease to the living. Death, therefore, is considered dangerous to the living. In Cambodia, for example, a dead person is carried from the house to the burial place feet first, in order that he cannot see the house; for if he did, sickness would attack the family. Other primitives build fires around the house, at the time when the deceased is removed, to keep away spirits which are attracted by the corpse and might bring sickness upon the survivors.

In this connection, a letter from a husband to his deceased wife, attached to a small picture of her, was discovered in Egypt during the latter part of the last century. The contents of this letter is of much interest and justifies reproduction.

In this letter the husband upbraids his departed wife's spirit for having afflicted him with disease as follows:

To the wise soul (Ka) of the Lady Anchera. What evil have I done thee, that I find myself now in this miserable state in which I am? What have I done unto thee, that thou shouldst lay thy hand upon me, though no evil has been done unto thee? From the time I became thy husband until now, have I done anything against thee that I had to keep it secret? Thou wast the wife of my youth, and I lived with thee. Then I filled all kinds of offices, and I lived with thee, and caused thy heart no sorrow. Behold when I ruled over the captains of Pharaoh's footmen and of his chariots I caused them to come to thee, to throw themselves on their bellies before thee, and they brought many good things and laid them at thy feet. When thou wast sick... Then when I had to go with Pharoah and his company to the South land my thoughts were with thee, and I passed the eight months without being able to eat or to drink. And when I returned to Memphis I besought Pharaoh, and came to thee, and made a great mourning for thee, and I and my people before my house. I gave bandages and stuffs for thy burial, and had much linen woven, nor was I lacking in making good offerings for thee. Since then I have past three years mourning, without entering my house, or acting as I might have acted; and lo! I did all this because it was for thee!

The Babylonians attributed death to a violation of a taboo by an early ancestor who insisted on partaking of a certain fruit prohibited by a deity. A similar account of death is given in the "Book of Genesis."

Legends of the Origin of Death: There are numerous legends with regards to the origin of death. Certain African tribes opined that death came about because one of their ancestors bathed in a stream which had been forbidden by a deity. The Australians blamed death on certain women who went to a forbidden tree where a bat was perched; suddenly the bat fluttered out and caused their immediate demise.[31] The Polynesians ascribed death to the fact that Maui, their divine hero, was not properly baptized.

According to Greek legend, Pandora, on whom all the gods and goddesses bestowed gifts, brought from heaven a box containing all human ills. She was under strict orders not to open this box. Her womanly curiosity, however, prompted her to peep inside of it; as a result, the ills and misfortunes escaped and spread all over the earth.

In the Solomon Islands, Koevari was the author of death because he allowed someone to view him casting off his skin. Koevari was informed by the messengers of the gods that he would cast off his skin when old and so renew his youth. The condition was imposed upon him, however, that no eye should witness the act of sloughing it off. He was imprudent enough to let himself be seen by his granddaughter; and as a result, mankind was denied the boon of renewed youthfulness forever. These and numerous traditions are widely spread among many peoples.

The chief reason why death is not understandable is that knowledge of it is purely objective; it always is seen to befall others but never oneself.

Because early man could not explain death as a natural phenomenon, it became personified as a wicked angel, the "angel of death." In the Old Testament, death is viewed under the form of an angel sent from God. The "angel of death" smites 185,000 men in the Assyrian camp. The destroying angel rages among the people in Jerusalem. The angel of the Lord is seen by David "standing between the earth and the heaven having a drawn sword in his hand stretched out over Jerusalem." The "angel of death" receives his orders from God. A Talmudic legend has it that when the "angel of death" appears, there is no remedy. There are two exceptions to this rule: a confessed sinner and one who has rescued himself from the "angel of death" by acts of benevolence. In the Palestinian city of Luz, the "angel of death" had no power; and when the aged inhabitants were ready to die, they went outside the city.

The "angel of death" plays an important part in the folklore of almost all peoples. It was easy to hoodwink him. The tricks played on this enemy of mankind are numerous. Sisyphus fettered death, keeping him prisoner till he was rescued by Aries. Venetian folklore had it that a certain Beppo tied him up in a bottle. In Sicily, an innkeeper corked him up in a similar way. A monk kept him in his pouch for forty years. Gambling Hansel kept death up a tree for seven years. The "angel of death" was not considered cunning, for changing the name or adding a new name to the person whom he was about to strike was sufficient to confuse him.

Such legends may be multiplied, but enough has been stated to show that the attitude of early man toward the riddle of his end has been in part dictated, and is even still influenced, by the savage belief that to die is unnatural. Frequently the cause of death is ascribed not to obvious causes but to subtle and mysterious arts of magic.

Relationship of Sickness to Death: Even if death follows a long period of sickness, it is not considered a sequel to the disease that preceded it. Early man could not see any casual relationship between these occurrences. He thought that sickness was caused by one act of malignity and death followed it by another act not necessarily emanating from the same source. This disinclination to admit that death is caused by sickness or from other natural causes is still widespread. It is a common belief in Melanesia, in Africa, and in the Andaman Islands that, even if one is murdered during a tribal feud or from the attack of a wild beast, death is still brought about by the agency of a magician or a deity.

Fear of the Dead: The dead were feared because they might afflict the living with diseases and misfortune out of revenge and jealousy. Even those attending the dead were feared. In Tahiti, embalmers are carefully avoided and are not allowed to handle food lest it be affected by the taint of death. Gravediggers, funeral directors, and shroud manufacturers are still looked upon with fear by superstitious persons. There is no respect or reverence for the dead involved in such concepts. On the principle of sympathetic magic alone, contagion of the corpse is considered to transfer disease to the living. Around this concept, developed a large number of religious customs, ceremonies, and rituals, most of which betray a common origin.

There can be little doubt that the customary clothes of solemn black worn by the relatives of the dead originated, not from grief or respect for the departed friend, but rather in the fear of being recognized by the returning spirit if the customary colors were worn. The ghost is supposed to come back to the house by the same route by which the corpse was taken away. Everything therefore is done to confuse the spirit if it tries to return to its accustomed haunts. Certain peoples let down the corpse through a hole in the floor and carry the corpse three times around the house before conveying it to the grave in order to confuse the spirit in finding its way back home by this circuitous route. For the same reason, the nearest relatives do not attend the funeral in order that the ghost, if it is hovering around, may not suspect that it is its own funeral that is taking place. The dark clothes and black hats and the custom of relatives' painting their faces black, by such races as the Minahassas, is a means of disguise so as not to be recognized by their departed kin. It is related that the Spaniards, at the time of the conquest of the Philippines, found that many of the inhabitants used white as a mourning color. Many of the races of Luzon and the Zulu Islands still use white instead of black, perhaps also so as not to be recognized by the ghosts of the dead.

Theory of Death as Slumber: Death is looked upon as a deep and prolonged slumber. Many persistent legends about famous "sleepers" that still survive appear to have originally been connected with the belief in the return of the dead.

Among the famous groups of sleeping heroes are the Seven Sleepers of Ephesus—the Christians who had been condemned to death by the Emperor Decius and concealed themselves in a cave where they slept for three and a half centuries. An eighteenth century legend tells of seven men in Roman attire, who tarried for a long period in a cave in western Germany. In Norse mythology, the seven sons of Miner sleep in the underworld awaiting the blast of the horn, which will be blown at Ragnarok when the gods and demons will wage the last battle. The sleepers of Arabia once awoke to foretell the coming of Mohammed, and their sleeping dog, according to Moslem belief, is one of the ten animals that will enter paradise.

This belief is still rooted among people even of the present time. Charlemagne, Frederick of Barbarossa, William Tell, and King Arthur are remembered as famous sleepers. French peasants long believed that the sleeping Napoleon would one day return to protect their native land from invaders; and during the Russo-Japanese War, it was whispered in Russia that General Skobeleff would suddenly awake and hasten to Manchuria to lead their troops to victory. In recent years, there were persons who refused to believe that General Gordon, Sir Hector MacDonald, and Lord Kitchener were really dead. The story of Rip Van Winkle is well known; stories like "sleeping heroes," die hard.

The evidence afforded by the Paviland and other Cro-Magnon burials indicates that they believed that death was but a prolonged slumber. They painted their dead red, before they were placed in the sepulcher, in order to infuse the vigor of life in them. Perhaps the loss of consciousness and vitality appeared to them to be due to the loss of vitalizing fluid which flowed in the veins. They observed that man and animals die in consequence of loss of blood, and those who were stricken with sickness grew pale because, as it seemed to them, the supply of blood was insufficient. They therefore painted their dead and sick red, believing that the active vitalizing principle in the blood was the substance that colored it red. This old practice still persists among Australians and some Indians who paint their bodies red for religious and magical purposes to gain vigor in their combat against enemies. The ancient Egyptians painted their gods red to make them healthy.

Fear of Death: The abhorrence of death is due more to its mystery than to the pain that accompanies dissolution. This fear gave rise early to an obstinate disbelief in the necessity of death and to the attempt in spite of all experience to escape it. Even the most natural causes were thought not beyond human control. The constant search for a fountain of eternal youth and the persistent refusal of mankind to accept death with resignation form one of the most pathetic factors in the history of mankind.

In all ages, man was eager to find the means of escaping death; he searched all four corners of the earth; he defied all kinds of peril to find the means of restoring youth. When he failed in his efforts to obtain physical survival, he set out on a long and winding journey to acquire spiritual immortality—a nebulous and fantastic survival with no material organs for expressing itself, not realizing the fact that the body is just as essential a component part of oneself as the soul. It is as hard to picture immortality of the soul without the body as to think of the life of the body without the soul. Energy cannot be separated from matter. No spirit can enjoy the pleasure of life without the organs of the special senses; indeed it is more reasonable to believe in the resurrection of both body and soul than the survival of the soul only.

Nature intended that, at fixed periods, men should succeed each other by the instrumentality of death. Man will never outwit nature; his death is as natural as his life. Disease may be a retribution of outraged nature, but death, never.

Landmarks of Existence: All organic beings pass four important landmarks during their existence, namely birth, maturity, decay, and death. If all vegetable and animal production of nature, from creation downwards, had grown, attained maturity, and there remained, the world would not have been capable of containing the thousandth part of them; so on this earth, decaying and dying appear indispensable if there are to be reproduction and growth. Viewed abstractly then, organized beings live as long as health and vigor continue, but they are subjected to a process of decay, which impairs gradually all their functions and at last terminates in their dissolution. The vernal bloom of spring changes gracefully into the maturity of summer and the decline of autumn. Death removes the old and decayed, and organic law introduces in their place the young, the gay, and the vigorous, to tread the stage with renewed agility and delight.

While the world is calculated to support only a limited number of living creatures, the lower animals have received from nature powers of reproduction far beyond those which are necessary to supply the waste of natural decay, and they do not possess intellect sufficient to restrain their numbers within the limits of their means of subsistence. Herbivorous animals in particular are exceedingly prolific, and yet the supply of vegetable food is limited. Hence, after multiplication for a few years, extensive starvation and the most painful and lingering deaths would inevitably ensue to the detriment of the race. With uncontrolled reproduction, all species would be multiplied beyond all limits, till even the globe itself could not contain them. Their food would fail them, and they would die of starvation, or, in their conflicts for the supplies that remain, they would destroy one another. The preservation of every individual produced would lead to ultimate destruction of the species.

Man is the only animal that has the conception that he is a mortal creature. It seems that nature, as a compensation, committed him to run the entire course of life, because, in this case only, can old age be useful to the race. Lower animals have not the slightest conception of death any more than a tree has. In consequence they live in as full enjoyment of the present as if every agreeable sensation were eternal. They count on no support in their old age from their offspring which instinctively leave them as soon as they are able to run, fly, or swim. Reflection would be to such creatures a burden which beasts are mercifully spared. Indeed death can hardly be a factor in the consciousness of lower animals.

Kinds of Death: There are several kinds of death which may be distinguished from one another under the heads of local and general.

Local: Local death is going on in the body all the time. Individual cells of the epidermis and other epithelium are incessantly dying and cast off, to be replaced by others which are as constantly coming into separate existence. The like is true of blood-corpuscles and probably of many other elements of the tissues.

This form of death is essential to the maintenance of life and is usually insensible. Occasionally, local death is on a larger scale, such as, for example, death of a part of the body due to injury, a burn, or disease where a part of the tissue may die or a portion of the skin may be destroyed. Regeneration may follow after local death. Muscles, nerve tissue, epidermis, and connective tissue may be reproduced.

General: General death consists of two kinds: death of the body as a whole and death of the tissues. By the former term is implied the absolute cessation of the function of the brain, and of the circulatory and the respiratory organs; by the latter, the entire disappearance of the structural constituents of the body. When death takes place, the body, as a whole, dies first, the death of the tissues not occurring until after an interval of some time. For example, the muscles of an executed criminal may be made to contract by the application of proper stimuli; the muscles are not dead, though the person is.

Suffering of Death: In natural decay there is reason to believe that death is attended with very little suffering to the lower creatures. The organs are worn out by age and the animals sink into gradual insensibility, unconscious that dissolution awaits them. Death always takes the individual by surprise, whether it comes in the form of violence or by the slow decay of age, and it really operates as a transference of existence from one generation to another without consciousness of the loss in the one which dies.

With reference to man, instant death is not attended with pain of any perceptible duration, and it is only when lingering death occurs in youth and middle age that the suffering is severe. Dissolution, however, does not occur at this period as a direct and intentional result of organic laws, but as a consequence of infringement upon them. Under fair and legitimate operation of these laws, the individual whose constitution has been sound and whose life has been in accordance with their dictates will live till old age fairly wears out his frame, and then the pang of expiration is but little perceptible. "And what thinkest thou," said Socrates to Aristodemus, "of this continual love of life, this dread of dissolution, which takes possession of us from the moment that we are conscious of existence?" "I think of it," answered he, "as the means employed by the same great and wise artist, deliberately determined to preserve what he has made."

Inevitability of Death: A man who sees disease occurring in youth or middle age, and whose mind is not capable of perceiving that it is the result of imperfect or excessive action in some vital organ, and that imperfect or excessive action is just another name for deviation from the proper healthy state of that organ, is not capable of reasoning on the subject.

The truth is that growth and maturity must be followed by decay and death in old age, as morning and noon are succeeded by evening and night, or spring and summer imply autumn and winter. Organic beings are so constituted because some must die so that others may live.

LIFE EXPECTANCY

But while death and old age cannot be abolished as long as man continues to be an organic being, premature death may be decreased in the exact ratio of man's obedience to physical and organic laws.

There is already some evidence of this process having actually begun.

With the knowledge of hygiene, sepsis, and antisepsis, some diseases have been almost completely exterminated. Surgery has been robbed of the worst of its dangers. Infant mortality has been more than cut in half. Cures or preventives have been discovered for some of the most deadly diseases, and the spread of most infectious diseases from person to person has been greatly checked. The average duration of human life is about 15 per cent greater than it was half a century ago. A large part of this great achievement of science has been the direct outgrowth of the discovery of the microscope.

Horace Walpole, a century and a half ago wrote: "About the time, or a little later, I die, the secret will be found of how to live forever." When enough time had passed to vouchsafe a reply, Helen Bevington answered:

> Horace, be comforted to die.
> One century has meandered by
> And half the next one since, it was true
> The temporal state eluded you.
> Now as I read your pensive letter,
> I wish myself that times were better
> And I might boast how men contrive,
> As you foretold, to stay alive.
> By now we should possess the key
> To fleshly immortality
> And, if we wanted to, endeavor
> To live forever and forever.
> This, to my infinite regret,
> Is not a custom with us yet.
> I write you Horace for good cheer.
> Life is about as usual here.

A century and a half ago, tables of the average duration of life compiled in England for the use of life insurance companies showed that the average life span was twenty-eight years. Tables at the end of the nineteenth century show an increase from twenty-eight to thirty-five years of age. At present, in consequence of hygienic rules, sanitary conditions, and particularly scientific medical care, the mortality has further markedly decreased. The duration of life should go on increasing and has already reached, in the United States, sixty-two years per man, and sixty-four per woman.

Mortality statistics show that, as a result of our success in conquering infection and some of the most deadly diseases of childhood, we now have an adult population that is larger in proportion than it has ever been before. It promises to grow even greater as the years roll by.

Our research has not scratched the surface of such problems as heart disease and coronary thrombosis, nephritis, arthritis, and cancer.

Some indication of the increasing advance of age may be gained from figures on the percentage of our population in the older age groups. According to United States census figures, and reliable estimates with respect to the future, the following represents the proportion of our population forty-five years of age and over:

1860—13.1 per cent
1880—16. per cent
1900—17.8 per cent
1920—20.8 per cent
1940—26.5 per cent
1960—33.3 per cent
1980—40.3 per cent

When we consider those sixty-five years and over, the following percentage distribution is reflected:

1860— 2.7 per cent
1880— 3.4 per cent
1900— 4.1 per cent
1920— 4.7 per cent
1940— 6.8 per cent
1960—10.0 per cent
1980—14.4 per cent

TRANSMISSION OF PARENTAL QUALITIES

There is one form of survival that is ever present in man and this is the qualities most active in the parents that the organic laws transmit to the offspring in an increasing ratio. The law of evolution and succession provides for a higher degree of improvement in the race than could have been reached if the permanency of a single generation possessed the present human constitution.

Oliver Wendell Holmes once remarked, "We are omnibuses in which all our ancestors ride." We carry the bodies and souls of our forefathers in our germ plasm, and we are resurrected in our progeny.

The English anthropologist and biologist, Francis Galton, stated, "An individual inherits on the average of one half in number, the qualities from his parents, one quarter from his grandparents, one eighth from his great-grandparents, etc. The series is $\frac{1}{2}$, $\frac{1}{4}$, $\frac{1}{8}$, $\frac{1}{16}$, $\frac{1}{32}$." This appears to be the sort of resurrection one transmits to his posterity.

There is perhaps no phenomenon in organic nature more remarkable or seemingly more miraculous than the transformation of a single and apparently simple egg cell into the complex and wonderful organized mechanism of the adult body. The germ plasm, according to Weismann, is supposed to be transmissible from one generation to the next by a continuous series of cell divisions. It is a thread that connects successive generations of individuals together, and these individuals resemble one another because they are all developed from one continuous substance.

The future of all living beings is vested in the ultramicroscopical "gene" which is so tiny that, if all of them contained in all living people of the world would be put together, there would be less than a thimbleful; yet these "genes" and their companions, the "chromosomes," govern every living cell and are the absolute keys to all human, animal, and vegetable characteristics. In such an infinitely small space, all hereditary and psychological characteristics of innumerable multitudes of ancestors are preserved.

Evolution begins in the cells, the entity of which carry the "genes"; how a thimbleful of "genes" can rule all life on earth is one of the greatest wonders which could only emanate from a Creative Intelligence.

References and Notes

1. Turner, E. G.: Samoa. London, 1884, p. 140.
2. Ellis, W.: Polynesia Researches. London, 1831.
3. Spencer and Gillen: The Native Tribes of Central Australia. London, 1889.
4. Ibid., p. 337.
5. Hose, C., and McDugal, W.: The Pagan Tribes of Borneo. London, 1912, Vol. II, p. 29.
6. Dr. Pichnel-Loesche: Die Loango Expedition, Vol. III, pp. 443-444.
7. Mackintosh, A.: An Account of the Tribes of Mhadeo-Kolies. 1864, Vol. I, p. 227.
8. Cummings: Sub-Tribes of the Gahi-el Ghazal Dinkas. J. Am. Anthropol. 156, 1904.
9. Boas, F.: The Northwest Tribes of Canada. Rep. Brit. A. Adv. Sc., 645-646, 1890.
10. Nassau: Fetishism in West Africa, p. 215.
11. Kingsley, M.: West African Studies, p. 169.
12. Smyth, B.: The Aborigines of Victoria. Vol. I, pp. 259-260.

13. Brooke: Ten Years in Sarawak. Vol. II, pp. 228-229.
14. Reed, W. A.: The Negritos of Zambales. Manila, 1904, p. 68.
15. "Fetishism in West Africa," pp. 81, 162.
16. Matthew 8:28.
17. Boas, F.: The Northwest Tribes of Canada. Rep. Brit. A. Adv. Sc. 557, 1890.
18. Mooney, J.: The Sacred Formulas of the Cherokee, p. 339.
19. "The Native Tribes of Central Australia," p. 531.
20. Shamanism. Hastings Encyclo., Vol. IX; p. 442.
21. Kuhn's ed.: Vol. IV, p. 775.
22. "The Native Tribes of Central Australia," p. 356.
23. Roscoe, J.: Manners and Customs of the Baganda. J. Am. Anthropol., 32:40.
24. "The Native Tribes of Northern Australia," p. 675.
25. "Manners and Customs of the Baganda." J. Am. Anthropol, 32:73.
26. deGroot, J. J. M.: The Religious System of China. Vol. 1, p. 464.
27. Ibid., Vol. 1, p. 348.
28. Ibid., Vol. 1, p. 763.
29. Ibid., Vol. 1, p. 802, et. seq.
30. See Levy-Bruhl, L.: How Natives Think, p. 275, etc.
31. Langlah, P. K.: The Enahlayr Tribes. London, 1895, Vol. 1, p. 148.

6

Nature Worship and Medicine

MAN, as we have seen, is comparatively a newcomer on the earth. Other creatures roamed about the globe perhaps millenniums before man made his appearance. Exactly how many years man has inhabited the globe is not known. The idea that it may be 500,000 or more years may seem to us staggering, but in the realm of nature it is but a second. Man started out on his way to civilization barehanded, with no mechanical means with which to protect himself against carnivorous beasts and the violence of nature; and by his own great efforts and experience, he slowly accumulated knowledge to dominate the elements of nature, and particularly to provide for his life and welfare.

AIR

He recognized at an early period the importance of the atmospheric air to life. He observed the first gasp of air in the newborn child and the labored breathing at death and naturally attributed these occurrences to the entrance and departure of the air into and from the body. He became aware that not only life and death depended upon the condition of the air but that his entire welfare throughout life depended upon it. He observed that, while certain diseases prevail during the hot and dry seasons, others are more frequent during the cold and rainy seasons. He naturally inquired into the question as to why his health should depend upon changes in the air, and the idea occurred to him that animistic forces of evil prevail in the air at certain times of the year to cause those ailments. The belief in the aerial spirits of evil became widespread, and these dreaded beings took on the aspect of an organized enemy of mankind carried by the winds or identified with the winds themselves.

139

In Korea and the rest of the Far East, it is still believed that demons of epidemics wander about in the air. In upper Burma, cholera and smallpox are thought to be real air devils which hover in the midst of fog and filthy air. The same belief is still held in India, Arabia, and even in some European countries. Among the Brazilian Botocudos, the air is alleged to be stocked with malevolent spirits which are said to come with the storm and thunder, and these are known as "storm" and "thunder" spirits.

EARTH

Next to air, the most important substance that excited the curiosity of early man was earth. Its wonderful productivity reminded him of his own mother. The earth assumed an anthropomorphic character. "Mother Earth" became, in the imaginative mind of the primitive philosopher, the spouse of "heaven" who is impregnated by drops of rain coming down from above, thus giving birth to limitless vegetation. The analogy between the fertilization of the earth and impregnation has been recognized by most ancient peoples. "Seed" and "semen" find a common expression; "field" and "furrow" are applied in many languages to the female generative organ. Among the Aztecs, the earth is depicted as a many-breasted woman.

Because of its miraculous fertility, the earth was worshipped. Thanksgiving offerings were made to the earth for her unlimited bounty. The offerings often took the form of human sacrifice; frequently a woman was buried alive. In primitive agricultural communities, "Mother Earth" has received religious rites. "Good Mother from whom all things come" has been one of the epithets applied to the earth. In Greece, the goddess, Demeter, represented the earth. She governed the production of grain, vegetables, fruit, herbs, and flocks. In ancient Mexico, the "Mother of All" was invoked by eating a morsel of earth, and was referred to as "the provider of nourishment for all creatures." At a festival which took place during the spring and summer seasons, homage was paid to her, and a woman representing the earth was sacrificed. In Japan, the earth is appeased before digging a well or erecting a building. In India, plowing is preceded by paying homage to the earth. The soil is mixed with human or animal blood to endow it with greater fertility. The Biblical narrative that the Creator molded man in his own image from earth appears to have been a common belief among many ancient peoples. Mexicans and Peruvians have similar traditions.

The earth is the womb and the tomb of mankind. Man returns to the womb of the earth from which he came; hence the belief that the shades of the unburied dead cannot rest and the customs among many ancient peoples to place the dead in the grave in the same folded position as that of the fetus within the mother's womb.

The earth was considered to be a kind of an underworld where men retired after their life above ground was finished. Their ghosts were believed to visit their relatives and friends and plague them with disease in order to facilitate their entrance into the world below. The earth also served as an underground habitation and as a hideout for the living while primitive man roamed the forests in quest of food before he was able to provide himself with a permanent home.

WATER

Assumed Cosmic Powers: Since water is essential to animal and plant life, it naturally also figured conspicuously in magic, religion, and medicine. From remote antiquity, water was considered to possess incomprehensible cosmic powers *(mana)*. When the idea of departmental deities developed, water too became the abode of spirits. The early Babylonians regarded water as possessing magical properties. The relation, existing between the growth of plants and water supplied by the Euphrates, led the Babylonians to associate water with the god, Tammuz. Religious rites were performed in midsummer, at the festival of Tammuz, at which time the god's image was washed with pure water. In Greece, the god, Adonis, was similarly worshipped to secure a good supply of rain for the crops.

When man observed that water promoted the fertility of plants, that deserts in the spring suddenly blossomed, he looked upon such phenomena as miracles. He could not perceive how the water *per se* could perform such changes, so he attributed these wonders to the *mana* within the water.

Assumed Spiritual Virtues: Because of the spiritual virtue contained in water, it was used to wash away disease, which was considered a product of religious defilement. Women employed water after menstruation and after childbirth, to cleanse themselves from their defilement. Birth, puberty, marriage, and death, the four most critical epochs so intimately associated with the mysteries of life, were consecrated with water.

Primitive man's deductions, although based on false premises, were nevertheless rational. He exhibited remarkable perspicuity in his observation of the healing virtues of water. He observed that bodily wounds heal by merely washing the injured parts with water. He logically concluded that the healing process was due to the beneficial spirit which is inherent in water. He did not think that healing was affected because of the fact that water washes away the impurities attracted by the wound. The same idea he applied to the healing virtues of mineral springs. He was not aware of the fact that these springs were impregnated with various chemical elements which have a beneficial medicinal value. He thought that the curative effect of such springs was effected by the spiritual virtue inherent in the fluid.

The primitive philosopher's reasoning was confined to the limits of his knowledge and was based on preconceived ideas. To him water was the source of all life.

Rain coming from the skies and wells bubbling from the ground he considered as sent by divine forces for the purpose of sustaining life. He looked upon the luxurious tree that was growing beside the well or near the stream with bewilderment, and upon the fruit it produces as sent purposely by the gods for his nourishment.

A rowan tree's red berries were supposed to contain a kind of blood which has an animating influence on the human body. They renew youth and protect those who use them from evil influence. A hazel tree's nuts were thought to be similarly healthful. An oak's acorns were regarded as bringing good luck.

Water, possessing such marvelous power to revive withering plants, was naturally considered very beneficial in treating persons stricken by withering disease or afflicted with the sequelae of old age.

In the Old Testament, baths were ordered as a prophylactic and as a cure against skin diseases.[1] Water was employed to cleanse menstruating and lying-in women, to purify those that had been defiled by touching unclean bodies,[2] to cleanse lepers,[3] and to treat gonorrhea (zab).[4] Sprinkling the body with water symbolized moral purity. Thus, Ezekiel said, "And I will sprinkle clean water upon you and ye shall be clean from all your uncleanliness, and from all your idols will I cleanse you."[5] The New Testament speaks of the water of life, "I will give unto him that is athirst of the fountain of the water of life freely."[6]

According to the "Book of Genesis," water was the first element. It existed before the world was created: "And the spirit of God hovered over the face of the waters."[7]

The present-day Aztec midwife, when washing an infant, recites the following prayer: "May this water purify and whiten thy heart; may it wash away all that is evil."[8] This concept assumed definite form in many religions and originated from the idea that water washes away defilement and sin, and bestows the newly born as it were with a clean bill of health.

In New Guinea, warriors are secluded for about a week after their return from battle, during which time they cannot come into contact with their wives nor touch food with their hands. On the fifth day of seclusion of one who has taken the life of an enemy, he walks solemnly down to the nearest source of water and washes himself.[9]

In the Pelew Islands, the young warriors, on their return from their first mortal combat, are shut up for three days; and then after smearing their bodies with charmed leaves and betel, bathe together as near as possible to the spot where the killing took place.[10] When a Pima Indian kills an enemy, he is taboo for sixteen days; then he retires to a grove along the river, or wanders about the adjoining hills. During this period, he is forbidden to touch his head or face. Before he returns to his home, he has to bathe in the river, no matter how cold the temperature of the water.[11] Contact with the dead is considered a potent source of impurity in primitive society, is the cause of taboo, and subjects the contaminated one to purification rites.

In the rite of Isis, in Old Egypt, baptism in water was thought to raise a mortal to divinity. In Babylonia, a sick person was sprinkled with water while the priest pronounced certain sacred formulas. The water was drawn from the Tigris or Euphrates. One or more springs or bath-houses were attached to every large temple, where purification rites were performed.[12] Details of the rites varied in different cities. There are indications that, even in later times, religious rites were performed on the banks of running streams.

The importance of water as a means of healing was greatly enhanced by the growth of Baal-worship, in which the deity, as the giver of life, was closely connected with life-giving waters. The indignation of Naaman when he was told to wash in the Jordan, and his confidence that the rivers of Damascus were better than all the waters of Israel, probably arose from the idea that the water of the Jordan was efficacious only for the Hebrews.[31]

The miraculous cure of Naaman reflects an ancient Semitic belief in the efficacy of water as a cure for leprosy. Of all remedial substances, water was thought to possess the most marked supernatural virtues among the Semites. It was known as "running water" or, as the Hebrews expressed it, "living water." It is, therefore, not surprising that certain wells and rivers were credited with the power of healing.

In the time of Antoninus Martyr, patients bathed by night in the thermal waters of Gadara.[14] In the Middle Ages, it was still believed that one who bathed in the Euphrates in the springtime would be free from sickness for the ensuing year.

Sources: Primitive man had to toil hard to get water. Those that led a nomadic pastoral life had to have water for their flocks and herds, and the chief source of supply came from the wells.[15] Wells thus became valuable property and in many instances tribal war was waged for their possession.[16] Well-diggers in those days were public benefactors, as is illustrated in the "Book of Genesis."[17] A well was the public forum of the village; all social and economic questions were discussed there. Young matrons went there towards evening to draw water for home and for the cattle; marriage ceremonies were celebrated there.[18] The pasturing of flocks was often the duty of young girls; and from the Biblical evidence, one is led to believe that the wells were attractive places for the young men of the village.

Rain-Making Rites: Water has been widely used by primitives in ceremonies for making rain. In southeastern Europe, even at the present time, rain is brought down by pouring a pail of water over a boy or girl who is attired in a garment made of grass, flowers, or corn leaves.[19] H. S. Moore records a practice at Poona, India: When rain is needed, the boys dress up one of their number in leaves and call him "King of the Rain." They then visit all the houses in the village. A householder sprinkles the rain king with water and makes offerings of food to the party. In Roumania, a clay figure is substituted for a living person in the rain-making rites. The image, which represents drought, is placed in a coffin and carried by children in a funeral procession with a burning candle before it. Finally, the coffin and the candle are thrown into a stream or well.[20] In France, images of saints, until recently, were dipped in water to procure rain. In Arcadia, in the classical period, the priests of Zeus dipped an oak branch into a certain spring on Mt. Lycaeus in time of drought to cause Zeus to send up a misty cloud, from which rain would soon fall.

As Preventive and Curative Agent: In Europe, water figures conspicuously in folklore as a means of preventing and curing disease. Thus, at Vitrolles, in the south of France, during the midsummer rites, young people bathe in a pond in order that they may not suffer from fever during the year.[21] In England and Sweden, certain springs are supposed to be endowed with wonderful medicinal virtues; many sick people resort to them for healing their infirmities. At Marsala in Sicily, the sick make pilgrimages to a spring, the "Grotto of the Sibyl," to be cured of their disease. On St. John's Day, the people of Copenhagen used to go on a pilgrimage to a neighborhood spring to heal and strengthen themselves in the water.[22] The famous grotto at Lourdes, which has been the reputed source of so many miracles since the alleged appearance of the Blessed Virgin to Bernadette Soubirous on February 11, 1858, belongs perhaps to a different category, since the existence of the spring was unknown to the inhabitants prior to the apparition.[23]

The Papuans of New Guinea hold it possible to ascertain the guilt or innocence of an accused person by the process of immersion in water; a similar method is employed by the Negroes of the Gold Coast.[24] In South Africa (where it extends from the Atlantic tribes to the Masai), trial by ordeal generally takes the form of swallowing a goblet full of *bundu* juice. If the poisonous beverage does not at once act as an emetic, the guilt of the accused is proved.

The importance of water to sustain life has always been recognized; for one can do for weeks without food, but a few days' deprivation of water is inimical to life. The reason for this is that the composition of the human body is almost 90 per cent fluid, which is lost very rapidly by evaporation, exhalation, sweating, and excretions, and this loss must be replenished. Dehydration leads to alkalosis, which is accompanied by a train of symptoms that include vomiting, muscle spasms, and in some cases, convulsions.

FIRE

Theories of Its Discovery: While the elements of air, earth, and water were essential to life and existed before animal life made its appearance, it is not known at what period fire was discovered. It has been calculated that fire has been known to man since the second interglacial period—approximately 400,000 years ago. The *Karpino man* possessed a knowledge of fire; this has been demonstrated from the remains in the cave-dwellings of France, Spain, and other European countries. Burned bones in hearths were discovered in these caves. It is known that cavemen of the Stone Age knew how to produce fire. Some of the flint implements dating from this period seemed to show traces of having been subjected to great heat, and burned stones have been found in the gravels at Ealing, along with calcined bones, ashes, and cinders.

Early man made fire by rubbing two branches of a tree together. The fact that fire came from the friction of two branches of a tree induced early man to believe that it was connected with lightning, and therefore with the sky god who thundered during the harvest. The red berries on the sacred trees were supposed to contain fire or the essence of fire. When early man made rowanberry wine, he regarded it as "fire water"; thus he introduced, into his blood, fire which stimulated him.

There are a number of theories which have been advanced to explain how man discovered fire. Some naturalists think that man first came to know fire when he observed volcanoes in action. Others believe that man first learned about fire by watching the effect of lightning as it struck a withered tree. Another theory is that man learned about fire as he observed the sparks produced in the manufacture of flint instruments. Again, the rays of the sun shining through a concave quartz crystal might have ignited combustible substances that attracted the attention of early man. Aristophanes mentions the "burning lens" in his comedy, "Clouds." Archimedes is said to have used a mirror to fire the ships of Syracuse. Garcilasso de la Vega relates that the "virgins of the sun" of Peru kindled the sacred fire with a concave cup set in a great bracelet.

The myths with regard to the invention of fire are numerous. One Chinese myth recounts how a great sage saw a bird peck a tree, with the result that fire issued forth from it. The sage, amazed by this phenomenon, took a branch of the tree and produced fire from it. Henceforth, this great personage was called Suy-Jun. Suy is the drill, or speculum. Suy-Jun is the first person who procured fire for man. In China, the burning glass is still commonly employed.[25]

Primitive Ideas of Its Evil and Good Properties: One can just imagine with what wonder and terror prehistoric man looked upon fire when he first saw lightning strike a tree, or when the flames of a forest fire spread for miles in the dark hours of the night. Early man, fearing supernatural forces, saw, in the ravaging fire, monstrous evil powers that came to destroy the world in which he lived. Gradually, however, he became accustomed to it and began to appreciate the manifold beneficial advantages fire brought to him. He enjoyed the warmth produced by the heat and the light engendered by the flame. He was gratified to behold that fire caused the terrors of the night to vanish, and he treasured the flames and kept them burning day after day and night after night. The extinction of his fire was indeed a catastrophe which he carefully tried to avoid.

Civilization has progressed more rapidly because of the discovery of fire. Without fire and proper clothing, man would have to confine his habitat to the tropical climates; without fire, he could hardly protect himself against the beasts and "evil spirits" that hovered about him in the darkness of the night; without fire, he would have no means of cooking food and smelting metals to be used as implements and instruments.

Perpetual Fires: It must be remembered that, before man learned the art of kindling fire, he expended great effort to keep the fire constantly burning in his home or at least in his community. A perpetual fire was always maintained when man began to live an urban life. It is recorded that the Egyptians had a perpetual light in every temple. The Greeks, Persians, and Romans preserved their fires in all towns and villages. In the western hemisphere, the Natchez, the Aztecs, the Mayas, and the Peruvians had their perpetual fires installed on large pyramids.[26] The eternal lamps in the synagogues, and in the Byzantine and Catholic churches, may be traced to the ancient practice of keeping up a permanent fire.

The extinction of the sacred fire in Rome was regarded as a national calamity. All civil and political interests grouped themselves around the pyrotenaum, which was employed as a temple, a tribunal, a town hall, and a gossiping center. All business was transacted before the warm communal fire. Fire grew into a religious institution.[27] If by chance the fire in the Roman temple was extinguished, all authority, all tribunals, and all private and public business had to stop immediately.

For ages, nomadic tribes carried fire with them. The Greeks and Romans always crossed a frontier carrying an altar with the fire taken from the pyrotenaum. There are still people who painstakingly keep a fire constantly alive, even though they possess the ready means of kindling a new fire. Travelers to Australia and Tasmania depict the typical native woman as still carrying burning brands; in fact, maintaining fire is considered one of her principal duties. According to Captain Cook, this is true, in spite of the fact that these natives have learned to produce fire with ease by manipulating two wooden sticks.[28]

Methods of Fire-Making: The Zambesi, according to Livingstone, carry with them, on their travels, two sticks, two or three inches long, with which to make a fire if they are obliged to spend the night away from home. Charles Darwin observed that African natives produce fire by friction in a few seconds, although it took his untrained hands a long time to perform this feat. Other methods employed to make a fire, before matches were invented, consisted of percussion (striking stones and metals, thus producing a spark for starting the fire) and concentration of sun rays through a concave glass. A possible reference to making fire by means of the friction of two sticks is mentioned in "I Kings" 17:12. The second "Book of Maccabees" refers to flint and iron.[29]

Hearn states that strictly orthodox persons in Japan consider it wrong to light a lamp with a match. They believe that a match is not always made with pure substance. They prefer to use the "light of Kami" (which is believed to be the purest fire), "that holy natural fire which lies hidden within all things."

Fire Worshippers: It is natural that such a fascinating phenomenon as fire, the character of which has been so little understood, should have been venerated and deified by early man. Fire worshippers are still present in various sections of the world. Frederick Starr states that a tribe of Indians in the state of Iowa (a remnant of the Sacs and Foxes) fear the god of fire and use "fire sticks" to make a fire in religious rites. The fire produced by the sticks is sacred and is believed to emanate from heaven. According to Hearn, the old Japanese primitive method of making fire by a drill is retained by religious conservatives. Each year the temple receives a new fire drill, thus upholding the traditional regulation as to the manner of producing fire.

Uses: The Brahmans considered fire as the first element and employed it routinely at marriages and at funerals. They believed that the spirit of the dead goes up to heaven with the smoke of the newly built fire. They also thought that the mechanism of the digestion operated through the action of fire.

Fire was looked upon as a purifier. The passing of children through the fire of "Molech" designates the burning of children as sacrifices. The ancient Greeks believed that burning renders one immortal.[30] There can be little doubt that fires of the *auto-da-fé* were kindled in consequence of the notion of purification.

Fire for domestic use was forbidden on the Sabbath day, perhaps to avoid any connotation of fire worship. "Strange fire," or the fire used for worship, was forbidden. There is a legend in the Talmud[31] that, when Adam was overwhelmed by darkness, the Holy One gave him two bricks and that he rubbed these together and fire came forth.

A concept that took such a strong hold on human imagination from the very day of its discovery was bound to make an immense impression on medicine. Anything that has played an important part in religion has always been applied to the treatment of disease. Fire, because of its spiritual virtues, has been used for curing many diseases since the dawn of history.

Australians perform the operation of circumcision by means of a fire stick.[32] Among many primitive tribes the newly initiated child is held by women over the fire.[33]

In Australia, fire is avoided by girls during their first menstruation period. Impregnation by fire was a common notion among natives of Australia.[34] Australian boys at their initiation to manhood receive a fire stick presented to them with great ceremony by their prospective mother-in-law.[35]

The Russian peasant carries his fire with him when moving to a new house; and while depositing it in the new premises, says: "Welcome, grandfather, to a new home." The old Norsemen marched around carrying fire from six in the morning to six in the evening.[36] The Calabrian takes an oath by nipping a flame between the fingers and swearing by the light of God. Iambilichus held that fire destroys all the mortal parts, leaving the immortal parts behind. In Germany, as late as the seventeenth century, when a murrain epidemic broke out among cattle, the farmers decided upon the use of a *nothfeuer* (need fire) which was supposed to avert the epidemic. On the day when the need fire was scheduled to be kindled, no fire was made in any of the houses; and from each house, brushwood, straw, and wood were brought.[37] A hole was bored through a heavy oak plank which was driven into the ground. Into this a windlass was struck, well smeared with tar and pitch, and turned around so long that it gave forth fire. The fire was fed by brushwood, straw, and wood until a large fire was made. Then the cattle and horses were driven through the fire with whips two or three times. This method of avoiding an epidemic was practiced as late as 1826 near Perth, Scotland. At Desau and Hanover, such a fire was last kindled in 1828 during an outbreak among pigs and cows.

Before there was any thought that syphilis was caused by a specific organism, the disease was assumed to be contracted through the air. A person who had the suspected "bad air" was advised to purify the air by burning all sorts of combustible material in the public highway and then protect himself by covering his face with a crude mask.

SEASONS AND CLIMATE

While superstition was unquestionably a controlling factor in ancient medicine, it must not be supposed that early man failed to observe the effects of change of seasons, climatic conditions, food, and drink on his body. He could not miss observing that epidemics of dysentery and cholera occurred primarily during the hot season, and severe colds during the winter season, and that violent gastric symptoms were related to the food he had just eaten—that most of the animal physiology is affected by the quality and quantity of food introduced into the system.

FOOD

The Quest for Food: Early man, particularly before he took to agriculture and raising livestock, had to search for his food and be satisfied with the plants he could find and animals he could kill. He could not always distinguish between those plants and vegetables suitable for nutrition and those which were unsuitable and poisonous. A countless number of poisonings, sicknesses, and deaths must have been caused by food before mankind learned what was edible and what was not. The quest for food, which began far back in prehistory, still continues in many places with all the energy and keenness of the past. Gastrointestinal disturbance, after eating a strange plant or poisonous root, undoubtedly brought to early man's attention the cause of the disturbance.

In the early stages of human life, man, like his anthropoid ancestors, depended solely on the vegetable kingdom for his nourishment, because it was best fitted for his mastication and digestion. Hunger drove him to add animal food to his diet. Once he became used to animal food, there was nothing too filthy which he did not use for food. Indeed one is horrified at the list of things that have passed through man's alimentary canal. The present natives of Australia, who have not changed in any appreciable degree from their early ancestors, still eat carion-kites, eels, bats, frogs, lizards, snakes, and worms.[38]

Negroes of Congo and Dor, according to Schweinfurth, allow no animal food except dogs and man to escape them. They eat rats, snakes, carion-kites, scorpions, ants, and caterpillars.[39] The Chinese consider trepangs a delicacy in flavoring soups. In Arabia, a flight of locusts is greeted as a feast dispersed by God. Judging from the food eaten by man, it would appear that the disgust caused by certain articles of animal food is merely conventional.

Cannibalism: Unlike the average beast who is averse to eating the flesh of his own species, early man did not even abstain from devouring the flesh of his own kind, at least in time of dire need and famine. As a matter of fact, cannibalism has prevailed in certain regions in historic times. In 1200 A.D., when a famine desolated the cities of Alexandria, Syene, and Damietta, cannibalism was practiced in Egypt on such a large scale that people engaged extensively in hunting men and especially children for food. All legal efforts to suppress this abominable practice were to no avail. The desire for human flesh was so great that burning at the stake did not deter the cannibals from their devilish practices, and those who had been punished with death were devoured by others. Schiller states that the Saxons, by the end of the Thirty-Year War, had become cannibals. Peschel recounts that, at the siege of Messina, flesh of captured soldiers was eaten and sold at a high price.[40] Letournean quotes a letter from Jerome to the effect that the Scotch were extremely fond of steaks made from young girls and boys.

Of course not all cannibals devoured the flesh of man because of the desire to partake of such as food. Many savages and barbarous tribes ate, and perhaps still eat, the flesh of the enemy, believing that, by so doing, they will draw into their system the qualities of the victim. Thus it is related that the Senecas, during the Revolutionary War, devoured two white Americans in order to gain bravery in warfare. In China, during the war with England, a merchant of Shanghai met his servant who was carrying to his house the heart of an Englishman which he was desirous of eating in order to secure the Britisher's courage.[41]

Primitive Idea of Food Value: Indeed it appears that the primitive idea of the value of food was not because of its nutritive value, but because of the benevolent spirit contained in it. Disease, following the eating of improper food, was ascribed to the evil spirit within the food.

All food, unless contaminated by an evil power, was considered sacred. Ancient man almost worshipped food. He blessed it before eating and kissed it when he picked it up from the ground; this practice still persists among present races of eastern Europe and Asia.

Bread: The most important article of food to man is bread. Measured by the length of time of human history, bread is a comparatively recent discovery — not over 6000 years old. Before that period, man roasted his grain, often while on the ear, on hot stones. The use of roasted corn for food was continued through Biblical times, as may be seen from the "Book of Ruth,"[42] "and they reached her parched corn and she did eat and was sufficed and left."

It is known that the Swiss pile-dwellers, after roasting their grain, mixed it with hot water to form a paste; and to avoid the decay of the porridge, they spread it on hot stones which formed a kind of flat bread. Such cake-like bread was eaten for ages. The porridge was made from various grains, such as peas, beans, and lentils. The last was considered a great delicacy. Esau sold his birthright for such a dish.[43] Pliny, who as a rule was careful in citing Roman tradition, states, "for a very long time, the Roman people lived on porridge, not on bread." The Greeks, until about 600 years B.C., depended upon flat cakes baked on charcoal for their sustenance.

Bread, as it is known at the present time, was discovered by chance in Egypt. The Egyptians, instead of exerting their efforts to prevent decay of their food by fermentation, permitted it to ferment.

. . . keeping the dough a certain time before putting it in the oven to bake, permitted the yeast-spores to mix with the tiny traces of sugar contained in the paste of the cereal and in the water of the Nile, which gave the yeast-spores time to break up the sugar into alcohol and carbon dioxide, and owing to the viscosity of the dough, the bubbles of the carbon dioxide could not escape, but by pressing against the resisting substances they puffed up the dough and loosened it. When the alcohol and the carbon dioxide did escape they left their stamp on the bread by giving it a porous texture.

The process of baking fermented bread was already common at the time when the Israelites left Egypt for we read, "and the Egyptians were urgent upon the people, to send them out of the land in haste . . . and the people took their dough before it was leavened."[44]

Of course, the Egyptians did not know the mechanism of this phenomenon. They ascribed it to some magic power having a hand in this strange occurrence. The belief in the magic power of bread induced the Egyptians to place breads in the tombs of the dead, or at least portray figures of bread in their graves. On the walls of Egyptian catacombs, are found paintings of various forms of bread. In the tomb of Rameses III, there is a picture of a bakery showing how the dough was prepared, and how it was molded into various forms and shapes before it was put in the oven.

Because of the spiritual virtue of bread, it has played an important part in the religious ceremonies of all faiths. Holiday bread and wedding breads are still in great demand.

In Rome, a baker was considered an artist, not an artisan; he was on the level with the writer, the painter, and the sculptor. He worked with his dough as the sculptor with his clay and wax. Bakers' guilds have existed since the year 1872 B.C. The Romans mixed all kinds of substances in their bread, such as honey, oil, cheese, nuts, almonds, anise, peppers, laurel leaves, rice and milk.

Bread was made of whole wheat or barley; the bran, containing minerals, vitamin B, and a rich store of calories, not only satisfied the hunger, but has been a source of strength. It was used as a vehicle to administer medicine. The very name of bread was personified and blessed before each meal.

In 1942, when the American soldiers landed in Morocco, they were instructed by their officers not to cut bread, but to break it into slices, in order to avoid offense to the natives who are averse of using a knife upon a holy substance such as bread.

Bakers in the Baltic provinces will avoid turning their backs to the bakeoven; while in the Middle East and Roumania, a piece of bread is kissed after it has fallen down.

Beliefs regarding Food Remnants: The Papuans, of the Island of Tanna in the South Seas, believe that a *nahak* (any neglected remnant of food) may inflict disease and death. The natives are careful not to throw waste foodstuffs away, but carefully and secretly burn or bury them. If a Papuan magician finds a banana rind which has been carelessly thrown aside, he rolls it up in a leaf, and when night falls, he sits down by a fire and slowly burns this *nahak*. If the whole is transformed into ashes, the spell has taken effect, and the person to whom the refuse belonged will die. News of such a dastardly nocturnal deed spreads rapidly. Hence, if there is anyone in the neighborhood whose conscience plagues him for neglecting the remains of his food, or who is already prostrated with illness, he gets his friends to blow a blast on the shell trumpet as a sign that the *shaman* is to cease his work of destruction. The next morning money is offered for the restitution of the *nahak*. The natives admit, however, that such countercharms have little effect on the illnesses introduced into the island by Europeans.

DRINK

Milk: Milk has been accorded a special place in ancient folklore. It has held an important place in religious rites, in ceremonies, and as a remedy for the sick. The healing properties of milk arose from the fact that it is the food that God, Himself, has provided for the helpless infant after it is separated from its mother's womb.

Before the domestication of milk-yielding animals, the human mother suckled her young for three years or longer, until the offspring was able to walk at her side and partially take care of itself. After the domestication of animals, milk of cows, goats, sheep, and camels became a substitute for mother's milk.

The Panjabis take the first five drops of milk drawn from a cow or buffalo after calving and allow them to fall on the ground in honor of the goddess.[45] Milk is also used as a protection against the evil eye and for magic and divination. Strong measures are taken in various parts of Europe to protect milch cattle from harm inflicted by witches.

Because of the spiritual qualities of milk, the Picts of Ireland, when struck by arrows, bathed their wounds in the milk of 120 white hornless cows. A story is told of the Irish Prince Bress, son of the Femorian Elatha, who allocated to himself the milk of all hairless dun cows in the land. He directed that a great fire of ferns be made and that all such cows in Munster be forced to pass through it. Following this, their milk became princely property.[46]

In preChristian times, the worshippers of the nymphs and Pan used milk and wine for baptism. In early Christian churches, milk was substituted for wine in the communion. The rite of bathing in milk was attributed to St. Bridget who is sometimes regarded as the patron of milk.[47] Milkmaids have, in many instances, been considered important personalities. The rite of bathing in milk was a form of baptism. In the early church, newly baptized children were given milk and honey to taste, symbolizing their regeneration through baptism.

There is in Bethlehem a cave called the "milk grotto." Legend has it that the Holy Family took refuge there and that, as the Virgin nursed the Child, a drop of her milk fell on the floor. Because of this circumstance, it is believed that the mere entrance into this cave will assuredly increase the flow of milk of women and animals. Going to this cave is also a cure for sterility.[48] The Hindus worship the cow daily for her possession of five essential products, three of which are her milk, curd, and butter.

Throughout antiquity, it was believed that a child cannot live without its own mother's milk. Next to the female generative organs, the ancients viewed the mammary glands with sacred curiosity as they watched them grow during pregnancy to provide, in advance, food for the future child. Animal milk was looked upon in early times with distrust as nutriment for the newly born child. They believed that the child so fed would develop the traits of the animal from whose milk it had been fed. However, the use of animal's milk for adults is an early practice and is frequently mentioned in Scripture.

The ancient Romans believed that cow's milk exerts an unfavorable influence on the character of the child. The brutal strength of Romulus and Remus, the twin sons of Silvia and Mars, who became the legendary founders of Rome, was ascribed to the fact that they were suckled by a she-wolf and fed by a woodpecker.

Among the early Israelites, milk, like wine, was a symbol of prosperity: "His eyes shall be red with wine and his teeth white with milk."[49] In Greece, in case of pestilence, milk, honey, and bread were offered to Hestia. Milk was a symbol of abundance and prosperity.

In modern times, when a milk diet is prescribed in disease, it is so recommended because of its nutritive elements. The ancients, however, used milk because of its spiritual animating properties.

Milk Substitutes: The famous Dutch chemist, van Helmont, was the first to contradict scientifically the notion that an infant cannot live on other food than its mother's milk. He proposed, as a substitute, bread boiled in beer and honey. He thought that milk was harmful to a child whose well-being had already been jeopardized under the influence of the mother's milk. Dr. Brouzet shared the same opinion and expressed a keen desire that at least undesirable mothers be prevented from suckling their children, lest they communicate immorality and disease to their children.

CONCLUSIONS

Ancient superstitions afford a glimpse of the world in which our ancestors lived and some idea of the incentives that caused them to undertake long and perilous journeys in search of articles of religious value. They were as greatly concerned therewith as were their descendants about health and fortune. Everything connected with the deity, or possessing the influence of the deity, was valuable as a charm or medicine.

Red earth, because of its color, was "blood earth"; it contained the animating principle of blood. Some herbs were specifics for certain disease; and in the course of time their precise qualities were identified. Many of them were used because of their color, others because of the shape of their leaves (resembling human organs) or of the position in which they grew. If one red berry was found to be curative, all berries of the same color shared this reputation.

References and Notes

1. Leviticus 14:8.
2. Ibid., 15:28.
3. Ibid., 14:8.
4. Ibid., 15:7.
5. Ezekiel, 36:25.
6. Revelation, 21:6.
7. Genesis, 1:2.
8. Schagun, B. de: Hist. Gen. de las casas de Nueva España, Mexico, 1829, Vol. 6, p. 37.
9. J. Anthropol. 1:213.
10. Kubary, J.: Die Socialen Einrichtungen der Pelawer. Berlin, 1885, p. 126.
11. Cited by James, E. O.: Hastings Encyclopedia, Vol. 12, p. 706.
12. Jastrow, M.: Aspects of Religious Beliefs and Practices of Babylonia and Assyria. New York and London, 1911, p. 312.
13. Kings 5:10.
14. De Locis Sanctis 7:52-54.
15. Genesis 26:18.
16. Ibid., 26:20.
17. Ibid., 25:11.
18. Ibid., 29:1-15.
19. The Magic Art. Vol. 1, p. 272.
20. Ibid.
21. Cited by James, E. O.: Hasting's Encyclopedia, Vol. 12, p. 70.
22. Ibid.
23. Gordon, B. L.: Romance of Medicine. F. A. Davis Co., Phila., 1945, p. 478.
24. Newton, H.: In Fair New Guinea. London, 1914, p. 89.
25. Tyler, E. B.: Early History of Mankind. London, 1870, pp. 231-239.
26. Elisée: Encyclopedia Brit., 11th ed., Vol. 10, p. 400.
27. Dion, H.: Antiquity of Rome. Vol. 2, p. 67.
28. Bonwick, J.: Daily Life and Origin of the Tasmanians. London, 1870, p. 20.
29. II Maccabees 10:3.
30. Spencer and Gillen: The Native Tribes of Northern Australia. London, 1889, p. 259.
31. Talmud Berochoth 12-a.
32. "The Native Tribes of Northern Australia," p. 259.
33. Frazer, G.: Totemism. 11:258.
34. Crowly, A. E.: The Magic Rose. London, 1902, p. 197.
35. "The Native Tribes of Northern Australia," pp. 250-349.
36. Grim: Deutschalterthumer. Gottingen, 1881, p. 195.
37. Perschel, O.: The Races of Man. D. Appleton-Century Co., New York, 1885, p. 144.
38. Lartsch, A.: Ausland. (Cited by Perschel, p. 159.)
39. Ibid. (Cited by Perschel, p. 163.)
40. Ibid., p. 165.
41. Tyler, E. B.: Early History of Mankind, p. 167.
42. Ruth 2:14.
43. Genesis 25:34.

44. Exodus 12:33-34.
45. Crowly, E. A.: The Mystic Rose. London, 1902, pp. 126-132
46. Ibbetson, D. C. J.: Ponjab Ethnology. Calcutta, 1883, p. 114.
47. Gomme, L.: Hasting's Encyclopedia, Vol. 8, p. 634.
48. Ibid.
49. Genesis 49:12.

7

Medicine in Assyro-Babylonia

SINCE medicine cannot be separated from general culture, the dawn of medicine must be looked for in the land most advanced in ancient civilization. Such a land, according to many archaeologists, is Assyro-Babylonia, which is said to have been the center of ancient civilization far back into the fourth millennium B.C.

THE SUMERIANS

An Ordered Civilization: The Sumerians, from whom the Assyro-Babylonians inherited their culture, at an early period achieved an ordered civilization. The cities of Ur, Erech, Lagash, and Kish had well-organized governments perhaps as early as the fifth millennium B.C. Sir C. Leonard Wooley, who excavated the city of Ur, is of the opinion that the Sumerian was a magnificent craftsman in metal, at a time when predynastic Egypt had not yet emerged from the Stone Age. He had a well-established government in many centers of the land. "The Death Pit of Ur," discovered by Wooley, shows that the Sumerians were advanced in arts and crafts. The rulers, with their gaily clad wives, attendants, concubines, and warriors, were buried in the same tombs together with their household belongings, horses, cattle, chariots, and charioteers, arranged in the subterranean resting places in the order corresponding to the position they occupied and the functions they performed during life. In this way, the kings were enabled to carry on in their customary way in the world below. Such mass funerals were evidently voluntary acts of self destruction, similar to the customs which persisted until the fourteenth century among the Mongols of Asia, and which were practiced by Hindu widows (suttees), who immolated themselves on the funeral pile of their deceased husbands in order not to be separated from their mates. Mr. Wooley has ventured the opinion that this wholesale death of the royal family and household was probably brought about by a special kind of a drug which rendered these persons senseless to the death that awaited them.

This practice, that prompted the royal knights, equipped with daggers and helmets, to follow the king and his grandees to the grave in order to protect him and his entourage from the evil spirits lurking in the world below, shows that the Babylonians made use of metals at an early period, and may have been familiar with soporific drugs which rendered themselves insensible to pain and suffocation.

A Cultured Dynasty: Since south Mesopotamia possesses no building stone, the Sumerians built great brick temples, beautifully decorated. They laid out spreading cities and provided what may be considered the earliest evidence of agriculture. Kish is among the most ancient of the Mesopotamian cities on record. There a wealthy and cultured dynasty reigned over Sumer and Accad before the rise of Ur.

Hygiene: Dr. Langdon discovered tablets relating to medicine, one of which is a physician's seal. According to Langdon, the Blundell-Field expedition discovered sanitary drains in strata of Kish, dating back as early as 3000 B.C.[1] Sir John Martial unearthed, at Mohenjo-Daro and Harappa, brick houses built according to sanitary principles, with bathrooms, waterproof brick floors, and drain pipes, by which the sewage was carried off into street tanks and thence removed by street cleaners.

Many lavatories were discovered in Sumerian courtyards, and balconies were found to have been constructed in the houses at Ur by 2000 B. C. Each house was provided with sanitary drains. One of these houses dates as far back as 3500 B.C.

Writings: The early Sumerian script, which according to Langdon originated in Kish, was invented about 4200 B.C. It was originally pictographic in form and ideographic in function. It gradually developed into cuneiform writing with increasing syllabic function. The Babylonian tongue, about 1500 B.C. was extensively used all over the eastern basin of the Mediterranean. It was the diplomatic language of antiquity. At Hammurabi's time (2285–2242 B.C.), a well-established system of laws, regulating the health and the welfare of the community, was enforced. Particular attention was paid to hygiene and prophylaxis. In the epilogue to the Code of Hammurabi, **the**

author prides himself on promoting the health of his subjects: "I brought health to the land, I made the populace rest in security." This famous code, which incorporates laws of a much earlier date, has a far-advanced system of legal and penal regulations. Surgeons,

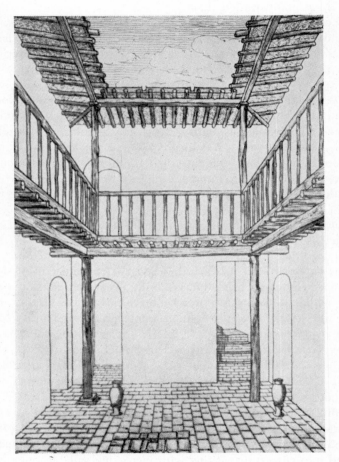

Fig. 51: Restoration of a private house at Ur. (From a drawing by A. S. Whitburn, A.R.I.B.A.)

particularly, practiced their profession without belonging to the priestly caste. Dr. Morris Jastrow pointed out that the physician and surgeon at that time were already, to some extent, differentiated from the magic healer, and perhaps not placed on the same level.

Lepsius, after studying many medical Mesopotamian tablets, formed an opinion that the first medical culture known was developed in this ancient land.

PHYSICIANS

Priestly Schools: Babylon and Nineveh were the homes of the famous priestly schools, where, in addition to religion, astronomy, mathematics, law, and principles of government, medicine was also taught. Medicine was practiced as a profession in Babylonia far back in the fourth millennium B.C. A gray seal cylinder of this period, unearthed at Lagash, bears the inscription, "O' Edig, Magie, servant of the god, Girra, who helps mothers in childbirth, Ur Luglendiad, the physician, is thy servant."

Priest and Lay Physicians: Early Babylonian medicine was associated with religion and magic and belonged to the domain of priesthood. In later times, a cast of layphysicians and surgeons were formed to practice the profession according to definite and natural regulations. The priestly "doctor" was known as the "assipu" priest. The layphysician was known as "asu" (Aramaic, *asya*). The *assipu* priest primarily dealt with internal diseases, and particularly with nervous and mental conditions, which were generally attributed to demonic possession and cured largely by religious and magical means. On the other hand, external pathological conditions, caused by injury and violence, belonged to the province of the *asu* and were treated by natural means. Sayce asserts that the term "asu" was applied to a physician, scribe, and seer. It was thus similar to the modern word "doctor" which applies to almost any learned person.

The Code of Hammurabi, which deals with practical problems of law and order, steadfastly ignores the *assipu* priest, whose practice was largely confined to internal diseases attributed to supernatural powers, such as the vengeance of the gods, demons, witches, unlucky stars, and the spiteful glance of the "evil eye." The "Book of Hammurabi" mentions only the *asu*, whose practice was largely confined to surgery. The etiologies of the ailments which the *asu* treated were perceptible even to the casual observer and such afflictions were treated rationally.

But even the *asu*, who usually adopted practical measures to counteract morbidity, could not tear himself entirely away from animistic medical conceptions; for the people at large believed in such practices, and he frequently was obliged to compound, so to speak, his natural methods of treatment with the "sugar-coated pills" of magic and divination.

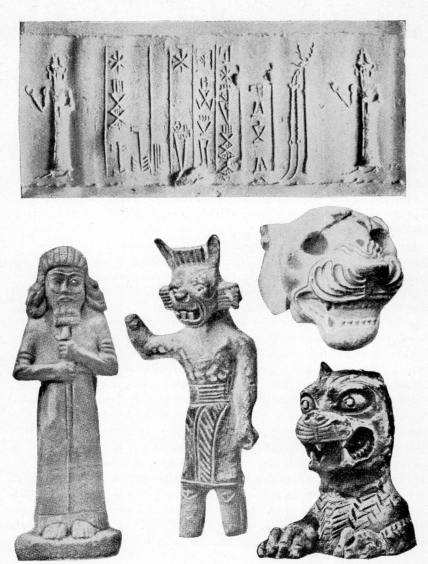

Fig. 52: *Upper:* Seal of a Sumerian Physician, c. 3000 B.C. The Babylonians signed their documents by rolling over wet clay an engraved cylinder, such as this, belonging to a physician from Lagash (original now in the Louvre). It represents Iru, a deity regarded as a form of Nergal, the god of pestilence and disease. The cuneiform characters are of an early type. (From a cast in the Wellcome Historical Medical Museum.) *Lower:* Ancient Mesopotamian religion and disease. Disease was largely of demonic origin, and consequently priests *(left:* from Nineveh, eighth century B.C.) were best qualified to combat it. Demonic figures were set up at the gates or buried beneath the thresholds of houses *(right)* to frighten demons away. The center figure, in bronze, was buried beneath the floor of a room and was supposed to be able to drive away the demons of sickness. (British Museum, London.)

162

DIVINITIES

The Assyro-Babylonians were nature worshippers, associating all natural phenomena with divinities. There was a divinity for every natural occurrence. Disease and other misfortunes were viewed as just punishments for disobeying the gods or violating religious taboos. Even if the religious violation was committed involuntarily or in ignorance, full responsibility was incurred by the offender. The sick person looked upon the disease that had overtaken him as positive proof that he had sinned.

Intermediary Task of Priests: The priests, belonging to the educated class, were the teachers of the schools of Nineveh and Babylon, the physicians, and the intermediaries between the common folk and the gods. They could ascertain the causes of disease; they knew how to interpret divine wishes; they knew how to predict the outcome of disease; and they were capable of propitiating the gods and expelling the evil spirits causing the disease. It was only through the priest that the layman could approach the deity and be led into the divine presence.

Gods of Healing: The principal god connected with healing was Ea, the god of the deep, and one of the triad that ruled the universe. The other two were Anu, the god of heaven, and Bel, the god of the earth. The Assyro-Babylonians unhesitatingly placed their faith in Ea to cope with the mysterious dangers and pitfalls which beset them on all sides. They turned to Ea particularly to rescue them from the evil demons which they fancied pursued them with malice and hatred. They did not have the effrontery to direct their prayers personally to Ea, for he was too mighty and exalted to be so addressed; they turned to his son, Marduk, to intercede for them with his great father. Marduk carried to Ea the suppliant's request. If illness was the trouble, a remedy was requested in the form of a charm or an incantation; if the victim was held under the spell of witchcraft, a counterspell was asked for.

The following text is often repeated on the clay tablets:

Marduk hath seen him [the sick man], and hath entered the house of his father Ea, and hath said, "Father, headache from the underworld hath gone forth." Twice he hath said unto him, "What this man hath done he knoweth not; whereby shall he be relieved?" Ea hath answered his son Marduk, "O my son, what dost thou not know what more can I give thee? O Marduk what dost thou not know what can I add unto thy knowledge? What I know, thou knowest also. Go, my son, Marduk...." [2]

Then follows the actual prescription for the patient:

Take a bucket, fill it with water from the mouth of the rivers: impart to this thy exalted magic power, sprinkle the man with it, son of his god. . . . . wrap up his head. . . . .and on the highway pour it out. May insanity be dispelled that the disease of his head vanish like a phantom of the night! May Ea's word drive it out! May Damkina heal him.

Associated with Marduk and his wife, were the chief deities of the principal cities, such as Nebo and Tashmit of Borsippa, Nergal, and Alatu of Kut, and Ninib of Lagash (the last was the physician of the gods). There was the goddess, Ninkharsag, who was aided by eight other divinities, each specializing over a different syndrome. There were also Adad and Shula, and there was Ninazu, the personal god of the physician. The most prominent healing-god was Ninurta (chief of the physicians) who was assisted by his spouse, Gula. Both were considered guardian patrons of the healing art. The seal of Gula had on one side a picture of the god, Ninurta, holding in one hand a cupping instrument and, on the other, the likeness of a healer. The symbol of the healing-god was a serpent.

When the priest appealed to the deities for help, he had to mention the particular god who governed or specialized on the particular disease which his patient had contracted. Thus:

When (a man) is smitten on his neck and his breast hurts him, it is the hand of Ishtar; when a man's temple pains him, and the neck muscles hurt him, it is the hand of a ghost. When a ghost seizes a man, mix (various substances together and annoint him with them) and the hand of the ghost will be removed. [3]

DEMONS

Seven Evil Demons (Maskims): The gods were opposed by seven evil demons *(maskims)*, sometimes called the "seven fiery phantoms," whose greatest delight was to undermine the orderly course of nature by causing earthquakes, inundations, tempests, and plagues.

Lesser Demons: In addition to the seven *maskims*, there existed a host of lesser demons which in every possible form assailed man. They waited in ambush for the unwary pedestrian. They compounded poison philters. They were out to harm man, not only bodily but also morally. They were devoted to Ishtar, the goddess of witchcraft and darkness, who seized her victims at night and particularly enjoyed slaying youths. Ishtar was dreaded particularly by the witches and streetwalkers, who undertook to minister to her and against whom all kinds of charms, such as small images of Lugalgirra, allama, and teraphim, were employed.

Fear of Demons: The fear of demons was peculiar not only to the early Babylonian, but it was common to all peoples as late as the fifth century B.C. The Greek poet, Aeschylus (525–456 B.C.), referring to demons, writes:

It is they who steal the child from the knee of its father, who drive the son from his father's house, who withhold from the wife the blessing of children; they have stolen days from heaven, which they have made evil days, that bring nothing but ill-luck and misfortune—and nothing can keep them out: They fall like rain from the sky, they spring from the earth—they steal from house to house—doors do not stop them—bolts do not shut them out—they creep in at the doors like serpents—they blow in at the roof like winds. Various are their haunts: the tops of mountains, the pestilential marshes by the sea, but especially the desert.

Disease-Demons: Disease-demons were among the most dreaded of these terrible fiends, and worst among those feared were Namtar and Dibbara, the demons of pestilence. Idpa was the cause of a certain mysterious disease of the head (perhaps insanity). This disease was said to effect the head and hold it tight like a tiara, so that the patient felt as though he was in a dark prison. The demon entered the body like a violent tempest; no one knew whence it came, nor what was its object.[4]

SORCERERS

As if all these terrors were not sufficient to make life miserable, the Assyro-Babylonians believed in wicked sorcerers, who knew how to compel the powers of evil to do their bidding and who could inflict sickness, death, or other disasters at their whim. They could bring on catastrophe in many ways: by a mere look, by uttering certain magical syllables, by drinks made of herbs prepared under certain conditions and ceremonies, and by the power of doing harm by a malicious glance (the last power was often ascribed to allegedly innocent persons who unintentionally inflicted disease by their evil eye).

When the Assyro-Babylonian Empire was conquered by the Persians, the secret arts (Chaldean wisdom) continued to be practiced. In fact the Persians introduced them to all the countries they conquered.

The Evil Eye: The belief in evil eye is of great antiquity. It is said to have originated in Babylonia and had for its object the explanation of the etiology of disease. The term has been applied to an eye believed to have the power of inflicting various diseases and evils on persons by a mere glance. An incantation against the evil eye, dating from 700 B.C., during the reign of Ashurbanipal, is found in an Accadian inscription at the British Museum.[5]

ASTROLOGY

Perhaps the greatest obstacle to medical progress in Chaldea was the pseudoscience of astrology,[6] the belief that the stars were divine beings, possessing supreme intelligence, and capable of ruling and

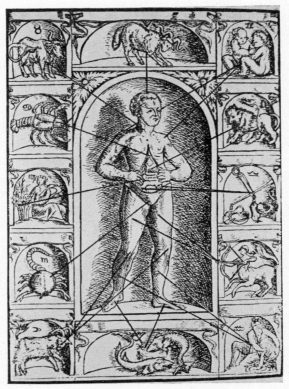

Fig. 53: The relation of the parts of the human body to the signs of the zodiak.

shaping the destiny of the universe and that of its hapless inhabitants.

Priestly Interpretations: The Chaldean priests interpreted the positions and movements of the stars in the sky, their rising and setting, their relations to one another, and their crossing each other's path, as determining the future of the nation and the destiny of the individual. The appearance of an eclipse was particularly taken as an ominous sign of an unusual phenomenon which was going to happen. Every future earthly occurrence was supposedly visible in the blue sky to the priest. This divine knowledge of the "hosts of heaven" was considered entirely out of reach to laymen. The priestly caste alone claimed to understand the language of the stars. They were the mediators of the gods, the teachers of the people, the scribes, the judges, the mathematicians, the astronomers, and the "doctors." To them, while gazing from the high towers of the temples of Babel, were revealed the secrets of each and every occurrence in the world below. They were the only possessors of divine revelation, thus being able to predict for the nation, the king, and the private citizen, what the gods had in store for them.

Astrologic System: The astrologic system included two groups of stars: planets, including sun, moon, Jupiter, Venus, Saturn, Mercury, and Mars; and constellations (*constella*, "stars together"), or fixed stars, usually appearing in clusters. There were sixty-four toward the south of the heaven and twenty-eight toward the north. The latter two groups were separated by a circle of clusters, the zodiac (Greek: "circle of animals"), corresponding to the twelve months of the year. The name of each cluster was based on fancied resemblance to an animal or object. The names of the divisions of the zodiac and the parts of the body they represented are as follows:

	SYMBOL	ASPECT *(Body)*
Aries, the Ram...........	♈	Head
Taurus, the Bull.........	♉	Neck and shoulders
Gemini, the Twins........	♊	Arms and hands
Cancer, the Crab........	♋	Chest and adjacent parts
Leo, the Lion.............	♌	Heart and mouth of the stomach
Virgo, the Virgin.........	♍	Intestines, base of the stomach, and umbilical region
Libra, the Balance........	♎	Kidneys
Scorpio, the Scorpion......	♏	Genitals
Sagittarius, the Archer.....	♐	Hips
Capricornus, the Goat.....	♑	Knees
Aquarius, the Water Carrier	♒	Legs
Pisces, the Fishes.........	♓	Feet

The signs of the zodiac formed an imaginary circle, or band of grouped stars, which encircled the heavens in the apparent path of the sun and planets.

Horoscopes: A horoscope was cast in the following manner: Having ascertained the exact time of birth of the person being studied, the astrologer traced the star that passed the diagram of the "house of heaven" at that particular hour. The astrologic observations were conducted within the confines of the temples of religion. The calendars compiled by the astrologers furnished hygienic and medical information. Astral medicine was not merely the pastime of a school of pedants; it exercised a great influence upon the Assyro-Babylonian—upon his health, his religion, his culture, his customs, and his way of life.

Star Worship: Just as the rivers and streams of Mesopotamia were recognized as the source of fertility, without which life was impossible, and were therefore venerated as gods, so were the stars worshipped because they determined the fate of the state, the king, and the people. It was not merely the sky, in the more general and abstract sense, that was worshipped but the individual stars that were adored as gods. Symbols drawn on seal-cylinders, discovered in the library of Ashurbanipal, show that the worship of the stars dates back to the oldest period of Babylonian culture, to the time when the cuneiform characters first evolved from the ideographic script. The elaborate system of astral medicine, of course, was an artificial creation. It gained its popularity from its connection with astronomy which was considered the science *par excellence*. Its relationship, of course, was purely fancied.

Because of its scientific pretenses, astrology attracted, not only the ignorant and credulous masses, but even the well-informed and cultured elements.

Prognostic Value of Astrology: From the Kouyunjik (Nineveh) medical texts in the British Museum, it may be inferred that astrologic medicine was originally limited to the prognosis of disease. Some of the texts read as follows:

1. Text 269. "If an eclipse of the sun occurs on the twenty-ninth day of the month of Iyyar, there will be many deaths on the first day."

2. Text 271: "If an eclipse takes place during the morning watch, and lasts throughout the watch, while the wind blows from the north, the sick in Accad will recover."

3. Text 69-a: "If the wind comes from the west upon the appearance of the moon, disease will prevail during this month."

4. Text 207: "If Venus approaches the constellation of Cancer, obedience and prosperity will be in the land . . . the sick of the land will recover. Pregnant women will carry their confinements to a favorable termination."

5. Text 79: "If a halo surrounds the moon and if Regulus stands within, women will bear male children."

6. Text 173: "If Mercury rises on the fifteenth day of the month, there will be many deaths. If the constellation of Cancer becomes obscured, a fatal demon will possess the land and many deaths will occur."

Diagnostic and Therapeutic Factors of Astrology: Later the stars were consulted, not only to foretell the outcome of the ailment, but also to diagnose and treat the disease. All the astrologic healer needed was a graph of the zodiac and a knowledge of the planet in conjunction when the patient was born or when he took sick. The graph of the zodiac was the principal diagnostic instrument in the astrophysician's medicine bag. The twelve signs were arranged in a circle around the figure of a man, "the grand man," in the center. Lines drawn from each sign of the zodiac indicate the part of the body governed by that sign. In case of disease, each sign, from Aries to Pisces, points to the weak or vulnerable part of the body, in the following manner:

Aries: Eyes, head, and stomach; also paralysis.

Leo: Lungs, heart, back, and kidneys; also continued violent fevers.

Sagittarius: Rheumatism, weakness of the lungs, and stomach trouble.

Gemini: Throat, stomach, nervous disease, worms, and eczema.

Libra: Nervous prostration and unusual stomach conditions, such as those brought about by excessive worry and impatience.

Aquarius: Brain trouble, poor circulation, and pain in the muscles and head.

Taurus: Morbid mental conditions, heart trouble, dropsy, tumors, apoplexy, and brain disorders.

Virgo: Certain nervous conditions and stomach troubles; also special reference to carelessness and neglect.

Capricorn: Indigestion and melancholia as a result of overwork, overambition, or poor judgment.

Cancer: Digestive and gastric troubles.

Scorpio: Lumbago, gout, and weakness of the back.

Pisces: Pain in the feet, back, head, and digestive organs.

The treatment of disease was also guided by the stars. Each planet represented the metals, plants, and drugs to be used.

Hippocrates' Interest in Astrology: In Greece, sidereal medicine surpassed the limits attained in Babylonia. No less an authority than Hippocrates accepted some of its doctrines. In the Corpus Hippocraticum, passages are found which show more than a passing interest in the astrologic art of healing. "Attention," said the father of rational medicine, "must be paid to the rising of the stars, especially to those of Sirius and Arcturus, the further, to the setting of the Pleiades, for most diseases reach a crisis during such periods." Hippocrates also stated:

He who knows how the change of seasons and the rising and setting of the stars take place will also be able to foresee how the year is going to be. If anyone should be of the opinion that the question belongs solely to the realm of astronomy, he will change his opinion as he learns that astronomy is not of slight but of essential importance in medical art.

Long Reign of Sidereal Medicine: Sidereal medicine reigned supreme well into the eighteenth century. Astrodiagnosis and astrologic remedies were held in high respect, being utilized by physicians in schools and institutions. Medical astrology had the support of leading physicians throughout the ages. Indeed, astrologists claim that Hippocrates designed the "grand zodiacal man." They point out that in modern times, Paracelsus, Van Helmont, and Kepler expressed themselves strongly in favor of sidereal healing, the first declaring: "A physician without the knowledge of the stars can neither understand the cause of, nor cure any disease, not even so much as a toothache."

DIVINATION

Man was always eager to know what the future has in store for him. To solve it, he not only looked towards the heavens but searched the phenomena of nature around him to obtain an answer. This intense desire to look into the future crystallized itself among the Babylonians in yet another concept which hindered the advance of medical progress. Divination was based on the belief that everything existing in nature and displaying activity possesses a certain native intelligence and purposeful plan.

Examination of Sacrificial Animals: Among the numerous objects used for divination were the organs of sacrificed animals. The organs of these animals were carefully examined in great detail by specially trained persons for the purpose of predicting future events. Any deviation from the normal color, shape, and form was interpreted as an omen for good or for evil, as the case might have been. The liver, particularly that of the sheep, was studied for oracular purposes. There is a clay model of such a liver in the British Museum dating from about 2000 B.C. This liver is divided into five quadrangular fields. Each field contains precise instruction on how to interpret the hepatic condition for divination. The model was evidently

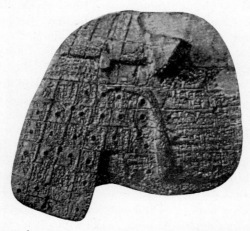

Fig. 54: Clay model of a sheep's liver for purposes of divination (c. 2000 B.C.). The individual fields of the model contain explanatory text. (British Museum, London.)

employed for the instruction of students. Another clay model of a liver, said to have been used for divination by King Sargon of Assyria (722–705 B.C.) reads: "If the gallbladder is filled with gall, it is a favorable sign. On the other hand, if the gallbladder is like an empty sack and a wedge projects from the liver to the right side of the gallbladder and seven depressions are seen in the liver in front of it, then it is an ill omen." On the strength of this oracle, King Sargon attacked Elam and destroyed the Elamites. Other clay liver models, dating from the days of Hammurabi, have recently been discovered at Mari at the middle Euphrates.

The prophet, Ezekiel, refers to the use of the liver by the Babylonians as a means of foretelling future events: "For the King of

Babylon standeth at the parting of the ways, at the head of two ways, to use divination; he shaketh the arrows to and fro, he inquireth of the teraphim, he looketh at the liver."[7]

Hepatoscopists: Those persons who occupied themselves with the foretelling of events from the appearance of the liver later became known as "hepatoscopists." Divination, like other oriental beliefs, had a religious basis. Animal sacrifices brought to the temple were closely observed by the priests. The liver was the organ generally used for divination because of the belief that it was the organ where blood was manufactured. Man has looked upon blood with great reverence from remote ages. Most of the emotions, which are at present ascribed to the brain, were attributed to the liver.

Beginning of Chaldean Anatomy: Divination, employing the liver and other organs, was the ancestor of the modern science of splanchnology and was the crude beginning of Chaldean anatomy.

Significance of Monstrosities: Most amazing is the significance attached to monstrous births. Human and animal monstrosities were considered ominous to the future welfare of the states. Every possible anomaly was registered as a means of foretelling the welfare of the king and the country. Ninety different abnormalities, ranging from an extra finger or toe to inequality in the size of the two ears, are listed. The most impossible monstrosities are seriously enumerated as having an important bearing on national affairs. A few may be cited as examples:

If a woman gives birth to a child with lion's ears a mighty king will rule the land . . . if a queen gives birth to a child with a lion's face the king will have no rival . . . if a woman gives birth to twins joined together back to back (Siamese) the country will be governed by one master and will not be controlled by another master; if joined by their sides, the gods will abandon the country, the king and his son will abandon the city.

Other malformations listed are the absence of two right hands of a twin Siamese monstrosity, or both left hands, as well as similar deformities of the lower extremities. Healthy twins were regarded as a favorable omen. Triplets and quadruplets, however, were always thought to be signs of evil.

Anomalies, such as the absence of a mouth, lip, or anus, or the presence of teeth at birth, supplied prized information to the Divinator. Premature births and abortions are described as having important significance. While such obstetrical irregularities were carefully observed, they were not considered from a medical point of view, but only as important prognostic indices for future events.[8]

CHALDEAN WISDOM

Each of the four major branches of Chaldean wisdom (i.e. religion, magic, astrology, and divination) were represented by "wise men"—priestly doctors—subdivided into various specialities; some were devoted to the interpretation of dreams; others to foretelling the outcome of disease or other important events; and still others occupied themselves with healing. All practiced in accordance with the rules laid down by authorities on these subjects, as noted in three great works written during Sargon's reign.

In a world filled with wicked metaphysical forces, medicine found little room for rational practice. The healing profession became a happy hunting ground of conjurors, enchanters, magicians, witches, and wizards.

The name "Chaldean wisdom" became synonomous in the New Testament with the practices of "the wise men of the East,"[9]

CONTRIBUTION TO MODERN SCIENCE

While it is evident that civilization has little reason to be grateful to the Assyro-Babylonians for the fantastic concepts which blocked scientific progress for thousands of years, one must not ignore the fact that, intermixed with these superstitious notions, were many important scientific facts relating to astronomy, mathematics, law, government, and medicine. Coexisting with these metaphysical ideas and practices were many medical principles, which at various periods were dominated by rational and keen observation. Hence, even if Babylonian medicine was not rational in the modern sense, it formed the basis of many scientific medical truths. For example, the idea that the various organs of the body were governed by a super deity, the all-powerful god, Ea, anticipates, so to speak, the principle of cerebral coordination of the various nerve centers; the doctrine of the demonic origin of disease, which superficially appears to be a base superstition, was in reality a progressive step over other existing ideas as to the etiology of disease. The mere fact that disease was conceived to be caused by external invisible powers and not through endogenous causes was a revolutionary advance. The relationship of the stars to medical science, which to the modern mind may seem far-fetched, stimulated the study of astronomy if it did not benefit the knowledge of medicine. The notion that physical ills were the result of violation of a taboo of uncleanliness carried with it the idea that diseases were caused by contagion, as is apparent from the following tablet from Ashur-banipal's library: "To go before a man under a taboo or to have a man under a taboo come before one, to sleep on the bed, sit on a chair or to eat or drink from vessels belonging to such a man is forbidden."

CONCEPTS OF CAUSES OF DISEASE

The Assyrian idea was that internal diseases were inflicted by invisible foreign bodies that entered the body with food, drink, or inspired air, much the same as external wounds were caused by out-side influences. These foreign intruders were thought to be malevo-lent spirits. What the modern psychiatrist would term "psychic trauma" was to the Assyrian healer a physical, although invisible, reality. To the early Assyrian, all aspects of life were real and material, possessing characteristic shape and form. Even a moving shadow was considered material. Sickness in its abstract sense was thought to be a material being. This being was addressed by name in the incantations as though it were a living entity. The arrow which flew through the air and the rock which fell from the cliff to cause injury acted, not because of the energy of the person who dispatched them nor because of their own density, but because of the inherent life within them. The regular rising and setting of the sun and moon were attributed to the life within them. The same was true of the planets which moved in the sky. It was life that gave them the power of movement. All that moved possessed life and all that was dead was motionless.

The measures adopted for removing visible weapons that had penetrated the body and caused wounds were simulated in dealing with internal invisible forces that caused internal diseases. There is no evidence, however, to indicate that the Babylonian exorcist pro-fessed, with his charms and incantations, to extract real objects from the body of his patient as is the custom of the medicine man of the American Indian and the Australian aborigine. He merely claimed to expel the spirit which caused the injury.

As the reader may have gathered, the Babylonian did not hold a very consistent theory about the origin of disease. On the one hand, all sickness was ascribed to demonic possession; the demon had been eaten with food, imbibed with water, or breathed in with inspired air; and until he could be expelled, there was no chance of recovery. But, on the other hand, a pestilence or epidemic, which swept over a whole country, was regarded with the same feelings of awe-struck veneration as the greater gods themselves. Such was believed to be an instrument in their hands for punishing the sins and shortcomings of mankind. The plague consequently was held to be a divine being who was sent by the gods, like the storm or the deluge, to take vengeance on men for their misdeeds and improprieties.

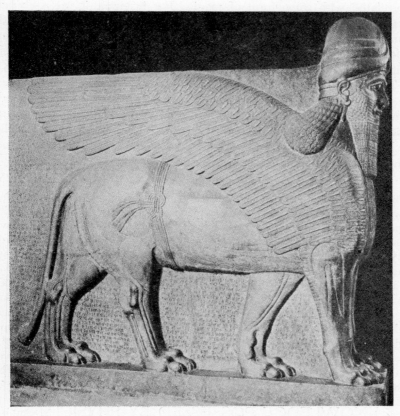

Fig. 55: Assyrian winged lion which once flanked the gateways of a royal palace to frighten off evil spirits. (Photograph in the Library of Congress from the original in the British Museum.)

RITUALS OF HEALING

The Babylonians also engaged in a large number of ritual performances, such as sprinkling the body of the sick with holy water, anointing the body of the patient with oil, and burning all objects with which the patient had come in contact. The patient himself had to take part in the ceremonies, some of which required kneeling or casting the sick person on the ground.

Numerology played an important part in Babylonian therapeutics. On certain days of the month, the physician was not permitted to touch the patient.

Even when drugs or plants were administered, these had to be correlated with some form of magic. For instance, it was specified that they were to be collected on a midsummer eve or during a midsummer night before sunrise. Blossoms were commonly hung on doorways and windows to preserve the house against thunder, witches, and evil spirits.

The healer was careful to observe regulations. When he was called to treat a patient, he made certain that his appearance was dignified. He was clad for the occasion and never failed to impress the patient with his authority and power. When he entered the house of the sick, he announced that he was empowered by Ea, Damika, and Marduk to heal him. Then he mumbled:

Shamash is before me, Sin is behind [me], Nergal is at [my] right hand, Ninib is at my left hand; when I draw near unto the sick man, when I lay my hand on the head of the sick man, may a kindly spirit, may a kindly guardian angel, stand at my side! Whether thou art an evil spirit or an evil demon, or an evil ghost, or an evil devil, or an evil god, or an evil fiend, or sickness, or death, or phantom of night, or wraith of night, or fever, or evil pestilence, be thou removed from before me, out of the house go forth. [For] I am the sorcerer-priest of Ea, it is I who [recite] the incantation for the sick man! The man of Ea am I, the man of Damika am I, the messenger of Marduk am I. The great Lord Ea hath sent me to revive the . . . sick man; he hath added his pure spell to mine, he hath added his pure voice to mine, he hath added his pure spittle to mine, he hath added his pure prayer to mine; the destroyer of the limbs, which are in the body of the sick man, hath the power to destroy the limbs—by the magic of the word of Ea may these evil ones be put to flight.[10]

KNOWLEDGE POSSESSED BY PHYSICIANS

A medical compendium discovered in the library of Ashurbanipal, comprising three cuneiform tablets, was deciphered by Frederick Kuchler, and shows that Babylonian physicians had a comprehensive knowledge of medicine. The author of this ancient medical document divided medical practice into three different groups: (1) cures, (2) achievements of the masters of the lancet, and (3) instructions for exorcisers. The first group appears to refer to the work of the *asu*, the second to the surgeon, and the third to the *assipu*, or medicineman.

Many prescriptions in this ancient medical work resemble those in a modern pharmacopoeia. Some are associated with charms and spells. For example, in the middle of a list of various medicines carefully

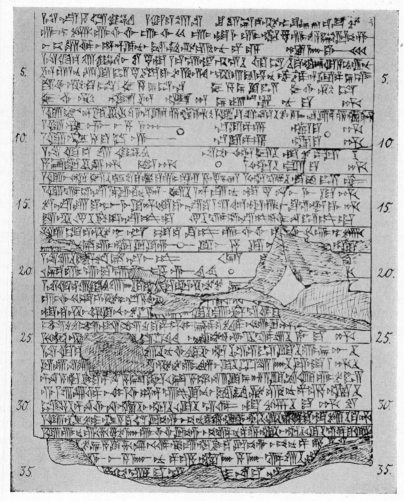

Fig. 56: Assyrian medical compendium. (Plate 1 from Kuchler, F.: Assyrian Medicine. It contains about thirty-five lines.)

prepared from different ingredients, and mixed in a group of vehicles including dates, wine, and water, may be found a charm to be chanted either while preparing the medicine or before administering the drug to the patient.

A line of demarcation must be drawn between the *assipu* (faith healer) and the *asu* (the physician). While it is true that the *asu* had to bow to the popular beliefs of the time and use religious and magic measures in addition to his rational medicine, he endeavored to depend mostly on legitimate medical methods.

The lay-physicians, or *asu*, of ancient Babylonia frequently ordered articles of diet which were considered unclean from a religious and esthetic point of view. Snakes, tongues of "black dogs," and ordure were all prescribed. The *asu* was occasionally accused of heresy because of such remedies. Perhaps the patient himself who swallowed these compounds had already lost faith in the old beliefs of his people.

It is not clear what kind of training the *asu* received before he was permitted to practice his profession. It may be assumed that he separated himself from theurgic therapeutics, did not belong to the priestly clan, and received his training by serving an apprenticeship with an older lay-physician.

The sum total of medical knowledge the *asu* possessed is not definitely established. In view of the fact that dissection on the human cadaver was taboo, it may be assumed that his knowledge of anatomy was derived from observation of sacrificed animals. The ideographic Sumerian pictograms, which resemble different parts of animal bodies, show that the Assyrians had only a rude knowledge of anatomy and that only the anatomy of the principal organs was known. According to their views of physiology, the Assyro-Babylonians considered the liver to be the location of the vital energy, where the blood that circulates through the body is generated.

According to the Babylonian myth of creation, man was created by mixing the blood of the decapitated god, Bel, with earth; this indicates that blood was considered the foundation of life. Reference to "day blood" and "night blood" are found in the cuneiform writings, perhaps alluding to arterial and venous blood. Respiration does not appear to have played an important part in the Assyrian scheme of physiology. Generally speaking, Assyro-Babylonian medicine was based first on practical experience, and secondly on traditions. These in turn were often harmonized with the religious beliefs of the day.

EXISTING DISEASES

It may be assumed that many diseases now prevalent in Mesopotamia existed in antiquity. Numerous known predisposing factors have existed since dark antiquity, and many ailments that affected the Babylonians three or four milleniums ago still prevail in modern Mesopotamia. Epidemics of *cholera* undoubtedly prevailed in the valley of the Euphrates throughout its entire history. *Dysentery* and *typhoid* are common to all countries where drainage is inadequate. *Smallpox* was common to all mankind, irrespective of locality, before the discovery of inoculation and vaccination. *Malaria* is a disease that prevails in warm swampy districts suitable as a habitat for the anopheles mosquito. *Skin eruptions* are common among all peoples where hygienic and sanitary conditions are at a low ebb.

Karl Sudhoff indicates that the Babylonians believed in the contagion of *leprosy* and took measures to counteract it.

In Babylonian mythology, there is always symbolic significance; Babylonian tablets show that these ancients attributed disease to some small animals as carriers. Nergal, the god of pestilence and destruction, appears in the form of an insect. This may be taken, at least as a hint, that even in this remote time insects were thought to play an important role in the spread of infectious disease.[11]

Baal-zebub,[12] the fly-god of Ekron, was perhaps a Philistine name for Nergal.

Diseases in the ancient Assyro-Babylonian texts discovered in the library of Ashurbanipal, for which remedies are prescribed, include those of the head, ears, mouth, lips, tongue, teeth, nose, heart, liver, kidneys, hands, feet, tendons *(saggulu)*, fingers, toes, hair, nails, and genital organs. *Rheumatism* and *arthritis* were common diseases. *Fevers, apoplexy, phthisis,* the plague called "*mutanu*," and *pestilence* were recognized. *Mental diseases* were thought to be due either to wounds or demons.

PROFESSIONAL LAWS

Code of Hammurabi: The Code of Hammurabi (c. 1950 B.C.) reveals that the Babylonian "physician" (referring to the surgeon in the modern sense), by virtue of the incessant wars of the Babylonian kings, occupied a high position in the state. His professional fees were regulated by law, on a scale corresponding to the rank of the patient, his ability to pay, and to the nature of the case.[13] His fee for opening an abscess was equivalent to about ten dollars in present American coin.

His high social standing, however, did not exonerate him from the responsibility of malpractice.

The Code of Hammurabi emphasizes that the professional fee was to be paid upon the cure of the patient, from which it may be in-

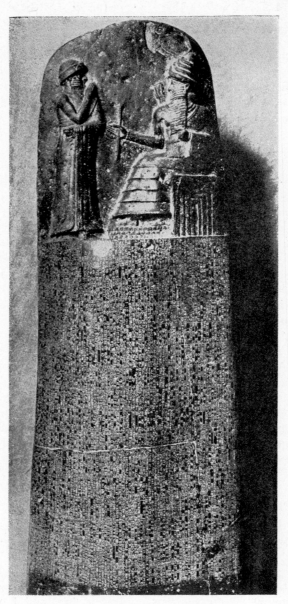

Fig. 57: The Code of Hammurabi. Hammurabi (2285-2242 B.C.) is identified by some with Amraphel (Gen. 14). His code is one of the most important monuments in the history of mankind. It contains the laws enacted by this king of Babylonia in the third millennium B.C. In this code, laws are found regulating the practice of surgery. On the obverse side, there are 1114 lines; and on the reverse side, there are 2500 lines of inscriptions. Thanks are due to the French government for carrying on explorations at Susa where the monument was discovered. The expedition was under the direction of M. J. Morgan.

ferred that, if there was no cure, the patient did not have to pay. In the event the patient died in consequence of the operation, the physician enjoyed a privilege denied to the average citizen. The law of *jus talionis* (life for life) was not imposed upon the physician. The extreme penalty in this case was not death but the cutting off of the physician's hand. The intention of the law evidently was to prevent repetition of such malpractice in the future. It is significant that the Code of Hammurabi refers only to surgical practitioners, ignoring internists altogether. This is probably due to the fact that the practice of internal medicine was largely in the hands of the priestly doctors and magicians who considered themselves messengers of the gods and, as such, could not be punished, since they were carrying out the will of the gods. The surgeon, on the other hand, who dealt with visible injuries and wounds generally due to natural causes and who used practical surgical methods without any secrecy or mysticism, was held strictly responsible for his actions.

The laws pertaining to the surgeon in the Code of Hammurabi are as follows:

215: If a physician operates with a bronze lancet on a [noble] man for a severe wound and saves the man's life or if he opens with a bronze lancet a *negabati* [perhaps an abscess] in the eye of a [noble] man and saves that man's eye, he shall receive ten shekels of silver as his fee [a shekel is equivalent roughly to ten dollars]. 216: If he be a free man he shall receive five shekels. 217: If he be a man's slave the owner of the slave shall give two shekels of silver to the physician. 221: If a physician set a broken bone for a [noble] man or cure his diseased bowels, the patient shall give five shekels of silver to the physician. 222: If he be a free man he shall give three shekels of silver. 223: It he be a man's slave, the owner of the slave shall give two shekels of silver to the physician.

As intimated, the physician's high social standing carried also a responsibility in the event that the patient was injured or died during the operation: "If an *asu* [physician] opens an *negabati* [perhaps an abscess] of the eye of a free man and causes the loss of his eye, the physician's hand shall be cut off; if he has caused the loss of an eye of a poor man or a slave, he shall pay one mina of silver."

With reference to *negabati* (generally translated "abscess") there is a difference of opinion among Assyriologists as to the meaning of the term, for the treatment of which the Babylonian *asu* was physically responsible. Johns stated that a *negabati* was an abscess (possibly of the lid or of the lacrimal canal). Magnus expressed the opinion that it was a cataract, because an abscess of the conjunctiva or of the canal would hardly cause blindness. Von Oefele, who agreed with Magnus, rendered the paragraph of text 218 of the Code of Hammurabi as follows: "If an *asu* opens a star (cataract) of a free man with a pointed knife of copper and causes the loss of a free man's eye, one shall cut off his hand." It should be pointed out that the fact that a knife was mentioned in connection with the cataract operation indicates that the Babylonian oculist favored paracentesis rather than *reclinatio lentis* (the couching, or expressing, operation practiced among ancient oculists). Because of the dislocation of the cataractous lens into the vitreous, ancient oculists seldom saw a cataractous lens, and they came to the conclusion that the impairment of sight was produced by injurious humors of the brain flowing through the hypothetically hollow optic nerve into the eyeball, where they settled between the iris and the lens. The density of the latter, observed in dead human beings and animals, was believed to be a post-mortem change.

Even the *gallabu* (barber), who performed only minor surgical procedures, such as for example, marking slaves on their bodies to indicate their masters, piercing ears, cupping, and perhaps pulling teeth, was regulated by law in the Code of Hammurabi.

The Babylonian Code of Hammurabi is of particular interest, for it reverses a much older Sumerian code of which fragments have been found. Incidentally, many Old Testament precepts can be traced to the older code.

MEDICAL TEXTS

Library of Ashurbanipal: Until 1849, few Assyrian medical texts had been discovered. About that time, Layard, excavating on the mound of Kouyunjik at Nineveh, discovered a large number of clay tablets[14] in the ruins of an ancient royal library. This turned out to be the library established by Ashurbanipal (668–626 B.C.), during whose reign Babylonian learning reached its climax. This monarch sent emissaries to all eastern countries to gather, for his library, documents which were customarily deposited in temples. These numerous and meritorious documents were inscribed on clay tablets to form a library covering almost every branch of knowledge.[15] About 12,000 fragments are preserved in the British Museum, 660 of which are of medical interest, have been published in the Assyrian language, and were partly translated by Dr. R. Campbell Thompson. To Thompson, more than to any other Assyriologist, medicine is indebted for our current knowledge of Assyrian medicine. In 1906, he began to collect, transcribe, and study systematically the medical texts, and in 1923 he published the text of 107 tablets and fragments. The results of his subsequent labors appeared in a number of volumes. Warren Dawson states:[16]

The modern student of Assyrian medicine is in a better position to investigate his subject, thanks to the labors of Campbell Thompson,[17] than the student of Egyptian medicine, for in the latter case, a great part of his

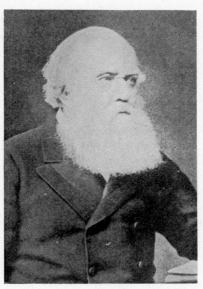

Fig. 58: Austen Henry Layard (1817-1894). Austen Henry Layard was born in Paris of Huguenot descent. His grandfather was a physician. His interest in archaeology originated in 1845 when the English Ambassador to Constantinople sent him to the Near East on a political mission. At that time, the ruins of Nimrod on the Tigris, were in process of excavation. The first of his discoveries was the ancient city of Nineveh, which he identified (1849) with Kuyunjik. His work "Nineveh" and the remains of that city are classical in the annals of archaeology. In 1852, he entered politics and was appointed Ambassador to Turkey. Layard is considered one of the founders of the science of archaeology.

preliminary work remains to be done. For apart from the translation of the more coherent and intelligible "Edwin Smith Surgical Text," no translation exists in which the slightest reliance can be placed.[18]

Symptomatic Treatment: It is to be noted that the Assyrians treated diseases symptomatically. Their prescriptions read as follows: "If a man's head has a scab, thou shalt do so and so"; "if a man's teeth hurt, thou shalt take such and such drugs and apply them"; and "if the accident of a blow has fallen upon him, thou shalt apply such and such a remedy," etc. The prescriptions often do not specify quantitatively the amount of the ingredients. The name of the ailment is usually not mentioned as is the case in the Egyptian prescriptions.

The work of identifying symptoms, diseases, and drugs in the Assyrian texts is a most difficult task. In most instances, symptoms were viewed as disease entities. Many broken tablets were difficult to match, and some of the names lost their original meaning. Dr. Morris Jastrow characteristically sums up the problem of identifying drugs presented as "the most formidable obstacle to a complete understanding of the medical texts." In most instances, only if we can find a corresponding term in one of the languages cognate to Babylonian, such as Hebrew, Arabic, Syriac, or Aramaic, can we solve the problem.

Notwithstanding the supernatural etiology and the magic treatment of disease, the symptoms of many diseases were correctly described. Legitimate drugs and many natural remedial measures were intermixed with the magical ritual. The magical means employed were often intended to reinforce the efficacy of the natural measures employed.

The following selection cited by Dawson may serve to illustrate the nature of Assyrian medicine:

If a man's eyes are sick and full of blood, unguents only irritating the blood, blood and tears coming forth from his eyes, a film closing over the pupils of his eyes, tears turning to film, look oppressing him; thou shalt beat leaves of tamarisk, steep them in strong vinegar, leave them out under the stars; in the morning [i.e. on the morrow] thou shalt squeeze them in a helmet; white alum storax, "Akkadian Salt," fat, cornflower, nigella, "gum of copper," separately shalt thou bray; thou shalt take equal parts of them, put them together; pour them into the helmet in which thou hast squeezed the tamarisk; in curd and sunis-mineral thou shalt knead it, and open his eyelids with a finger and put it in his eyes. While his eyes contain dimness, his eyes thou shalt smear, and for nine days thou shalt do this.

In the text quoted, the symptoms of ocular infection are correctly described, and the treatment is almost entirely therapeutic; the only magical element is the direction to leave the medicine under the stars (i.e. to expose it to the magical influence of the stars).

In the following text, the symptoms of alcoholism are graphically described, and the treatment is therapeutic in character; the only occult element is the administration of the remedy before the divinity, Gula:

When a man has drunk fermented drink and his head aches and he forgets his speech and in speaking is incoherent and his understanding is lost and his eyes are fixed; bray [eleven plants], drink them in oil and fermented drink before the approach of Gula in the morning before dawn before anyone kisses him.[19]

In some texts, after the symptoms are enumerated and the diagnosis of the case is given, the disease is easily recognized. For example: "If a man has a pain in the pit of his stomach accompanied by heartburn when he eats, and if he vomits bile, this man is attacked by a serious *tugatu* [gastrohepatic disease]." "If a man eats and drinks until he is satisfied and he then has a pain in his stomach so that his viscera seem to be on fire and he has colic, this man is attacked by *musbekmu* [gastritis]." It is to be noted that many texts deal with gastrointestinal disease; no less than fourteen recipes are recommended for stomach trouble.

Another instance where the ailment (heat exhaustion) is lucidly described by the symptoms is as follows:

If a man has heartburn and his stomach holds "fire," his chest rendering him, that man is suffering from the heat of the day....hellebore, lupons, calendula, chrysanthemum, segetum....gum of Andropogon, manna, ricinus, lolium....together thou shalt pound in beer without a meal, let him drink and he shall recover.

It is to be noted that these prescriptions have many ingredients.

The following text is homeopathic in nature—the "bitter," or gallbladder, is being treated with bitters, "for diseased gallbladder: milk, water, and strong wine; drink quantities of calf's milk, calf's milk and bitters, drink in palm wine, garlic and bitters drink in palm wine." The Babylonians were forbidden to use medicine on the seventh day (Sabbath). The signature on many of these recipes specifies their use on an empty stomach.

In the following text, the diagnosis of jaundice is given after a description of the symptoms:

If when a man's body is yellow, his face is yellow and black, the root of his tongue, black *ahhazu* is its name. [The therapy then follows.] Thou must take great wild musdimgurinna, he shall drink it in fermented drink, then will the *ahhazu* which is in him be silent. [20]

Incidentally, the term *ahhazu* ("to be seized") probably signifies a disease caused by an evil spirit. The word "ahhazu," in the cognate languages such as Hebrew and Aramaic, signifies seizure; in the Talmud it is generally applied to disease ascribed to demons.

Toothache was attributed to worms. It is curious that the Arabs of Mesopotamia still believe worms to be the cause of toothache. They treat it by fumigation with smoke of dried *Withania solonaceae*. The mixture of medical and magical treatment in the texts is illustrated

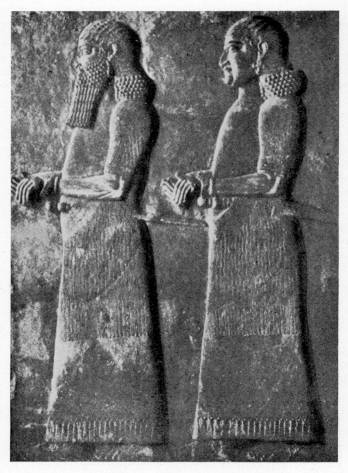

Fig. 59: Assyrian eunuchism (eighth century B.C.). Eunuchs were often entrusted with the administration of medicine. In wall reliefs of this type, the beardless figure is conceived to represent a eunuch. Here two bodyguards of the king are shown. (Louvre.)

by the following: "Mix beer, saki plant and oil together"; then repeat an incantation "three times three"; put the remedy on the tooth, "and the worm will drop out of his mouth."[21]

It is interesting to note that the physicians of Ashurbanipal ordered the removal of the royal teeth in order to cure pain in a distant part of the body. This offers a premonition of the concept of focal infection among the Babylonian doctors as early as the seventh century B.C.

The symptoms of pulmonary phthisis are correctly described:

The sick one coughs frequently, the sputum is thick and sometimes contains blood; his respiration gives the sound like a flute; his skin is cold but his feet are hot; he sweats greatly and his heart is much disturbed. When this disease is extremely grave, his intestines are frequently open.

The cause of consumption was áscribed to the entrance of the demon, asakku, into the system.

Occasionally an entire syndrome was observed. In this case the symptoms are enumerated at the beginning or at the end of the prescription:

If a man's belly unexpectedly is irritated, he holding wind in his anus, food and water being returned, and he being affected with constriction of the anus and while it hurts him he cries out and it is grievous to him...thou shalt reduce lion's skin, mix with lion fat...let it dry again, mix with cedar oil, make into a suppository, put it into his anus.

As another example of a syndrome, the following text may be cited:

If the patient has colic and his stomach will not retain food and there is flatulence, the treatment is to bray up together one half *ka* of date juice, one half *ka* of cassia juice, with oil and wine, three shekels of purified oil, two shekels of honey and ten shekels of the ammi-plant.

The patient is instructed to drink this preparation on an empty stomach before the rising of the star Sin. A charm is then recited.

Doctrine of "Signature": The doctrine of "signature," based on the belief that the creators stamped all objects medically beneficial to mankind and that there is a connection between every part of the human body and the parts of the world of nature, was recognized by the Assyro-Babylonian *asu.* According to this concept, diseases readily respond to remedies bearing some real, symbolical, or fanciful resemblance to the diseased part either in appearance or structure. This doctrine presupposes that there are specifics for all pathologic conditions if man can only recognize them. Thus, in one of the texts translated by R. Campbell Thompson, a mixture of an eviscerated yellow frog, gall, and curd were applied to the eye, for the treatment of leukoma (an ocular disease characterized by the formation of a yellowish film upon the cornea of the eye). The yellowish colors of the frog and bile formed a signature with the yellow color of the leukomatous eye.

The concept of signature was applied for the cure of gray hair. The recipe includes one gall of a black ox, a gall of a snake, a gall of a scorpion, a gall of a pig, punpulla. ". . . Thou shalt reduce, bray these five drugs in equal parts, thou shalt mix . . . Take up and

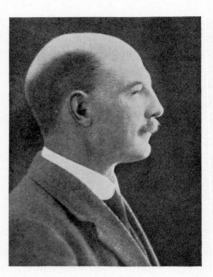

Fig. 60: R. Campbell Thompson, M.A., F.S.A. R. Campbell Thompson is perhaps the greatest contributor to our present knowledge of Assyro-Babylonian medical texts. Most of the texts belong to the Kuyunjik collection of the British Museum. Thompson, for a long period, devoted much time to the study and the translation of these texts. When he was called to military service during the first World War, his work was interrupted. In the spring of 1924, after twenty years of hard work in reading and translation of the texts, he published his corpus, which contains 660 tablets and fragments. Since then, Thompson has issued a large number of articles containing facsimiles of texts and identifications of medicines, both vegetable and mineral. For the first time, the student may avail himself of accurate copies and translations of these medical tablets. Indeed, many conclusions reached by Oefele, Kuchler, Ebbeling, Maisner, and others need to be revised in the light of evidence produced by Thompson.

together mix in the oil of cypress of the cemetery, press in his head seven times and the grey hair will turn black."

Forms of Remedies: Medical remedies were made in the form of powders, pills, poultices, plasters, philters, and enemas. Splints and bandages were applied. A bronze tube is mentioned in a medical text; perhaps it was used as a catheter in the urethra to relieve retention of urine. The eye received careful attention; eye medicine was administered with a bronze spatula. Various equipment was carried along by the *asu* in his medical chest *(takaltu)*. The physicians were organized in special guilds. Each group regulated their practice according to accepted standards. Venesection, cupping, and massage were known to the Babylonians; these were not regarded as direct remedies but as means of ridding the patient of the demon. Seven strokes were administered by the masseur (seven was a magic number).

In case of pain, the healer laid the head of his patient lower than the feet and kneaded or struck the back gently, repeating the formula, "it shall be good."[22] This manipulation was to drive the evil spirit out of the system. The conjuration was accompanied by a mixture of "salt of the mountain" and amanu-salt, pounded together and put in fermented liquor, which was to be drunk on an empty stomach. This medicine was also used as an enema or sprinkled upon the patient.[23] A mixture of the *nuhurtu* plant and seven corns of *si-si* was also considered efficacious. This too could be administered as a draught or as an enema.[24] A simpler method was to sit the patient down and let cold water flow on his head.[25]

"When a man's right temple hurts him and his right eye is swollen and lacrimates, it is the hand of a ghost or the hatred of a goddess against his life." The following is the recipe: "Mix *sihu* [tree], *arganu* [tree], *bariratu* [tree]. One shekel of 'river foam' *ditbat*-plant, ginger in ground meal, steep it in beer and bind on as a poultice. When the left eye or temple is afflicted, the physician must bray together dates from *Dilmun*, Thyme and cedar sap in oil of *gir* and apply them before the patient breaks his fast." If the patient, in addition to his neuralgia, vomits and his eyes are inflamed, it is the hand of a ghost and the remedy to be employed is calcined human bones: "bray them and rub them on the place with oil of cedar."

Many preparations containing a number of ingredients bore secret or sacred names, i.e. "Simgod," "skin of yellow snake," "dog's tongue." As flavoring agents, date syrup and honey were used. Sesame oil was used as the chief basis for ointment.

As previously mentioned, remedies for gastrointestinal ailments abound. For example, "When the patient's internal organs burn and he is constipated, let him drink a medicine of garlic and cumin,[26] or the pounded rind of green *il* [a plant] mixed with swine-fat." Other remedies are prescribed when "garlic, leeks, beef, pork and beer are unretained by a man, and in his belching the gall is with-

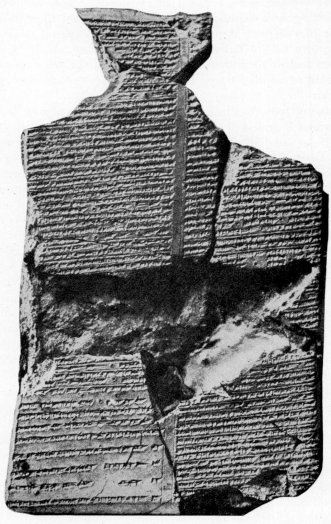

Fig. 61: Cuneiform tablet K 191. Medical compendium from the library of Ashurbanipal at Nineveh, restored from many fragments. (British Museum, London.)

held[?]." For constipation, the patient drank a mixture of green garlic and *kukru-rind* in fermented milk, followed by dates in swine-fat or oil. Garlic appears to have been used frequently in gastro-hepatic dysfunction. Another prescription is cypress cones pounded up and mixed with fermented drink. If, in addition to constipation, internal gastrointestinal inflammation prevails, a decoction of *haltappanu-plant,* sweet red *ballukku-plants,* and cypress is administered as an enema. An enema is also prescribed when a man is consti-pated after heavy eating and drinking, and his inside is "angry" *(borborygmus).*[27]

When a man's inside eats him, he is to be given *haltappanu-plant* and salt, pounded up and dissolved in water or fermented drink or plain *haltappanu, diyatu,* or *si-si.*[28] For liver complaints, garlic was prescribed,[29] or cassia in beer, or large draughts of beer, wine, or water.

Other diseases, for which prescriptions are presented, are diarrhea, anorexia, bulimia, cough, poisoning, ophthalmia, icterus, and pro-lapse of the rectum.

Venereal diseases are prescribed for, in various medical tablets, the color of the urine being observed in ascertaining the diagnosis.

The Assyrian medical texts treat of diseases pertaining to the special senses. Thus, "If a man's nose and mouth hold *foretori* . . . thou shalt roll up a linen pledget, bray salicerina, alkali [glass-worth], powdered alum . . . ami alum, sprinkle the pledget of linen without . . . mana-green, thou shalt brew five shekels of . . . thou shalt let him drink it, thou shalt reduce, bray mixed in oil let him drink and be healed."[30]

For a scorpion sting, oil of cedar mixed with various substances was advocated locally. For snake bite, the victim was urged to peel mellow roots and eat or drink them, then a potion of *si-si.*

The ancient Babylonians used a large variety of medical plants and remedial substances in their practice. V. Oefele identified 250 different medical plants, 120 mineral substances, and 180 miscel-laneous drugs among the Babylonian remedies.

Jastrow is of the opinion that animal substances in Babylonia were mostly used to drive out the demons of disease by virtue of their vile character. According to Jastrow's translation of the Ashurbanipal text (p. 141), as a general rule herbs predominated. In Assyro-Babylonian medical texts, animal substances were rarely employed and were used more as vehicles than as medicaments.[31]

Among the drugs employed were turpentine, oils, and products obtained from juniper, cypress, myrtle, cedar, cactus, and laurel trees. Resins were used, such as galbanum, myrrh, asafetida, and ambra. Other plants were camomile, mustard, windflowers, and numerous alkalies. The juices and skins of certain fruits, such as apples, lemons, oranges, and pomegranates were employed extensively as remedies. As narcotics, mandragora, opium, and hemp were used. Milk, honey, oil, and wine were used as vehicles as well as remedies.

CONJURATION AND RITUAL: While drugs were extensively used, they were accompanied by conjuration and religious ritual, both prophylactically and therapeutically. The following charm was intended to be a prophylactic or a cure for all ailments:

Conjure, O spirit of heaven! conjure, O spirit of earth!...that which is misformed, that which is diseased, that which is racked [with pain], even a diseased muscle, a constricted muscle, a swollen muscle, an aching muscle, a painful muscle, a broken muscle, an injured muscle,—conjure, O spirit of heaven! conjure, O spirit of earth! the sickness of the entrails, a sick heart, faintness of the heart, disease of the bile, headache, violent vomiting, a broken blood-vessel [?], disease of the kidneys, difficult micturation, painful sickness which cannot be removed, a dream of ill omen,—conjure, O spirit of heaven! conjure, O spirit of earth! him who is the possessor of the likeness of another, the evil face, the evil eye, the evil mouth, the evil tongue, the evil lips, the evil breath,—conjure, O spirit of heaven! conjure, O spirit of earth! the painful fever, the virulent fever, the fever which quits not a man, the fever-demon who leaves not [the body], the fever unremovable, the baleful fever—conjure, O spirit of heaven! conjure, O spirit of earth! the painful plague, the virulent plague, the plague which quits not a man, the plague-demon which leaves not [the body], the plague unremovable, the baleful plague,—conjure, O spirit of heaven! conjure, O spirit of earth! [32]

The following Assyrian incantation for toothache is particularly interesting, both from the medical and mythological points of view:

Charm. After Anu made the heavens, the heavens made the earth, the earth made the rivers, the rivers made the canals, the canals made the marsh, the marsh made the Worm. The Worm came weeping unto Shamash, Shamash came unto Ea, her tears flowing: What wilt thou give me for my food, what wilt thou give me to destroy? I will give thee dried figs and apricots. Forsooth, what are these dried figs to me, or apricots? Set me amid teeth, and let me dwell in the gums, that I may destroy the blood of the teeth, and of the gums chew their marrow. So shall I hold the latch of the door. Since thou hast said this, O Worm, may Ea smite thee with his mighty fist.

Incantation for a diseased eye:

This is for red wool, a thread thou shalt spin, tie seven knots, as thou tiest them recite the charm, bind on his sick eye. Charm. O failing eyes, O painful eyes, O eyes sundered by a dam of blood! Why do ye fail, why do ye hurt? Why has the dust of the river come nigh you, or the spathe of the date-palm whereof ye have chanced to catch the pollen which the fertilizer hath been shaking? Have I invited you, come to me? I have not invited you, come not to me, or ever the first wind, the second wind, the third wind, the fourth wind cometh to you!

Surgical Treatment: Surgical diseases were seldom treated magically, as the following correspondence of the royal physicians of the Sargonid period will show:

With regard to the patient who has a bleeding from his nose, the Rab-Mugi reports: Yesterday, towards evening, there was much hemorrhage. These dressings are not scientifically applied. They are placed upon the alae of the nose, oppress the nose, and come off when there is hemorrhage. Let them be placed within the nostrils, and then the air will be kept away, and the hemorrhage restrained. If it is agreeable to my lord, the King, I will go tomorrow and give instructions; (in the meantime) let me hear how he does!

Letters of Arad-Nana: Several letters from a certain physician, Arad-Nana (c. 681–669 B.C.)[33] dating from the seventh century B.C. and written to the king, have been discovered. This Arad-Nana is assumed to have been the court physician who was permitted by the king to treat certain members of his staff. One report states: "Bel-epus, the Babylonian magician, is very ill; let the King command that a physician come and see him."

The following report will throw some light on the professional skill of Arad-Nana.

To the King, my lord, thy servant, Arad-Nana, a hearty greeting to the King, my lord! May Adad and Gula grant health of mind and body to the King, my lord! All goes well in regard to that poor fellow whose eyes are diseased. I had applied a dressing covering his face. Yesterday, towards evening, undoing the bandage which held it [in place], I removed the dressing. There was pus upon the dressing about the size of the tip of the little finger. If any of thy gods has put his hand to the matter, that [god] must surely have given express commands. All is well. Let the heart of my lord the King be of good cheer! Within seven or eight days he will be well. [34]

Other Cuneiform Letters: The important role the physician has played in the seventh century B.C. in Mesopotamia may be seen from the following cuneiform letters, now in the British Museum.[35] A certain Kudurru wrote to King Ashurbanipal: "Ikishaaplu, the physician, whom my lord the King sent to save my life has cured me." In another letter in the British Museum, an official informs the king that a lady named Bugamillat is seriously ill and cannot eat and that the king should order a physician to visit her. According to this document, the Assyrian physician appears to have been in the service of the king.

An inscription on a clay tablet, found in the British Museum, refers to a certain astrologer who reported to the King of Synd the existence of a skin affection similar to the present skin disease known as "Baghdad boil" or "Aleppo Button": "Concerning this evil of the skin, the king, my lord, has not spoken from his heart; the sickness lasts a year; those who are sick will all recover." (Baghdad boil is still popularly believed to last for a year.)

WIDESPREAD REPUTATION OF ASSYRO-BABYLONIAN ASU

The Assyro-Babylonian *asu* was well known beyond the boundaries of the valley of the Euphrates. The Hittite emperor Hattusil (about 1280 B.C.) sent a request to the Babylonian king to send an exorcist and a physician. In granting the request of the Hittite emperor, the king picked out one of the best of his medical talents. The Babylonian healer was away from his native land a few years. King Tushratta of Mitanni sent the wonder-working statue of the goddess, Ishthar of Nineveh, to the court of Pharaoh Amenophis III who was sick. The statue was accompanied by a court physician. Thus it is seen that even the Egyptian monarchs availed themselves of the medical knowledge of the Babylonians.

It is apparent from the texts cited that there was no scarcity of physicians in Assyro-Babylonia. Both the medical texts and magical series show that the medical profession was well organized. This appears to contradict the statement of the historian, Herodotus:

They bring out their sick to the market-place, for they have no physicians; then those who pass by the sick person confer with him about the disease, to discover whether they have themselves been afflicted with the same disease as the sick person, or have seen others so afflicted: thus the passers-by confer with him, and advise him to have recourse to the same treatment as that by which they escaped a similar disease, or as they have known to cure others. And they are not allowed to pass by a sick person in silence, without inquiring into the nature of his distemper.

(This scarcity of physicians, at the time Herodotus visited Babylonia, may well have been due to wars and other local conditions.)

Montaigne goes so far as to state that "the entire nation was skilled in medicine." Assyro-Babylonian medicine, of course, was a branch of general culture. What the patient desired was not theory but the practical experience of those who had coped successfully with similar diseases.

These is no record that the Assyro-Babylonians brought their indisposed people into the temples to be treated as was customary among the ancient Egyptians and Greeks who were taken to the temples of the gods for ablution of their sins.

The practice of attending the sick in open-air places seems to have been a custom, not only among the Babylonians of the fifth century B.C., but also among the Jews of Palestine as late as the second century A.D. The mild climate of the Middle East was most conducive to recovery.

INFLUENCE OF ASSYRO-BABYLONIAN MEDICINE

It is clear from the texts in our possession that, although the trend of Assyro-Babylonian medicine toward magic detracted much from its science, enough was accomplished in practical medicine to influence posterity. Out of primitive notions arose a real medical science. When the ailment could be located and the natural remedy determined, a more materialistic rational view of therapy was taken. Many herbs and drugs, originally used for supernatural reasons, when tried and found effective lost their magical significance and were viewed in a natural light. It is curious to note that magical formulas and amulets were employed in ailments considered incurable, such as epilepsy and snake bite, but in curable disease, recourse was had to natural remedies.

References and Notes

1. Neuburger, M.: History of Medicine. Oxford University Press, London, 1910, p. 14.
2. Thompson, R. C.: The Devil and Evil Spirit of Babylonia and Assyria. London, 1903-1904, Vol. IV, 746.
3. Ibid., Vol. IV, p. 741.
4. Ragozin, Z. A.: Chaldea. G. P. Putman's Sons, New York, 1901, pp. 156-261.
5. For a more detailed description, see "The Romance of Medicine" by the present author: F. A. Davis Company, Phila. 1944-1945, pp. 228-257.
6. Ibid,. pp. 253-289.
7. Ezekiel 21:26.
8. Leix, A.: Ciba Symposia, 1940.
9. See New Testament.: Matthew 2:7.
10. Utukku series: Tablet III, Vol. 1, 65. Thompson, R. C.: The Devil and Evil Spirit of Babylonia and Assyria. London, 1903-1904, Vol. I, p. 9.

11. Castiglione: A History of Medicine. New York, 1941, p. 41.
12. II Kings 1:3.
13. Gordon, B. L.: The Romance of Medicine. F. A. Davis Company, Phila., 1944, p. 520.
14. The earlier medical tablets belong to the time when the kingdom was divided into two parts, a northern, called "Akkad" and a southern, "Sumer." At the extreme north was Assur, and between them was Chaldea.
15. These tablets, interpreted by Oefele, Sayce, Layard, and Thompson, present a complete medical work in serial form. One such composition is made up of twelve tablets detailing a series of remedies of magic medicine. It begins with the words with which the conjuror enters the house of the sick one. An obstetrical compendium is composed of twenty-five tablets and begins with the words: "When the woman is sick."
16. Dawson, W.: Magician and Leech. London.
17. Assyrian Medical Texts. Luzac, London, 1926. Assyrian Herbal. Luzac, London, 1924. Sect. Medical History, 17:1, 1923-24, 1929, 1925-1926.
18. Breasted, A.: Preface to Edwin Smith Papyrus.
19. Kuchler, F.: Beitr. und Kentnis der Assyr. Bab. Medizin, 2:22; 1:55 ff.
20. Ibid., 1:61; 2:26-27.
21. "The Devil and Evil Spirit of Babylonia and Assyria," Vol II, 160. Cuneiform texts, Bab. Tab., 1903.
22. Kuchler, F.: Beitr. und Kentnis der Assyr. Bab. Medizin, 2:14-16.
23. Ibid,. 2:5; 1:31.
24. Ibid., 1:32.
25. Ibid., 1:3; 1:13.
26. Ibid., 1:23; 2:17-18.
27. Ibid., 2:7, 11; 10-11; 15-16; 17-20.
28. Ibid., 1:5; 1, ff.
29. Ibid., 1:53; 1:70; 1:55; 1:71.
30. Dawson, W.: The Beginnings in Egypt and Assyria. Paul B. Hoeber, Inc., New York, 1930, pp. 62, 65.
31. Jastrow, M.: The Medicine of Babylonia and Assyria. Proc. Roy. Soc. Med. 7:158, 141, 1913-1914.
32. Sayce, A. H.: Hibbert Lectures. Williams and Norgate, Edinburgh and London, 1888, pp. 329-330.
33. Many of his writings have been preserved, including his prescriptions and letters.
34. Breasted, A.: The Edwin Smith Papyrus, 1:476.
35. Harper: Assyrian and Babylonian Letters. London, 1909, No. 392. (See Thompson, R. C.: Late Babylonian Letters. London, 1906, No. 114.)

8

Medicine of Ancient Egypt

It is difficult to draw a parallel between Babylonian and Egyptian medicine; while it is true that both medical systems were associated with religious mysticism and priestly magic, they essentially differed one from the other. The Babylonians were more systematic in their studies, applying their knowledge of mathematics and astronomy to their medical erudition. The Egyptians, on the other hand, were compilers of knowledge and folklore, frequently failing to discriminate between fact and fancy. They gathered their medical knowledge from the old traditions of their own people as well as from the Nubians that preceded them.

They differed also in the method of treatment. The Babylonians treated ailments symptomatically, such as, for example, "If a man's head has a scab, thou shalt do so and so," or "if a man's teeth are painful, thou shalt apply this or that remedy." The Egyptians, on the other hand, applied their remedies to the disease itself. Thus the prescription reads: "For driving away ophthalmia, administer such and such a drug." In ordering a drug, the Babylonians were satisfied in mentioning the name of the drug, leaving the quantity to the judgment of the healer. On the other hand, the Egyptians stipulated in their prescriptions the quantity of each drug. The records left by the Babylonians were generally brief and inscribed on clay tablets; those of the Egyptians were long and written on papyrus scrolls.

EARLY EGYPTIAN PHYSICIANS

King-Physicians: If the Egyptian priest-historian, Manetho, can be believed, medicine was cultivated in Egypt as early as the fourth

of medicine. His reputation as a healing god did not equal that of Serapis, to whom divine honors were paid by the Egyptians and Greeks as a celestial healer, and to whose memory many temples were dedicated.[6]

Priests: The chief methods of treatment employed by the priests were magic and divination. The priests were assisted by the pastophori, or image bearers, who held a subordinate office in the order of the priesthood. To them was assigned the application of the remedies prescribed in the sacred volumes of Thoth. Moses refers to the priests and magi in the seventh and eighth chapters of Exodus when he mentions "the wise men, the sorcerers, and the magicians."

The office of the Egyptian priest-physician was hereditary. He was particularly concerned with botanical drugs, but his pharmaceutical remedies extended also to the animal and mineral kingdoms. Squill was prescribed in dropsical conditions as a diuretic, and an iron salt was employed to restore the tone of the system.

Kings' Interest in Medicine: Early Egyptian kings, like the Ptolemies of later days, were keenly interested in medicine. King Nachepsus of Sais (1700 B.C.), grandfather of Pharaoh Necho (mentioned in the Bible),[7] according to Galen and Pliny, wrote on medicine. Galen relates that this monarch was the first to observe the marvelous value of green jasper, a stone which, when engraved with a dragon "with rays" and hung around the neck, was a capital cure for digestive diseases. Galen's experiments with the stone showed him that the dragon face was not necessary; it worked as well without the dragon. If Galen had experimented a little longer, he might have discovered that his patients would have recovered without his green jasper stone altogether.

Imhotep: The most celebrated physician of ancient Egypt was Imhotep[8] (I-em-hetep, "he that comest in peace") (c. 2980 B.C.). He flourished during the reign of King Djoser of the third dynasty. Because of his medical fame, he was deified, like Aesculapius of Greece, and became the patron god of Egyptian medicine, "whose protection of life was dealt out to all men" and "who gave a son to him who had none." The hermetic literature attributes to him great healing powers. Sanctuaries and sanatoriums were erected in his honor at Memphis. His promotion to a full deity occurred about 525 B.C. when Egypt was conquered by the Persians. He then replaced Nefertem to form with Ptah and Sechmet the great triad of Memphis. Jamieson B. Hurry notes the location, the day and month, and approximately the year of his birth (3000 B.C.) and gives the name of his parents and his activities. Imhotep occupied the position of grand vizier. He was an architect, sage, astronomer, physician, and scribe.

Discoveries of Egyptian University Expedition: In 1930, the Egyptian University Expedition discovered a stele whereon is mentioned the name of a high priest and those of his father and mother. His mother was described as "chief physician"—perhaps the first woman of the old kingdoms to occupy such a position. The same expedition

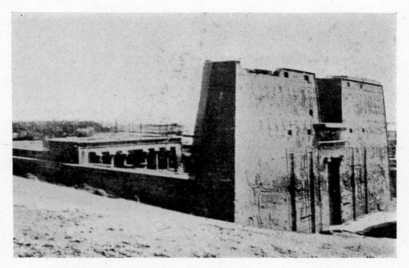

Fig. 65: Temple of Edfu. Portions of this temple are supposed to have been built by Imhotep. (Caton.)

discovered that there was a high priest named "Ra-Ouer," who occupied the position of barber to the King Neferika-re (c. 27 B.C.); two flint razors were found in his tomb.

EARLY EGYPTIAN CONCEPT OF ETIOLOGY

As an indication of the early Egyptian concept of the etiology of disease, a letter from a husband to his deceased wife, attached to a small image of her, discovered during the latter part of the last century, is of much interest. The husband upbraids his departed wife's spirit for having afflicted him with disease and reproachfully calls to mind his kindness to her during her life and illness. This document[9] has been reproduced in Chapter 5.

EGYPTIAN MEDICAL DOCUMENTS

The papyrus on which the Egyptian medical documents were written was obtained from a tall weed which grew in ancient Egypt but which is now extinct. The medical texts are written in hieratic, the priestly script (hier-"sacred"), since medicine was both a sacred and a secret science, knowledge of which was confined to the priestly caste.

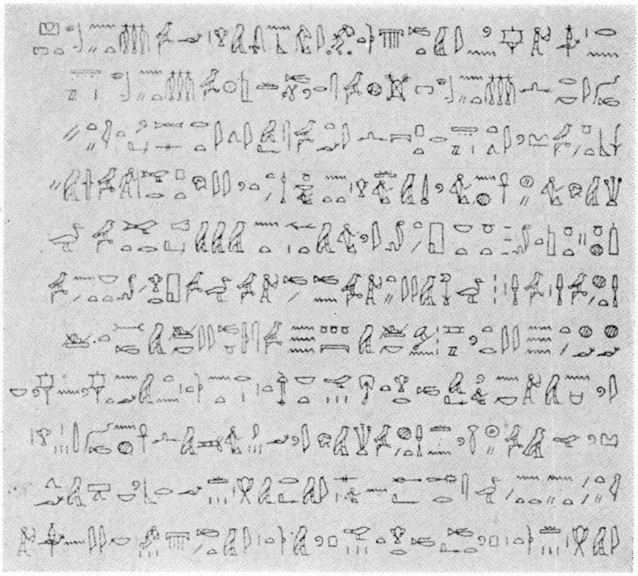

Fig. 66: An Egyptian incantation for warding off an epidemic. (Breasted, J. H.: The Edwin Smith Surgical Papyrus. Oriental Institute of University of Chicago, Vol. II, Plate XVIIIa.)

The two most important documents, the Edwin Smith and Ebers Papyri were discovered about the same time in the year 1862. In 1895, scientific papers concerning these manuscripts began to appear. Dawson is of the opinion that these documents are a miscellaneous collection with extracts from at least forty different sources. The contents deal mainly with prescriptions of plants and drugs, the methods of their administration, and the quantity of each ingredient. Only one of the papyri (the Edwin Smith Surgical Papyrus) may lay great claim to scientific attributes.

The papyri date from 2000 to 1700 B.C. and are perhaps transcriptions of original texts written as long as a thousand years before. The papyri are named after the discoverer, the donor, or after the place where they were discovered.

Kahun Papyrus: The oldest of these is the Kahun Papyrus (fragment) discovered in 1889 by Sir Flinders Petri. It is sometimes known

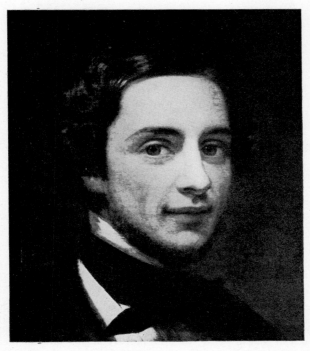

Fig. 67: Edwin Smith (1822-1906). Edwin Smith was born in Connecticut in the year that Campollion first deciphered the Egyptian hieroglyphics. Smith was perhaps the first American to learn the Egyptian language. He studied hieroglyphics in London and Paris. In 1858, he moved to Luxor, Egypt, where he remained for nearly twenty years and where he acquired the papyrus that bears his name (1862). He knew enough hieroglyphics to recognize that this document dealt with medical subjects. He made no effort to publish it while he was alive. On his death, his daughter presented the papyrus to the New York Historical Society. In 1920, the Society requested Henry James Breasted to translate it. (From a painting by F. Anelli, 1847; Courtesy of New York Historical Society.)

as the "London Papyrus" because of its location at the Edward College Library of the University of London.

The Kahun Papyrus contains thirty-four gynecological sections dealing with uterine disorders, dysmenorrhea, prolapsus uteri, vaginal diseases, scanty lactation, pregnancy, sex determination, and cessation of lactation in nursing women. It was written in the twelfth or thirteenth dynasty (c. 2000–1800 B.C.). The prescriptions are essentially magical in character.

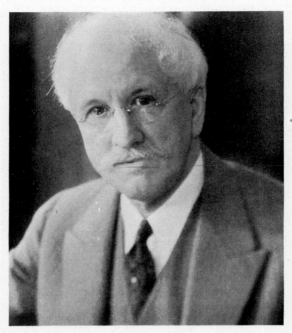

Fig. 68: Henry James Breasted (1865-1935). Henry James Breasted, American orientalist, was born at Rockford, Ill. He was first interested in theology, and in 1886, entered the Theological Seminary of Chicago. He also attended lectures in Yale and in Berlin. In 1894, he gave up the study of theology in preference to Egyptology, and he was appointed Assistant Egyptologist at the University of Chicago. Nine years later, he became Professor of Egyptology and Oriental History and Director of the Oriental Museum of the University of Chicago. The same year, he directed an archaeological exploration in Egypt and in the Sudan. In 1919, with the aid of the Rockefeller Foundation, he organized the Oriental Institute of the University of Chicago. As director, he led a number of expeditions in Egypt, the Near East, and Palestine. Among his numerous contributions to oriental science was the translation and publication of the Edwin Smith Papyrus in 1920. (Courtesy of the Chicago Oriental Institute Museum.)

Edwin Smith Surgical Papyrus: By far the most important Egyptian medical document is the Edwin Smith Surgical Papyrus. It was compiled about the beginning of the new Egyptian kingdom in the seventeenth century B.C., from an original text which was perhaps 1000 years older. The text is written on both sides of the papyrus.

The subject matter on the front side deals systematically with forty-eight different wounds. It gives the case histories, discusses the diagnoses and treatment in a systematic manner, and comments upon the nature of the wounds and the organs affected in conjunction with the anatomy and physiology. Rational methods of treatment are suggested in treating wounds inflicted by human agencies.

Originally this surgical papyrus was approximately fifteen feet long and one foot wide and dealt with surgery of the entire body. The present text is abruptly interrupted when it reaches the breast. There is evidence that the scribe copied his manuscript from two older works and, in a number of cases, added glossaries which furnish additional information on the idioms, text, and terminology. The treatment in general is rational and not magical. In his brilliant analysis of the Edwin Smith Surgical Papyrus, the late Professor James H. Breasted expresses the opinion that the Edwin Smith Papyrus is the earliest known truly scientific writing. The surgical papyrus was purchased at Luxor in 1886 by Edwin Smith, an American, who presented it to the New York Historical Society where it is now exhibited.

Ebers Papyrus: Next in importance, the largest and probably the best known document of the early history of Egyptian medicine, is the Ebers Papyrus.[10] The Ebers Papyrus begins, "I came forth from On (Heliopolis)," but there is a contradiction in the very next line, which reads, "I came forth from Sais." Evidently the compiler of this papyrus made extracts from works produced by sages of the two great medical temple libraries.

It was compiled about the year 1550 B.C., perhaps from several other medical works as much as 1000 years older. One prescription is associated with a queen of the sixth dynasty indicating its older origin. Another passage points the origin of the papyrus to be about 3400 B.C. The best evidence of the origin of the papyrus is philological; the language of the papyrus elucidates the fact that the author had before him several earlier works. Dawson pointed out that the fact that an ancient work claims a still earlier date is by no means sufficient proof of its great antiquity, for ancients were accustomed to ascribe books to an earlier origin in order to enhance the value of the work in the estimation of the public that believed the older the work, the better.

The Ebers Papyrus comprises about 800 prescriptions arranged in sections in accordance with organs and diseases. It gives directions for the use of the drugs and the quantity to be given. Some prescriptions offer explanations and comments on the remedies prescribed.

Only in a few instances, were the symptoms pointed out. As a rule there are no descriptions; the diseases only are named.

The text in the original roll is twenty meters long, covering 100 large columns. In the present printed form, it comprises 877 prescriptions. The text is interspersed with incantations and charms and closes with a short section on surgery. The names of the diseases have remained only partly identified up to the present time. On the back of the roll is a calendar which proved useful for the study of Egyptian chronology.

Clement of Alexandria perhaps includes this papyrus among the six books on medicine which are included in the forty-two hermetic books of the Egyptians.[11] The Ebers Papyrus was found by an Arab in the year 1862 at Thebes. It was lying between the legs of a well preserved mummy. The finder subsequently sold it in 1872 to George Ebers, a German Egyptologist. The latter deposited it in the museum of the University of Leipzig.

That the origin of Egyptian medicine is bound up with religion and magic may be seen from the prologue to the Ebers Papyrus:

Here begins the book of the preparation of medicines for all parts of the body of a person. I was born in Heliopolis with the priests of Het-Aat, the lords of protection, the kings of eternity and of salvation. I have my origin in Sais with the maternal goddesses who have protected me. The Lord of All has given me words to drive away the diseases of all the gods and mortal sufferings of every kind. There are chapters for this my head, for this my neck, for these my arms, for this my flesh, and for these my limbs, to punish the supreme beings who allow disease to enter into this my flesh, placing a spell on these my limbs, so that (disease) enters into my flesh, into this my head, into these my arms, into this my body, into these my limbs, whenever Ra has taken mercy and has said, "I protect him against his enemies." It is his guide Hermes, who gave him the word, who created the books and gave glory to those who know everything and to the physicians who follow him to decipher that which is dark. He whom the god loves is made alive; I am the one whom the god loves, me he makes alive, to pronounce words in the preparations of medicine for all parts of the body of a person who is sick. As it should be a thousand times. This the book of the healing of all diseases. May Isis heal me as she healed Horus of all his pains which his brother, Seth, inflicted on him because he killed his father, Osiris. I, Isis, thou great enchantress, heal me, deliver me from all wicked, evil, typhonic influence, from the demonic and mortal diseases and impurities at all times which are precipitated upon me, just as thou didst free and save thy son Horus. [12]

The Ebers Papyrus mentions the heart, vessels, liver, spleen, kidneys, uterus, and bladder. The blood vessels are said to arise from the heart. Other vessels are described: some carrying air, some mucus, two going to the right ear carrying the breath of life, and two to the left ear conveying the breath of death.[13]

The Ebers Papyrus concludes with a brief chapter on tumors. Tumors are to be palpated to ascertain if they fluctuate. If they do,

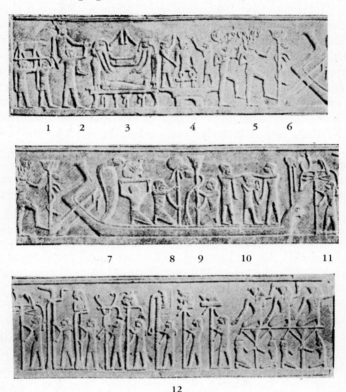

Fig. 69: These three figures deal with the mystery of birth. (From Stele C. in the Louvre.) 1: Animal to be sacrificed. 2: The Tikenou. 3: Isis and Nephthys making incantations. 4: Reconstitution of the body. 5: Crowned dancers. 6: Flaying of the sacrificed animal. 7: The uraeus (?) crown in the barque. 8: The Symbol of the Tikenou under the skin. 9: The skin exhibited. 10: The dead Osiris reborn. 11: Anubis (?) and the shedshed. 12: The gods hail the reborn Osiris.

they are considered to consist of fluid or fat, and are treated by the knife, phlebotomy or cautery. But there is one tumor, the most terrible of all, which becomes covered with pustules, discolors the skin, "makes figures," and causes sharp pains; to such a tumor say, "It is a tumor of the god, Chensu; do nothing at all to it."[14]

Other Papyri. *Hearst Papyrus:* Another important Egyptian medical document is the one known as the "Hearst Papyrus." It was discovered near Deir-el-Ballas in upper Egypt in 1899 by an Arab. He sold it in 1901 to the late Dr. Reisner of Harvard University who was excavating in the district. It was afterwards acquired by Mrs. Phoebe Hearst for the University of California. Because the Arab kept it tightly bundled up in a head cloth, three columns of the text were badly damaged, but fifteen closely written columns are left in a fairly good condition. Its medical content in the main resembles that of the Ebers Papyrus, thus indicating that the material used in both papyri are taken from the same sources. Both of these documents were produced at about the same time. This papyrus is divided into 260 sections. The arrangement of the material shows that the author of the papyrus intended his work to be used by students and young practitioners as a formulary.

London Medical Papyrus: The London Medical Papyrus was written in about 1600 B.C. It bears resemblance to the other papyri, but is probably much older. It contains more magical treatment. It belongs to the latter part of the eighteenth dynasty, and contains this statement, "This medical book was found at night in the hall of the Temple at Tebmut in the sanctuary of the goddess, by priests of the temple. Behold! the darkness of night enveloped the earth, but the moon cast her beams upon all pages of this book, and it was brought to the treasury of His Majesty King Khufu."

Brugsch Papyrus: Still another medical work of a later origin is the Brugsch, or the Berlin, Medical Papyrus. The text of this document is divided into 204 sections. On the back roll, there are passages which deal with matters of sterility and prenatal diagnosis of sex. The Berlin Papyrus dates from the nineteenth dynasty and contains a statement that the content of the document "was found in an ancient script in a coffer with writing materials under the feet of the god, Anuba, in Leontopolis, in the reign of His Majesty the Egyptian King Usaphis."

Leyden, Turin and Westcar Papyri: To the above-mentioned documents may be added a few minor medical works, such as the Leyden, Turin, and Westcar Papyri.

Thanks to the dry soil of Egypt, the medical documents, which led many investigators to believe that the land of the Nile is the original home of medicine, have been preserved.

Queen Mentuhotep's Pharmacy: In the Berlin Museum is found Queen Mentuhotep's (c. 3000 B. c.) medicine chest made of palm fiber and containing five straight alabaster vases and one serpentine-shaped vase. The latter was probably used for magical purposes.[15] The vases contained various substances, perhaps drugs, to be dispensed among her sick subjects. Warren Dawson believes that the

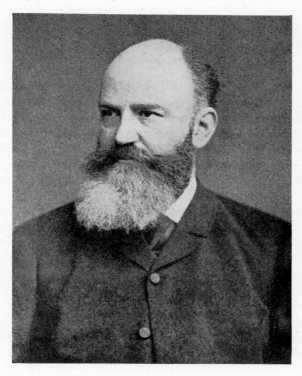

Fig. 70: George Ebers (1837-1898). George Ebers devoted much time to the study of Egypt and her hieroglyphics, and he took delight in making that country the scene of his novels. He made several journeys there; and on one of his trips, he discovered the valuable papyrus that has been named after him. In his first novel, the heroine is the daughter of King Amasis. "Die Schwestern" ("The Sisters") carries the reader back to the year 64 B.C. Its locale is Memphis, and the scene alternates between the temple of Serapis and the castle of the Ptolemies. "Der Kaiser," in which the heroes are Hadrian and his favorite, Antonius, is laid in Alexandria, midway between the East and West, and shows how Christianity made its way into the king's home. In "Arachne" (1897), the author returns once more to Egyptian life, taking his readers among the weavers of the Nile Delta and to Alexandria and the art-loving Pergamos.

contents of the chest were used for cosmetic purposes. Prescriptions have been found in the chest for painting the eyes and for restoring fallen hair. This indicates that the chest was a sort of traveling pharmacy employed by the royal family when attending to their subjects. Among other formulas were perfumes for keeping the skin soft and smooth, for improving the complexion, and for perfuming the female genitalia.

Divine Origin of Formulas: Many formulas in the Ebers Papyrus carry statements of divine origin. One headache cure composed of wormwood, juniper berries, and honey, to be applied externally to the head, is prefaced by the statement that it was "made by the goddess, Isis, herself for the god Ra, himself," in order to drive away the pains in his head.

From the medical papyri, it is apparent that an important element in the healing power of Egyptian medicine was the suggestive force incorporated in the cures rather than the medical value of the prescriptions. The beliefs that the formulas had been recited under supernatural circumstances, that the prescriptions had been prepared and used by the gods, and that supernatural influences had been invoked during the preparation of the drugs and during their administration, were no doubt of great pyschotherapeutic value.

Evaluation of Egyptian Medicine: Pliny asserts that the Egyptians were the founders of medicine. He even credits them with postmortem studies for the purpose of investigating the nature of disease. Clement of Alexandria maintains that Moses was educated in all the wisdom of the Egyptians, thus conveying the idea that Hebrew medicine might trace its origin to Egypt. The same author states that the medical science of the Egyptians was contained in forty-two Hermetic books whose authorship is ascribed to the god Thoth (Hermes of the Greeks). Herodotus related that medical specialists were abundant in the land of the Pharaohs.[16]

This medical evaluation pertains perhaps to the old and middle kingdoms when the knowledge of medicine was more or less scientific; for notwithstanding the frequent association of medicine with religion and magic, the therapeutics were rational. During the new kingdom and in still later periods, medicine received a setback and again became dominated by magic.

Reading the two principal medical documents of ancient Egypt, one is struck by the fact that the Ebers Papyrus, dealing with internal ailments, attributes diseases to supernatural causes and resorts to religion and magic for their treatment. On the other hand, the Edwin Smith Papyrus, dealing with surgical diseases patent to the eye and healed by skilled hands, ascribes surgical ailments to natural causes, such as injury and external influences. A similar distinction was made by the Greeks. Homeric surgery was devoid of occult elements; the treatment consisted of natural methods. The classification of medicine into "supernatural" and "natural" prevailed down to the Middle Ages. There is a similar division in the Talmud; diseases are classified into those caused by human agencies, *bidei-adam* (natural causes) and those inflicted by the hand of Providence, *bidei-shamayim*.

EGYPTIAN HEALING GODS

Thoth: The Egyptians brought a number of deities into close relationship with medicine. First among the healing gods of Egypt was the moongod Thoth (Duhit or Hermes). According to mythology, Thoth cured Horus from the sting of a scorpion; and in the struggle between Horus and Seth, he treated the wounds of both. In later times, he became identified with Hermes Trismegistus, the master of secret science, the discoverer of reckoning and measurements, and the founder of religious and scientific writings, hence the founder of medical science. He particularly specialized in diseases of the eye, the most common ailment of Egypt. Thoth was symbolized by a dog-headed man and by the ibis. To him was ascribed the discovery of an enema, his invention being based on the observation of the ibis who injects sea water into its rectum with its long beak.

Neith: The goddess Neith was considered the patroness of the physicians and the helper of women in childbirth. She had the reputation of possessing the power of bringing pestilence and other grave disasters to the land through the winds of the torrid desert. She was also credited with the power of turning away evil demons from sleeping persons. Her temple was in Sais. She was symbolized by a figure of a lion.

Isis: Another Egyptian healing divinity was the wonder-working Isis (earth), whose temples were at Koptos (upper Egypt) and at Anubis (lower Egypt). She was considered a great enchantress. Her motto was, "Bring life to him who is no longer living."

Ra, Seth, and Sechmet: The sungod Ra was the discoverer of medicine. The god, Seth, had the function of spreading as well as healing epidemic diseases. He was the special incarnation of a malignant spirit. Sechmet was another famous goddess and she specialized in gynecology. She was court physician to King Sehura of the old kingdom. Her slogan was, "Sechmet is, for me, life."

Lack of Immunity of Gods: The Egyptian gods were not exempted from disease. Isis herself suffered from an abscess of the breast after the birth of Shu and Tefnut. Ra was troubled from the effect of a serpent bite in his heel cured by Isis. Horus had dysentery and anal weakness. Seth and Horus inflicted each other with wounds which were treated by Thoth. Indeed the skygod himself saw his eyes— the sun and the moon—affected by sudden diseases which he attributed to the attack of an evil spirit, and this was one of the numerous ways in which the appearance of an eclipse was explained.

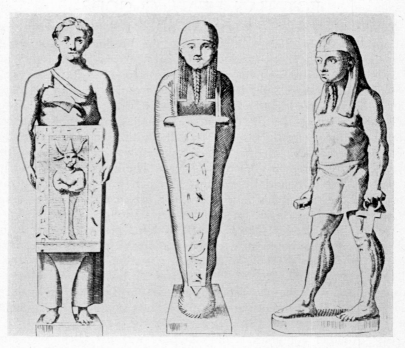

Fig. 71: Renaissance representation of ancient Egyptian healing divinities. *Left:* The Egyptian goddess Isis was of human form. She was the devoted sister-wife of Osiris (at *right*), and she was the mother of Horus. Isis was known for her magical powers of healing and protection. She is often depicted as watching the body of her murdered spouse Osiris, who was killed by his brother Seth. She cured the god Ra from snakebite. Among the Greeks, the cult of Isis spread with that of Serapis during the third century B.C. Horus, according to Greek legend, was the father of Apollo, the god of medicine. Apis Conditus (*middle* figure) is referred to in the present text. (From an old print.)

The literature of the temples preserved prescriptions used for the indisposition of the ailing gods. A remedy of this kind had been composed by the invalid Ra. Thus it was commonplace for the highest beings to be troubled with the ills of the common folk.

PRIEST-PHYSICIANS

Schools: The physician belonged to the priestly caste which was entrusted with all learning as well as religious worship. Medicine, in common with all branches of knowledge, was taught in the priestly schools which were connected with the temples. The most celebrated schools were On, Sais, Memphis, Thebes, and Letopolis. These houses

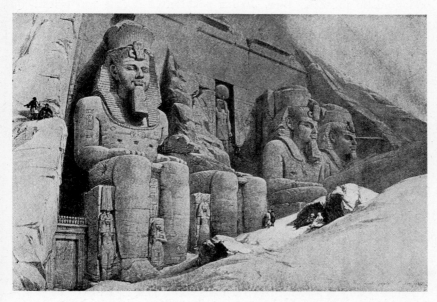

Fig. 72: The great temple of Aboo Simbel. (Lithography by L. Haghe from drawing by David Roberts, R. A. [From Roberts, D.: Egypt and Nubia].)

of learning were under the direct supervision of the learned priest-hood who were the acknowledged leaders of civilized Egypt in antiquity and for centuries later. To be learned in the wisdom of the Egyptians meant to be in possession of all knowledge.

Sacred Libraries: The sacred libraries of the Egyptian temples were the depositories of lists of diseases and their alleged cures. Numerous prescriptions were found in the libraries of Heliopolis (the Hall of Rolls) and in the temple of Ptah at Memphis. In the library of the temple of Edfu, an inscription was found referring to books that teach of abating the causes of disease.

Concept of Divine Intervention: Egyptian medical science never completely suppressed the primitive notion of direct divine intervention in case of illness; the great scourge of plague and other epidemics were recognized as sent from the gods. The historian, Manetho, mentions that the plague which devastated his country in the reign of Semempse was thought to be connected with the great sins committed by man. The Egyptians did not produce an Alcameon, a Pythagoras, and certainly not an Hippocrates.

Duties of Priests: In Egypt, science, religion, and magic were not antagonistic to each other. In his position of doctor and priest, the physician discharged duties outside his professional field. He inspected sacrificial animals and passed judgment upon other ecclesiastic matters.

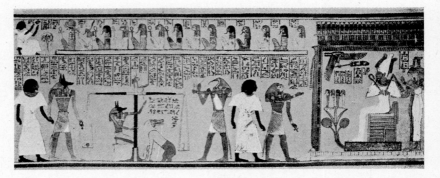

Fig. 73: Anubis, with the head of a jackal, leads the deceased into Osiris' judgment hall. His heart is weighed in a scale by Anubis to Ammit—who is one-third crocodile, one-third lion, and one-third hippopotamus—with the feather of truth in the other tray. The ibis-headed Thoth, the scribe of the gods, records the result. If the weighing proves favorable, the deceased is brought in by Horus to Osiris, who sits on his throne by the river in the Other World. Behind him stand Isis and Neftys. On the lotus blossom before him stand the children of Horus. The inscriptions contain (from the *left*) the prayers of the deceased, as he is brought into the judgment hall, Thoth's notes, and Horus' report to Osiris. In the small register above, the deceased appears kneeling before the gods, headed by Ra. (From the Hunefers Papyrus in the British Museum.)

As minister of the gods, the priest-physician was supposed to know better than any other person how to protect the people against disease and how to cure disease. He had an exclusive monopoly on magicomedical cures as revealed by the gods. The observation of disease and the supposed knowledge of the names of forces to be adjured or driven off, were acquired from early medical records attributed to six books of medicine by Hermes Trismegistus. These were later ascribed to Thoth as the god who invented the medical formulas against disease.

ANIMISM

Clement of Alexandria states that when any part of the body was sick the demon to which that member belonged was invoked. This tends to explain the traditional view of the Egyptian on the nature of disease. Always it was the work of demons, spirits, jinns, ghouls, vampires, or spirits of the dead, which insinuated themselves into the patient through the nostrils, mouth, or ears and devoured the vital substance.

Out of such primitive notions, however, arose a real medical science. When the ailment could be located and its nature roughly determined, a more naturalistic view was taken. Many herbs and drugs that were originally used for magical reasons, once they had been found to be actually effective therapeutically, lost their superstitious significances and were viewed as natural remedies. It is interesting to note, that in the papyri, natural remedies were employed for the more curable diseases while magical formulas and amulets were reserved for those that were harder to cope with, such as epilepsy, snake bite, and scorpion sting.

Even in these latter conditions, the formulas recited for such purposes were not purely mystical; although since mystery is the very essence of magic, foreign words and outlandish names occurred in them by preference. The magician often recited a mythical case in which a god had been afflicted with a disease similar to that of the patient and had finally recovered. A number of such tales had been told of Horus who was usually treated by some device of his mother, Isis, who was regarded as a great enchantress. The mere recitation of such, or similar, cases was supposed to be effective. Such magical words held great psychological values. Almost unlimited power was supposed to be inherent in a mere word. The demon could be directly invoked and commanded to come forth. The gods were often threatened with privation or even destruction if they refused to aid the healer. The Egyptian found little impiety in the use of profanity against the divine name. For instance, a magician declared that, if his spell proved ineffective, he would cast fire into Mendes and burn up Osiris. The verbal spells were usually accompanied by some manual performance, such as, for example, the tying of a magical knot or the preparation of some amulet. Particular importance was attached to the sevenfold knot. Often the formula was written down on a strip of papyrus tied around the neck of the person whom it was intended to cure. Beads and all kinds of amulets were infused with magical power so as to appear potent to those who wore them.

The accumulation of the magic formulas, the conjuring recitations of the magi, and the experience of the physician were mixed and at an early period compiled in "handbooks" for future reference and to be used in the schools for aspiring students of the medical arts. These developed in the course of time into a rather extensive literature, a considerable part of which was preserved in the papyri manuscripts. They were written down during the first half of the new kingdom about the middle of the second millennium. The textual material, however, is considerably older, some of it reaching as far back as the beginning of the pyramid era.

EARLY EGYPTIAN SPECIALISTS

As early as the period of the pyramid builders (about the middle of the third millennium), one reads of eye specialists who confined their practice to the visual organs. Ocular disease has evidently prevailed in epidemic form in the valley of the Nile from time immemorial. Bowel specialists ("shepherds of the anus") who concerned themselves with the egestive faculty, assisted in the administration of enemas.

The stele of Pepi-ankb (Ery), discovered by H. Junker in 1926, when excavating in the empire cemetery near the great pyramid of Gizah in the tomb of a court physician of the sixth dynasty (c. 2600 B.C.) (referred to at the beginning of this chapter), reads, "the physician of the belly of the Pharaoh, the guardian of the anus (i.e., he who has supervision of the clysters and purges), the surveyor of the Pharaoh, the chief magician who prepares the bm. (an important remedy) and knows the liquids of ntnt.t. (bladder)." This passage adequately demonstrates that 2000 years before Herodotus, Egyptians specialized in various branches of medicine.[17]

There was the dentist who filled cavities and provided patients with durable dentures. In a grave dating to about the pyramid era, a skull was found which presents evidence of the drainage of an abscess at the root of a first molar. Another skull exhibits two teeth skillfully tied together with gold wire. Thus the statement of Herodotus that the Egyptians were specializing in the various fields of medicine applies not only to the time of his visit to Egypt but even as far back as the days of the pyramid construction. One record refers to a certain doctor "who knows the hidden invisible disease (internist)." During the time of Herodotus, Egypt was swarming "with medical practitioners; some undertake to cure diseases of the eye, others of the teeth, others of the head, others of the intestines and some others which are not localized."

POLITICAL HISTORY OF EGYPT

The era of the highest medical development was about 2000 years B.C., as is evidenced from the Ebers and Brugsch Papyri. By the time that the land of the Nile was opened to the Greeks (about 700 B.C.), Egyptian medicine was on the decline.[18]

There has been a tendency among writers to appreciate Egyptian medicine as if the land of the Nile passed through a short period of history and as if the Egyptians were a homogeneous people located in a small territory. It is indeed idle to speak of the Egyptians as a whole, with reference to any kind of culture. The political history of ancient Egypt shows the country divided into two kingdoms, often at war with each other, and dominated by kings belonging to different races, worshipping various gods, and speaking different languages.

Chronological Outline of Egyptian Dynasties: A brief chronological outline will show how erroneous such a view is and may help to understand the status of ancient Egyptian medicine.

1. Predynastic: Covering up to 3400 B.C. and including the paleolithic, neolithic, and chalcolithic (copper and stone-using) periods.

2. Old kingdom: Beginning with the first dynasty, including the great pyramid age (2900–2750 B.C., or fourth dynasty), and ending in 2430 B.C.

3. Middle kingdom: Including the eleventh and twelfth dynasties (2160–1788 B.C.).

4. The Eighteenth dynasty: The new kingdom and the first empire (after 1580 B.C.). This lasted for 500 years, until a century after the fall of Troy, and until the death, in 1094 B.C., of the last of the Rameses.

5. Begins with the conquest of Egypt by Persia when Sais was overpowered by the Persian conqueror, Cambyses who ordered the destruction of the school of Sais. King Darius I, however, called the high priest of Asis, who also was a physician, to rebuild the great institution of learning, which he fully equipped. Many students of noble birth who had been dispersed, were brought back to the school, and students of the lower strata of society, who had previously been welcomed by the Egyptian rulers, were rejected. The next conqueror was Alexander the Great (322 B.C.) who was succeeded for the next 300 years by the liberal Ptolemies who ruled until Egypt became a province of Rome.

Available Records: The written records of Egypt go back to about 3500 B.C., and the archaeological remains enable us to trace Egyptian history for one or two thousand years beyond this date.

Effect of History on Disease and Medicine: A country having such a long existence undoubtedly underwent many changes. The long narrow Nile Valley was cut up into numerous municipalities, warring continuously with one another and suffering the usual consequences of war, marked by all kinds of injuries and diseases. The torrid desert on both sides of the valley seemed to nurture many eye complications and gastrointestinal disturbances. The fertile valley, and especially the delta, frequently changed into marshes by the inundation of the Nile, often became a hotbed of growth for the malarial germ and a fertile soil for rheumatic and arthritic conditions.

Considering the long historic period of the Egyptians, the vicissitudes of fate, and the many religious beliefs, one has to expect different views on a vital subject like medicine. Rawlinson believed that the Egyptian physician was not under priestly domination, as is generally thought. Sayce[19] thought that, during the eighteenth dynasty, medicine was almost as advanced in Egypt as in the days of Galen. Various diseases were carefully distinguished from one another and the symptoms, as well as the treatment, were minutely described. On the other hand, later writers are not so favorably impressed with Egyptian medicine. Breasted holds that, with the exception of the Edwin Smith Surgical Papyrus, the other documents are irrational, incoherent, and a senseless mixture of magic, incantation, superstition, and empiricism.

Dr. Max Meyerhof of Cairo, a keen student of ancient Egyptian medicine, appears to be in accord with this statement:

Their works are rarely illuminated by a spark of deeper thought. There is a lack of knowledge pertaining to the human heart and blood vessels. The largest and the best known Papyrus, that of Ebers, in the section dealing with the mysteries of the physician, shows how lamentably crude their notion was on the structure of the body.

PHYSICAL ATTRIBUTES OF ANCIENT EGYPTIANS

Before presenting a summary of the anatomy and physiology known to the ancient Egyptians, it may be of interest to know what the Egyptian was like physically.

Two Types: Maspero,[20] in his interesting "Dawn of Civilization," attempts to reconstruct two physical types among the ancient Egyptians:

The highest type of Egyptian was tall and slender, with something that was proud and imperious in the carriage of his head and in his whole bearing. He had wide and full shoulders, muscular arms, a long fine hand,

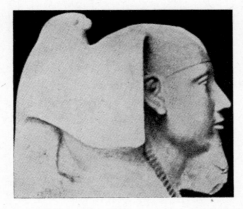

Fig. 74: Chephren (IV Dynasty). Chephren was perhaps the noblest example of the Egyptian Pharaohs. He was one of the pyramid kings. At the back of his head is a falcon which represents Horus, the god of kingship, whose incarnation the Pharaohs claimed to be. His diorite statue was discovered by Mariette in the "Temple of the Sphinx" near Gizeh.

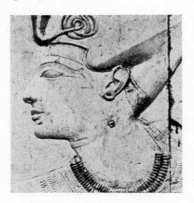

Fig. 75: Seth I (XIX Dynasty). The statue of Seth was found near Gizeh. It conveys a fair idea of the appearance of the Egyptians of the pyramid period. Incidentally the personal and court physician of this Pharaoh was named Rhuj. He was also the chief of physicians in upper and lower Egypt. He described himself "at the hand of the Pharaohs." He was the superior of the priests of the pyramids. He had the reputation for being learned in the sacred script.

slightly developed hips and sinewy legs. The head is rather short, the face oval, the forehead somewhat retreating. The eyes are wide and fully opened, the cheekbones not too marked, the nose fairly prominent, and either straight or aquiline. The mouth is long and the lips full. The hair was inclined to be wavy.

The common type was squat, dumpy, and heavy. The chest and shoulders seem to be enlarged at the expense of the pelvis and hips, to such an extent

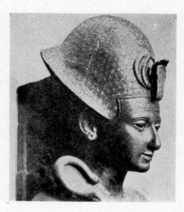

Fig. 76: Rameses II (XIX Dynasty). Rameses II was the son of Seth. He was identified by Lepsius with the Pharaoh of the Exodus. Petrie found a sculpture at Tel Rotab, west of Pithom, and concluded that this was Rameses II. (Black granite figure at Turin.)

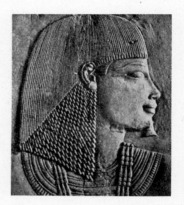

Fig. 77: Kha-em-hat. This is a relief of an Egyptian Pharaoh who flourished in the pyramid period. His features convey an idea of the appearance of the Egyptians at that time. Smith was able to define to some extent, from the human remains discovered in lower Egypt, that its population had better cranial and muscular development than that of upper Egypt.

as to make the want of proportion between the upper and lower parts of the body startling and ungraceful. The skull is long, somewhat retreating, and slightly flattened on the top; the features are coarse, and as though carved in flesh by great strokes of the roughing-out chisel. Small eyes, a short nose, flanked by widely distended nostrils, round cheeks, a square chin, thick, but not curling lips—this unattractive and ludicrous physiognomy, sometimes animated by an expression of cunning, which recalls the shrewd face of an

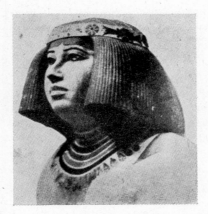

Fig. 78: Nefert. The portrait of a lady of rank from the statue chamber of a tomb near Gizeh. (IV Dynasty [about 2700 B.C.].)

old French peasant, is often lighted up by gleams of gentleness and of melancholy good nature.

The external characteristics of these two principal types, whose endless modifications are to be found on the ancient monuments, may still be seen among the present Egyptians.

EGYPTIAN KNOWLEDGE OF ANATOMY

Having these two types in mind and reading the different opinions quoted by authorities, one might be interested in gaining an insight into the knowledge of the Egyptian physician on such medical subjects as anatomy, physiology, diagnosis, pathology, and treatment. It has already been pointed out that, as far back as the first dynasty, a certain king-physician was the author of a manual of anatomy, but nothing is known of the contents of this book.

Knowledge Gained from Embalming: That the Egyptians possessed at least a superficial knowledge of the structure of the human body may be assumed from the technique of the Egyptian embalmer. He appears to have been acquainted with the gross anatomy when performing his work. He knew the position of the internal organs, and of the blood vessels and their relation to each other. He took care not to injure the internal organs, particularly the heart, while manipulating blindly in the interior of the body, for the heart was viewed as the abode of the soul and the seat of the intellect, without which resurrection was thought impossible. The brain was removed by forcing a passage with a chisel through the nostrils and the ethmoid bone into the cranial cavity; a bronze hook was then inserted and the brain tissue extracted piecemeal. The intestines were removed carefully and placed in four vases (Canopic jars).

The other internal organs were removed in their entirety, after which the body cavity was filled with preservatives such as natron and asphalt to keep the skeleton and muscular walls of the body from decaying. After this post-mortem operation, which had to be done with the utmost care and required skill and the knowledge of at least the gross anatomy of the organs, the body was bound in a copious swathing of linen bandage, with a mask of linen and stucco on the face. The *mummy* thus prepared was then laid on its side as though asleep, the head supported by a headrest, in a sarcophagus of wood or stone. The operations, in connection with the mummy, grew more and more elaborate towards the end of the Pharaonic period. By the time of the new kingdom, the wealthiest persons had their deceased laid in gaudily painted coffins depicting mythological scenes with inscriptions. The costliest process of embalming lasted no less than seventy days. Many superstitious rites had to be observed in the course of the process; a late book has preserved for us the magical formulas that were repeated by the wise kher-heb priest (who in the necropolis performed the functions of *taricheutes,* [embalmer]) as each bandage was applied. The Egyptian physician appears to have presided over the process of embalming.[21] The practice, however, might have been entrusted to temple servants.

Diodorus Siculus (212 B.C.) related that the one who made the post-mortem incision had to flee to avoid being stoned or as a gesture to acknowledge his offense against the dead.

The special treatment of the viscera familiarized the Egyptian physicians with the appearance and position of the organs and enabled them to recognize the homologies between the internal organs of the human body and those of animals, the latter having been long familiar to them through the practice of cutting up animals for sacrifice and for food. It is a noteworthy fact that the various hieroglyphic signs represent pictures of the organs of animals and not of human beings, thus showing that the Egyptians' knowledge of the internal structure of animals is older than their knowledge of the visceral anatomy of man. This also demonstrates that the Egyptians had a knowledge of comparative anatomy, recognizing the essential identity of structure between man and higher animal; for in some instances they borrowed the signs based upon the organs of animals and used them unaltered when speaking of the corresponding organs of the

human body. Thus the sign for "heart" is the heart of an ox, not
that of a man, and the word for the human "throat" or "gullet" employs the structures of the same animal. The sign "womb" is a configuration of the bicornate uterus of a cow, for "ear" a nonhuman
mammalian ear, and for "tooth" a mammalian tusk. Other hieroglyphic
signs borrowed from mammalian anatomy include those for the liver
and the mammae of a hoofed animal.

Ancient Anatomical Terms: In the ancient Egyptian language,
there are over 100 anatomical terms. On the whole, the gross anatomy of the body is fairly accurate. However, there is failure to differentiate between nerves, muscles, arteries, and veins. One word *metu* denotes these structures, and the Egyptians appear to have regarded them
as a single system of branching and radiating channels arising from one
source. The same term was applied to the vessels communicating with
the heart.

The Egyptian conception of the dynamics of the human mechanism is complicated and confusing; for aside from being governed
by a number of deities, it was assumed to be controlled also by three
other spiritual forces.

Anatomical Divisions: The "Book of the Dead" divides the human
body into thirty-six parts, the functions of each part or organ being controlled by a special deity. The eyes, for example, are governed by
Hathor, the ears by Asud, the lips by Amibus, the growth of the
hair by Nei, and the face by Ra. All these individual powers were
coordinated by Thoth, who supervised the function of the entire
body. This last divinity was, so to speak, the center of coordination, which we now locate in the brain. There was the *ka*,[22] which
governed perception and enjoyment, and was supposed to go with
the body into the tomb and remain there as long as the body was intact or mummified. The *ka* retained consciousness after death. This
spiritual entity was represented by the shadow that follows a human
being and was supposed to be born at the same time as the newborn infant. On the sarcophagus of Panahemisis is inscribed, "The
ka is thy god, he parted not from thee and saw thy soul live eternally."
Here the *ka* has become a divine principle, parallel with the doctrine of the *Logos* in its early development; the *ka* was believed to
go to Osiris to join the company of the gods.

Another spiritual phenomenon was *ba* or *bai* which was symbolized
by a bird with a human head. It was the nearest approach to the
Greek conception of a disembodied soul. The ba was assumed to
go to Hades after death. For a time, it would wander about in the

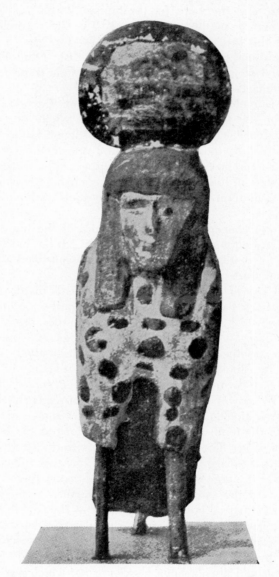

Fig. 79: The Egyptian *ka,* or soul. (From a statuette.)

cemetery requiring food. It was associated with the mummy *(sabu),* as the ka was with the body in the grave *(khat).* Certain Egyptian drawings show the ba at the side of the mummy at the bier, seeking to reenter its former habitation. The idea of the bird-like soul was perhaps derived from the owl, which is pictured as haunting the tomb pits and flying noiselessly around the grave.

The third spiritual entity was the *ab.* She controlled the will and intuition, which were thought to come from the heart. *Ab* was frequently used in the same metaphoric sense as heart. The physical heart was known as *hati.* A scarab frequently was used to replace the heart in the body of the mummy.

Hostility to Post-mortem Examination: Like all ancient and some modern nations, the Egyptians considered dissection as hostile to their belief in the resurrection of the entire body. Members or organs of the body that had been severed during life had to be restored before the body had been put to rest. No mutilated person could enjoy the blissful life of the future world. Numerous bodies with artificial legs, arms, teeth, and obsidian eyes have been discovered, which indicate that post-mortem replacements were made. Some authorities hold that these findings argue against the belief that the Egyptians practiced mechanical dentistry or inserted artificial eyes for cosmetic purposes during life.

EGYPTIAN KNOWLEDGE OF PHYSIOLOGY

Heart and Vascular System: Egyptian physiology recognized the heart as the center of the vascular system and believed it to be connected with the other organs of the body by a system of twenty-four or thirty-six nerves, extending to the little fingers; hence the custom of dipping fingers during the ceremony of libation.

A detailed account is given of the number of vessels which serve every part of the head, limbs, and body. The "vessels" of the nose, for instance, are four in number; two of these convey blood, and two, mucus. There are four vessels within the temples which convey blood to the eyes, and a glossary adds that, when the eyes water, the moisture comes from the pupils or from the eyelids (i.e. they knew that the water is produced locally and is not conveyed by the vessels). They did not recognize the existence of the lacrimal system.

The vessels described are not all blood vessels; some convey air and other secretions. Thus, the vessels of the nostrils convey air to the heart and to the lungs; those of the testicles convey semen; and those of the liver carry moisture and air. The vessels of the ears are also a part of the breathing system, "There are four vessels for the two ears, two on the right and two on the left. The breath of life enters by the right ear and the breath of death enters the left ear.

The heart was recognized as the origin of the blood vessels. The heart and stomach are designated in hieroglyphic writing as the "cooking pot"—a double system in which the blood was prepared for the digestion of food. The Egyptians recognized that the heart can be detected, not only in the region of the heart itself, but also all over the entire body when placing the finger on the head, the hands, the arms, and the legs.

The Thebeth Papyrus (1522 B.C.) states:

There is in the heart a vessel leading to every member of the body. If the physician places his finger on the head, neck, arms, hands, feet or body, everywhere he will find the heart, for the heart leads to every member and speaks in the vessels of every member.

The Ebers Papyrus, quoting Pharaoh Usaphias, states:

Man hath twelve principal vessels proceeding from his heart which extend to his body and limbs; two to each arm; two vessels go to the eyes and two to the nose; two branches go to the right ear through which the breath of life goes; two go to the left ear; through them pass the breath of death; they all proceed from the heart.

The concluding sentence is in keeping with the widespread belief that the left side of the body is sinister and ill-omened.

As among many other ancient nations, the heart was regarded as the seat of consciousness and of character among the Egyptians. The importance of the heart as the organ of consciousness and character may be seen in the "Book of the Dead," which described the weighing of the heart, in one pan of a scale, and the emblem of truth in the other. The heart was carefully left in situ by the embalmers and was not removed with the other organs during the process of mummification, for the person could not do without his heart in this or the next world.

Other passages describe the abnormal behavior of the heart during illness and its effect upon various parts of the body. The heart was supposed to get smaller with age. Death was caused by complete atrophy of that organ. Beneath this mass of physiologic concepts, which are manifestly erroneous, there is a nucleus of correct observations which indicates that, at very early times, a serious attempt was made to understand the structure and working of the body.

Respiration: Respiration played an important part in the working of the human mechanism. The entrance of the air into the body through the respiratory organs was well described. The arteries were thought to be air channels through which the pneuma circulates throughout the system. In the Ebers Papyrus, a distinction is made between good and bad air—air of life and air of death—which may possibly have counterparts in inspired air and expired air.

Organs of Reproduction: The Egyptians had a curious notion concerning the uterus. The organs of reproduction were believed to be a separate entity, independent of other organs, and subject to frequent fits of wandering about in the pelvic cavity. The patient suffering from a uterine disorder was made to stand over hot coal on which scented wax was sprinkled. The perfumed smoke rising to the genitalia was then expected to lure the errant uterus back to its normal place. In the light of our modern knowledge that the womb is not bound down by bony attachments, that it is frequently subject to retro- and anteflexion and version, that it moves up from the pelvis into the abdominal cavity during pregnancy, and that douches, intravaginal medications, Elliott therapy, and intravaginal diathermy are useful treatments for uterine and adnexal disorders, such concepts are not altogether without merit.

It is noteworthy that this method of treatment was practiced in ancient Greece. Both Hippocrates and Plato recommended the use of perfumed fumigation in uterine disorders. Galen, who surely was opposed to many of the ideas of the Egyptians, nevertheless followed the time-honored treatment of fumigation. Throughout the Middle Ages, physicians of Western Europe continued to treat most women's diseases by fumigating the external genitalia with scenting drugs. A seventeenth century dispensatory recommends the fumigation of the genitalia of hysterical persons with musk, givet, storax, and benzoin.

Traces of this ancient practice are still observed in the folk medicine of many countries. In certain rural districts of the midwestern states, young girls troubled with menstrual pain are advised by elderly women to seek relief by standing over rising steam produced by urinating into a bucket or scuttle of red hot coal.

Digestive System: The stomach and the digestive system prepared the food before being changed to blood by the heart. The most important natural cause of illness was thought to be overeating; other causes were the entrance of spirits or worms (real or imaginary) into the system. The parasitic theory of disease was a natural conclusion in a subtropical climate where all sorts of parasites cause so much annoyance to man and animal life.

Body as a Microcosm: The old conception that the human body is a miniature world (microcosm) had a great influence on Egyptian medicine. The human body (like the universe) was believed to be composed of four elements: earth, water, fire, and wind. The bodily solids (bones and flesh) represent the earth; the fluids of the body are carried by vessels, like water by the channels of the Nile, to all parts of the body; the pulse throbs, like the rise and fall of the Nile; the heat of the body represents fire and warms the body, like the sun warms the earth; and the human respiration is like the wind in the universe.

EGYPTIAN DIAGNOSIS, PATHOLOGY, AND TREATMENT

Diagnosis: The Egyptian physicians of the papyri period appear to have had fairly advanced methods of diagnosis. They knew the importance of the pulse, they estimated the height of fever of a patient by touch, and employed the practice of palpation to diagnose many diseases. The art of inspection of the body to elicit physical changes was highly developed. Indeed some have concluded from the phrase of the Ebers Papyrus, "here the ear hears beneath," that the Egyptian practiced direct auscultation.

Pathology: Because of linguistic difficulties, it is hard to get a clear idea from the papyri as to the pathology of the ancient Egyptians. There are words for which no closer equivalent can be found than "swelling" or "lump," although each term had a specific pathologic meaning to the ancient Egyptians. Some of these swellings are undoubtedly boils[23] and carbuncles of various kinds, which were in ancient times, as today, a source of distress to the inhabitants of Egypt.

About 250 different maladies can be distinguished in the Egyptian papyri. The Ebers Papyrus itself enumerates 170 varieties. The Edwin Smith Papyrus lists a number of surgical diseases. Diseases of the stomach, the bowels, the bladder, the heart, the respiratory organs, the head, the sinuses, the eyes, the skin, and the teeth are still common among the Egyptians and, for that matter, among people of other countries.

Treatment: Herodotus and Diodorus stated that the Egyptian physicians looked upon excessive consumption of food as the main cause of disease. Ailments due to dietary excesses were cured chiefly through fasting, emetics, and purgatives.[24] Diodorus remarks that the physician was under obligation to treat soldiers and travelers without fee. The unsuccessful termination of a course of treatment, conducted upon recognized and prescribed lines, was not held to be the fault of the physicians. However, independent procedure, going outside the bounds of the tradition and recognized practice, carried the death penalty with it if a fatality ensued. The principle of recognized practice is still the basis of malpractice laws in a large part of the modern civilized world.

Remedies are prescribed in the Ebers Papyrus for headache, coryza, migraine, fever, epilepsy, and nervous ailments. Other diseases seem, by comparison with modern Egypt, to have been particularly prevalent. Asthma, anemia, angina pectoris, and hematuria fall into this category. Some diseases were due to lack of hygiene, others to intemperate and improper food. Skin diseases, numerous boils and blains, parasitic diseases,[25] elephantiasis, worms, and pyorrhea alveolaris were described.

According to Elliot Smith, investigation of mummies showed the prevalence of smallpox among early Egyptians.[26]

Surgical diseases referred to include ulcers, Nile boils, and carbuncles on the breast and legs. Egyptian women were subject to a long list of ailments as described in the gynecologic papyrus (dating from the twelfth dynasty), including dysmenorrhea, menorrhagia, and metrorrhagia, erosions, pustules, prolapsus uteri, and cancerous tumors.

A large variety of ophthalmic disorders are mentioned in the Ebers Papyrus, including styes, vitreous opacities, ectropion, blepharitis, trachoma, lippitude, hydrophthalmia, staphyloma, conjunctivitis, purulent ophthalmia, and other eye ailments. This long list of diseases does not necessarily indicate that the climate of the land of the Nile was unhealthy, but rather shows the degree of diagnostic and therapeutic acumen of the Egyptian physician.

In the 875 prescriptions itemized in the Ebers Papyrus for abnormal conditions, forty-seven cases are diagnosed. Among these are twenty different cases of disease of the stomach, where the symptoms, diagnosis, and treatment are given for each. According to Dawson, these mark a great advance in real scientific medicine. Each case begins, "if you examine a man who suffers in the stomach." After describing the symptoms it continues, "thou sayest concerning it; it is so and so" (diagnosis). Then follows the treatment, with a prescription of drugs, "treat him with something that cools heat and opens his bowels, especially with drought of sweet beer poured upon dry *neqaut* fruit; four times shall he eat and drink." Other forms of dis-

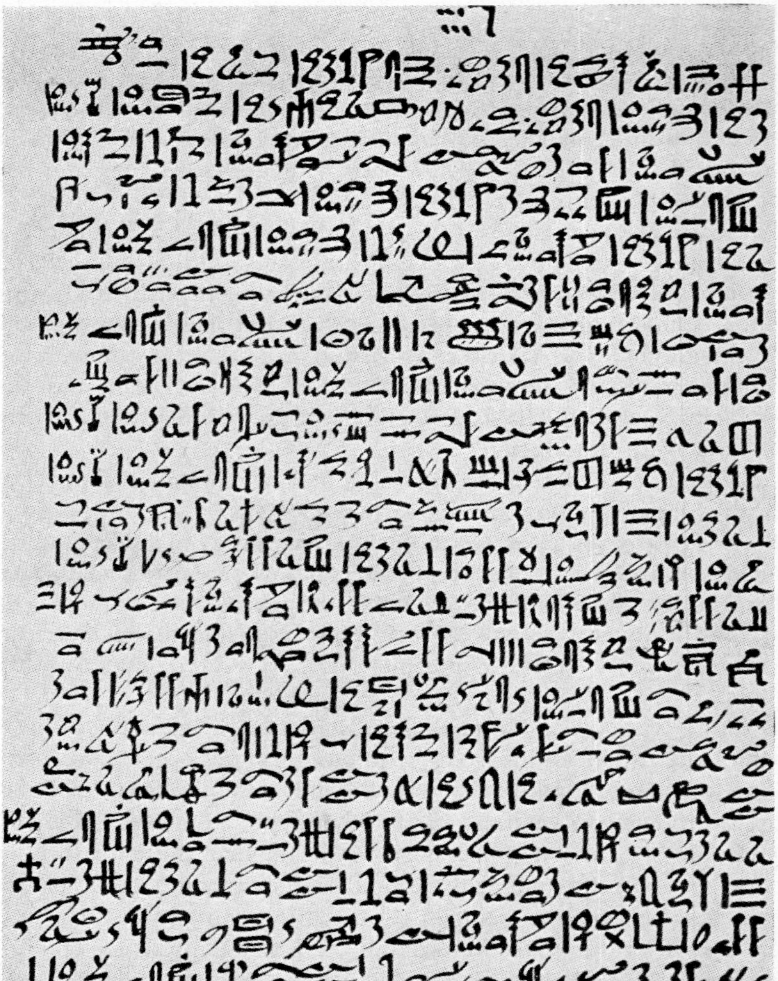

Fig. 80: A page from the Ebers Papyrus on ophthalmic remedies.

ease are "that where the patient vomits and feels very ill" and that in which the belly is "hot and swollen." For each of these, different treatment is required. The following passage by Maspero gives an idea of how a medical subject is discussed:

If you have to deal with a patient (attacked) by an obstruction....if he feels heaviness after eating, if his stomach is full of wind, if his heart troubles him while walking, as it does in the case of a patient suffering from anal fissure—examine him lying on his back, and if you find his stomach warm and some obstruction in the intestines, say something is wrong with the liver.

Then he is given the secret remedy of herbs which the doctor must mix himself:

Take the pulp of walnuts, and dates, mix, soak in water, make the patient drink it four mornings consecutively, to relieve and empty the stomach. If after having done this you find the two hypochondria, that on the right warm, that on the left fresh (clear), say (about it): "The internal juices are fighting the evil which is destroying them!" If on examining him a second time you find all the stomach clear, say "His liver is cured, it is cleansed, he has taken the remedy well."

Study of Mummy Tissue: The Egyptian technique of mummification aided in identifying certain diseases of the predynastic and dynastic periods, which the medical papyri do not convey to us because of linguistic difficulties. The study of Egyptian paleopathology was first introduced by the French scientist Fouquet and was followed by Elliot Smith, F. Wood Jones, and Sir Marc Armand Ruffer. The last scientist particularly deserves the credit for devising a technique by which the desiccated tissues of the mummies, dead for three or four millenniums, are restored to a condition sufficiently soft to examine under the microscope and thus detect pathologic changes which have taken place in their bodies during life.

Ruffer's studies disclosed among the ancient Egyptians and their predecessors, the Nubians, many diseases which are still prevalent in the land of the Pharaohs. He detected a case of smallpox in a mummy of the twentieth dynasty (1200–1090 B.C.). The body showed vesicles or bulbous eruptions. He found in one case evidence of an abscess in the right psoas muscle. He also established the existence of arteriosclerosis among the Egyptians of the twenty-first dynasty (c. 1000 B.C.). His microscopic examination proved that young, as well as old, Egyptians suffered from hardening of the arteries. The arterial lesions were identical with those found among twentieth-century patients, which have been variously (but not quite scientifically) ascribed to the use of tobacco, alcohol, and heavy meat diet. It is questionable whether syphilis plagued the ancient Egyptians.

Shattock and Ruffer studied the pathological anatomy of the aorta of King Merneptah, the Pharoah of the Hebrew exodus. The mummy was found in Thebes in the tomb of Amenehotep II, who reigned in Egypt from 1449 to 1420 B.C. Merneptah was unwrapped by Dr.

G. Elliot, who subsequently sent the aorta to the Royal College of Physicians of London. Shattock made a microscopic study of the aorta and demonstrated a section of it. This Pharoah of the exodus was the thirteenth son and successor of Rameses II (1292–1225 B.C.). His old age was recognized by his baldness, by the whiteness of the few hairs left, by the complete ossification of the thyroid cartilage and the first rib, and by the calcareous patches of the aorta. Only

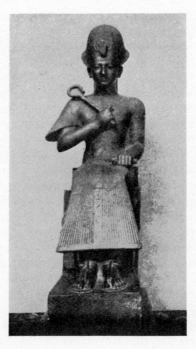

Fig. 81: Rameses II. Rameses II was a mighty warrior, even though his conquests were not so great as represented in his inscriptions. (Statue of black granite in Karnak, now in the Museum in Cairo.)

one tooth, the upper right medium incisor, was found. Arteriosclerosis was widely disseminated among young and old, 3000 years ago at the home of the Pharoahs, and presented the same anatomical pathological signs as today.

Marc Armand Ruffer found evidence of arthritis deformans in upper and lower Egypt, from predynastic times to the third century A.D., a period of at least 8000 years during which arthritis was both chronic and common. He even records a case in a Miocene-Period skeleton,

going back 900,000 years. Thoma believes that the majority of bony
lesions in the Egypt of 3000 years ago were typical of chronic arthritis. The spinal colum was mostly affected, the bones of the hand
and feet being next in order to be involved.

Dr. John K. Mitchell of Philadelphia diagnosed the ailment of an
Egyptian mummy at the University of Pennsylvania Museum as polio-
myelitis. This mummy was discovered by Sir Flinders Petri in Dash-
ashe and dates from about 3700 B.C. Dr. G. Elliot Smith reported
a case of chronic appendicitis evidenced by the presence of adhesions.
Douglas E. Dorry, in 1930, described a case of hydrocephalus in an
early Egyptian mummy. Rickets appears to have been common.
Pneumonia, renal abscesses, all forms of fractures, necrosis, tumors,
ostitis, and arthritis were frequently met with. Ruffer located a
tuberculous lesion in the vertebrae of a mummy. Smith and Jones reported several cases of tuberculosis of the spine, discovered in a cata-
comb at Thebes dating from the twenty-third dynasty. Ruffer and
Elliot Smith found Pott's disease in a mummy of about 1000 B.C.

It is difficult to discuss ancient Egyptian medicine without making
a few personal remarks concerning Sir Marc Armand Ruffer, that illustrious investigator of the paleohistology and paleopathology of the
ancient mummmies. Ruffer was born in Lyons, France, in 1859. The
son of Baron Alphonse Jacques de Ruffer, he was educated at Bra-
senece College, Oxford, where he received his B.S. in 1883. In 1889
he received the degree of Bachelor of Medicine from the University
College of London. He then joined Pasteur and Metchnikoff at the
famous Pasteur Institute, devoting his studies to phagocytosis. His
description of diphtheritic membrane is well remembered. He pictures
it as a battlefield "in which pathogenic bacteria and amoeboid leuco-
cytes contend for supremacy."

In 1891, Ruffer became the first director of the British Institute of
Preventive Medicine. At Metchnikoff's suggestion, he took up the
study of cancer and established the provisional status of the quasi-
parasitic formation of cancer cells. While testing the new diphtheritic serum at the Pasteur Institute, Ruffer was so severely
smitten with diphtheria and paralytic sequelae that he was compelled to resign his directorship. He left for Egypt to recuperate
and subsequently made Ramleh his permanent home. He later became professor of bacteriology at the Cairo School of Medicine, and
was appointed president of the Sanitary, Maritime, and Quarantine
Council of Egypt (1901–1917), in which office he was instrumental
in ridding Egypt of cholera by adopting strict hygienic regulations

and by policing the route of the pilgrims and the railroad stations. Ruffer made a great impression on the study of the medical history of ancient Egypt by his articles on the paleopathology and paleohistology of the lesions he found in mummies of the eighteenth and twenty-seventh dynasties.

At the opening of the First World War he was head of the Red Cross in Egypt. He left in the winter of 1916–1917 for Salonica to reorganize the sanitary service of the Greek provincial government. He died a tragic death at the hands of an assassin in the spring of 1917, as he was returning from Salonica. Thus his scholarly researches were rudely interrupted. After his death, Lady Ruffer collected his manuscripts, which were eventually edited by Roy L. Moodie and published by the University of Chicago Press under the title "Paleopathology of Egypt."[27]

Hygiene and Prophylaxis: Herodotus, describing the life of the Egyptians, stated:

> Their manner of life is this. They purge themselves every month, three days successively, seeking to preserve health by emetics and clysters; for they suppose that all diseases to which men are subject proceed from the food they use. And, indeed, in other respects, the Egyptians, next to the Libyans, are the most healthy people in the world, as I think, on account of the seasons, because they are not liable to change; for men are most subject to disease at periods of change, and, above all others, at the change of the seasons. They feed on bread made into loaves of spelt, which they call cyllestis; and they use wine made of barley, for they have no vines in that country. Some fish they dry in the sun, and eat raw, others salted with brine; and of birds they eat quails, ducks, and smaller birds raw, having first salted them; all other things, whether birds or fishes, that they have, except such as are accounted sacred, they eat either roasted or boiled. [28]

Diodorus Siculus states that the Egyptians, in order to prevent sickness, practiced drenching and fasting and used emetics and enemata, sometimes every day and sometimes at intervals of three or four days: "For they say that the larger part of the food is superfluous, and that from the superfluous part, diseases are engendered."

In no other branch of medicine did the Egyptians excel more than in hygiene and prophylaxis. Even viewed from the standard of present-day knowledge, their hygienic measures deserve the fullest recognition. The statement of Herodotus that "the Egyptians are, with the Libyans, the healthiest of nations" was due largely to their hygienic regulations.

The greatest stress was laid upon cleanliness of the body, care of dwellings, proper diet, and suitable dress. The priests set the example in carrying out the strictest rules of cleanliness: They bathed twice daily and twice nightly. Because hair attracted dirt, they shaved their entire bodies every third day. In the epoch of the new kingdom, their heads were always shaven clean. They wore white linen while performing their temple duties. In the choice of food, they carefully avoided pork, beans, and onions on account of flatulence. In later times, they drank only boiled or filtered water, their favorite drink being a kind of beer ("the gift of Osiris") which they brewed from barley. The belief in moderation may be seen from the following exhortation to a student: "Thou forsakest thy books, thou givest thyself up to pleasure, goest from tavern to tavern,—the smell of beer makes man shun thee." Excess in this direction, as well as in sexual intercourse, was forbidden by priestly orders, and stringent penalties were applied to such offenses.

Birth control and abortion were severely punished; intercourse during menstruation was forbidden; self-abuse was named as a vice in the "Book of the Dead." Priests were allowed but one wife. Circumcision was practiced as a rite, and was performed upon boys of the priestly and warrior caste between the sixth and tenth years with a flint knife. Marriage between brother and sister was practiced only in the royal families (down to Ptolemaic times).

The highly developed hygiene of the Egyptians overshadows their medical knowledge. There can be no doubt that Egypt exercised a powerful influence upon the social hygiene of Judea as well as upon the scientific medicine of Greece.

"The whole manner of life," says Diodorus, "was so evenly ordered that it would appear as though it had been arranged according to the rules of health by a learned physician, rather than by a lawgiver." This description seems to corroborate the picture of the Egyptian as penned by Maspero.

Dentistry: Sudhoff, upon examining Nubian and Egyptian craniums, was astounded to find their teeth well preserved, although the masticatory surfaces showed abrasions. This suggested to him that the early Egyptians used simple food, mainly of a vegetable character and rich in cellulose, with perhaps a generous adulteration of sand particles.

In later times, when more refined food was used, signs of dental decay, such as simple caries, alveolar abscesses, and tartar formation appeared more frequently. In some 5000 skeletons of the wealthier classes of the third and fourth dynasties, excavated at the Gizeh pyramids, dental diseases were more noticeable among the richer classes and less so among the poorer classes. Dental surgery, it appears, was not developed at that period. "It is impossible," said Ruffer, "that Amenhotep III would have endured the agony which he must have gone through if the court dentist knew how to pull out teeth."[29]

Prevalence of Eye Diseases: Among the most prevalent diseases of Egypt must be included those affecting the eyes: of the 875 prescriptions in the Ebers Papyrus, ninety-three are intended as therapy for eye ailments. Only the names of the diseases are mentioned; and owing to the lack of knowledge of the terminology, many of these names are still not sufficiently identified. Dr. B. Ebbell of Norway deserves much credit for identifying many ancient names of ocular diseases. The delicate soft structures of the eye, which could not resist the ravages of thousands of years of decay in the dry sand and rocky caves, have removed all pathologic traces of ancient Egyptian ocular disease. Investigation of mummies, therefore, furnishes no evidence as to the nature of eye affections.[30] For such evidence one has to rely entirely on inscriptions on stone or on the papyri which the dry sand helped to preserve.

Cataract, for example, is known in the Ebers Papyrus as "mounting of water in the eye"; a similar term also was applied to the same condition by Hippocrates, Celsus, and Galen. Cataract was believed to be caused by a fluid running down the head and lodging itself between the iris and the lens; accordingly, a flow of tears was considered a good omen because, by releasing the fluid from the eye, the cause of the cataract might be obviated.

A letter from an Egyptian painter named Poi (who had lost his eyesight) to his son Rahatep (during the reign of Rameses II, about 1250 B.C.) reads:

Do not abandon me; I am in distress: Do not cease to deplore, for I am in darkness! My god Amon has abandoned me, bring me some honey for my eyes and some fat. . .and real eye paint (Mesdemet re stimmi, stibium) as soon as possible. Am I not your father? Yes, I am weak. I want to have my eyes and they are missing.

"This," stated Max Meyerhof, "is almost the only document about blindness from papyri or similar vehicles." However, blindness in Egypt was, and still is, frequent. It is often represented on the ancient Egyptian monuments. The most famous painting was discovered in the temple of Tellel-Amarna, which represents a blind harpist accompanied by seven blind choristers. The Ebers Papyrus refers to blear-eyedness (lippitude), the treatment of which was an ointment composed of resin, malachite, stibium, myrrh, and burned papyri, Another prevailing eye affection was trachoma *(nebat* [dripping eyes]), a disease which "always attacks both eyes."[31] Remedies of a corrosive nature, such as red and yellow ochre, stibium, and red natron, were used. Leukoma, resulting from corneal ulcer, is still seen in Egypt, and was treated with the bile of a tortoise, a treatment which was also used by the Greeks, Arabs, and Hebrews.[32] The bile of many animals has been used for leukoma and nightblindness (nyctalopia). "Little grain" or "ball" was the name for a chalazion cyst. It was treated by an ointment applied to the eyelids.

The term *adyt* was applied to a pterygium. *Bt nt mu* was a term used for cataract and means "rising of water" in the eye. The Greeks used the expression "pouring down of water." Many medical remedies were recommended for cataract, but no surgical measures are suggested. Lacrimation was known as *k. le not.*

A number of remedies were suggested for pain and extravasation of blood from the eye. For pain, external applications to the temples were used. Nightblindness was treated with a diet of ox liver (still in use by ophthalmologists). Drooping of the lids (ptosis), ectropion (ectropium), and trichiasis were diagnosed and treated. Epilation was recommended for trichiasis, a treatment still used by modern physicians. Other remedies used in eye diseases were the blood of a lizard or bat, verdigris, natrum, malachite, milk and urine. Another popular remedy used by the Egyptians was elderberries, which also came from Phoenicia.

Circumcision: Circumcision was practiced in Egypt at an early period. Elliot Smith showed that this operation was performed at least 2000 years before Rameses II. One of the best representations of the operation is depicted in a bas-relief discovered in the temple Khonus at Karnak. It has been suggested that this bas-relief represents the circumcision performed on one of the children of Rameses II. This operation in Egypt was first limited to priests; later it was adopted by royalty and nobility; and still later it became a universal practice. It is recorded that Pythagoras (sixth century B.C.) had to submit to the operation before being permitted to study at the Egyptian schools.

Egyptian Therapeutics: Egyptian therapeutics may be divided into five classes: (1) magical, (2) empiricomagical, (3) empirical, (4) empericorational, and (5) rational. The magical method of treatment has already been discussed in this chapter. Now the other methods of treatment will be dealt with. In the empiricomagical method, the physician yielded to popular belief in prescribing remedies. An amulet was left with the patient; a charm was recited when the prescription was prepared; or the drug was ordered to be taken at a particular time, such as before sunrise. The empirical method of therapeutics was purely traditional, irrespective of physiological drug action. The empiricorational method of treatment included the use

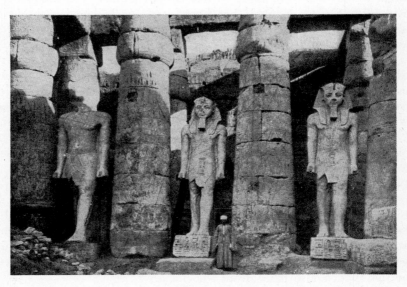

Fig. 82: The portrait statues of Rameses II at Luxor. Rameses II, who came to the throne of Egypt some 125 years after Tutankhamen and ruled for sixty-seven years, has been facetiously called the "father of mural advertising." He erected colossal portrait statues of himself in many parts of Egypt, and one eminent archaeologist charges that "he stole the works of better men and battered his own eternal cartouche in upon their inscriptions, the most valuable records being ruthlessly falsified to the vainglory of the sublime egotist."

of a mixture in the prescription wherein the effectiveness of some of the ingredients was on a physiological basis and some not. As an example, the following may be cited, "To cure granulations of the eye, you will prepare a collyrium of verdigris and onions; mix it all and apply it to the eye of the sick person." The rational method of therapeutics is mainly confined to the Edwin Smith Surgical Papyrus where the general attitude was largely one of cooperation with nature, putting the patient on a diet, and ordering strict hygienic regulations.

The papyri prescriptions include both those that specify accurately the quantity of the drug and those which simply call for certain ingredients without specifying the quantity.

Judging from the surgical papyrus, the ancient Egyptians seem to have had a sound method of treating surgical disabilities, such as fractures, dislocations, and injuries resulting from falls or blows.

The Edwin Smith Surgical Papyrus describes methods of reducing dislocations of the jaw and setting fractures of the collarbone; the latter follows:

If thou examinest a man having a break in his collarbone...thou shouldst place him prostrate on his back, with something folded between his two shoulder blades; thou shouldst spread out his two shoulders in order to stretch apart his collarbone until that break falls into its place. Thou shouldst make for him two splints of linen, thou shouldst apply one of them both on the inside of his upper arm and the other on the under side of his upper arm. Thou shouldst bind it...treat it afterwards (with) honey every day until he recovers.

The author of the Edwin Smith Papyrus knew that one may sustain a depressed fracture of the skull without wounding the scalp, and that such a trauma might result in loss of speech and paralysis of the limbs if it involves the brain. The depth of wounds was explored with the finger; those that did not require suturing were closed by a plaster and bandaged. Splints were made of wood or of linen steeped in glue. A clinical record of every case was kept. The pulse was carefully studied as a gauge of the patient's reaction to the injury or the operation. Attention was paid to diet, especially the patient's customary food. Very few drugs were recommended. "Put the patient on his finger" was the idiom expressing proper diet and medical regulation. Thus it is evident that the Edwin Smith Papyrus is organized along a system which may be considered rational and almost modern. Each case usually begins with the history and continues with the physical findings, diagnosis, treatment, and prognosis. Thus, for example, History: "Instruction concerning a wound." Physical Finding: "If thou examinest a man having a wound in his ear, cutting through his flesh, the injury being in the lower part of his ear and confined to the flesh." Treatment: "Thou shouldst draw off together for him with stitching behind the hollow of the ear." Diagnosis: "Thou shouldst say concerning him, 'a sufferer having a wound in his ear.'" Prognosis and general considerations: (1) "It is an ailment I will treat." (2) "An ailment I will contend with." (3) "An ailment I will not treat." This papyrus repeatedly emphasizes that the

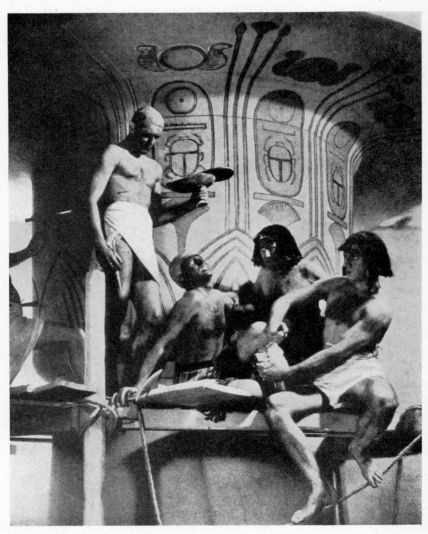

Fig. 83: Surgeons of ancient Egypt were well advanced in knowledge of anatomy and wound treatment. The Edwin Smith Papyrus, though written nearly four thousand years ago and constituting the oldest medical work in existence, describes methods and appliances surprisingly modern. The cautery was known but was seldom used. Wounds were approximated with adhesive plaster made from strips of linen and were closed with sutures. (Courtesy of Davis and Geck, Inc.; as depicted by an artist.)

patient should do nothing medically but place himself on a normal diet and await results.

On the back of the famous Edwin Smith Surgical Papyrus, there is an incantation for preventing epidemics. At the end of the incantation are the following instructions: "Speak the words (of the incantation) over two vulture feathers with which man has covered himself, place as his protection in every place where he goes; it is a protection (against) the year expecting sickness in the year of pests." This magic formula shows that, although the Edwin Smith Papyrus does not indulge in magic when it deals with surgery, it resorts to superstition when dealing with epidemics.[33]

Prescriptions: The oldest medical prescriptions known may be traced to hieratic writings. There is, in the British Museum, one attributed to the age of Cheops (about 2700 B.C.) and another one in the Metropolitan Museum in New York which are inscribed on stone tablets. These prescriptions mention a certain ground green stone which is to be burned and the smoke inhaled for the purpose of fumigation and inhalation.

Many of the prescriptions in the Ebers Papyrus are supposed to have been concocted by the gods, although there is little mystery about their ingredients. Invocations were made to the gods, Ra, Isis or Horus, while swallowing or applying the remedy. Some of the prescriptions are rational, as, for example, the use of opium for pain. The use of this drug was thought to hark back to Isis who cured the headache of Ra with medicine containing the berry of the poppy plant. This is one of the earliest records of the use of opium in medicine. Opium was also used as an ointment, having the fat of an ass as its base. Some of the prescriptions are pharmacologically sound. Many of them are for cosmetic purposes, such as for baldness, removing wrinkles and moles, dyeing the hair and eyebrows, tattooing, sweetening the breath, and relieving excessive perspiration.

DRUGS USED: Of the three classes of medicines those derived from vegetable substances have been most used. Next came remedies derived from animal substances, and lastly those prepared from minerals. Mammalian medicine contained material even from human beings, including blood, brain, and heart tissue which are frequently used to imbibe vigor, courage, and wisdom respectively.

Seven hundred different drugs, including plants, minerals, and animal substances are mentioned in the Ebers and Hearst Papyri, but not all of them, recommended for healing purposes, have been identified. Some have been identified from Coptic derivations of old

Egyptian words, others from the determinatives in the hieratic script, which indicates whether or not the healing material used is granular, gummy, or liquid in character and whether the drug is derived from a tree, root, bud, leaf, or other part of the plant. Often the use to which the plant is put proves its identity. After Ebers and Wreszinski, Dr. Ebbell of Norway deserves the most credit for identifying many names of diseases. He based his proof on careful philological and technical investigation. Failure to identify accurately a large number of abnormal conditions by lack of terminology comprehension, makes it difficult to discuss the rationality of many medical agents.

Animal Drugs: The remedies of animal derivation consist of fat, flesh, blood, testicles, horns, hoofs, hide, and bones. For example, the testicles of a black ass in wine are recommended for obscure diseases. The tissues of the vulva and phallus, mixed with a black lizard, are recommended for baldness. A face cream, composed of bullock's bile and ostrich egg beaten up in fresh milk, is prescribed to improve the complexion of a school girl.

Animals, identified for medical use in the Ebers Papyrus, include the ass, ox, hippopotamus, pig, lion, goat, oryx, bat, and mouse. Birds so employed are geese, ducks, swallows, and other species which have not been identified. Frogs, lizards, snakes, tortoises, and many kinds of fish appear in the prescriptions. Animal excretions, such as urine, dung, mucus, and saliva were used. Even flyspecks were used to combat colic in babies, and one might add that this substance is probably as effective as numerous modern preparations.

Hoefler estimated the proportions of the various kinds of animal matter used in ancient medicine. Out of 1254 cases, 870 were of mammals, 255 of birds, 103 of amphibians, and 89 of fish. Of birds, the hen came first with 46, the hawk 39, the partridge 23, the crow 21, the swallow 19, and the pigeon 12. Of the internal organs of birds, the brain was used in 90 cases, the gall in 70, the heart in 54, the liver in 32, and the lung in 3.[34]

Vegetable and Mineral Drugs: The number of vegetable drugs is very large. The entire plant, or its fruit, bark, seeds, leaves, or juice, was employed. The mineral drugs are even harder to identify than the plant and animal drugs. Included in the medical writings are references to such remedies as alum, copper, feldspar, iron oxide, limestone, red ochre, sodium carbonate, sodium bicarbonate, salt, stibium, sulfur, and possibly arsenical compounds. These are usually recommended as applications to the skin or for such conditions as boils, felons, and burns.

Plant remedies in the papyri are acacia, anise, barley, cassia, castor beans, worm seeds, coriander, cucumber, cumin, dates, figs, gourd, juniper, lotus, peas, poppy seeds, saffron, sunflower, styrax, thyme, myrtle, hyocyamus, mustard, cinnamon, terebinth, willow buds, wheat, white thistles, and others.

While a large number of different types of drugs from animal sources are recommended in the medical papyri, their use was apparently not as extensive as plant and mineral drugs. According to Dr. Singer, some 30 per cent of the crude vegetable drugs in the modern official pharmacopoeia were known to antiquity. Among the household remedies frequently used by the Egyptians were water (specified as plain water, well water, salt water, spring water, water from the bird pond, water from the rain of heaven [most potent of all was the water in which the phallus has been washed]), milk (milk was the favorite vehicle and the animal to be used was specified; human milk was considered most valuable), honey, beer of various kinds (beer was a favorite vehicle and was variously prescribed as plain beer, sweet beer, bitter beer, flat beer, cold beer, froth of beer, yeast of beer, or beer which had been brewed from many ingredients), yeast, oil, fennel, flaxseed, garlic, onions, and leeks. Others included myrrh, aloes, castor oil, lettuce, turpentine, and various lead preparations.

USE OF DRUGS: Fat and grease from various animals are frequently mentioned in the prescriptions both for oral administration and for application to the skin. Thus goose fat is found in prescriptions for internal use to relieve pain, and to be applied to the body externally for relaxation. Blood, bone marrow, bile, liver, and spleen are all recommended for various disorders, but with little evidence of rationality in the light of modern knowledge. Liver is incorporated in prescriptions to prevent hair from turning gray, and blood is advised for baldness. Excrement of various animals is incorporated in prescriptions for the relief of throbbing limbs and for the applications to promote relaxation. These materials have been employed among other peoples, especially among primitives, for driving out evil demons causing such conditions.

Wax is extensively recommended in Egyptian medical papyri for use as a vehicle in various ointments and in preparations for application to the skin or wounds. A number of alkaline powders are recommended, derived from such sources as wall brick, limestone, builder's lime, clay, and gravel. Soot and charcoal are recommended for skin applications in cases of burns or itching.

Abrasions, lacerations, or inflamed areas on the skin seem to have

been treated by the application of soothing mucilaginous preparations made from gummy plant materials such as frankincense and
acaia. A large number of mild alkaline and mucilaginous materials
seem to have been recommended for oral administration, for the
relief of "pain in the left side" and other similar conditions which
suggest gastric hyperacidity or peptic ulcer.

The Ebers Papyrus suggests "to cool a head that suffers pain" that
hart's horn be combined with other ingredients, ground up, mixed
with water, and applied to the head. "To drive out painful swelling
which affects a man in winter and summer," an ointment made of
hart's horn, ground up with incense and flour and mixed with sweet
oil, was to be taken. Hart's horn, administered by fumigation, was
recommended for ear diseases and to drive out the demon which
caused diseases. In the latter case, it was mixed with the legs of a
bird, the hair of an ass, and the dung of swallows and geese.

Douches of wine and garlic were used for amenorrhea. Anointing
a virgin with a mixture of dried liver of a swallow and sour milk
was prophylaxis against leukorrhea. To facilitate labor, peppermint
in one form or another was employed. The mold, gathered on the
wood of a ship, rubbed in yeast or fermented beer, and taken internally, was a remedy for uterine displacement. There were also
abortionists in old Egypt who, like their modern counterparts, often
profited from the gullibility of the multitude; they claimed to accomplish abortion by the application of onions and dates to the
vulva.

A drug used frequently by the Egyptians was castor oil which was
cultivated extensively in the valley of the Nile. The plant obtained
from the seed was known as *kiki* (similar to the Hebrew *kikoayn*).
The later Egyptian name for castor oil was *degam*. *Ricinus* seeds,
chewed up or taken in beer, were recommended by the Ebers Papyrus
as a purgative. An oil prepared from the seed was employed as an
ointment for sores and boils. (The oil was also used for lighting.
One of the inscriptions stated, "I have given oil of Degam for the
lighting of the temples.")

Many of the substances owed their supposed virtue to alleged
magical powers, such as their supposed relationship to a certain god
or spirit. The original virtues associated with them were based on
the concept that spirits cause as well as protect from disease. The
belief that certain drugs had magical power to harm and cure was
general in Egypt as in other countries.

In all cases, the quantity of the drug is carefully specified in the prescription, and minute directions are given as to how the drug is to be mixed and when it is to be taken.

Surgical Diseases: Surgical diseases are dealt with occasionally in the Ebers Papyrus. To cope with a tumor in the flesh, the surgeon was instructed to use a knife and then check the hemorrhage by means of red hot cautery. Discussing the diagnosis of obstructions in the abdomen, the writer states, "It is the blood that has got itself fixed and does not circulate."

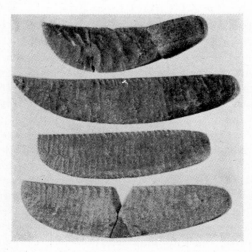

Fig. 84: Prehistoric Egyptian flint knives. The top knife has a wooden handle. (State Museum, Berlin.)

When dealing with fatty growths in the neck, the surgeon says, "I will treat the disease with the knife, taking care of the blood vessels the while"; in connection with a fluid swelling, "I will try to heal it with fire, like the cautery heals." Tumors in the head, tumors of blood vessels, and lipomas (fatty tumors) were treated with the knife.

For "stinking ulcers," take thorns, ostrich eggs, and tortoise shell, and "warm and anoint therewith, but don't get tired doing it."

Egyptians had sound methods of handling fractures (one of the Pharaohs himself suffered from a fractured leg) and injuries resulting from falls or blows.[34] Surgery was apparently free from magic and superstitious procedure. Only internal disorders with an insidious onset and having no obvious cause inspired the concept of supernatural etiology, with resultant magical methods of treatment. In this connection, it may be of interest to quote an old Egyptian text cited by Gaston Maspero:

Whoever treats a sick person has two equal important duties to perform. He must first discover the nature of the spirit in possession and if necessary to name and then attack it, drive it out. . .he can only succeed by powerful magic so he must be an expert in reciting incantations and skillful in making amulets. He must then use medicine (drugs and diet) to contend with the disorder which the presence of the strange being has produced in the body.

CONCLUSIONS

Von Oefele[35] and Schneider are of the opinion that Egyptian medicine was first purely empirical and became magical through the influence of the Babylonian priests; later, they claim, their magical concepts again declined and medicine once again became empirical. They based their opinion partially on the fact that the gynecological text, which is of the later period, is practically free from magic. This, however, may be disputed. In the first place, the later text consists of only short fragments (three columns), while the Ebers Papyrus contains 120 pages. Furthermore, magic in this text is met with sporadically, and large portions of the text have none of the magical treatment at all. It is reasonable to suppose that a people with such an intense belief in the supernatural as the Egyptians, whose cults for the dead were completely permeated by magic, would, even as far back as the ancient empire, cultivate occult methods of treatment.

Learning among the Egyptians was not always pursued for its own sake, as it was among the Greeks. Often it was merely a means of receiving material benefits as is seen from this letter of a father who writes to his son: "My son, apply yourself to learning, that thou may be a scribe. The old people are heavily laden asses, but the scribe is the driver. The scribe is never hungry; he sits at the farest table and his belly is filled by reason of wisdom."

While the medical concepts of the Egyptians are not in harmony with modern medical thought, they must be credited with furnishing the foundation upon which the Greek medical structure was based. As Plato declared, "whatever we received from the barbarians (Egyptians) we improved upon." The Greeks recognized their debt to the Egyptians and, indeed, they identified Aesculapius, their patron god of medicine, with the Egyptian Imhotep. As late as the period of the Odyssey,[36] the Egyptians carried their medical fame beyond the confines of their country.

The Persian admiration of Egyptian medicine at a still later date is graphically set forth by the father of history.[37]

References and Notes

1. A story probably due to the similarity to the name Thoth. Ebers believed that his Papyrus was nothing else but the Hermetic Book on drugs.
2. Die Stele des Hoffarztes Iry. Ztsch. f. Egypten Schprache u. Alterthumkunde, 69:53, 70, 1928.
3. Withington, E. T.: Medical History from the Earliest Times. The Scientific Press, London, 1894, p. 15.
4. Mayers: Der Alten Aegyptens. Berlin, 1885, 2:95.
5. Clemens Alexandrinus: Stromateis (patchwork). Potters ed., Lib. 6:4.
6. Cited by William Hamilton: Colburn, H., and Bentley, R.: History of Medicine, Surgery, and Anatomy. London, 1831, Vol. 1, pp. 5-15.
7. II Kings 23:29.
8. Hurry, J. B.: Imhotep. Oxford University Press, 1928, 2d ed.
9. Maspero, G.: Etudes Egyptiennes. 1:145. Cited by Edward T. Withington p. 24.
10. The Joachim Translation, Berlin, 1890, has often been consulted.
11. Stromateis (patchwork). Potters ed., Lib. 6:4.
12. Ztsch. f. Egypten Schprache u. Alterthumkunde, 65:53, 70, 1928.
13. Macalister: Archaeologia Anatomica (Anatomy & Physiology). Vol. 32, p. 775.
14. Ebers: Report of the Oriental Congress. London, 1874.
15. Genesis 43:2-5.
16. Herodotus: Henry Cary Trans.: Euterpe, 2:85, Oxford, 1874. "The art of medicine is thus divided among them; each physician applies himself to one disease and not more. All places abound in physicians; some physicians are for the eyes, others for the head, others for the teeth, others for the parts about the belly, and others for internal disorders."
17. Der Alten Aegyptens, 2:95.
18. Herodotus: Rawlinson's Trans,. 2:84.
19. Sayce: Ancient Empires of the East. London, 1884, p. 76.
20. Maspero, G.: The Dawn of Civilization, Egypt and Chaldea. Eng. Trans., 1894, p. 47.
21. Genesis 50:2.
22. Maspero, G.: (Translates it "the double." Historie ancienne des peuples de l'orient). 4th ed., pp. 55-56.
23. Boils and blains were included in the ten plagues with which the Egyptians were punished. (Exodus 9:10)
24. Herodotus: Henry Cary Trans., p. 124.
25. Ztsch. f. Egypten Schprache u. Alterthumkunde, 65:53, 70, 1928.
26. Smith, E.: Egypt. 8:14-17.
27. The writer is indebted to R. L. Moodie's manual, Paleopathology, University of Illinois Press, 1923, for valuable information pertaining to the medicine of ancient Egypt and for the sketch of the life of Ruffer.
28. Herodotus: Henry Cary Trans.: Euterpe; 2:77, American Book Co., N. Y. 1874.
29. Ruffer, Sir M. A.: Studies in the Paleontology of Egypt: Ed. R. L. Moodie, University of Chicago Press, 1921.
30. Spiegelberg found that the Egyptian name for oculist was *svanw-iv-ty*. The Egyptian oculist was famous in the time of Herodotus. King Cyrus of Persia asked King Hmasis (c. 560 B.C.) to send him the best Egyptian oculist.

31. Ebers: Report to the Oriental Congress. London.
32. Tobias 3.
33. See Introduction: Breasted, H. J.: Edwin Smith Surgical Papyrus. University of Chicago Press, 1920.
34. Hoefer, M.: Die Volksmedizinische Organotherapist. Pp. 279, 280.
35. Cited by Max Neuburger: Gesch. der Medizin. Jena, 1901, p. 75.
36. Homer: Iliad. 4:229.
37. Herodotus: 3:7, 32. For further references see Ermann: Life in Ancient Egypt. Trans. by Tirard, London, 1894. Kulter und Denker der Alten Egypter, 1907.

9

Ancient Hebrew Medicine

For the purpose of evaluation, the subject of this chapter may be conveniently divided into three periods: (1) The period of the Old Testament, dating from the time of Abraham (2000 B.C.) to Ezra (450 B.C.); (2) from Ezra to the beginning of the present era; and (3) the period of the New Testament. It should be borne in mind that the Old Testament, which is the main source of information under discussion, is primarily a religious anthological and chronological document and is in no sense a medical work. One should not expect to find there more than a casual reference to medicine and then only when it pertains to religious or civil laws, or when important characters are thereby affected.

The ancient Hebrews have not left any extant medical documents. They have not bequeathed any medical inscriptions on clay tablets, medical papyri, or votive tablets on the temple walls. The ancient Hebrews did not have a prehistoric period: their antiquity is limited to the period of Abraham (c. 2500 B.C.), a period when history had already begun to be recorded. But, if the Hebrews cannot boast of being first in point of time, they can be proud of having preserved many old medical practices and traditions which throw light on ancient medicine in general and on Hebrew medical practices in particular.

OLD TESTAMENT PERIOD

Disease as Sequel to Sin: The Hebrews, like other contemporary peoples, entertained a supernatural concept regarding medical phenomena, differing only in the fact that they, being a monotheistic people, attributed health and disease to one divine source. Disease

251

and premature death were considered as emanating from God. Everyone who suffered from any bodily ailment was thought to have previously violated a religious ordinance for which his bodily affliction was an atonement. As examples may be cited the case of Miriam who was punished with leprosy for slandering her brother Moses,[1] and the cases of Gehazi[2] and Uzziah,[3] who were punished with the same disease for sins committed by avarice and presumption respectively. For similar reasons, Jehoram was inflicted with intestinal disease and prolapse of the rectum.[4]

Epidemics were brought on a community for trespassing certain regulations by the people themselves or by the leader of the community. The Sodomites were smitten with blindness for their attack on Lot.[5] The Egyptians were punished with pestilence for the sins of Pharaoh.[6] The Philistines were attacked with emerods because their chiefs had committed a gross offense against the Israelites.[7]

Pharaoh was punished with a peculiar skin eruption for the abduction of Sarai, the wife of Abraham, and, for the same offense, Abimelech and his household were punished with barrenness.[8] Shameful or grave violations were punished with death as in the cases of Er and Onan;[9] and in the case of Bathsheba, whose firstborn son died,[10] and in the case of Achiyah,[11] son of Jeroboam, whose death meant destruction of Jeroboam's dynasty. Death was also the punishment for gluttony at Kiryath Hattaaba.[12]

Treatment of Disease: Healing, in the Old Testament, is clearly a divine attribute as may be seen from the following passages, "If thou surely harken to the voice of the Lord . . . the disease which I put on the Egyptians I will not put on thee, for I am the Lord that healeth thee."[13] Another passage shows that both the disease and its cure emanate from God, "I kill and I make alive" . . . "I have wounded and I heal."[14]

Prayer and Repentance: Since disease was considered the natural sequel to sin, only prayer and repentance could heal or prevent its occurrence, once some wicked deed was perpetrated. In the case of Miriam, her brother Moses cried out, "Heal her now, O God, I beseech thee."[15]

In II Chronicles, the Lord says to Solomon:

If I shut up heaven that there be no rain, or if I command the locust to devour the land, or if I send pestilence among My people; If My people, upon whom My name is called, shall humble themselves, and pray, and seek My face, and turn from their evil ways, then will I hear from heaven, and will forgive their sin, and will heal their land. [16]

Mutilation: Mutilation of the bodies of wrongdoers was naturally anathema to the ancient Hebrews who looked to God to mete out all punishment. It was sinful to maim or torture anyone, for such deeds thwarted the divine will. Apart from the *lex talionis,* in deliberate murder there is only one Biblical law exacting mutilation:

If men are fighting together, one with the other, and the wife of one draws near to save her husband from the hand of the smiter, and she sends forth her hand and seizes his privates, then shall you cut off her hand; your eye shall have no pity. [17]

Analogous laws have been discovered in the Old Assyrian Law Code dating from about the twelfth century B.C. and in the Nuzi tablets which date from about the fifteenth century B.C. Since punishment by mutilation is quite characteristic of the Assyrian code, it would seem that one has to look toward Assyria for the source of the above passage which is conspicuous in the Old Testament by its incongruity.

Restrictions of Lay-Physicians: The restriction against lay-physicians in the Old Testament, however, appears to have applied only to internal diseases where the cause was not manifest, as, for example epilepsy or malaria, but did not apply to cases of trauma, where the etiology is self-evident; in the last, lay-physicians were legitimately used as is evident from the "Book of Exodus," "and he shall cause him to be healed."[18]

Physicians were looked upon as messengers of the Divine Power. The case of Asa (915–875 B.C.) reveals that lay-physicians have been employed as early as the tenth century B.C. in internal diseases. It is related that King Asa was "diseased in his feet. . . . Yet in his disease he sought not to the Lord but to the physicians."[19] (The sickness was either podagra or paraplegia.) .

Human Agencies: At a later period, human agencies were added to religious rites in treating disease. Thus the prophets Elijah and Elisha, when called upon to administer to children who were at the threshold of death, resorted also to physical devices. In the case of Elijah,[20] the child could not breathe: the prophet took him to the roof of the abode into the open air and "stretched" himself upon the child. ("Stretching" was perhaps an ancient method of artifical respiration.) Then he resorted to prayer and supplication. Elisha, when called to treat a supposedly dead child, after prayer and supplication, put his mouth to the mouth of the child, possibly for the purpose of blowing in air, a form of artificial respiration presently employed soon after birth when the newborn does not breathe.[21]

Elisha followed this treatment by stretching himself upon the child, "and soon the flesh of the child waxed warm." He repeated the same process: the child sneezed (which probably dislodged the mucous plug or foreign body) and opened its eyes. Still later, Isaiah did not resort to any religious rites at all: he is recorded to have administered a cataplasm (a cake) made of figs to the inflamed parts of King Hezekiah.

Duties of Lay-Physicians and Priests: King Asa appears to have been the first patient on record to separate religion from medicine, "and in the thirty and ninth year of his reign, Asa was diseased in his feet; his disease was exceedingly great; yet in his disease he sought not to the Lord, but to the physicians. And Asa slept with his fathers and died in the one and fortieth year of his reign."[22] The outstanding implication with regard to Asa (915–875 B.C.) is that 450 years before Hippocrates, the people of Judea had professional physicians who separated priesthood from magic.

In the days of Jeremiah (sixth century B.C.), there appears to have been many lay-physicians in Palestine. Jeremiah thought it unbelievable that there should be no physicians. "Is there not balm in Gilead?" he asked. "Is there no physician there? Why, then, is not the health of the daughter of my people recovered?"[23]

Job mentioned physicians, but he had no confidence in them. He characterized them as *rophe elil* (physicians of no value).[24] The practice of healing among Hebrews was not, as it is generally understood, in the hands of priests as it was among Egyptians, Babylonians, and Persians. According to the Old Testament, priests had no authority to treat internal diseases. To them were assigned the duties of health warden, such as, for example, the supervision of patients suffering from leprosy, plague, gonorrhea *(zab)* and spermatorrhea *(shichbath zera)*,[25] the enforcement of the laws pertaining to social hygiene, isolation of contagious diseases, contact with dead bodies, and ablution of those who were near them.

The Hebrew priests had no jurisdiction over disease in general. Indeed, according to a later tradition, priests themselves called on lay-physicians in case of sickness. Temple physicians *(medicus viscerus)* were appointed to treat priests who were often troubled with abdominal pain and probably also arthritis, in consequence of their being obliged to undergo daily ablution in cold water and to perform their services while barefoot on cold stones. It is related that a certain physician, Ben Achiyah, was appointed to treat priests who suffered from intestinal troubles.

Social Hygiene: The distinction of medicine in the Old Testament does not lie in the diagnosis of disease nor in the therapeutics but in social hygiene; five centuries before the Greeks visited the land of the Pharaohs (1200 B.C.), Israel was in possession of a document containing laws and regulations, the realization of which was bound to promote the welfare of the ancient Israelites and the preservation of the future nation.

The precepts that physical and mental purity are interdependent was the keystone of the Mosaic law. Prevention of epidemics, suppression of prostitution and venereal disease, frequent ablution, care of the skin, regulation of sexual life, dietary laws, regulation of labor, the observation of the Sabbath day, measures with regard to menstruation and lying-in women, circumcision, isolation of those suffering from gonorrhea, and many other laws have tended to prevent disease from spreading through Palestine. "And ye shall be unto me a kingdom of priest and holy nation,"[26] was the cornerstone upon which those laws were founded.

It is entirely immaterial whether the hygiene and prophylaxis as promulgated by Moses in the Pentateuch were intended as religious rituals or as health measures. The fact is they were scientifically sound; nor does it matter whether these doctrines were original with Moses or selected and edited by Moses from old traditions and/or manuscripts. The fact is that neither the old Egyptian medical documents nor other early medical codes have been so thoroughgoing on subjects of hygiene and prophylaxis as the Mosaic Code.

The recognition that "an ounce of prevention is worth a pound of cure" accounts for the absence in the Old Testament of many diseases which prevailed in Egypt at that period. The strict sanitary and dietetic regulation and the balmy climate of Palestine were destined to eliminate many diseases prevailing in the neighboring countries.

Moses: If Moses was not the father of Jewish medicine, he certainly was an apt pupil. According to the New Testament, Moses was instructed in "all the wisdom of the Egyptians,"[27] which included medicine, for medicine in Egypt was a branch of general culture. It was taught in the temples of On, Sais, Thebes, and Memphis by the priests attached to these sanctuaries. Philo (20 B.C.–40 A.D.) of Alexandria repeats the tradition that Moses was educated in the fashion of the Egyptians and Chaldeans. Clement of Alexandria (160–215 A.D.) had the same tradition that Moses was trained in all the wisdom of the Egyptians which included medicine and alchemy.[28] Thus,

Moses, in addition to being a codifier, was also the father of ancient Jewish medicine.

King Solomon: After Moses, tradition credits King Solomon (reigned 971–931 B.C.) with a knowledge of medicine. The "Book of Kings" refers to him as a wise monarch, particularly learned in botany and natural history.[29] From the scriptural books ascribed to him, it is evident that he had a knowledge of the bodily organs and their functions.[30] His long peaceful reign and his friendly relationship with neighboring countries, particularly Egypt, offered him added opportunities to study the wisdom of the Egyptians where medicine was highly developed at that period.

Babylonian Influence: The dissolution of the Jewish state marks the second epoch of medicine. Great changes took place in the cultural aspects of the Hebrews. The captivity in Babylon brought the exiles into contact with a new sphere of thought which, in a measure, had a wholesome influence on them: when they returned after seventy years to their homeland, they brought with them also, in addition to their own intellectual store of knowledge, the Babylonian culture. They had their *soferim* (scribes),[31] their *maskilim*[32] (enlightened ones), and their *mevinim* (men of understanding). Daniel extolled scholarship, "They that be wise shall shine as the brightness of the firmament." A learned man was considered greater than a prophet.[33] Schools and academies were established in the larger cities of Palestine.

Hellenic Influence: Later, when Palestine came under the political supremacy of Greece, the Hellenes exercised a great cultural influence upon the Judeans, as is evident from the "Book of Sirach" (written during the early part of the third century B.C.). This apocryphal author, who extols medicine in the highest terms, lived during the reign of the first and second Ptolemies at a time when Alexandria was the greatest medical center of antiquity and when Herophilus and Erasistratus spread their medical wisdom all over the ancient world. Alexandria, having the largest Jewish population next to Jerusalem, undoubtedly exerted a cultural influence upon the Hebrews of Palestine.

The high esteem in which the physician was held is proved by the beautiful words of Jesus, the son of Sirach (written c. 210 B.C.) (R. V., Chapter 37):

> Show the physician due honor, in view of your need of him,
> For the Lord has created him;
> Healing comes from the Most High,

And he will receive presents from the king.
The skill of the physician exalts him,
And he is admired among the great.
The Lord has created medicines out of the earth,
And a sensible man will not refuse them.
Was not water made sweet by wood,
So that he might be glorified for his wonderful works.
And he has given men knowledge
So that he might be glorified for his wonderful works.
With them he cures and takes away pain,
The druggist makes a mixture of them.
His works will never end,
And from him, peace spreads over the face of the earth. [34]

The book "Ecclesiasticus" ascribes sickness to excesses:

And do not be carried away with food,
For sickness comes with excessive eating,
And greediness leads to severe illness.

The Hellenic influence upon the Jews of Palestine is evident from the fact that an important section of Palestine Jewry (the Sadducees) emulated the Greeks, not only in their cultural activities, but also in their physical practices. Athletic games, similar to those performed on Mt. Olympus, were established in Jerusalem and other cities of Palestine. If Hellenism was not accepted in the academies as a part of the curriculum, it was studied indirectly to illustrate certain points of law.

Biblical Anatomy

That the Hebrews had more than a passing knowledge of anatomy can be demonstrated by the following: (1) From passages concerning the methods of sacrifice and (2) from passages of poetry where the names of organs and structures are used metaphorically. As an illustration of the first type of passage, Exodus may be quoted, "And thou shalt dissect the ram and wash its inwards, and its legs and put them with its pieces and with its head."[35] (Incidentally, in this passage the Hebrew term *nituach*, signifying dissection, is used for the first time.) Illustrations of the second type of passage are as follows, "He poureth out my gall *(mererah)* upon the ground."[36] "And the marrow of his bones *(moah 'asmotav)* is moistened."[37] "I am weary with my crying; my throat *(garon)* is dried."[38]

Terms for the visible parts of the body were naturally well known to the early Israelites, such as "eye," "tooth," "hair," "nails," "brow," "earlobe," "hand," "leg," "finger," "thumb," "neck," "breast," "mouth," "nose," and "shoulder."[39] In Solomon's "Song of Songs," "temple," "palate," "cheeks," "neck," "breasts," "head," "hands," "fingers," "eyes," "lips," "legs," "mouth," "navel," "belly," "nose," and "hair" are all mentioned. *Rehm*, meaning womb, possibly includes the entire birth canal. The word *'orlah* refers to the prepuce.[40]

Basar, literally translated as "flesh," includes muscle tissue. In "Job," special mention is made of the abdominal and thigh musculature. *Serire bitno* (sinews of his belly), is the term for the former, and *gide-gahadaw* (lit., sinews of his thighs), the expression for the latter. This passage illustrates the fact that the Hebrews well understood the relationship between muscular development and strength. Two words for "bone" *('ezem)* also occur in this passage. The structure of bones is compared to "pipes of brass" and "pipes of iron." Here follows the quotation:

> Lo now, his strength is in his loins,
> And his force is in the stays of his body (lit., sinews of his belly).
> He straineth his tail like a cedar;
> The sinews of his thighs are knit together,
> His bones are as pipes of brass;
> His gristles (really bones) are like bars of iron. [41]

The analogy of the bones to pipes suggests that the Hebrews well knew the gross anatomy of the long bones.

The word for "blood" *(dam)* is frequently mentioned in the Bible. The early Israelites considered the blood to be the seat of the soul. It is stated, "Only flesh with life thereof which is the blood thereof shall ye not eat."[42] The heart *(leb)* is frequently mentioned in the Old Testament[43] as the seat of emotion and intellect. The function which is now ascribed to the brain was thought to emanate mainly from the heart, and no word for brain is mentioned.[44] The animal heart was differentiated from the human heart by the fact that the former was considered devoid of intelligence, "Let his (Nebuchadnezzar's) heart be changed from man's, and let a beast's heart be given unto him."[45] The heart was recognized as a vital organ, "Above all that thou guardest keep thy heart; for out of it are the issues of life."[46]

The ancient Hebrews had a good knowledge of the abdominal viscera, even understanding the function of the omentum as the "policeman of the abdomen":

And Ehud put forth his left hand, and took the sword from his right thigh, and thrust it into his belly. And the haft also went in after the blade, and the fat closed upon the blade, for he drew not the sword out of his belly; and it came out behind. [47]

The liver *(kabed)* is mentioned many times in early Hebrew literature. The term *yoteret hak-kabed* occurs in six Biblical passages, It refers to that part of the organ which had to be sacrificed, as a fatty piece.[48] The Authorized Version, following Jerome, renders it "the caul above the liver," and "Rashi" does the same. The "Septuagint" renders it "the lobe of the liver," which indicates that the sacrificed portion was an integral part of the liver itself. The ancient Hebrews knew that the liver is a vital organ, trauma of which would lead to uncontrollable hemorrhage. Only a fool would have "an arrow strike through his liver . . . and knoweth not that it is at the cost of his life."[49] They also recognized the fact that the liver manufactured a fluid. In "Lamentations," we read, "My liver is poured upon the earth."[50]

In the English translations, the word "caul" has been used far too promiscuously. According to Dorland, the caul is either the great omentum or a piece of amnion which sometimes envelopes a child's head at birth. Nowhere in the Bible does it have either of these meanings. Most often, the word "caul" is employed to translate *yoteret*, a word which often occurs in connection with the liver in discussions of priestly regulations. It is discussed in the preceding paragraph, and the tendency now is to take it to mean the fatty mass surrounding the liver which was included in the burnt offering.[51] *Segor libbam*, usually translated as "caul of their heart," probably refers to the pericardium.[52] The word "caul" is also referred to as an article of jewelry.[53]

The early Hebrews were well aware of the structure of the kidneys and of the renal fat. Most of the references given for *yoteret* also make mention of *ste hak-kelayot* (the two kidneys) and *haheleb 'aser'alehen* (the fat which is upon them). The visceral fat in general is referred to as *kol-haheleb hamekasseh* (all the fat that covereth the inwards).[54] *Peder* is believed by some to be the fat that covers the intestine under the omentum.[55] In "Leviticus," *mur'ah* refers to the "crop" of fowls.[56]

Biblical Physiology

The Old Testament attributed all bodily function, both in health and disease, to divine guidance, "Who hath made man's mouth? Or who maketh a man dumb or deaf or seeing or blind; is it not I, the Lord?"[57] The idea of a soul that was supposed to govern the human mechanism is of Greek origin not known in the Pentateuch, and the Hebrews adopted it at a later period.[58] There is scarcely any mention of a soul in the Pentateuch and in the Early Prophets. The term *nephesh* in the Bible, rendered "psyche" (not immortal soul) is applicable also to animal life,[59] *ruach* (spirit) applies to vital energy which also refers to lower beings;[60] *neshamah* (breath), which was later applied to the soul, is defined as normal breathing. The principle that every human action or impulse is governed by Providence remained the firm belief of Jews throughout posterity.

Hygiene in the Bible

According to ancient Hebrew tradition, even before Moses' time, cleanliness of the body was so inextricably tied up with purity of the soul that the Old Testament, without any question, assumes that the two go hand in hand. Before one could communicate with God, or purify himself after disease, he had to cleanse himself thoroughly. Thus we read:

Then Jacob said unto his household, and to all that were with him: Put away the strange gods that are among you, and purify yourselves, and change your garments; and let us arise, and go up to Beth-el; and I will make there an altar unto God.... [61]

In Exodus, it is noted that before the Israelites were permitted to obtain the commandments, "the Lord said unto Moses: go unto the people, and sanctify them today and tomorrow, and let them wash their garments . . ."[62] So deeply was this idea of personal cleanliness ingrained that it was often used symbolically, "for though thou wash thee with nitre, and take thee much soap, yet thine inquity is marked before Me, . . ."[63]

Now, this spirit of cleanliness is more remarkable if it is realized that water in the orient was, and for that matter in most places still is, considered a "luxurious necessity," so to speak. Natives today are hesitant about "wasting," for washing purposes, water that they need for the more important function of drinking.

Unclean influences put the body in a state of taboo until thorough cleansing was accomplished. Elaborate sanitary precautions were exercised by persons having communicable diseases and by persons coming into contact with them.[64] When a person was exposed to a corpse, a bone, or a grave, he was required to bathe in water.[65] Anyone eating carrion was likewise obliged to cleanse himself.[66]

Types of Ablution: The Bible, by inference, designates two types of ablution. The most common type requires immersion of the entire body in water, as in the following passages: (1) When a person was healed of leprosy, he was required to shave off his hair, wash his clothes, bathe his entire body, and thus become clean.[67] (2) No leprosy priest was permitted to eat the flesh of a sacrificed animal until he had washed his whole body in water.[68] (3) Anyone coming in contact with the body of, or with objects used by, a person having a discharge from his flesh or sexual organs was forced to cleanse his body and his garments.[69] (4) Any person suffering from a discharge from his flesh or sexual organs had to wash his entire body and clothing.[70] (5) Anyone touching a menstruating woman, or any particle used by her, required immersion of the entire body.[71] (6) Any person eating unclean flesh of a beast which had died of itself was obliged to cleanse his whole body.[72] (7) Whoever came into contact with a corpse was unclean for seven days, after which he washed his whole body and all of his clothes in water.[73] (8) A menstruating woman required immersion, as is demonstrated by II *Samuel*.[74] The menstrual bath is ordained in "Leviticus,"[75] and was punctually observed with running water in sufficient volume. This law survives among modern orthodox Jews in the communal pool for women, which is known as the *miqwah*.

The second type of ablution is washing of the hands and feet. Before any priest could enter the tabernacle, he had to wash his hands and feet with water from the laver which stood between the tabernacle and the altar.[76] The dusty soil of Palestine in conjunction with the open shoes worn, necessitated frequent washing of the feet.[77] That washing of the hands was considered fundamental for purity and cleanliness can be seen from the following passages, "Surely in vain have I cleansed my heart, and washed my hands in innocency."[78] "I will wash my hands in innocency; so will I compass Thine altar, O Lord, . . ."[79]

The spirit of cleanliness was carried by hospitality beyond the defined limits of the Pentateuch. Thus a good host had his guest's feet washed. We note that Abraham's servant obtained "water to wash his feet and the feet of the men that were with him" before entering Rebekah's house.[80]

As a logical consequence to the fact that one had to cleanse himself before engaging in so many details of ancient Hebrew life, particularly of a religious nature, it naturally followed that one would wash himself and his clothing thoroughly before visiting a person of note.

Hebrew Diseases: A list of several diseases prevalent in Biblical times is presented in the twenty-third chapter of "Leviticus" and in the twenty-eighth chapter of "Deuteronomy," and these include *shahepheth* (consumption), *kadahath* (fever) that will consume the eyes (evidently it refers to malarial cachexia, a severe form of chronic malaria that affects the eye), *daleketh* (inflammation), *harhur* (the meaning of which is not clear),[81] *yerokon* (jaundice)? Egyptian boils, emerods (tumors or plague boils), scurvy, scab, itch, insanity, blindness, and sore boils of the knees and legs.[82] Other pathological conditions mentioned in connection with the priestly code, which render the priest ineligible to attend to his priestly duties are the following: fractures of the arms and legs,[83] rickets, scurvy, supernumary or missing organs, and some eye diseases which will be described later.[84] The incurability and hopelessness of these ailments are stressed over and over again. However, it is foolhardy, on the basis of the Biblical description, to recognize modern clinical entities, for no clinical pictures are given.

The two great diseases considered communicable and discussed in the Old Testament are leprosy and gonorrhea. According to the priestly code, the priesthood is given exclusive control only over these diseases. The statutes concerning these dreaded plagues are obviously directed, not only to impart a knowledge of the symptoms and thus make diagnosis comparatively easy, but also to pevent spread. Quarantine was rigidly enforced, especially for leprosy.

For the discussion of leprosy, the reader is referred to "Leviticus."[85] The Biblical passages should be read in toto because the precise detailed and scientific account presented in the Pentateuch could not be improved by addition or subtraction. The method of obtaining a differential diagnosis is amazing, the knowledge of the dormant and necrotic stages of the disease is spectacular, and the careful regard for minute detail and clinical observation is noteworthy.

However, it does not seem likely that this Hebrew leprosy is to be always identified with modern leprosy. In the first place, Biblical leprosy was considered a curable disease, whereas present-day leprosy is, except in isolated and doubtful instances, incurable. Then too, the Biblical description does not even vaguely allude to rotting of the limbs and facial deformity which are present-day features of leprosy. Lastly, today's leprosy is an extremely chronic disease, and the Biblical priests certainly would not be able to note its progress in seven-day intervals.

The Hebrew word for leprosy, *zara'at,* probably was a general term for a number of skin ailments. The white spots so often mentioned as a diagnostic sign probably were caused by the tropical disease, *leukoderma* (also called "piebald skin" and "vitiligo"). This disease is characterized by bright white spots on which the hairs also become white. The white patches enlarge and are especially conspicuous on persons of dark complexion. Cutaneous syphilis might also have been included under the classification of leprosy.

The laws of quarantine were rigidly enforced in Biblical times. Even kings were not exempted, as is seen in the following passages:

> Now there were four leprous men at the entrance of the gate; and they said one to another: Why sit we here until we die? If we say: We will enter into the city, then the famine is in the city, and we shall die there; and if we sit here, we die also. Now therefore come, and let us fall unto the host of the Arameans; if they save us alive, we shall live; and if they kill us, we shall but die. [86]

> And Uzziah, the king, was a leper unto the day of his death, and dwelt in a house set apart, being a leper, for he was cut off from the house of the Lord. [87]

Evidently the leprosy of Uzziah was fatal and incurable and may well have been identical with, or similar to, the modern type.

This isolation of lepers demanded by the Old Testament is of less importance as a hygienic measure than as an influencing factor on medical history. It must be borne in mind that leprosy is a much less actively communicable disease than several other well-known affections not requiring segregation. Yet, because of Biblical influences, lepers, to this day, dwell "in a house set apart."[88]

It is interesting, in passing, to note that the Old Testament considers mildew of clothes and of house walls as forms of leprosy. This further bears out the contention that the word *zara'at* was a general term, loosely used.

It is possible that the Biblical *magepho* refers to syphilis. According to the account in "Numbers,"[89] Balak, king of the Moabites, feared that his kingdom would be overrun by the Israelites on their sojourn from Egypt. He sent emissaries and thrice built altars to induce Balaam, the holy man, to curse the Hebrews, but to no avail. Many of the Israelites, however, took up with Moabite women and began worshipping the pagan Moabite gods, especially Baalpeor. It is likely that promiscuous sexual rites were an integral part of this pagan worship. One Israelite actually had the audacity to bring a Moabite woman home to the Hebrew camp. In all, it is recorded that 24,000 Hebrews died of the plague that ensued following contact with the Moabite women. Might this plague not have been lues? Surely the predisposing factors were present. Medieval times saw syphilis strike a similarly deadly blow under similar circumstances.[90] Incidentally, from the description "fallen down with open eyes," it would appear that Balaam was afflicted with epilepsy.

Gonorrhea is believed to be the dominant venereal disease of antiquity. According to the priestly code, whenever there was an intermittent or continuous discharge from a person's sexual organs, that person was declared unclean and anyone engaging in coitus with him or touching him or anything with which he had come in contact (i.e. his bed, chair, saddle, saliva) had to wash his clothes and bathe in water. Earthen vessels used by the infected person had to be broken and wooden ones washed. After the discharge had stopped for seven days, the infected person was required to wash his clothes and bathe in running water, after which the taboo was removed. These statutes, given completely in "Leviticus,"[91] are excellent hygienic measures to hinder the spread of gonorrhea, and the precautions exercised for venereal disease might well have been applied to a purulent discharge from any part of his body.[92]

Materia Medica

From various Biblical passages, one can deduce that the ancient Hebrews were well aware of the apothecary's art:

The Lord spoke unto Moses saying: Take thou also unto thee the chief spices, of flowing myrrh five hundred shekels, and of sweet cinnamon, half so much, even two hundred and fifty, and of cassia, five hundred, after the shekel of the sanctuary, and of olive oil a hin. And thou shalt make it a holy anointing oil, a perfume compounded after the art of the perfumer;....
Take unto thee sweet spices, storax, and onycha, galbanum; sweet spices with pure frankincense; of each shalt there be a light weight, and thou shalt make of it incense, a perfume after the art of the perfumer, seasoned with salt, pure and holy. And thou shalt beat some of it very small, and put it before the testimony of the tent of meeting where I will meet thee; it shall be unto you most holy. [93]

Aside from the drugs, the explicit directions to the compounder is of interest. Among other remedies mentioned is mandrake (*dudaim*), which was considered to possess aphrodisiac properties.

It is natural that among a people who viewed sterility as the greatest misfortune, effort should be made to search for remedies that would promote conception. This drug was efficient for Rachel when all else failed.[94] According to the Biblical narrative, Leah's son found mandrakes in a field, so he brought them to his mother

Leah. Rachel, who wanted them badly made a deal with Leah to turn over the mandrake in return for Jacob's company. As a result of the bargain, Rachel became impregnated. Mandrake has been praised for its aroma in the "Song of Songs."[95]

Balm of Gilead is mentioned many times in ancient Hebrew works.[96] The hills of Gilead, located in central Transjordania, were famous for their medicinal herbs. According to Jeremiah, balm of Gilead (which may or may not have been a definite compound) was used as a palliative.[97]

Niter (Hebrew *neter*) is used in parallelism to the word for soap (*borit*).[98] This indicates that niter as well as soap was employed as a cleansing agent and surface antiseptic.

Fruits and saps of certain trees were available, such as, for example, *tsri* (balsam), *nchoth* (tragacanth), and *lott* (laudanum). Certain poisonous roots, characterized by a bitter taste, are mentioned, such as, for example, *pore*,[99] *rosh*, and *v'laanah; gofrith* (sulfur) is noted with reference of the destruction of Sodom.[100]

Oil was employed to dress wounds, bruises, and festering sores.[101] Wine was employed as a mental depressant: the daughters of Lot drugged their father with wine until he was in deep stupor.[102] Pharmaceutical substances were quite numerous in Biblical days; Jeremiah declares, "In vain dost thou use many medicines; there is no cure for thee."[103]

Penetrating Wounds in Biblical Days

Many of the wounds mentioned in ancient Hebrew literature were fatal. Joab "took three darts in his hand, and thrust them through the heart of Absalom."[104]

He also smote Amasa "in the groin, and shed out his bowels to the ground," thus killing him.[105] Abner "with the hinder end of the spear smote Asahel in the groin, that the spear came out behind him; and he fell down there, and died in the same place."[106] Phineas killed a man and woman by thrusting a spear through their abdomens.[107] Ehud killed a man by thrusting a sword through his abdomen.[108] Jael murdered Sisera in the following manner: "Her hand she put to the tent-pin, and her right hand to the workman's hammer; and with the hammer she smote Sisera, she smote through his head, yea, she pierced and struck through his temples. At her feet, he sunk, he fell . . . dead."[109]

It must have been quite common indeed for wounds to become infected. "My wounds are noisome, they fester" is the plaintive cry of the psalmist.[110] The common treatment for wounds and bruises was oil and bandages, as may be inferred from the following passage:

> From the sole of the foot even unto the head
> There is no soundness in it;
> But wounds, and bruises, and festering sores;
> They have not been pressed, neither bound up,
> Neither mollified with oil. [111]

This reference also shows that drainage was accomplished by pressure around the infected area. Various forms of wounds are mentioned: *makkah* (the general term for a wound), *makkah triyah* (a festering wound), *makkah machlah* (a grievous wound), *makkah anusa* (weak wound, a wound that would not heal), *petzah* (a stab wound), *habburah* (hematoma or boil), and *mazor* (a boil, containing septic matter).

Cutaneous Diseases

Furunculosis appears to have been a common ailment among the ancient Hebrews. The boils mentioned seem to have been of a virulent variety occurring epidemically. Perhaps cutaneous leishmaniasis (oriental sore, aleppo boil, delhi boil) is the condition referred to when "Exodus" speaks of a boil breaking forth with blains upon man and beast, throughout all the land of Egypt.[112] The fact that animals to this day may be naturally infected with cutaneous leishmaniasis seems to lend weight to this contention.

Various forms of skin disease are referred to in "Deuteronomy":

The Lord will smite thee with the boil of Egypt, and with the emerods, and with the scab, and with the itch, whereof thou canst not be healed. [113]

The Lord will smite thee in the knees, and in the legs with a sore boil, whereof thou canst not be healed, from the sole of thy foot unto the crown of thy head. [114]

In this case, cutaneous leishmaniasis is ruled out, for it is specifically stated that the plague was incurable, whereas oriental sore usually leads to spontaneous recovery in three to twelve months.

Infections of the Bones

Infection and necrosis of the bone were not uncommon among the early Israelites, as may be seen from the following metaphorical passages taken from "Proverbs":

> A virtuous woman is a crown to her husband;
> But that doeth shamefully is as rottenness in his bones. [115]
> A tranquil heart is the life of the flesh;
> But envy is the rottenness of the bones. [116]

"Rottenness of the bones" may refer to osteomyelitis.

Intestinal Parasites

Intestinal worms were common among the ancient Hebrews who inhabited subtropical climes. One of the reasons why the ancient Israelites were forbidden to eat meat from animals not having a cloven hoof might well have been the fact that Trichinella spiralis was present in the muscles of pigs, and caused trichinosis when eaten by man.

Like other peoples, there is evidence that the ancient Hebrews also practiced sympathetic magic. When fiery serpents bit the Israelites with numerous fatalities, Moses made a serpent of brass. Henceforth, anyone bitten by the said serpents, who looked at Moses' model, survived.[117]

Surgery

The only surgical operations mentioned in the Old Testament are circumcision and castration, the former being mandatory[118] and the latter forbidden.[119]

The first Biblical record of the instruments used in circumcision is found in "Exodus," "Then Zipporah took a flint, and cut off the foreskin of her son."[120] Flint, however, was not necessarily the usual instrument of circumcision, for Zipporah was forced to act quickly to stave off God's wrath, and she probably availed herself of whatever was handiest. It is highly probable that metal knives were also employed. It should be remembered that the manufacture and use of brass and iron implements are so ancient that Hebrew tradition ascribes to them an antediluvian date.[121] The technique of circumcision as practiced among the early Hebrews is unknown. That it was a painful operation can readily be discerned,[122] for so great was the weakness and pain of the circumcised adults, even on the third day following circumcision, that two men were able to slaughter all the males of the entire town without so much as a finger raised in self-defense.

The concept of the spread of disease by direct contact with minute pathogenic particles in the air has been attributed to Moses. He was instructed to "take handfuls of ashes (or soot) and disseminate it through the air in Pharaoh's presence."[123]

Fractures are referred to as *sheber yad* (hand or arm fractures) and *sheber regel* (foot or leg fracture);[124] dislocation of the hip joint, *kaph yerech*, is alluded to in the case of Jacob.[125] Ezekiel gives ample evidence that he has more than a passing knowledge of the art of reducing fractures when he says, "Son of man, I have broken the arm of Pharaoh, king of Egypt; and lo, it hath not been bound up

to be healed, to put a roller, that it be bound up and wax strong, that
it hold the sword . . ."[126]

Eye Diseases

The eye *(ayin)* is alluded to in the Bible many times.[127] The pupil
is known as *babat ha'ayin* (door of the eye).[128] The eyelids *(af appayim)* are referred to in "Jeremiah,"[129] in the passage, "and our
eyelids gush out with waters," which indicates the belief that the
lacrimal apparatus is located in the lids.

Foreign bodies in the eyes are frequently referred to in the Old
Testament. For instance, in "Joshua" we read, "and pricks in thy
eyes . . ."[130]

Blepharitis ciliaris appears to have been a common disease among
the ancient Jews of Palestine. An interesting case is that of Leah.
The passage reads, "and Leah's eyes were weak; but Rachel was of
beautiful form and fair to look upon."[131] From the text, one is led
to believe that the weak eyes of Leah spoiled her appearance: they
were red and swollen about the lid margins with perhaps the loss
of eyelashes and the formation of concretions on the margins. Her
case could not have been that of tender eyes as rendered in the King
James version, for such eyes could hardly be called ugly and give
rise to complaint by Jacob.

Exophthalmos appears to have been attributed to an increase of
fat in the orbital cavity. The psalmist sets forth, "their eyes stand
forth from fatness . . ."[132]

Gonorrheal ophthalmia undoubtedly existed because gonorrhea of
the genital organs was prevalent in both sexes. As seen from the
excellent account of the symptomatology and of the sanitary precautions observed,[133] the visual organs were frequently infected by
contact with the discharge.

The Hebrew words for blindness *(sanwerim*[134] and *iwwaron*[135])
used in the Bible are extremely vague terms; they cover all types
of partial and complete blindness of a temporary or permanent nature. The prevalence of blindness is well illustrated in II Samuel,
"The inhabitants (of Jerusalem) complained to David: Except thou
take away the blind and the lame, thou shalt not come in hither;[136]
thinking David cannot come in hither." In fact, blindness was so
prevalent that special laws were necessary to protect the blind. In
"Deuteronomy," we read, "cursed be he that maketh the blind to
go astray in the way."[137] Whereas diagnosis was not made, there
can be but little doubt that such diseases as *retrobulbar neuritis,*

albuminuric neuritis, optic neuritis, and other forms of organic diseases existed.

Senile cataract has always been a prominent cause of blindness, and probably occurred frequently among the ancient Hebrews. The most suggestive passage is the following, "now the eyes of Israel were dim for age so that he could not see."[138] Both age and race are predisposing causes of cataract. The "dimness" of his sight rather than blindness is indicative of cataract. However, this case might have been the early stage of glaucoma.

Four cases of Old Testament amaurosis present the possibility of glaucoma:

1. And it came to pass when Isaac was told that his eyes were dim so that he could not see. [139]

2. Now the eyes of Israel were dim for age so that he could not see. [140]

3. Now Eli was ninety and eight years old and his eyes were set; so that he could not see. [141]

4. Now he (Ahijah) could not see; for his eyes were set by reason of his age. [142]

In case (1), the word "dim" is confusing, for according to the Biblical narrative, Isaac suffered from total loss of sight. The patriarch, it will be remembered, could distinguish his two sons Esau and Jacob only by the sound of their voices and by his sense of touch. In each case, the writer gives old age as the cause of blindness. Cases (3) and (4) are most significant. The Hebrew word *qamu* literally means "they stood still." The English version "eyes were set" practically expresses the same idea. In other words, the blind eyes of Eli and Ahijah were at a standstill. They could not fix on objects in front of them, as is characteristic in amaurosis following glaucoma, in which perception of light is gone; there is a peculiar stare, and the eyes either do not move or do so aimlessly. This peculiar stare could not be mistaken for senile cataract, for in this condition there is usually some light perception, and the ocular muscles keep working in all directions to find a fixation point in order to locate luminous objects in front of the eye or to recognize dark objects in daylight.

The etiologic factors in all the cases cited bear a striking similarity: old age is given as the main cause of blindness. It is now generally agreed that the cause of glaucoma lies in those degenerative processes which are inseparable from the wear and tear of the living organism occurring in old age. In all of the above cases, there is a history of mental and physical strain, which is recognized as a predisposing factor to ocular trouble. All these Biblical persons were living in the same environment and climate. Two pursued the life of shepherds, exposed to the hot sun during the day and to the cold and damp Palestinian air at night. The contrast between the glare of the sun by day and the cold, damp night air is considered a factor in causing glaucoma. All four of the affected persons were members of the Semitic race, among whom glaucoma is especially prevalent. In cases (1) and (2), each showed a hereditary predisposition to glaucoma; in cases (1), (3), and (4), each suffered total loss of vision; in case (2), sight was only partly impaired, and in all the cases, the loss of vision was bilateral. If unilateral blindness, as well as amaurosis not contingent on old age, is barred, and senile cataract is eliminated for the previously mentioned reasons, the clinical history in the four cases cited is strongly suggestive of glaucoma.[143]

Another disease of the eye mentioned in the Old Testament is *jabeleth*,[144] a hard wart situated beneath the skin of the lid (also found in animals). According to the Mosaic Law, when an animal is troubled with a *jabeleth* on the eye, it is not fit for sacrifice because *jabeleth* is a permanent defect. *Dak*, described as a gray spot on the pupil interfering with the vision, is noted in "Leviticus" 21:22. *Thebalul*, etymologically speaking, is a mixture of colors of the iris and sclera, and is understood to represent two congenital conditions: a *coloboma* of the iris and sclera and also a condition in which the sclera covers a part of the entire pupil.[145] Among other pathological conditions that disqualify a priest from attending to his priestly duties are the following: *meroach ochesh* (hydrocele),[146] *ptsua dakkah* (crushed testicles),[147] *chrooth shafcho* (hypospadias),[148] *horutz* (harelip), and *shabur* (hernia).[149]

Functions of the Heart

Most functions which are now ascribed to the brain were considered by the early Israelites to emanate from the heart. Such thoughts as joy, gladness,[150] fear,[151] pride,[152] and sorrow[153] spring from the heart. Memory is attributed to the heart.[154] Knowledge is stored up in the heart;[155] the heart knows and understands.[156] The man devoid of understanding is the man "without heart."[157]

The heart is the organ concerned with all moral and spiritual functions, such as a pure heart and a good heart. The heart is the seat of all conscious resolve. Ahasuerus says to Esther, "Who is he, and where is he, that durst presume in his heart to do so?"[158] The phrase "with all your heart"[159] denotes conscious resolve, in which the whole being consents.

Insanity

Insanity was not unknown among the ancient Hebrews ("The Lord will smite thee with madness"[160]). David, when visiting the Philistines, feigned insanity. An interesting feature of his guise was that he slobbered at the mouth. Saul seems to have been more furious than insane in his fits of passion against David, who, after all, from Saul's point of view, was an upstart and eventually a usurper.

The simple life led by the children of Israel, however, was certainly not one to bring mental disturbances to the fore by taxing the intellectual capacities of the people.[161] There probably were village idiots just as there are today among the clans and townfolk of the Near East, but these were few in number. To characterize ancient Hebrews as neurotics because they cried, rent their hair, and donned sackcloth and ashes in time of distress is just as ill-founded as saying that westerners are neurotic because they clap their hands and shriek with laughter when a radio humorist tells a funny story or when they are at a ball game. Different people have different customs and traditions. The Semites, inhabiting the Near East today, act very much like the ancient Hebrews, without being neurotic in the least.

The fact that many of the Biblical persons married within the clan[162] and often within the family is no sound reason for thinking that insanity would crop up. There is really an absence of bonafide cases of insanity in ancient Hebrew literature.

Obstetrics and Gynecology

Intercourse: Because intercourse does not necessarily lead to pregnancy, ancients were ignorant of the cause-and-effect relationship existing between intercourse and pregnancy. From the story of Onan, it is evident that the ancient Hebrews were well aware of the fact that coitus was prerequisite for pregnancy. Thus, Onan, when he did not wish to impregnate his brother's widow, since his brother would be the legal parent of the child, "when he went in unto his brother's wife . . . spilled it on the ground, lest he should give seed to his brother."[163] Incidentally, this is the first recorded case of *coitus interruptus* and birth control in history. Such a procedure was evidently frowned upon, for Onan was killed for this act. Since the Israelites realized that intercourse was necessary for, but did not invariably lead to, pregnancy, they felt that successful fertilization was in the hands of God. Thus it is noted, "and the man knew Eve his wife; and she conceived and bore Cain, and said: I have gotten a man with the help of the Lord."[164]

A similar instance may be cited in the case of Abraham, "and Abraham prayed unto God; and God healed Abimelech and his wife, and his maid servants; and they bore children. For the Lord had fast closed up all the wombs of the house of Abimelech, because of Sarah, Abraham's wife."[165]

Barrenness: The very derivation of the Hebrew word for "barren" (*aqar*) gives us an insight as to how the ancient Israelites regarded the condition of childlessness. This word signified "uprooted," and the family that was left childless certainly was torn away from the root of Abraham. Strength and wealth among the ancient Hebrews were considered in terms of children, for he who had the most numerous children had the greatest security in life. No happier man could be depicted than that mentioned by the psalmist:

> Thy wife shall be a fruitful vine, in the innermost parts of thy house;
> Thy children like olive plants, round about thy table.
> Behold, surely thus shall the man be blessed
> That feareth the Lord. [166]

And how unhappy was the woman who could not give her husband much wanted children! "Give me children or else I die,"[167] begged Rachel. The very fact that she gave her handmaid Bilhah to Jacob shows how keenly she suffered because of her barrenness. Hannah's rival, Peninnah, "vexed her sore, to make her fret, because the Lord had shut up her womb."[168]

It must be remembered that the presence of an heir [169] was needed for the continuance and the solidarity of the clan.

The first barren woman[170] mentioned in the Bible was Sarah, Abraham's wife. The fault certainly did not lie with Abraham, for he had a son with Hagar. "And Sarai (Sarah) was barren: she had no child."[171] And when Isaac was born, Sarah cried out in amazement, "Who would have said unto Abraham that Sarah should give children suck? For I have borne him a son in his old age."[172] It should be pointed out that Sarah had definitely undergone menopause when all this took place, "it had ceased to be with Sarah after the manner of women."[173]

Since birth control was considered sacrilegious, the number of children which a woman bore depended solely on her physiological limitations. Thus while Leah bore seven children with Jacob, Sarah gave birth to only one.

Labor and Delivery: The Old Testament gives minute obstetrical details in the passage concerning Tamar, who was impregnated by Judah, her father-in-law:

And it came to pass in the time of her travail, that behold, twins were in her womb. And it came to pass, when she travailed, that one put out a hand; and the midwife took and bound upon his hand a scarlet thread, saying, This came out first. And it came to pass, as he drew back his hand that behold, his brother came out; and she said: Wherefore hast thou made a breach for thyself? Therefore, his name was called Perez (a breech).. And afterward came out his brother that had the scarlet thread upon his hand; and his name was called Zerah. [174]

The return of the fetus with the prolapsed hand with the delivery of its twin first should be noted.[175] It should also be pointed out that the identification bands, employed to identify the babies, rival the technique used in our modern obstetrical nurseries, where bracelets of beads on threads are attached to the infants at birth. And the fact that the colored threads were applied before delivery indicates that a diagnosis of twins had been made in advance—by no means a simple feat even today.

The following seems to be a breech delivery, for how else could the midwife know the sex of the child before delivery was complete, "And Rachel travailed, and she had hard labor. And it came to pass, when she was in hard labor, that the midwife said unto her; Fear not; for this also is a son for thee."[176]

Rachel gave birth to a living child, but died during this delivery.

When Rebekah was pregnant, great significance was placed on the fact that her twin fetuses "struggled together within her." The Lord said unto her:

> Two nations are in thy womb,
> And two peoples shall be separated from thy bowels;
> And the one people shall be stronger than the other people;
> And the elder shall serve the younger. [177]

In recording the delivery, besides describing a prolapsed hand, "Genesis" also points out that Esau had much lanugo. This latter fact was taken as an omen that Esau would be hairy throughout life, no doubt, for later we find Isaac distinguishing between his two sons by touch, since Jacob was smooth-skinned and Esau hairy. Let us quote from "Genesis":

And when her (Rebekah's) days to be delivered were fulfilled, behold, there were twins in her womb. And the first came forth ruddy, all over like a hairy mantle; and they called his name Esau. And after that came forth his brother and his hand had hold on Esau's heel; and his name was called Jacob (i.e. "one that takes by the heel"). And Isaac was threescore years old when she bore them. [178]

In Egypt the daughters of Israel bore quickly with a minimum of labor. During delivery,[179] they sat erect on a birthstool, resembling a toilet seat, under which the hands of the midwife received the infant.[180] This was the Egyptian method of delivery.

The method of delivery practiced among the Hebrews before and after the Egyptian bondage is most interesting, but unfortunately it is not well understood. We frequently come across passages such as the following, (1) "And she (Rachel) said: Behold my maid Bilhah, go in unto her; that she may bear upon my knees . . ."[181] (2) ". . . Why did the knees receive me?"[182] Evidently, the parturient woman reclined in a semi-erect position, and the child was born upon the knees of the midwife. Further than this, we can only guess at the obstetrical procedure.

While it is true that the ancient Hebrews were keen observers of obstetrical detail, it is only fair to point out that they were not totally free from superstition. They believed in the doctrine of maternal impression, as is evident from the following passage:

And Jacob took him rods of fresh poplar and of the almond and of the plane tree; and peeled white streaks in them, making the white appear which was in the rods. And he set the rods which he had peeled over against the flocks in the gutters in the watering-troughs where the flocks came to drink; and they conceived when they came to drink. And the flocks conceived at the sight of the rods, and the flocks brought forth streaked, speckled, and spotted.[183]

Menstruation: The priestly code ordains that a menstruating woman is unclean for one week from the beginning of the period, no matter how long it lasts. During the time of the taboo, her defilement is communicated to every object with which she comes in contact.[184]

When Rachel made off with her father's (Laban's) household gods, (*Terafim*, which constituted title to his property)[185] and he pursued until he caught up with her, she sat upon the Terafim and she said to her father, "Let not my Lord be angry that I cannot rise up before thee; for the manner of women is upon me."[186] Laban believed her and did not make her arise. The belief that a menstruating woman is defiling to those that come close to her was also believed by the Arameans. Laban feared to come in contact with his own daughter because of her condition.

Infant Care: Weaning probably took place between the ages of two and three. It was the occasion of great joy and feasting, for the child had passed through the most precarious years. According to "Genesis," Abraham made a great feast on the day Isaac was weaned.[187] It can be inferred that Samuel was weaned at the end of his third year, for only from that age were children admitted to the service of the temple.[188]

Very few infant deaths are mentioned in the Bible. Furthermore, no stillbirths or miscarriages are recorded. There is one case of a prostitute accidentally killing a newborn babe.[189] Practically all recorded births survive the trials of childhood. Rather than ascribe this to super medical care, or super stock, the answer probably lies in the fact that only important persons are noted at all in the Bible, and the births of the multitudes that doubtless died at a tender age are left unrecorded. This idea gains further credence when it is noted that the prophets several times revived presumed dead children,[190] thus indicating that many others must have perished unheralded. Then, too, the following lament certainly indicates that miscarriage, stillbirth, and death during infancy must have existed:

> Why died I not from the womb?
> Why did I not perish at birth?
> Why did the knees receive me?
> And wherefore the breasts, that I should suck? [191]

Complications: In the book of "Numbers," Miriam was smitten with leprosy. Aaron beseeched Moses in her behalf saying, ". . . Let her not, I pray, be as one dead, of whom the flesh is half consumed when he cometh out of his mother's womb."[192]

That abortion and miscarriage are connected with improper dietary intake may be inferred from the following:

And ye shall serve Jehovah your God, and he will bless thy bread, and thy water; and I will take sickness away from the midst of thee. There shall none cast her young, nor be barren, in thy land: the number of thy days I will fulfill.[193]

Midwives: Midwives are mentioned in the Old Testament as far back as "Genesis": Rachel was assisted by one.[194] Tamar also had a midwife.[195] While not explicitly stated, the duties of the midwife after delivery were probably those mentioned in Ezekiel, "And as for thy nativity, in the day thou wast born thy navel was not cut, neither wast thou washed in water for cleansing; thou wast not salted at all, nor swaddled at all. No eye pitied thee, to do any of these unto thee . . ."[196]

It seems as though midwives were not employed in normal cases. Rachel's delivery was definitely a hard one;[197] and Tamar, who gave birth to twins, also had an unusual delivery. Only two midwives *(hoyoth)*, Shiprah and Puah, were employed in a community of 600,-000 Jews in Egypt.[198] Usually friends or relatives aided in the delivery.[199]

Male Births: An interesting feature of the Bible is the fact that recorded male births tremendously exceed female births. This is probably due to the fact that only the births of the great were recorded; and women as a rule, were not permitted to attain any greatness except that which might be reflected from their husbands. This point of view seems to be upheld by the fact that there is no dearth of wives for the excess of men mentioned in the Bible.

Among the Israelites, the firstborn son was considered to possess the best hereditary makeup. This is demonstrated by the following passage:

> Reuben, thou art my first born,
> My might, and the first fruits of my strength;
> The excellency of dignity and the excellency of power. [200]

Therapeutics in the Bible

The early Hebrews realized that water could be a source of disease. When the men of the city said unto Elisha, "Behold, we pray thee, the situation of this city is pleasant . . . but the water is bad . . . he cast salt in the well, and said: Thus saith the Lord: I have healed these waters; there shall not be from thence anymore death . . . So the waters were healed unto this day . . ."[201] The disease contained in the water, since it was fatal, was probably typhoid, or some other water-borne plague, and evidently Elisha's salt solution killed off the organisms in the putrid water.

Anesthesia and the art of grafting, which are the acknowledged achievements of modern times, are anticipated in the Old Testament, as the following passage demonstrates, "And the Lord, God, caused a deep sleep to fall upon the man, and he slept; and He took one of his ribs, and closed up the place with flesh instead thereof."[202]

Elijah and Elisha can be considered the first ones in history to use artificial respiration. When Elisha revived the "dead" child, he lay upon him and placed his mouth upon the child's mouth, probably blowing into it. The child, as he was coming to, sneezed seven times and opened his eyes. The fact that Elisha "stretched himself" upon the child (as did Elijah)[203] indicates that he probably employed a mechanical procedure to stimulate the lungs, as well as one of aeration.[204]

Death

Causes of Death: The causes of death are very seldom given in the Old Testament. It should be remembered that many Biblical characters lived to a ripe old age and probably died of "causes incidental to old age," such as cardiovascular or renal failure. Many also died of traumatic causes. Then, too, since only important persons are mentioned in the Bible, they were usually able to take better care of their health than the average.

By gathering material from here and there, one may ascertain some of the diseases which caused death. The following fatal case is evidently one of chronic dysentery, probably amoebic, as this is prevalent in semitropical climes and is often epidemic:

. . . Behold (said Elijah to Jehoram because he has been an ungodly king who slew his brethren), the Lord will smite with a great plague thy people, and thy children, and thy wives, and all thy substance; and thou shalt have great sickness, day by day. [205] And after all this the Lord smote him in his bowels with an incurable disease. And it came to pass, that in process of time, at the end of two years, his bowels fell out by reason of his sickness, and he died of sore diseases. [206]

This is a case of prolapse of the bowel caused by dysentery.

Another cause of death was a severe disorder of the legs which ended the life of King Asa, "And in the thirty and ninth year of his reign, Asa was diseased in his feet; his disease was exceedingly great . . . and Asa slept with his fathers, and died in the one and fortieth year of his reign."[207]

Embalming: Whereas the art of embalming is not strictly a medical pursuit, it would not be out of place to discuss it at this point. All of the embalming mentioned in the Bible[208] occurs in the land of Egypt among Hebrews high in Pharaoh's esteem, and previous to the period of servitude. There is reason to believe that the method employed was that of the Egyptians. It should be noted that the "forty-day" period of embalming should be interpreted as embalming "many days."[209] When Herodotus visited Egypt, he jotted down the methods employed at that time. These probably were basically the same as those used in Joseph's day.[210] Joseph and his father were embalmed as men possessing great prestige and wealth in the land of Egypt.

Influence of Neighboring Nations on Biblical Medicine

It is difficult to ascertain how far Biblical medicine was influenced by healing arts of neighboring nations. It is known, however, that, during the years of bondage, Egypt was a great medical center. A number of medical papyri were written during that period or sometime earlier, especially in the middle-kingdom times.

According to these papyri, both surgery and medicine made phenomenal strides in Egypt. Amputations of the legs and arms were performed; the bladder was opened for stones; cupping and bloodletting were prevalent practices; couching for cataract was performed; and ancient Egyptian mummies revealed that decayed teeth were filled and artificial teeth of gold were employed to replace missing teeth. This being the case, it is difficult to conceive that the Hebrews, during the centuries of the Egyptian bondage, should not learn some of their medical practices which concerned their health.

If we are to believe Manetho, as quoted by Josephus, the Egyptians universally acknowledged Moses to have been a man of singular wisdom and integrity.

Medicine in the Apocrypha and the Pseudepigrapha

The second period of ancient Hebrew medicine includes the books of the Apocrypha and the Pseudepigrapha. The Apocrypha is a compilation of books similar, and largely supplementary to, the volumes that comprise the Old Testament. The Apocryphal works are a product of the period following the Babylonian exile. The entire corpus, with the exception of Esdras II, was included in ancient copies of the Greek version of the Old Testament (known as the "Septuagint").

Book of Jubilees: The "Book of Jubilees" traces the start of the healing art and the authorship of the first medical text to Noah:

And all the healing of their diseases we told to Noah, together with the means of administration thereof; so that he might cure through the trees of the earth. And Noah wrote everything as we had taught him, in a book, concerning all kinds of healing. And the evil spirits were fended off from the children of Noah. And he gave everything he had written to Shem, his oldest son, for he loved him more than all his sons. [211]

Wisdom of Solomon: In the Apocryphal book, the "Wisdom of Solomon," a plaster and herb are spoken of as a means of healing. Tobias, whose father Tobit had a white film over his eye, roasted the heart and liver of a large fish that leaped out of the Tigris River and employed the smoke from this fire to effect a cure.

Book of Tobit: The "Book of Tobit" mentions a case of leukoma secondary to infection from fecal material. Tobit declares:

I knew not that there were sparrows on the wall, and mine eyes being open, the sparrows muted warm dung into mine eyes, and a whiteness came in mine eyes; and I went to the physicians, but they helped me not.... (Upon the advice of an angel, Tobit's son took the gall of a fish)....and he strake of the gall on his father's eyes....and when his eyes began to smart, he rubbed them; And the whiteness peeled away from the corners of his eyes....and Tobit's sight returned. He was afflicted altogether eight years. [212]

The Maccabees: The "Maccabees" refers to sickness as a result of grief, "And he fell sick with grief, for matters had not gone as he intended. He was sick for a long time, for grief was intensified and he concluded he was going to die."

Book of Enoch: The "Book of Enoch" records the tongue as the organ of speech and the moving tongue and breath as the physiological mechanism involved in the production of speech. The heart is referred to as the organ of understanding: Enoch declares, "I saw in my sleep what I will now say with a tongue of flesh and with the breath of my mouth; which the Great One has given to man to converse therewith and understand with the heart."[213] Evidently disregarding the vocal cords, speech was considered to originate from the passage of inspired and expired air about the moving tongue. This is an early concept of the anatomy and physiology of the speech faculty.

The "Book of Enoch" traces numerous earthly ills and, by inference, unquestionably disease, to the giants which resulted from the forbidden union of the "watchers of heaven and the daughters of men":

And now, the giants, who are produced from the spirits and flesh, shall be called evil spirits upon the earth, and the earth shall be their dwelling. Evil spirits have proceeded from their bodies....And the spirits of the giants afflict, oppress, destroy, attack, do battle, and work destruction on the earth, and cause trouble. [214]

Michael, one of the angels escorting Enoch on his sojourn, showed him the tree of life which was reserved for the righteous on Judgment Day. Its fruit assured certain protection against "sorrow or plague or torment or calamity."[215]

The "Book of Enoch" records the healing virtue of water. God declares to Enoch's grandson Noah, "But those waters shall in those days serve for the kings and the mighty and the exalted, and those who dwell on the earth, for the healing of the body . . ."[216]

Enoch attributes miscarriage, snakebite, mental derangement, heat exhaustion, and demonic attacks to one of the fallen spirits, named "Kasdeja." It was he "who showed the children of men all the wicked smitings of spirits and demons, and the smitings of the embryo in the womb, that it may pass away, and the smitings of the soul, the bites of the serpent, and the smitings which befall through the noontide heat . . ."[217]

The close association between healing and virtue and lack of healing and sin can be inferred from the following, "Healing shall therefore be far from you because of your sins."[218] "But for the righteous, . . . healing shall be your portion."[219] "Barrenness has not been given to the woman, but on account of the deeds of her own hands, she dies without children."[220]

Odes of Solomon: The therapy of draining the milk from overfilled lactating breasts is recognized in the "Odes of Solomon" ". . . the Holy Spirit milked Him; because His breasts were full, and it was necessary for Him that His milk should be sufficiently released."[221]

Third Book of Maccabees: The pseudepigraphical "Third Book of Maccabees," concerning the punishment of Philopator, states, "The God . . . scourged him who was greatly uplifted in violence and insolence, shaking him to and fro as a reed by the wind, so that lying on the ground powerless and paralyzed in body he could not so much as speak, being smitten by a righteous judgment."[222] This description of a cerebral accident, starting with a convulsive seizure and ending with paralysis and aphasia, did not finish the wicked king or deter him from his villainy. He recovered sufficiently to carry on his evil designs.

THE ESSENES AND THE THERAPEUTAE

These two preChristian Jewish mystical orders (the healers) are of interest because of their influence on the medicine of the New Testament. They thrived during the second and first centuries B.C.

The Essenes were an offshoot of the Pharisees. They dwelt in pious seclusion in villages in the vicinity of Jerusalem, where they maintained themselves by the work of their hands, devoting their leisure time to study and devotion. They lived in a state of communal life, eating from the same table, and deriving their livelihood from a common community chest. Philo,[223] who was a contemporary of this sect, states that it had 4000 members. The Essenes shunned city life, because of the following:

. . . its lawlessness might contaminate their souls, and the tainted air might infect their bodies with deadly diseases. They leave physical science to theorists; they consider it too deep for ordinary man . . . They devote all their time to ethics under the guidance of their ancient laws which came to them by divine inspiration. The sect is formed not by family descent, for descent is not reckoned among one's choice, but in zeal for virtue and philanthropy. If any one of them should fall sick, he is treated medically from the common resources.

After pointing out their relationship to the Persian magi and the Indian gymnosophists, Philo quotes many examples of their customs and practices.

Josephus[224] admired their benevolence:

They take great interest in healing the sick and attending to the aged. . . . they take great pains in studying the writings of the ancients and choose of them what is most advantageous to the soul and body, and they inquire after such roots and medical stores as may cure their distempers.

The Essenes claimed the power of invoking the good spirits and conjuring the evil ones who took possession of the person. They believed the very contemplation of God enables one to acquire divine power to ward off misfortune and restore health to incurable persons, even to the blind, deaf, and lame. Prayers, incantations, charms, and mystic symbols were the principal measures employed when disease overtook a member of their order. They denied to man any control over his destiny. Everything was predestined. They used physical measures, such as herbs and drugs, only as an adjunct to spiritual treatment.

There is a striking similarity between the principles of the Essenes and the teachings of the New Testament: both were averse to conjugal relationship; both had the same system of organization; both had the same rules for traveling brethren; both were delegated to benevolence and charity; both had love feasts or brotherly meals; both lived in a communal state;[225] both practiced frequent bathing; both believed in the powers of prophesy; and both dedicated their lives to healing the sick by spiritual means.

The New Testament admonishes the Sadducees for their denial of the existence of demons.[226]

The Order of the Therapeutae was probably an Alexandrian branch of the Order of the Essenes. The members of this group settled on Lake Mariotis in the vicinity of Alexandria: hence the adoption of the Greek translation of Essenes which signifies "healer" in the Aramaic dialect.

MEDICINE IN THE NEW TESTAMENT

Miracle Cures: The medicine mentioned in the New Testament[227] falls entirely within the province of miracle cure. No medications are needed. Abiding faith is all that is necessary to effect a complete and immediate cure. Jesus, himself, declares, "thy faith hath made thee whole; go in peace."[228]

The only New Testament author who is reputed to have been a physician was Luke. In the Epistle of Paul to the Colossians, Luke is referred to as "the beloved physician."[229] It is only natural, then, that Luke should be the New Testament author par excellence to record Christ's medical miracles with professional skill.

To restore a man with a withered right hand, Jesus merely commanded him to stretch forth his hand. Immediate restoration of structure and function ensued.[230] He caused the centurion's servant to be cured at once without even seeing him, even though he "was sick and at the point of death."[231] He brought the widow's only son back from death by merely touching the bier and commanding, "Arise."[232] Likewise, he revived a dead maiden.[233]

The fascinating story of the demoniac of the Gerasenes is told by Luke.[234] The victim of demonic possession "had demons: and for a long time he had worn no clothes, and abode not in any house, but in the tombs . . ." Demonic attacks "oftentimes . . . had seized him: and he was kept under guard, and bound with chains and fetters; and breaking the bands asunder, he was driven of the demon into the deserts." Upon the command of Jesus, the demons were exorcized from the demoniac (who was at once cured "and in his right mind") into a herd of swine who thereupon "rushed down the steep into the lake, and were drowned."

This passage gives an insight into the methods employed in handling the mentally deranged and also illustrates the principle of the scapegoat in medicine.

Jesus gave the twelve apostles "authority over all demons and to cure diseases. And he sent them forth to preach the kingdom of God, and to heal the sick."[235]

The Great Healer brought succor to women afflicted with "evil spirits and infirmities."[236] He cast seven demons out of Mary Magdalene.[237] He expelled the "dumb" demon from a man who had aphasia.[238] Jesus cured a Syrophoenician woman's daughter by casting out the demon that afflicted the child.[239]

Jesus restored the sight of Bartimaeus, the blind man near Jericho, with the curt admonition, "Receive thy sight; thy faith hath made thee whole."[240]

In the first days of Jesus' career, while giving a Sabbath sermon at Cape Naum in Galilee, he cast out a demon from a member of the congregation.[241] Following the service, he visited Simon's mother-in-law who was afflicted with a violent fever. "He stood over her, and rebuked the fever; and it left her: and immediately she rose up and ministered unto them."[242]

The evening of the same day "all they that had any sick with divers diseases brought them unto him; and he laid his hands on every one of them, and healed them. And demons also came out from many, crying out, and saying, 'Thou art the Son of God.' And rebuking them, he suffered them not to speak . . ."[243]

He "stretched forth his hand" upon a leper and "straightway the leprosy departed from him." He then bade the cured man to cleanse himself according to the Mosaic Code.[244]

A paralyzed man who, recumbent on his couch, was lowered from the housetop through the tiles to Jesus' presence was completely cured when told to "arise, and take up thy couch, and go unto thy house."[245]

Luke records that a woman who had persistent uterine bleeding for twelve years and "who had spent all her living upon physicians," to no avail, was cured as soon as she touched Jesus' garment, even though he did not know who had touched him.[246] The lament of the patient who has spent all her earnings on medical attention to no avail strikes a familiar note to Luke, the physician, and to modern physicians as well.

Jesus was greatly perturbed after curing the ten lepers that only one gave thanks to God. It should be noted that he insisted that the lepers go to the priests, according to the Mosaic hygienic regulations, and be cleansed.[247]

Interesting is the case of the "woman that had a spirit of infirmity eighteen years; and she was bowed together, and could in no wise lift herself up." As soon as Jesus "laid his hands upon her . . . she was made straight."[248]

In the "Acts," reference is made to a man with a birth palsy, ("lame from his mother's womb"). Peter, in the company of John, "took him by the right hand, and raised him up: and immediately his feet and his ankle bones received strength. And leaping up, he stood and began to walk; and he entered with them unto the temple, walking, and leaping, and praising God."[249]

Luke mentions "sick folk and them that were vexed with unclean spirits." By the hands of the apostles and in the name of Jesus, such cases "were healed every one."[250] Believers "carried out the sick into the streets, and laid them on beds and couches that, as Peter came by, at the least his shadow might overshadow some one of them."[251]

Paul's healing prowess is illustrated by his cure of Publius' father who "lay sick of fever and dysentery." When this was accomplished, "the rest also that had diseases in the island came, and were cured."[252] Fascinating is the story of the epileptic child. His father pleaded with Jesus to cure his only son because "a spirit taketh him, and he suddenly crieth out; and it teareth him that he foameth, and it hardly departeth from him, bruising him sorely. And I besought thy disciples to cast it out; and they could not." As the son was "coming, the demon dashed him down, and tore him grievously. But Jesus rebuked the unclean spirit, and healed the boy, and gave him back to his father."[253]

This description of the epileptic cry, the foaming at the mouth, the epileptic seizure, and the ensuing bruises conveys a classical picture of the grand mal syndrome that could only have been written by Luke, the physician.

Jesus performed a surgical miracle on Malchus, a servant of the high priest, who had his ear cut off with a sword. He effected complete healing.[254]

According to Mark, there was brought to Jesus "one that was deaf, and had an impediment in his speech . . . he . . . put his fingers into his ears, and he spat, and touched his tongue; and looking up to heaven, he sighed and saith unto him, Ephphatha, that is, Be opened. And his ears were opened and the bond of his tongue was loosed, and he spake plain."[255]

The placing of his fingers in the patient's ears evidently cured the deafness, and the fact that he touched the tongue "and the bond of his tongue was loosed," may indicate that he broke the membrane which had caused tongue-tie.

Luke makes mention of the miracle cure of a dropsical man.[256] John relates the narrative of the Bethesda Pool in Jerusalem. In its five porches:

. . . lay a multitude of them that were sick, blind, halt, withered, and a certain man was there, who had been thirty and eight years in his infirmity. When Jesus saw him lying, and knew that he had been now a long time, he saith unto him. Wouldst thou be made whole? The sick man answered him,

Sir, I have no man, when the water is troubled, to put me into the pool: but while I am coming, another steppeth down before me. Jesus saith unto him, arise, take up thy bed, and walk. And straightway the man was made whole and took up his bed and walked. [257]

Thus the pitiful soul who sought hydrotherapy in the pool but could not obtain it because of the greedy invalids who pushed him aside to rush into the pool whenever the water was turbulent was cured by Divine aid. This use of turbulent water in the treatment of disease may be considered the forerunner of our modern whirlpool bath.

Causes of Disease: The medicine of the "Gospels" and the "Acts" shows three different beliefs as to the cause of disease. The most advanced is the belief that all disease comes direct from God as a punishment for sin, "Behold, thou art made whole: sin no more, lest some worse thing happen to thee." (John 5:14.) And again, "Rabbi, who hath sinned, this man or his parents, that he should be born blind?" (John 9:2.) In the second place, there is the view that disease is due to the indwelling of an evil spirit, "There met Him a certain man, who had a devil now a very long time." (Luke 8:27.) And, "They brought to Him a dumb man possessed of the devil." (Matthew 9:32.) It is hardly possible to read into the many accounts of possession a description of lunacy and to hold that all the possessed of the New Testament were maniacs. That would constitute far too high a percentage for the small population of Palestine. It seems clear that one view of the pathology of disease in general was that the evil spirit had for the time being taken up its dwelling within the body of a human subject. As illustrating the third belief, many of the medical stories savor of pure magic. "They brought forth the sick into the streets, that when Peter came, his shadow at least might overshadow any of them and they might be delivered from their infirmities." (Acts 5:15.)

Now, these views are alien to the views of orthodox Jewry and the views of the Old Testament. The nearest approach is the description of the sufferings of Job. But, even here, there is no suggestion that he is being punished for his sins and no evidence that he is possessed. His treatment is certainly not magical. The sole instance of possession in the Old Testament is the case of Saul. (I Kings 16:14.) Magic, of course, there was. But the strict monotheistic and hygienic doctrines of Moses prevented the superstitions of the Jews from even approximating those of their neighbors.

These doctrines were not inherited from the Christian forefathers, the Hebrews. They came from Persia, where dualism, magic, and possession are all found.

Healers: It is evident that healing of the sick is one of the most sacred duties in the New Testament. The method, however, is distinctly religious in character as is particularly shown in the "Book of James" (5:14-15), "If any is sick among you let him call for the elders of the church and let them pray over him anointing him with oil in the name of the Lord and the prayers of faith shall save the sick and the Lord shall raise him up. Pray for one another and you shall be healed."

Gibbons, in his "History of Rome," says that one of the most powerful factors contributing to the spread of Christianity was the supposedly miraculous powers of the primitive church, among which he named the expulsion of demons from the sick. Gibbons, of course, scoffs at exorcism and at superstitious practices but he states that the great masses of people at that period were sunken in superstition.

Indeed the healing powers of the church became so famous that the third century A.D. witnessed a special order within the church, the function of which was to cast out demons from sick persons. Healing of disease was one of the few noble deeds that elevated members of the church to sainthood. This is reminiscent of the practice that existed in ancient Egypt, Greece, and Rome, where it was the custom to elevate distinguished physicians to the position of godhood.

Among the first healers who were elevated to sainthood were Cosmos and Domean: they dispensed medicine to the poor from a monastic cell at Sicilia. When Rome succumbed to the onslaught of the northern barbarians, medicine was compelled in the stress of time to find asylum in the monastic cells. In the cells of Mt. Cassino Monastery, for example, the members of the Order of St. Benedict became famous for their knowledge of the medical classics. They collected the medical works of Greek and Roman physicians and studied them diligently. Of course, they attempted to harmonize the scientific medical doctrines of the Greeks and Romans with the teaching of the church. For example, the Galenic theory of pneuma was identified with the Christian idea of the soul. Be this as it may, the church on Mt. Cassino must be credited with preserving many a manuscript that might have been lost were it not for the interest and zeal of these monks in medicine. Aside from the medical help offered to the poor in the monasteries, infirmaries were erected in the vicinity of cloisters where young clerics were taught medicine and pharmacy.

The works on medicine left by the monks in the monasteries are of course of little value to modern medicine, but they were widely read by physicians during the Middle Ages.

In the year 391 A.D., after numerous and bloody contests in the streets of Alexandria, a fanatical mob headed by Bishop Theophilus took possession of the Serapeum Temple, which was the mecca of diseased people from all over Egypt, demolished it because of its pagan practices, such as incubation and votive offerings, and erected a church on its ruins. As fate would have it, the monks who replaced the priests of the ancient temple restored the same pagan practices they condemned. They emulated the practice of incubation, exhibited models of healed limbs, and instituted dream oracles at the shrines. In other words, they invoked all the practices in vogue in the temples of Aesculapius and Serapis. The Aesculapian practices were also instituted in the convents of Italy and the churches of Rome.

"Surgeries": At the beginning of the Christian era, open "surgeries" (*iatria* or *taberna-medico*) existed in Alexandria and Rome. According to Galen and Placetus, many towns built them at their own expense. The *iatria* attended largely to outpatients. No establishment appears to have been founded for relief of the bedridden until the time of Constantine. The law of Justinian, referring to various institutions connected with the church, mentions the nosocomia which corresponds to the modern idea of the hospital.

Origin of Hospitals: In the year 370 A.D., St. Basil built a hospital for the lepers at Caesara. Incidentally, St. Basil, who was of a delicate constitution and susceptible to illness, paid much attention to medicine which he declared to be the noblest profession. The bishop, who evidently read the works of Hippocrates, did not agree with the father of medicine, however, when he stated:

Not all diseases are produced by nature; some are sent directly from God as trials of our faith or as punishment for some forgotten scene, [258] and when we are conscious of this we should not go to a physician but bear it patiently for chastising of the Lord until he sees fit to remove the disease. [259] Some diseases come from Satan as in the case of Job. [260]

Returning to the origin of the hospital, St. Jerome, who was instrumental in the formation of the first sick house in Rome and the first inn for sick strangers in Ostia (through the generosity of a rich Roman lady, a convert to Christianity, named Fabiola, who even became a nurse there herself) said that he was happy to see a branch of Abraham's terebinth brought from the East. Thus he credits the hospital to the patriarch Abraham.

The house set apart in which the leprous King Azariah passed his last days[261] is believed by some to have been an infirmary. The hospital is an old institution. In Egypt and Greece the custom of placing the sick in the temples was an old practice.

Ebers, of the papyrus fame, is of the opinion that Heliopolis had a clinic united to the temple, as did the Temples of Thebes and Memphis. The Aesculapian Temples, such as Epidaurus, Cos, and Trikka, had hospices connected with them. The Buddhists had their hospitals as early as 260 B.C. Emperor Asoka founded many hospitals.

PHOENICIAN MEDICINE

In reviewing the medical culture of the Phoenicians, it is important to remember that, in the Ebers papyrus, it is stated that one of its books is the work of a physician of Byblos. What is known of this book permits the conjecture that much more important medical knowledge than has been heretofore suspected was possessed by this Semitic race. Not only was it distinguished for its technical, nautical, and meteorological knowledge, its activity in colonization, its commerce, and its luxury, but also for exercising an important influence upon the Greeks, which is evident in Greek medicine. That the Phoenicians indulged in an extremely sensual religious worship is known. It is also known that their supreme deity, Baal-zebub (the god of flies), the Baal-zebub of the Bible, was a god of medicine and was interrogated as an oracle of health and disease. His priests were clad in red clothing, possibly the earliest example of the red garments of the physician. The Carthaginians, as Phoenician colonists, differed but slightly in their medical customs from the parent stock.

References and Notes

 1. Numbers 12:10.
 2. II Kings 5:27.
 3. II Chronicles 26:21.
 4. II Chronicles 21:18-19.
 5. Genesis 19:11.
 6. Ibid. 12:17.
 7. I Samuel 15:12.
 8. Genesis 20:18.
 9. Ibid. 38:7.
10. II Samuel 12:14.
11. I Samuel 42.
12. Numbers 11:34.
13. Exodus 15:26.

14. Deuteronomy 32:39.
15. Numbers 12:10.
16. II Chronicles 7:13-15.
17. Exodus 21:18-19.
18. Ibid. 21:9.
19. II Chronicles 16:12.
20. I Kings 1:17-22.
21. II Kings 4:32-34.
22. II Chronicles 16:12-13.
23. Jeremiah 8:22; II Kings 8:29; II Chronicles 16:12, etc.
24. Job 3:4.
25. Leviticus 22:24.
26. Exodus 19:6.
27. Acts 7:22.
28. Libre 1:419.
29. I Kings 5:13.
30. Proverbs 3:8; 6:15; 12:18; 17:22; 20:30; 19:1; Ecclesiasticus 3:3.
31. Sanhedrin 87-a; Sukah 20-a; Meg. 19-b.
32. Daniel 12:3.
33. Sanhedrin 87-a.
34. Sirach 38:1-4.
35. Exodus 29:17.
36. Job 16:13.
37. Ibid. 21:24.
38. Psalm 69:4.
39. Exodus 28:29.
40. Genesis 17:11.
41. Job 40:16-18.
42. Genesis 9:4.
43. Song of Songs 8:6; Proverbs 4:23.
44. The word Moach (Job 21:24) stands for marrow.
45. Daniel 4:13.
46. Proverbs 4:23.
47. Judges 3:21-22.
48. Exodus 29:13-22, etc.
49. Proverbs 7:23.
50. Lamentations 2:11. The Hebrew root "kbd" has a double meaning: "glory" and "liver"; it was believed that the liver was the seat of intellect.
51. Exodus 29:13-22.
52. Hosea 13:8.
53. Isaiah 3:18.
54. Exodus 29:13. The belief that the kidneys are the seat of intellect is repeatedly manifested in the Old Testament: Job 38:36; Psalms 16:7; 26:2.
55. Leviticus 1:8.
56. Ibid 1:16.
57. Exodus 4:11.
58. Ecclesiasticus 12:7; Proverbs 2:27; Job 12:8.
59. Genesis 1:24-30.
60. Ecclesiaticus 3:21.

61. Genesis 35:2.
62. Exodus 19:10.
63. Jeremiah 2:22.
64. Leviticus 13:14-15.
65. Numbers 19:19.
66. Leviticus 17:15-16.
67. Ibid. 14:8-9.
68. Ibid. 22:4-6.
69. Ibid. 15:5-10.
70. Ibid. 15:16-18.
71. Ibid. 15:19-27.
72. Ibid. 17:15.
73. Numbers 19:19.
74. II Samuel 11:2-4.
75. Leviticus 15:19-33.
76. Exodus 30:19-40.
77. Genesis 24:etc.
78. Psalm 73:13.
79. Ibid. 26:6.
80. Genesis 24:32.
81. Deuteronomy 28:22.
82. Ibid.
83. Leviticus 21:19.
84. Ibid. 21:20.
85. Leviticus 13.
86. II Kings 7:3-4.
87. II Chronicles 26:21.
88. It is taken from the Evening Bulletin, Philadelphia, Wednesday, Sept. 21, 1938, p. 21, columns 7-8.
89. Numbers 25:1.
90. Gordon, B. L.: The Romance of Medicine. F. A. Davis Co., 1944, p. 344.
91. Leviticus 15.
92. Ibid. 15:2-14.
93. Exodus 30:22-26.
94. Genesis 30:14.
95. Song of Songs 7:14.
96. Jeremiah 8:21-22; 46:11.
97. Ibid. 51:8-9.
98. Ibid. 2:22.
99. Deuteronomy 29:17.
100. Genesis 19:24.
101. Isaiah 1:5-6.
102. Genesis 19:32.
103. Jeremiah 46:11.
104. II Samuel 18:14.
105. Ibid. 20:10.
106. Ibid. 2:23.
107. Numbers 25:8.
108. Judges 3:21-22.

109. Ibid. 5:26-27.
110. Psalm 38:6.
111. Isaiah 1:5-6.
112. Exodus 9:9-10.
113. Deuteronomy 28:27.
114. Ibid. 28-35.
115. Proverbs 12:4.
116. Ibid. 14:30.
117. Numbers 21:6-9.
118. Genesis 17:10-11.
119. Deuteronomy 23:2.
120. Exodus 4:25.
121. Genesis 4:22.
122. Ibid. 34:24-25.
123. Exodus 9:8-11.
124. Leviticus 21:19.
125. Genesis 32:24-33.
126. Ezekiel 30:21.
127. Genesis 29:17.
128. Deuteronomy 32:10.
129. Jeremiah 9:17.
130. Joshua 23:13.
131. Genesis 29:17.
132. Psalm 73:7.
133. Leviticus 15:3-6.
134. Genesis 19:11.
135. Deuteronomy 28:8.
136. II Samuel 5:6.
137. Deuteronomy 27:18.
138. Genesis 48:10.
139. Ibid. 27:1.
140. Ibid. 48:10.
141. I Samuel 4:15.
142. I Kings 14:4.
143. See Ophthalmology in the Bible and the Talmud. Arch. Ophth. May, 1933.
     pp. 751-788.
144. Leviticus 22:22.
145. Ibid.
146. Ibid. 21:20.
147. Deuteronomy 23:2.
148. Ibid.
149. Leviticus 22:22.
150. Zephaniah 3:14.
151. Jeremiah 32:40, Apocrypha Baruch 3:7.
152. Apocrypha Tobit 4:13.
153. Psalm 13:3.
154. Apocrypha Tobit 1:2.
155. Apocrypha II Esdras 9:31, and II Maccabees 2:3.
156. Deuteronomy 29:3; Job 34:10.

157. Proverbs 10:13.
158. Esther 7:5.
159. Deuteronomy 6:5.
160. Ibid. 28:28.
161. Today, with the problems and anguish of the Jews at an all-time high, such is not the case.
162. Genesis 20:12.
163. Ibid. 38:9.
164. Ibid. 4:1.
165. Ibid. 20:17-18.
166. Psalm 128:3-4.
167. Genesis 30:1.
168. Samuel 1:6.
169. Gordon, C. H.: Biblical Archaeologist III. 1940, p. 116.
170. The ancients did not reckon with the possibility that a man might be sterile though not impotent.
171. Genesis 11:30.
172. Ibid. 21:7.
173. Ibid. 18:11.
174. Ibid. 38:27-30.
175. Primogeniture was important because of the laws of inheritance.
176. Genesis 36:16-17.
177. Ibid. 25:23.
178. Ibid. 25:24-26.
179. Exodus 1:15-30.
180. The Egyptian birthstool was like a toiletseat. The parturient woman sat erect and the child was received (by the attendant) under the circular hole in the seat. We know this because the Egyptian hieroglyph "to bear" depicts this vividly. See the Hieroglyph in G. Roered: Aegyptische Grammatik, C. H. Beck, Munchen, 1926, p. 65, No. A-15, "gebaren".
181. Genesis 30:3.
182. Job 3:12.
183. Genesis 30:37-39.
184. Leviticus 15:19-30.
185. Gordon, C. H.: The Story of Jacob and Laban in the Light of the Nuzi Tablets. Bulletin of the American Schools of Oriental Research, No. 66, April, 1937, p. 26; also note 24, p. 30.
186. Genesis 31:35.
187. Ibid. 21:8.
188. II Chronicles 31:16.
189. Kings 3:19.
190. Kings 17:17-22; II Kings 4:18-35.
191. Job 3:11-12.
192. Numbers 12:12.
193. Exodus 23:25-26.
194. Genesis 35:17.
195. Ibid. 38:28.
196. Ezekiel 16:4-5.
197. Genesis 35:18 tells us that Rachel died during delivery.

198. This point is also sometimes adduced to show that actually the Hebrews in Egypt were fewer than is generally supposed.
199. I Samuel 4:20.
200. Genesis 49:3.
201. II Kings 2:19-22.
202. Genesis 2:21.
203. I Kings 17:17-22.
204. II Kings 4:34-35.
205. II Chronicles 21:14-15.
206. Ibid. 1:18-19.
207. Ibid. 16:12-13.
208. Genesis 50:2-3.
209. The number "forty" was used idiomatically to mean "many." Thus, the flood lasted for forty days and forty nights; the children of Israel wandered in the wilderness for forty years; Moses received the commandments on Mt. Sinai after forty days.
210. Cary, H.: Herodotus; A New and Literal Version. American Book Company, New York, 1848; Enterpe II, Sec. 85-91, pp. 125-127.
211. The Book of Jubilee 10:12-14.
212. Tobit 2:10.
213. The Book of Enoch 14:2.
214. Ibid. 15:1-12.
215. Ibid. 25:3-7.
216. Ibid. 65:11-8.
217. Ibid. 59:12.
218. Ibid. 95:4.
219. Ibid. 96:3.
220. Ibid. 98:5.
221. The Ode of Solomon, Ode 19.
222. III Maccabees 1:21-24.
223. Hastings Encyclopedia; Letters Essenes.
224. Josephus, Flavius: Antiquities.
225. Acts 4:34.
226. Ibid. 23:8.
227. The version of the New Testament most frequently quoted in this work is the New Testament, standard edition, edited in 1900 by the New Testament Members of the American Revision Committee, Thos. Nelson and Sons, New York.
228. Luke 8:48.
229. The Epistle of Paul to the Colossians 4:14.
230. Luke 6:10-11; Matthew 12:10-13.
231. Luke 7:2-10.
232. Ibid. 7:12-14.
233. Ibid. 8: 49-56.
234. Ibid. 8:26-39.
235. Ibid. 9:1-2.
236. Ibid. 8:2.
237. Ibid.
238. Ibid. 11:14.

239. Mark 7:25-30.
240. Luke 18:42; Mark 10:46-52.
241. Luke 4:33-37.
242. Ibid. 4:38-39.
243. Ibid. 4:40-41.
244. Ibid. 5:12-14.
245. Ibid. 5:18-26.
246. Ibid. 8:43-48.
247. Ibid. 5:12-14.
248. Ibid. 13:11-13.
249. Acts 3:2-8.
250. Ibid. 5:16.
251. Ibid. 5:14-15.
252. Ibid. 28:8-9.
253. Luke 9:38-43.
254. Ibid. 22:50-51.
255. Mark 7:32-36.
256. Luke 14:2-4.
257. John 5:2-9.
258. I Cor. 11:30.
259. Micha 7:9.
260. Job. 2:6-7.
261. II Kings 15:5; II Chronicles; 26:21.

10

Medicine in Ancient Persia

Three Periods of Medical History: The medical history of ancient Persia may be divided into three distinct periods. The first period dates from the reign of Jamshid, the first king of Persia (c. 1400 B.C.) (according to the poet Firdausi). The sixth book of the *Zend-Avesta* refers to the medicine of this period. The *Vendidad*[1] devotes most of the last chapters to the art of medicine. The second epoch covers the period of the *Pahlevi,* a name given by the followers of Zoroaster to the language in which is written the ancient traditions of the sacred books. In the later *Pahlevi* literature, the entire subject of medicine was systematically treated in an interesting tractate incorporated in the encyclopedic work the *Dinkart.*[2] The third period begins with King Achimenes (c. 700 B.C.) and covers the reign of Darius I.

Darius: The most reliable information concerning Persian medicine is associated with the name of Darius (died 486 B.C.). It is related that his interest in medicine was so great that he reestablished the medical school of Sais in Egypt, which previously had been destroyed, and restored to that school the books and equipment that had been removed when Egypt was conquered by the Persians. The advance of Greek scientific medicine naturally had a great influence upon the physicians of Persia. As a matter of fact, many Greek physicians settled in Persia and introduced the new science into the land of Zoroaster.

Period of Greatest Development: The greatest medical development took place after the Arabian conquest following the year 650 A.D. Many Arabic physicians of Persian origin became celebrated for their originality and scholarship. The most important of these were Ali ibn Abbasi (Hally Abbas; died 994 A.D.), Ibn Sahl al-tabari, Sinan bin sabit qurrah (died 942 A.D), Al-Rhazi (850–932 A.D.), Bar Judeus, and above all, Avicenna (980–1037 A.D.). But these belong to the modern period and cannot be discussed here.

Extent of Medical Knowledge: The extent of medical knowledge in Persia during the first period is largely a matter of conjecture. Unlike Babylonia and Egypt, Persia has left no medical texts, no medical papyri, and no mummified remains suitable for disease identification, and certainly not any medical writings comparable to those of Susruta and Charaka of India. Persian rulers, with the exception of King Jamshid and other semimythical rulers, such as Hushang and Feridun (whose reigns date back as far as 4000 B.C.), were not associated with medicine as were the early Egyptian potentates.

RELIGION AND MAGIC

The medicine of ancient Persia was associated with religion and magic and was administered by priests. Medicine was practiced by the priests on the supposition that the *daeva* had created 99,999 ailments which should be treated by a combination of magic and hygiene. They resorted more frequently to spells than to drugs on the grounds that, although spells might not cure the disease, they at least would not kill the patient.[3] The very origin of the art of medicine as recorded in the *Avesta* is of a mythological nature. The sixth book of the *Avesta*, the *Vendidad*, which devotes most of the last three chapters to medicine, attributes the origin of medicine to a certain rich, benevolent, intellectual, and powerful hero named "Thrita." He is stated to be the first of the *Paradhata* race to possess magic power to combat sickness and death. In answer to his fervent prayers, Ahuramazda (or Ormuzd), the god of light and of everything good, caused Ameretop, the goddess of long life, to plant at the center of the garden, where a thousand health-giving trees grew, the tree of all seeds (*vouruksha*) near the miraculous tree *gookrarena* (the tree of eternal life) which cures all ills and gives immortality.[4] This divinity presented to Thrita a metal operating knife with a gold point and base, by which he was enabled to practice the surgical art. Thus, Thrita, in Persian mythology, is the patron saint of medicine, much as Imhotep is in Egyptian mythology and Aesculapius in Greek mythology.

According to the *Avesta*, bodily ailments like spiritual ills (such as sin) are treated by religious exercises; both are regarded as abnormalities and both are derived from the same source.

Zoroaster: The religion which Zoroaster preached was the creation of a single man, who, having pondered long and deeply over the problems of existence and the world, found the solution in divine revelation. Naturally he starts from the old views, and is indebted to them for many of his tenets and ideas; but out of this material, he builds a uniform system which bears throughout the impress of his own intellect. In this world, two groups of powers confront each other in a truceless war, the powers of good, of light, of creative strength, of life and of truth, and the powers of evil, of darkness, destruction, death, and deceit. In the van of the first, stands the holy spirit, or the "Great Wisdom," Mazda. His helpers and vassals are the six powers of good thought, of right order, of the excellent kingdom, of holy character, of health, and of immortality, and a host of subordinate angels are ranked with them. The powers of evil are in all points the opposite of the good, at their head being the evil spirit *Angra Mainyu*. These evil demons are identical with the old gods of the popular faith, the *daevas*.[5]

Midway between the camps of the powers of good and evil, man is placed. He has to choose on which side he will stand; he is called to serve the powers of good; his duty lies in speaking the truth and combating the lie. And this is fulfilled when he obeys the commands of law and order, when he tends his cattle and fields (in contrast with the lawless and predatory nomad *[dahae]*), when he wars on all harmful and evil spirits and on the devil-worshippers, when he keeps free from pollution the pure creations of Ahuramazda (fire foremost, but also earth and water), and, above all, when he practices the good and true in thought, word, and deed.

Cause of Disease: In the Persian dualistic conception of the universe, disease as well as sin is caused by the power of evil and darkness Angra Mainyu (or Ahriman) who, with six subordinate malignant spirits or *devas*, seeks to harm the believers in the good and merciful god Ahuramazda, the protector of the health and life of his followers. Thus the state of health and sickness was considered to be a condition representing a struggle between two spiritual forces.

Assyro-Babylonian Influence: There is no doubt that the inhabitants of Medes and Fars, that form what is known as Persia, were largely influenced in their concepts by the Assyro-Babylonians whose elaborate system of medicine connected its etiology and treatment with spiritual forces. In Persia, as in Assyro-Babylonia, health was considered a reward dispensed by the gods for obedience of the law. On the other hand, disease was looked upon as caused by the vengeance of the deities whose commandments were violated. The punishment of disease was effected through evil messengers sent by Angra Mainyu to take possession of habitual sinners.

THE AVESTA

The *Zend-Avesta* frequently mentions the healing art which it ascribes to Zoroaster. This work is said to have originally consisted of twenty-one books, containing no less than 2,000,000 verses written upon 1200 cowhides. Pliny, who had seen an abstract of a Greek translation of the *Zend-Avesta* wrote that the Persian religion is founded on medicine. Little of the *Avesta* has survived except the nineteenth book (the *Vendidad*) which is a code of purification (literally "The Law Against Demons").

In strict accordance with the dualistic conception of the universe, bodily disease, and its treatment by medical art, corresponds exactly with sin. It is regarded as a spiritual malady, and its treatment by religious exercise is conceived as ethical or spiritual medicine. All bodily diseases are expressly declared to be the creation of the evil spirit.

In the *Vendidad,* Ahuramazda declares that his adversary Angra Mainyu plagued mankind with not less than 99,999 ailments. This fantastic figure was changed by the commentator and translator of the *Avesta-Gujarati* to 90,000 and Bund lowered the quota to 4,333 diseases.[6]

Geiger, the foremost authority on the *Zend-Avesta,* collected in his *Ostiran Kultur,* the names of a considerable number of diseases in the various parts of the *Avesta;* most of the names, however, are not identified. The mixture of the old Iranian dialect with the idioms of the Zoroastrian scripture renders interpretation of medical terms difficult, for no descriptions of the diseases are available. The same is true of the remedial substances. The names of drugs are particularly difficult to identify.

The cause of illness in the *Avesta* is attributed to an evil and defiled genius (Ganak Manoi) who enters the person and afflicts him with disease. The concept that sickness and death are brought about by a wicked and unclean spirit, and the fear that the sick will contaminate those that touch them, prompted the isolation of unhealthy persons. The dread that the polluted dead may defile those near them restrained the Persians from burying or cremating their dead. They believed that a corpse might make the earth unclean if buried, and that cremation was an offense against the purity and sanctity of fire; consequently they left the dead to be consumed by crows and other scavengers.[7]

According to the *Avesta*, the bodies of the dead fall to the share of the evil spirits which take possession of their prey in the guise of flies. Uncleanliness spreads from the corpse into the house in which it lies, contaminating all within it. The evil influence extends to all the relatives and is greater the nearer the relationship. Laying out the dead was the work of bearers who made this their trade and were therefore utterly despised. The defiled relations of the deceased had to withdraw for a time from all association with their neighbors.

Incidentally, it should be noted that the Zoroastrians laid stress upon immortality and resurrection. Death signified a separation of the soul from the body. The Iranian recognized that the vital force guides bodily function, which comes into being with the body and which perishes with it. Associated with the vital force, and united to the body, are faculties, such as consciousness and spirit or soul (will-power), which do not perish with the body.

As intimated, the dualistic concept of the universe invested the governing of the normal function of the body in the state of health to a benevolent spirit or soul, and correspondingly the abnormal function of the body in a state of disease to an evil spirit *(Ahriman)*.

Whatever worthwhile ideas of medicine the Persians possessed were borrowed from the Babylonians and Egyptians. They themselves left but little impression on medicine. Their falacious concepts were bound to prove retrogressive to the art and science of Persian medicine.

Classification of Disease: The *Avesta* classifies medicine in accordance with the means employed to combat disease: (1) knife *(kereta)*, (2) herb *(urvara)*, and (3) formula *(manthra)*. In other words, the early Persians divided medicine into surgery, remedial measures, and prayer. A similar classification was ascribed by Pindar to Aesculapian medicine. "The Avesta" appraises the medical cure by means of conjuration or prayer as the best of all classified methods. The physician who cures by prayer was known as the physician of physicians *(manthra beechaza)*. "When physicians compete," says Ormuzd, "knife doctor, herb doctor, and word doctor, then shall the believer go to him who heals by the holy word for he is a healer of healers, and benefits the soul also," thus indicating the triple division of Persian medicine. The sacred formula *(manthra spenta)* is personified and invoked as a genius. The *manthra* is considered more than a prayer. The latter is personified and appealed to as in the following ritual, "Heal me.

O, Manthra Spenta, O, brilliant one." In the *Vendidad* 20:7, disease is personified as is seen in the following magic formula, "I conjure thee, disease! I conjure thee, death; I conjure thee, burning; I conjure thee, fever; I conjure thee, headache; I conjure thee, smallpox!"

Method of Healing: Conjuration and the magic art as a method of healing the sick are perhaps as old as man himself. The very word "magic" was coined in Persia, originating from the Zend word *mah* (pronounced *mag*), meaning great or excellent. *Mah* or *mag* was applied to Persian priests. They were divided into three classes: *Erebis* (novices), *mobebis* (masters), and *disturis* (perfect masters). All three classes were governed by an Arch-magus who resided at Bactra, "Mother of Cities." The Arch-magus was regarded as the successor of Zoroaster. There were a large number of magi in every section of Persia. It is related that thousands were present at one of their councils, when the monarchy of the Parthians fell, and when the former religion was restored to Persia (226 A.D.).

Water: The *Avesta* stresses the physical and spiritual virtues of water and recommends it both as a therapeutic measure and as a method of religious purification. The sick as well as the sinful were cleansed and treated with water. Zoroaster was against everything that was unclean in thought, word, and action and insisted on physical and spiritual cleanliness. Physical cleanliness symbolized moral and spiritual purity. Cleansing with water not only purified the surface of the body but also entered the nine portals or openings of the body (i.e. the eyes, ears, nostrils, mouth, genital opening, and anus). Water was considered sacred. The *Avesta* strictly forbids spitting or urinating in a river or even washing in it.

The *Avesta* states that all diseases, except those due to trauma, are demonic in origin. Consequently treatment was directed to cast out the demon that caused the disease through purification of the body with water supplemented by herbal and other therapeutic means.

Herbs, Trees, and Words: Many cures were effected by water, others through herbs and trees, and still others through words, "By the divine word are the sick certainly healed." Ahuramazda, in order to curtail the destructive actions of the demons, endowed herbs—particularly poisonous ones—with healing powers.

Milk: Next to water, milk was regarded as a divinely purified provision in the breast of the female. A prosperous woman was one who had many children and much milk. A cow was regarded as a sacred animal, but in no sense a heavenly animal, personally guarded by Ahuramazda as he guarded other things upon which the prosperity of the people depended.[8]

Rules for Practice of Surgery and Medicine: The *Avesta* lays down rules governing the training, examination, and fitness of those who desired to practice surgery and medicine. The qualifications of a medical and surgical practitioner were based on practical experience. One passage of the *Zend-Avesta* reads:

> O, Maker of the material world, Thou holy one, if a worshipper of God wishes to practice the art of healing, on whom shall he first prove his skill— on the worshippers of Ahura Mazda, or on the worshippers of the Daevas (the evil spirits)? Ahura Mazda made answer and said; on worshippers of the Daevas shall he prove himself, rather than on the worshippers of God. If he treats with a knife a worshipper of the Daevas and he die, if he treats with a knife a second worshipper and he die, if he treats with a knife a third worshipper of the Daevas and he die, he is unfit forever and ever; let him never cure any worshipper of God. . .if he heals with a knife any worshipper of the Daevas and he recovers; if he treats with a knife a second worshipper of the Daevas and he recovers; if he treats with a knife a third worshipper of the Daevas and he recovers, then he is fit forever and ever; and may at his will treat worshippers of God and heal them with a knife. [9]

If in spite of his failure, he dared practice on a Zoroastrian and the latter, as a result of unskilled surgery or medicine, died, the would-be healer was held guilty of a crime equivalent to homicide.[10]

After three successful operations, the embryo physician was considered a fully qualified medical man.[11] A serious view was taken of a physician's obligations. He was required to rush when called to visit his patient, "If he were called to treat a patient towards night, he was required to arrive by the 'second watch'. If he were called during the 'second watch', midnight was the deadline for arrival. If called past midnight, it was required that the call be made by daybreak." Darmestater cites a recent Parsi commentator[12] who naively stated, "the doctor may not cure, but he would do no harm."[13] In other words, the duties of the physician were strictly regulated. He could not postpone his visit to his patient too long. "If an illness commence in the morning, proceed to a cure with the day; if during the day, it should be undertaken at night; if in the night, the physician's treatment must follow the daybreak."[14]

Fees: The fees of a physician were also regulated by the *Avesta* on a definite scale and in accordance with the means and rank of the patient. A priest enjoyed clerical courtesy. His blessing and prayer were held in higher esteem than monetary gain:

A priest, he (the doctor) shall cure for a pious prayer, the head of a household for the price of a small draught animal, the head of a family for the price of a moderate-size draught animal, the head of a race for the price of a most excellent draught animal; the lord of a province he shall cure for the price of a four-span wagon.

For the treatment of their wives, female animals of the same kind were required. Later it appears that these fees were changed into monetary payments.

A *Pahlavi* commentator, estimating the comparative value of these fees, states that prayer paid by the priest is equal in value to 3,000 stirs, while the wagon with four horses, the fee paid by the lord of a province, is only worth seventy stirs.

Veterinary Medicine: Incidentally it should be noted that the Avestan physician also practiced veterinary medicine. A regulated scale of fees was also fixed for the treatment of cattle; even the fee for the cure of a rabid dog was regulated.[15]

For treating animals, the physician received the value of an animal next in rank. In the case of a sheep, which was considered the lowest animal on the list, his payment consisted only of the price of a "good meal." To Zoroaster's inquiry as to what is to be done if a dog refuses to take his medicine, Ormuzd replies that in such a case it shall be lawful to bind him and force open his mouth with a stick.

Qualifications of a Persian Physician: The following description, as quoted by L. C. Casartelli, represents the ideal qualifications of a Persian physician:

He should know the limbs of the body, their articulations; remedies for diseases; should possess his own carriage and assistant; should be amiable without jealousy, gentle in word, free from haughtiness; enemy of disease but friend of the sick; respecting modesty; free from crime, from injury, from violence; expeditious; the right hand of the widow; noble in action, protecting good reputation; not acting for gain but for spiritual reward, ready to listen; having become a physician by favor of Aryaman; possessed of authority and philanthropy, skilled in preparing health-giving medicine in order to deliver the body from disease, to expel corruption and impurity, to further peace and multiply the delights of life. [16]

PROPHYLAXIS

Generally speaking, the prophylaxis of ancient Persian medicine was well advanced. Cleanliness was a religious duty. The degree of purity was minutely laid down. Frequent ablution and sterilization of soiled clothes, vessels, and implements were scrupulously observed. All precautionary measures were taken to prevent the transmission of defilement. Sexual vices, such as adultery, prostitution, masturbation, pederasty, and criminal abortion were threatened by the *Avesta* with the severest punishment in this world and eternal damnation in the next. The punishment of the pederast was severe. It is stated that "before death he is a devil and after, he is an unbelievable monster."

Feminine Hygiene: Particular stress is laid on female hygiene. Rules for the care of women in menstruation, pregnancy, and childbirth were enacted. Cohabitation with a woman during menstruation and late pregnancy was prohibited. Criminal abortion was severely punished. Miscarriages were treated with cow's urine *(gomez)*, both by mouth and as a douche. Food and wine were to be given but not water; "If she has fever on the fourth day, water is to be allowed because the best thing for her is to have her life saved." To this day, fire worshippers in Persia wash their bodies at least once a year with gomez.[17]

TREATMENT

But while stress was laid by the masters of Persian medicine on ethics, prophylaxis, and hygiene, the medical art proper was neglected. Anatomy, which is the first fundamental step in the science of medicine, and which can only be mastered suitably by dissection of human cadavers, was prohibited. The taboo placed on persons touching a dead body precluded dissection. In view of the low state of the art of medicine, one is inclined to believe that the prophylactic and hygienic measures were not to guard against physical abnormalities by aseptic or antiseptic measures but rather to prevent violations of religious doctrines. The priest, for instance, after purifying the patient, sprinkled him with cow's urine. This being the case, one is not surprised to learn that the Persian kings and nobility did not trust their own physicians but preferred Egyptian or Greek physicians. The demand for these foreign physicians was so great that they were taken by force as happened to an Egyptian oculist. When Cyrus was stricken with an eye affection, he asked Emasis, the Egyptian monarch, to send him an eye doctor; the latter picked out the best physician in his domain and sent him to the king of the Persians.[18] Darius I (521–485 B.C.) dislocated his astragalus as a result of leaning from his horse when hunting. His local physicians attempted to reduce the dislocation by twisting his foot, but their manipulations merely served to aggravate the condition. As a result,

"Darius lay seven days and seven nights without sleep." He sent
for the Greek physician Democedes, whose care was as follows,
"using Grecian medicine and applying moderate after violent remedies, he caused him to sleep and in a little time restored him to
health, although he had before despaired of ever recovering the use
of his foot."[19]

Darius was a liberal monarch. He restored the medical school of
Egypt which was destroyed by Cambyses. The director whom he
appointed for this work states:

On the order of Darius, I founded the school with all its students, men
of good birth and not of humble condition; over them I set a wise man of
every order, for their work. His majesty caused them to be given all kinds
of things suitable for doing this work. I supplied them with everything that
was useful, with every instrument according to the basis just as they were
before. His majesty did this because he knew what was useful for the arts
to make every man live and to establish the name of every god in every
temple.

Persian medicine developed along with the growing wealth of
the nation, and in the time of Artaxerxes II, there was a well-
recognized guild of physicians and surgeons whose fees, like those of
the Babylonians in the period of Hammurabi, were fixed by law,
according to the social rank of the patient.[20] Novices practiced a
year or two upon the bodies of immigrants and the poor. The *Ahura
Mazda* (lord of light) decreed that a young physician was expected
to begin his career by treating infidels and foreigners.

Artaxerxes II[21] employed a Greek physician named "Ctesias" who
had been taken prisoner in the Battle of Cunaxgin (401 B.C.). He
was the author of *Commentarii Medica*. Only fragments of this work,
as quoted by other writers, are extant.

Democedes also cured "Atossa, daughter of Cyrus, and wife of
Darius, who had a tumor on her breast; after some time it burst,
and spread considerably. As long as it was small she concealed it,
and from delicacy informed no one of it; when it became dangerous,
she sent for Democedes and showed it to him."[22]

Incidentally, Herodotus made a curious observation with reference
to the skulls of the Persians:

The skulls of the Persians were so weak that if you should hit them
by a single pebble, you would break a hole in them; whereas those of the
Egyptians are so hard that you scarcely fractured them with a stone. The
cause of this they told me is as follows: and I readily assented; that the
Egyptians begin from childhood . . . shave their heads and the bone is

thickened by exposure to the sun; from the same cause they are less subject to baldness for one sees fewer persons bald in Egypt than in any other country . . . and the reason why the Persians have weak skulls is this; they shade them from the first, wearing tiaras for hats. [23]

The same author quotes an Egyptian official who states that the Egyptians do not live as long as the Ethiopians because "they live on wheat" and that those that live longer have to be thankful to their delightful wine.[24]

HISTORY

To the Persian poet, Abu'l Kasim Mansur (or Hasan) who took the nom de plume of Firdausi[25] (born in 941 A.D. at Shadab, a suburb of Tus), medical history is indebted for bringing to light many historical facts relating to Persian medicine. In his epic poem *Shah Nameh* or "The Epic of the Kings," he describes in nearly 60,000 verses, the genuine traditions of Persia of his day. He gives a pen picture of the Zoroastrians as they were known at that period. He delves deeply into the *Pahlevi* or Middle-Persian literature, especially the ancient historical records which existed in that tongue. *Shah Nameh*, which was completed in the year 999 A.D., refers to surgical physicians as well as to healers who cure with herbs and the holy word.

In his *Shah Nameh*, Firdausi states that Jamshid discovered the art and means of healing:

Jamshid thus spent
Another fifty years and did much good,
He introduced the scents that men enjoy,
As camphor, genuine musk, gum Benjamin,
Sweet aloe, ambergris, and bright rose-water.
Next leechcraft and the healing of the sick,
The means of health, the cause of maladies,
Were secrets opened by Jamshid.

Cesarean Section: Most interesting is the case of Cesarean section, after rendering the patient insensible to pain with wine, recorded in *Shah Nameh:*

His birth could not be natural;
So willeth He who giveth good, Bring thou
A blue-steel dagger, seek a cunning man;
Bemuse the lady first with wine to ease
Her pain and fear: then let him ply his craft
And take the lion from its lair by piercing
Her waist while all unconscious. Then imbruing

Her side in blood, stitch up the gash.
Put trouble, fear, and care aside, and bruise
With milk and must and herb that I will show thee,
And dry them in the shade. Dress and anoint
Rudaba's wound, and watch her come to life. [26]

The same author describes the birth of the legendary hero[27] Rustam by Cesarean section as follows:

A skillful mobed arrived and intoxicated Rondabeh, the moon-faced beauty. Then he ripped open her side without her feeling it, and turning the child's head toward the opening delivered it without harming the mother ....she slept for a day and a night; they sewed up the wound and gave her treatment for pain. When she saw the child she said, "I am delivered and my pain is finished." [28]

Firdausi's description reveals three medical facts: (1) The Persians had a knowledge of surgical anatomy; (2) they used an anesthetic; and (3) Cesarean section was employed or at least comprehended at an early period.

Firdausi's reference to Alexander the Great is of medical interest. While he was in Persia, he relates that an Indian rajah presented the Macedonian with four gifts: a girl, a philosopher, a magic cup, and a physician:

A youthful leech who diagnoseth disease by making an uroscopy,
So long as he is at court the Shah will never ail.[29]

Firdausi used the word *ozar* to describe the cause of Alexander's death. The meaning of this term is uncertain. Aristotle gave, as the cause of Alexander's death, a "poison damsel"—possibly the girl, to whom reference has just been made, was infected with syphilis.

Cure was ascribed to the influence of good spirits; "rain from heaven produces plants and trees whose properties are to prevent and cure disease."[30]

The Dinkart: The *Dinkart* following the *Avesta*, lists, in a somewhat altered form 4333 diseases. Interesting is the division of ailments into corporal and spiritual categories. Corporal diseases are subdivided into voluntary sicknesses, such as venereal disease, and involuntary sicknesses, such as fevers. Spiritual ailments are subdivided into sins tending forward, such as passion and anger, and those inclined backward, such as idleness. The author of this work speaks of bodily and spiritual abnormalities. An analysis of these two conditions is presented as follows: The soul's inclination is toward mercy, justice, and righteousness; the bodily impulses are towards physical pleasure leading to evil. The first is under the control of *Ahuramazda;* the second is governed by *Ahriman.* The constant struggle going on between these two forces forms an interesting chapter in moral philosophy. The reciprocal action between soul and body is discussed with considerable skill and corresponds with the idea of a sound mind in a sound body: *mens sano in corpore sano.*

The difference between a spiritual and physical healer is stated by the *Dinkart* as follows: to the spiritual physician, "the human soul is endowed with a body," and to the corporeal physician, "the human body is endowed with a soul."

In the third part of the work, the author treats of two fundamental maladies which seem to indicate forms of moral evil. Every kind of vice and evil passion is ascribed to the evil spirit. To him is also attributed colds, dryness, bad odor, corruption, hunger, thirst, old age, pain, and various other physical maladies and death.

The fourth part of the *Dinkart* deals with therapeutics. The number of remedies derived from the vegetable kingdom are listed as seventy. These are divided into those which are by nature beneficial and those which are injurious (poisonous) but may become medicinal if properly administered. As an example of the former is mentioned the *myrobalan* of Cabul. The miraculous trees *Gokart* and the white *Hom* are referred to as sources of healing. The Persians possessed an extensive knowledge of poisons. The *Houma*-drink (a drink prepared from the plant *Houma,* which possessed almost divine powers) was prescribed by the physicians for pains in the limbs, catarrhal obstructions, and urinary diseases.

The subject of medicine during the later *Pahlavi* period received a more systematic and rational treatment in the *Dinkart.* In this encyclopedic work, the general subject of medicine is discussed under four headings: (1) medicine; (2) the physician; (3) diseases; and (4) remedies. The last is classified into prophylaxis, or preservatives of health, and therapeutics, or curative medicine. For healing of disease, two kinds of practitioners are distinguished: the master, or officer, of health *(druistopat)* and the healer, or doctor *(bijishak).*[31] The former was the forerunner of the modern public-health service physician.

In the section on the physician, this work defines the basis and importance of medicine and then ascribes the etiology of disease to the demon. Next the work distinguishes between spiritual and material medicine and again between general and individual medicine. General medicine evidently applies to public health patients and individual medicine to prviate patients. The supreme chief of corporal or general medicine is the emperor. The chief regulator of spiritual medicine is the supreme high priest *(garathustrotema).*

The *Dinkart* describes five means of healing instead of the three measures pointed out by the *Avesta.*

Division of Diseases: The division of diseases into hot and cold, and moist and dry, common among modern occult healers, also existed in ancient Persia. A "hot" disease was combated by the use of a "cold" diet, and vice versa.

Many of the ailments prevailing in modern Iran undoubtedly existed in ancient Persia, and many remedial measures of antiquity are still employed in Persia. Blowing upon, expectorating on, and stroking a sick or injured part of the body are methods of therapy which were inherited from ancient Persia. The ancient widespread belief in the spiritual virtue of blood is still common among the peasants. A sheep is often killed so that its blood may be sprinkled on the foundation or the doorstep of the house occupied by the patient. One sick with fever, instead of using antifebrile drugs, may swallow water wherein a paper with a charm written on it has been soaked.

Many diseases, such as relapsing fever, malaria, sunstroke, and ophthalmia, have unquestionably prevailed in Persia since deep antiquity. The oriental boil (lieshmaniasis), scabies, favus, typhus, and many forms of dysentery have also been common for untold centuries, primarily as a result of unsanitary conditions. Owing to the use of raw food and polluted water, half of the population suffers from tapeworm and hookworm; children particularly are kept emaciated from worms within their alimentary canal. Smallpox, until recent years, has been considered a necessary illness for a child. Phthisis and tuberculous bone diseases have always existed in Persia. Epilepsy was a common ailment. Cambyses, according to Herodotus, was troubled with "the sacred disease (epilepsy)."[32]

Every variety of ocular disease has prevailed in Persia, resulting, in a large percentage, in blindness. Some of these ocular diseases may be attributed to the blowing of dust from the desert, others to filth and infection through flies. The most frequent serious eye affection is trachoma. Other common eye diseases are entropion, corneal ulcer, and cataract. Smallpox and gonorrhea are responsible for a large number of eye affections. Religious purification, such as ablution in municipal wells where all people bathe in the same water, has been the cause of the spread of many epidemic diseases.

Superstitions: Ailments were often attributed to the evil eye—a superstition which probably originated in Babylonia and which the Persians adopted. This fallacy is based on the idea that the spirits of some persons are magically superior to those of others and that the superior spirits possess the power to influence, control, and subdue the weaker ones by merely staring at them. This superstition passed quickly from one country to the other in remote antiquity. It has been recognized by sacred writers, by classical thinkers, and by ancient physicians. The Old Testament refers to the evil eye mostly in a figurative sense. The "Book of Leviticus" is outspoken against "enchantment and observations."[33] It is often referred to in the New Testament.[34] The implication by St. Paul that the "foolish Galatians" had been "spellbound" probably refers to the evil eye (i.e. the malicious glance had blighted them).[35]

Naturally an erronous idea conceived by superstition must also be combated in a similar manner; evil eye specialists were, and are still, found selling charms to treat disease caused by the evil eye.

One may observe, attached to private houses and factories, desert-grown berries and Dashtel plants *(esfant)*, sacred to Zoroastrians, combined with bits of blue and pink material to ward off the evil glance. If a stranger looks at a person and the latter happens to become sick or stumbles thereafter, the disease or injury is ascribed to the stranger's evil eye. Consequently no one stares even for a moment at another person, and everyone guards against being considered prying or envious or possessing any quality which is thought to predispose toward evil eye. Amulets are carried to counteract the possible effect of the evil glance. Plants are burned every morning in some homes and are used at weddings and funerals to drive away spirits. Women still tie a large padlock and two or three keys around their waists in the hope of repelling evil influence—particularly that evil influence which prevents pregnancy and the birth of sons.

A charm is thought to be of more benefit than hygienic precautions or natural remedies to cure disease. It is customary to write a charm on paper and sew it into a child's hat, or even to insert it under the skin as protection against evil.[36]

Influence of Other Countries: There is no doubt that many Persian occult medical ideas have been borrowed from Egypt and especially Babylonia. The Persians, like the Accadians, personified disease. One conjuration begins, "I conjure thee, Disease; I conjure thee, Small-pox; I conjure thee, Burning; I conjure thee, Headache; I conjure thee, Fever."[37] But there can be no doubt that during the fourth and third centuries B.C., Persia was also influenced by Greece; at least the courts of the kings and princes were dominated by Greek physicians. Persia was not always the borrower. She also made contributions. Prior to 700 B.C., when the Greeks themselves had not yet reached their peak of culture, they borrowed medical knowledge from the neighboring countries including Persia and India. It is known that Persia displayed great cultural activity during this period, and contributed, in common with Babylonia, Egypt, Phoenicia, and India, towards Greek thought. One particular concept, the humoral theory, is claimed to have been evolved in Persia.

Concept of Microcosm: Another concept said to be of Persian origin is that of "microcosm," a philosophical term applied to man when contrasted with the universe, which in this connection is termed "macrocosm." The idea that there is an analogy between man and the universe was expressed by the ancient Greek philosophers, Pythagoras, Pedocles, Heraclitus, Plato, Aristotle, and especially the Stoics who developed this concept in connection with their doctrine of pneuma.

They considered the universe to be an animated being resembling man and, like him, made up of a body and a soul. According to this idea, man is a miniature universe and conversely the universe is man in great degree. The soul of man, which forms a part of the universal soul, is in the same relation to his body as the universal soul (God) to the universe, and the rational part of the human soul performs in man the same function as the universal intellect in the universe. From this analogy of man to the universe evolved the doctrine that there is a mutual influence of one upon the other.

Here are some of the comparisons made by the Persian philosophers:

The Back is like the sky, the Tissues are like the Soil, the Bones like the Mountains, the Veins like the Rivers, the Blood in the body like the Water in the Oceans, the Liver like the Vegetation, the Places where the hair grows profusely like a thicket, and the Marrow of the body is like Liquid metal within the Earth.

This concept gained new impetus among the Scholastics and the Talmudists, and particularly among the scholars of the Middle Ages. The Talmud finds this analogy between man and the universe, "The hair represents the forest, the bones the wood, the lungs the wind, the stomach the mill; when erect, man resembles the mountains, when recumbent, the valley." Less fantastic analogies between man and universe are given by Jewish, Middle-Ages philosophers, such as Israel, Saadiah, and Donolo; they find in the universe the four elements and the four humors.

Perhaps through the influence of the Cabalah, the doctrine of microcosm came into great favor among the philosophers of the Renaissance, like Bruno, Paracelsus, and Leibnitz, who held that in man's nature is found the sum total of all cosmic forces. He is able to understand the material world because he unites in his body the finest essence of all the material things, and as an intellectual being, he has the faculty of conceiving the world of intellectual forms through the spark of the divine infused in his nature. The idea of microcosm in Persia is perhaps an outgrowth of the concept of dualism, the sinful man as opposed by the righteous universe. It would seem probable that the Persian lore, modified in Mesopotamia and linked to the superstition brought from Egypt, was the chief source of the views of sickness and death that prevailed in Palestine during the years of the formation of Christianity.[38]

References and Notes

1. For The Vendidad and Persian Medicine generally, see Darmesteter: trans. of The Zend-Avesta, Part I, Sacred Books of the East, Vol. 4. Geschichte des Alten Persians, 1897. Dinkart: History of Antiquity. Vol. 1.
2. Printed since in two Vols., 1874 and 1910.
3. Maspero: The Dawn of Civilization. London 1897, p. 57, p. 491.
4. The Vendidad. Vol. 20, 1:17.
5. Meyer, E.: Encyclopedia Britannica, Ed. 11, Vol. 21, p. 205.
6. Dinkart: Peshotan ed., Bombay, 1874 and 1910, Vol. 4, Chapter 157.
7. Herodotus 1:141.
8. The Vendidad 5:20.
9. Deodorus 1:81. Mencken, H. L.: Treatise on the Gods. p. 117.
10. The Vendidad 7:95-104.
11. Ibid.
12. See Darmesteter: trans. of The Zend-Avesta, Part I, Sacred Books of the East, Vol. 4.
13. Ibid.
14. The Vendidad 21:9-11.
15. Ibid. 13:97-99.
16. Casartelli, L. C.: Hasting Encyclopedia, Vol. 2, p. 259-a.
17. Elgood, C.: Medicine in Persia. Paul B. Hoeber, New York, 1934, p. 21.
18. Herodotus 3:1, p. 370.
19. Ibid.
20. Cf. Code of Hammurabi, John's. ed.
21. Artaxerxes is the son of Xerxes of Biblical fame, known in the Bible as "Ahasueros" in The Book of Esther.
22. Herodotus, p. 225 (131-133).
23. Ibid. 3:174 (11-13).
24. Ibid.

25. Firdausi (940-1020) worked thirty-five years to produce his gigantic task. Sir W. Jones calls the Shah Nameh a "glorious monument of eastern genius and learning" which, if ever it should be generally understood in its original language, will contest the merits of invention with Homer itself.

26. Shah Nameh of Firdausi: Tübner's Oriental Series. London, 1905, Book 5:1, 33. Warner's trans.

27. Rustam is the Persian Hercules. His seven labors remind one of the twelve labors of Hercules. Some writers think that the Persians adopted the Greek legend of Hercules as their own.

28. Aesculapius: 1938, p. 68. Cited by Castiglione.

29. Shah Nameh, Book 20:8.

30. Darmesteter: Sacred Books of the East. Vol. 23.

31. The Dinkart. Book 3: Chapter 157. Printed in Vol. 4 of Peshotan's ed. (Bombay, 11 Vol., 1874-1910).

32. Herodotus 3:32-34, p. 184.

33. Leviticus 19:26; Deuteronomy 18:10.

34. Matthew 6:23; 10:13; Mark 7:22; Luke 11:34.

35. Galatians 3:1 .

36. For more details with reference to the evil eye, see the author's Romance of Medicine, pp. 228-252.

37. Leuormont: Chaldean Magic. English trans., 1877, p. 4, 20, 260.

38. Elgood C.: Medicine in Persia. Paul B. Hoeber, New York, 1934, p. 13.

11

Antiquity of Indian Medicine

HISTORIANS who have been accustomed to trace all sciences to ancient Greece, have in recent years undergone a change of mind. The dry land of the province of Sind in India, has, like the desert of Egypt, yielded to the efforts of the archaeologists, elucidating numerous remains of a civilization that had been concealed 6000 years or more. Recent researches of Vedic scholars have also given a new outlook to ancient Indian history. The revelation has come that a great Aryan civilization flourished in India in remote antiquity.

The excavations of Sir John Marshall and his Indian coworkers have uncovered buried cities, well-constructed houses with adjoining bathrooms, and a remarkably well-developed system of drainage. They found many articles, such as ornaments and fineries, made of gold, silver, copper, and iron, which betray a well-advanced civilization. It has thus been definitely established that the Hindus in very remote antiquity enjoyed a civilization comparable to that of Mesopotamia, Egypt, and Phoenicia.

The studies of Indian Sanskrit scholars, such as Bannerjes, Sircar, Tilak, and others, disclose that at an early historic period, Aryans migrated from India and established colonies in Egypt, Babylonia, Phoenicia, and Persia and, in later years, also in Greece and Rome. According to "Beal's Record," the Druids (who settled in Britain at an early period) and the Scandinavians originated from Buddhist Brahman castes.

Since religion was an important part of the daily life of the Hindus, they developed those sciences that helped them in their worship, such as, for example, the science of astronomy. Other subjects cultivated were mathematics, geometry, gross anatomy, and medicine. The art of writing has been known to the Hindus from at least 4000 B.C. According to Björnstjerna, the Hindus possessed written books on religion before 2800 B.C. or 800 years before Abraham. They invented a language of unequalled richness—Sanskrit—one of the world's great classical languages. They invented fairy tales that have become children's nursery stories, translated into almost every language of the world.

In the time of Solomon (who reigned 971–931 B.C.), India was already accessible to the West. Indian merchants exported gold, silver, salt, cotton, silk, pearls, and rubies. The navies of Hiram and Solomon brought back from India gold, silver, ivory, ebony, apes, and peacocks.[1]

The Hindu system of medicine, known as *Ayur-Veda* (the science of life), said to have originated from Brahma, the fountainhead of all learning, may be traced back to 6000 B.C. A Bactrian document found in Cashmir proves that India enjoyed, far back in antiquity. a splendid civilization in which medicine formed an important part.

PERIODS OF HINDU MEDICINE

Hindu medicine may be divided into three different periods: the Vedic, the Brahman, and the Buddhic.

Vedic Medicine

The first period may be traced from the early migration of the Hindus into the Punjab, perhaps to the eighth century B.C. The term *Vedic* applies to a certain period of Indian civilization represented by the four Vedas (the holy writings, consisting of religious hymns and dogmatic principles).

VEDIC HYMNS

The earliest medical utterances which have been preserved in Aryan literature are *Vedic* hymns consisting of songs or invocations addressed to different Aryan deities in the language of praise and prayer. These hymns are not the outcome of a single generation, but the growth of centuries. The earlier hymns represent the religious ecstasy of a childlike people. The later hymns are more thoughtful and lofty and represent the ideas of children or savages, expressed in the language of sages and divines. The poetical feelings and imagery of a more advanced civilization, with spiritual and moral sentiment, resulted from later Braham teaching. The four elements, earth, water, air, and fire, supposed to constitute matter, are mentioned in these hymns.

VEDIC RELIGION

Since the *Vedic* medicine was associated with religion, a brief review of the *Vedic* religion is pertinent to understand the medicine of that period.

Gods: The element of fire was personified. It was known as *Agni,* the god who cooked the food, warmed the dwelling, and frightened away beasts of prey. *Agni* thus became the divinity of the homestead. Water was personified as *Varuna,* the god of the sea, and Varuna was gradually invested with divine attributes as a deity powerful to destroy, but mighty to save, who engulfed the wicked man in the drowning depths, or mercifully bore the repentant sinner over the surging billows in safety to the shore. The wind and breezes were personified as *Vayu* and the *Maruts. Vayu* roared among the trees. The firmament was personified as *Indra*:

He was king of the *Vedic* gods; he healed the sick, struck the sky with his thunderbolts, pierced the black clouds with his spear and brought down the earth-refreshing showers. He was the national deity of the Aryan invaders; he slew his enemies by thousands and destroyed their cities by hundreds; he brought back the spoil and recovered the cows that were carried away; he majestically remained enthroned in his heaven of Swarga on the Himalayas, like Zeus among the deities of Olympus. [2]

Surya, or the sungod, the Persian Mithra, was originally the deity who journeyed through the sky and measured the days and nights, but he was eventually invested with attributes more divine than those of *Indra.* In later *Vedic* literature, he was elevated in the pantheon as the creator of the universe, and the divine soul that illuminated the universe. Eventually the worship of the sun developed into that of *Vishnu,* the supreme spirit, whose incarnations as *Krishna* and *Rama* were glorified in the *Mahabharata* and *Ramayana.*

The *Vedic* hymns contain no distinct reference to a future state of reward and punishment; but there are numerous allusions to a judge of the dead, who is personified as the god *Yama* and who consequently may be regarded as presiding over the entrance to the world of departed souls.

In *Vedic* literature, all the more prominent gods are extolled in turn as the supreme being; but in the modern belief of the Hindus, three different deities stand out as representatives of the One God: *Brahma, Vishnu,* and *Shiva.* Each of these gods is worshipped in different localities as the creator and ruler of the universe, the divine spirit who is above all and in all. One important sect of Hindus worship *Brahma* as the creator, *Vishnu* as the preserver, and *Shiva* as the destroyer of the universe; but more frequently all these attributes of creation, preservation, and dissolution are assigned to one supreme being, who permeates the universe and is the universe; and all the endless emblems, incarnations, and idols are revered as so many vehicles through which the supreme spirit receives the adorations and offerings of his worshippers.

Brahmans: The growth of the Brahmans in power and influence is one of the most important elements in Indian history. Every rajah or ruler had his own Brahman priest, preceptor, or *purohita.* So had every family, group of families, and village community. Priests and laymen have been subject to inquisitorial forms of Brahmanical government, of which many traces are still to be found.

Laws of Manu: A further development of the religious teaching of the Hindus is to be found in the Brahman code, known as the "Laws of Manu." The life of Manu is unknown and he has no personality whatsoever. A mythical being, a reputed son of Brahma, he is lord of all living creatures. The sacred character of the code of Manu is acknowleged and revered throughout India.

Manu taught belief in endless transmigrations of the soul. According to this concept, the soul of every individual being, whether man or animal, passes at every successive death into a newly born body, rising or falling in the scale of life at every successive birth according to the sum total of its merits or demerits in all past lives.[3] Thus the belief in a future state of rewards and punishments was associated by *Manu* with a chain of existences without beginning or end, running up and down the scale of animal life from the meanest vermin to the highest order of intellectual man.[4]

While the code of Manu enforced the worship of the gods, it further developed those conceptions of the supreme spirit which finds expression in the *Vedic* hymns:

All gods are in the Divine Spirit; all worlds are in the Divine Spirit; and the Divine Spirit produces the connected series of acts which are performed by embodied souls. Him some adore as present in the element of fire; others as present in Manu,—lord of creatures; some as present in Indra; others as present in pure ether; and others as present in the most high Eternal Spirit. It is He who, pervading all beings in five elementary forms, causes them by the gradations of birth, growth, and dissolution to revolve in this world like the wheels of a car.

But Manu pointed out that there was a way of deliverance or emancipation of the soul from the endless chain of transmigrations, whether on earth or in heaven or hell. The soul would at such a time enter upon a term of pure contemplation, during which it would behold the supreme soul present in all things, and would finally be absorbed in the divine spirit.[5]

Manu thus fashioned a universe of beings, driven by an artificial law of merits and demerits along a chain of endless transmigrations. He next mapped out the life of man into the four terms of student, householder, hermit, and devotee, with the view of enabling each person to work out his own deliverance or emancipation. As a student, each person of the twice-born castes would learn the divine law; as a householder, he would marry a wife and thereby derive merits as a husband and a father; as a hermit, he would perform strict religious functions; and as a devotee, he would contemplate the supreme soul until his own soul was absorbed in the divine spirit. The duties which each person must fulfill within the four terms are duly set forth in the code of *Manu*, and still make up the ideal of the Hindu.

VEDIC LITERATURE

The *Vedic* literature consists of four *Vedas:* the *Rig-Veda* (c. 4000 B.C.), consisting of hymns; the *Sama-Veda*, containing chants; the *Yajur-Veda* (secret formulas); and the *Atharva-Veda* (a collection of later hymns); they constitute the first medical period.

The second, or the Brahman Period, is considered the middle age of ancient India; medicine was then entirely under the authority of priestly castes. The third period was that of Hinduism, dominated by the writings of Susruta and Charaka (second century B.C.), whose books were considered standard works of Hindu medicine for many centuries. They were revised and reedited by many Indian physicians down to the time of *Bhava Misra* (1550 A.D.) and, through the efforts of Arab physicians, left a strong impression on European medicine.

The four *Vedic* texts, or *Samhitas*, are the Hindu scripture; each of them has attached to it a number of Brahman commentators who explain the importance of the sacrificial rites and other religious worship for which these holy books have been composed. Two of the *Samhitas*, owing to the fact that many of their verses were taken from the *Rig-Veda* and deal mostly with religion, are only of secondary importance to the present inquiry and will not be discussed.

The Rig-Veda: The *Rig-Veda* was not written on papyrus scrolls as the Egyptian medical documents were, nor on clay tablets as was the custom among the Babylonian writers. It was transmitted from generation to generation orally; but because of its sacred character, it lost virtually nothing during the long ages.

The *Rig-Veda* (knowledge of praise), the oldest and most important of the four *Vedas*, from which a considerable portion of the other books took material (composed from 2000 to 1000 B.C.), is a collection of metrical hymns containing a number of mythological elements. The hymns are invocations to the gods, intended to accompany the oblation of *soma* juice and the fire sacrifice of melted butter to the gods. The *Rig-Veda* mentions a special class of physicians; it contains passages in praise of the healing powers of herbs and water; and it notes at least two diseases, phthisis and leprosy.

The later hymns of the *Rig-Veda* contain data of a well-developed civilization near the modern Punjab, where the Indo-Aryans settled and built towns and villages. They domesticated animals, such as the cow, the sheep, the goat, the horse, the ass, and the elephant. The elephant was trained for burden and transportation. The pious Hindus worshipped the cow for possessing five essential and life-sustaining products. In health, they depended upon her for milk, curds, and butter; and in disease, they took advantage of her dung and urine. Some devotees lived and slept in the cow pen and followed the cow wherever she went.

The early Hindus cultivated rice, barley, and millet and used various kinds of metals for domestic and ornamental purposes. Their physicians lived in houses surrounded by gardens of medicinal plants which they dispensed to the sick of the community. The *Rig-Veda* praises certain plants for having a purifying effect upon the air. Surgeons were employed on the battlefield and to attend patients suffering from injuries resulting from clan warfare: they extracted arrow shafts, amputated limbs, and substituted artificial ones. They removed eyes blinded by injury and assisted women in labor, prescribing the *soma* plant to relieve pain.[6] The *Rig-Veda* contains hymns to combat diseases. One hymn against a lung condition presents a fairly good description of pulmonary tuberculosis.

The Atharva-Veda: The chief source of *Vedic* medicinal knowledge, however, is the *Atharva-Veda* (a knowledge of spells) compiled at about 700 B.C. This *Samhita* never reached as high a degree of sanctity as the other *Vedas*. The *Atharva-Veda* contains 100 hymns intended as cures for as many or more diseases. The hymns served as charms against certain diseases and are the embryonic tissues from which later Hindu medicine is derived.

Anatomy: The knowledge of anatomy found in the *Atharva-Veda* is rather primitive. It is largely confined to the gross structures of the human body, such as the limbs, the external part of the head, the ears, the nose, and the mouth. It also refers to the anatomy of some internal organs. Beyond this basic knowledge which is really prehistoric, the *Atharva-Veda* does not go. It does not distinguish between hard bone and cartilage, nor between arteries and veins. The rude knowledge of anatomy represented in this work is derived from the examination of sacrificed animals.

Etiology: The etiology of disease is ascribed to the action of supernatural powers. The popular mind was ever ready to look upon disease as a manifestation of the will of such forces. The thoughts of primitive man were largely controlled by fear; for the primitive lacked the means of explaining the workings of nature which to him represented inscrutable phenomena which were more often hostile than amicable. Like modern man, he tried to counteract the powers of nature; but not having science at his disposal, he developed supernatural methods to achieve his goal. Primitive man, if he wanted anything to happen, gave solemn expression to the wish or represented the object of his wish pictorially, supporting this procedure by ceremonies meant to endow it with supernatural strength. Although the means he adopted did not yield concrete results, it nevertheless satisfied his fancy.

While pains were taken to recognize diseases, and frequently identification of them was effected by the careful use of their special senses, when it came to determine the cause of disease, and the special senses were not of any help, resort was made to imagination and intuition. The causes of death and disease, when brought about by violence, were readily understood but there could be no grasp of death and disease attacking man without any traumatic cause. For want of a rational explanation of morbid conditions, the inference was made that an offended, jealous, or evil force from without entered the sick man's body to seek vengeance.

In the *Atharva-Veda,* no distinction is made between disease and the supernatural power that causes the trouble. Diseases in the *Atharva-Veda* ascribed to worms were looked upon as demonic in origin. In one of the hymns, the god *Indra* is invoked to destroy the worms in a child, praying that all the *Arati* (certain female demons) be slain. *Takman* was the name of "fever" and also the name of the demon that caused fever. An invocation against Takman reads, "May refusal meet Takman who has glowing weapons, O Takman, go to the Tunjavant or farther. Attack the Sudra (low caste) woman, the teeming one; shake her, O Takman."

The most select remedies seem to have been preserved for princes; thus when the son of Bimbesara, king of Magadha (about 600 B.C.), fainted, he was placed in six tubs of fresh butter and afterwards in a seventh filled with the most costly sandalwood oil. It is interesting to know that the prince survived and succeeded his father after such treatment.[7] *Apachit,* a disease marked by scrofulous sores, was similarily personified. Disease itself was believed to come of its own volition through the air to hover over and settle upon its victim.

Occasionally, the *Artharva-Veda* ascribes a disease to one of the greater gods as a punishment for sin. Diarrhea is connected with the raingod *Pargania.* Sharp pains are imputed to the spear of *Rudra.* The arrows of *Rudra* cause tumors. *Agni* is recorded as the producer of fever, headache, and cough. Some diseases, like dropsy, are recognizable from the description and some from the very name attached to the syndrome (i.e. "water in the belly" [ascites]). The most dreaded disease in the *Atharva-Veda* is malaria *(takman).* It prevailed largely in the autumn and is known as the "King of Diseases." The symptoms are "alternations between heat and cold," delirium, the return of the fever daily or every third day, its association with jaundice, and a certain red eruption followed by headache, cough, spasms, and itch.

Venereal diseases, characterized by tumors, are treated in the *Atharva-Veda* by a hymn. Constipation is attributed to sexual excess. The cure of scrofula and leprosy are effected by two hymns. A certain disease known as *ksetriya* was supposed to be hereditary.

Interesting is the fact that the *Atharva-Veda* associates dropsy with heart disease. In the same hymn prescribed for dropsy is mentioned swelling of the heels and the front part of the foot (puffiness) which is so characteristic of cardiac dropsy. Constipation and retention of urine are the subject of another hymn. There are hymns for colic, rheumatism, intercostal neuralgia, and ocular pain; the last was ascribed to worms. There are special charms against the flow of blood (external, internal, or menstrual) and against wounds and fractures. There are charms against epilepsy, convulsions, and lockjaw. Owing to the fact that India was always a snake-infested country, there are three charms against snake bite.

Though the incantations of the *Atharva-Veda* were undoubtedly recited by Brahmans, it is important to note that the physicians of the Vedic age did not belong to this priestly caste. They are classed in the ancient laws of *Manu* among those unclean persons who are excluded from the funeral feasts, and their origin is attributed in the Brahmanic writings to intermarriages between men and women of the different castes. The majority, however, probably belonged to the great Hindu middle class, the *vaisyas* (agriculturists and traders). In later times a physician was permitted to take, as a pupil, a member of any caste except *Sudra*.[8]

Not all the diseases which prevailed in Vedic times have as yet been identified, but those that have show that the pathologic conditions of India have not changed materially since remote antiquity. Supernatural treatment was frequently reenforced by healing substances.

Remedies. WATER: First on the list of all remedies was water. It was personified by the goddess *Varuna*. Because of its cleansing and cooling properties, water was considered the essential and official remedy in the ancient East; it purified both body and soul. It was employed not only because of its own medical virtues but also as a vehicle for other remedies. One of the *Atharva-Vedic* hymns praises the medicinal virtues of water for expelling disease.[9] Water was employed as a panacea for many diseases, particularly for dropsy. The fact that water was used as a cure for disease caused by the presence of water in the system, indicates that the *Atharva-Vedic* physician believed in the homeopathic theory of medicine.

PLANTS: Next to water, plants were considered effective remedies. Because their growth depended on water, they were considered to possess the curative properties of water. Many hymns in the *Atharva-Veda* are addressed to plants, imploring them to serve as remedies.

One of the most efficient therapeutic plants, which were considered holy, was the *soma* tree, spoken of as the "lord of plants" or the "lord of the forests." The tree symbolized the god Soma, the third most important Vedic deity.

This plant, which yielded a mild acidulous milky juice, played an important part in the sacrifice being offered, especially to the god *Indra*, and was always before the eyes of the Vedic priest as he sang praises to the god that personified the plant.[10] The mental stimulation produced by drinking *soma* juice is expressed by one of the poets of the *Rig-Veda* as follows, "We have drunk Soma; we have become immortal; we have entered into the light; we have known the gods." Soma juice was regarded as a drink which bestows immortality. Hence the god who personified the drink, Soma, placed his worshippers in the imperishable world of eternal life and glory. A plant possessing such merits was sure to become important as a therapeutic agent. It became known as the "all healer; it heals the sick, it makes the blind see and the lame walk."

Many plants in the *Atharva-veda* owe their medicinal virtues to fanciful, symbolical, or etymological concepts. They were employed in medicine because they, in some way, resembled the part of the body affected. For example the leaves of a *parasu* (axe) tree were applied to an abscess in the belief that the axe-shaped leaf would open the sore. The wood of the tree known as *karunka* (a bow) was applied to cure wounds produced by a poisoned arrow. Growth of hair was promoted by the *nitatni* ("she that takes root") plant in the hope that hair would take root. Fractures were healed by a root *aha* ("to set"), under the premise that such a plant applied to the fracture would set the bones in their proper places. This method of therapeutics, later known as "signature," is probably the earliest healing method in the history of medicine. It is based on the assumption that the Creator stamped all objects medically beneficial to mankind and that there is a connection of every part of the human body with a corresponding part of the world of nature. This concept is founded upon the doctrine that the human being is a microcosm (little world) and each of his anatomical parts has a counterpart in the macrocosm (large world). The system of color signature played an important part in the *Atharva-veda* pharmacopoeia. Lotus root, because of its yellow color, was prescribed for jaundice, a concept still persisting among certain peoples. The writer recalls cases of *icterus neonatorum* (jaundice of the newborn) in his early practice, which were treated by midwives with gold coins on the umbilicus or yellow ribbons suspended from the neck. Other remedies mentioned in the *Atharva-Veda* are colorifolia, pepper, black beans, grass pollen, and camphor. The offensive odor of pritika grass led to its use in treating constipation.

OFFENSIVE SUBSTANCES: Offensive substances, such as dog saliva, slime from teeth, spittle, rock salt, and rotten fish were employed therapeutically. These were not intended to cure the patient but to disgust the demon within the patient and induce him to leave its victim.

DRUG VEHICLES: Many kinds of foods were used as vehicles for the administration of drugs. Rice, porridge, milk, honey, and fat were so employed. The best vehicle for infant remedies was recognized to be its own mother's milk.

SCAPEGOATS: Diseases were occasionally transferred to birds and frogs. Frogs were thus used as "scapegoats" to cure fever and yellow birds to combat jaundice. The porcupine, an animal considered unlikely to be bitten by snakes, served as an antidote for snake poison. Many kinds of amulets were employed as preventative and curative measures.

PREPARATION AND ADMINISTRATION: *Atharva-vedic* medicine also concerned itself with the preparation and administration of various remedies. Some remedies, to be effective, had to be prepared in a cow horn and others in a red copper vessel, or a vessel of reed. Some had to be stirred with a reed or poisoned arrow. The place where the remedy was prepared was also important: a crossroad was frequently selected. Fire in a forest was specified to be employed in boiling the ingredients when preparing a remedy for dropsy. The position of the patient, the time when the medicine was to be administered, and the patient's food and clothing were all important to the cure. Therapeutic hymns were chanted either at sunrise, noon, or sunset, and frequently as the stars faded away. The *Atharva-veda*, in a hymn, offers an explanation for selecting the proper time, "when the constellation fades away and when the dawn fades away then shall he shine away from us every evil and the *keystrya*."

NATURE OF REMEDIES: While the ceremonies associated with the cure of morbid conditions varied, the treatment had one object in view: to expel from the body of the sick the intruding spirit that caused the trouble. This was first attempted by propitiation and then by certain rituals or exorcism. When resort was had to other remedial measures, these were not intended to cure the patient but were directed against the demon, either as a bribe (in which case the drug was made palatable), or as a threat (in which case the drug was made repugnant and offensive).

It is apparent that *Atharva-vedic* therapeutics was largely magic veneered with religion. The hymns and prayers were addressed to the gods, to the demons, or to the remedy itself. There are, however, many instances in Vedic medicine which have a rational aspect although the original intention might have been magical. To cite only a few examples: the use of a probe in cases of retention of urine as in the following hymn, "I split open by Pasas like the dike of a lake and relaxed is the opening of thy bladder"; another hymn, associated with relieving an overdistended bladder, refers to pouring of water to induce urination, a practice still exercised with beneficial results; still another hymn implies cauterization of snake bite with a torch. Many measures in the *Atharva-veda*, designed to relieve pain and suffering, are practical, even though they originated symbolically.

Status of Physicians: In later Vedic times, medicine became an independent profession. The physician separated himself from the Brahman priest healer and to a certain extent opposed him. His aims were not altogether ethical, as may be gathered from the following aphorism, "The wagoner desires wood; the doctor, sickness; and the priests, libation." A passage in the *Rig-Veda* refers to a physician who hopes to be remunerated with horses, cattle, and clothing.

Upa: Besides the four great Vedas, the Hindus have certain supplementary *Upa* (Vedas) of a later date which deal with secular subjects, such as medicine, music, or architecture. The first, known as *Ayur-veda* (knowledge of life) is a term that includes all books on medicine thought to have been revealed by the gods, not any particular book, although a later legend credits an original *Ayur-veda* to Brahma himself, containing 100 sections and 100,000 stanzas *(slocas).* The term *Ayur-veda,* however, applies more to the works of Charaka, which are said to have been revealed by *Indra* himself through the medium of a *rishi,* or sage, and to those of Susruta, dictated by the divine healer *Dhanvantari,* who became the patrongod of Indian medicine.[11]

Buddhic Period

As a revolt against the Brahman system of religion came Buddhism. It ignored the existence of the popular deity, denied the efficacy of prayers and sacrifices, broke up the bondage of the caste system, and declared that goodness and loving-kindness were the only merits by which the soul could rise in its successive transmigrations. It laid down five commandments which must be observed—against murder, theft, adultery, drunkenness, and falsehood—and it taught that the slightest infringement of any one of these commandments, in thought, word, or deed, constituted a demerit which would detract from the happiness of the soul in a future state of being.

But as regards the deliverance or emancipation of the soul, the teaching of Gautama Buddha coincided (with one important exception) with that of Manu. Gautama Buddha taught that a life of goodness and divine contemplation would quench the fires of affection, passion, and desire, and bind the soul to the universal being. But he denied the existence of a divine spirit, and was thus driven to accept the dogma of annihilation. Consequently he taught that when the soul was delivered from the chain of existence, it sank into the eternal sleep, or annihilation, known as *nirvana.*

Miraculous Cures: The third period of Indian medicine, which began with Buddha (600 B.C.),[12] gave rise to the canonical books of Buddha. These include some medical statements, most of them referring to miraculous cures, particularly in diseases of children. Buddha himself is said to have treated, with a spell, a young pupil who had been bitten by a cobra. The ancient Indian physician, Jivaka, a contemporary of Buddha, is alleged, in Buddhist scripture, to have cured a patient by making an incision in his head and pulling two worms out of the wound.[13] Except for the fact that they erected hospitals for men and animals in various parts of the country, the Buddhists cannot claim any credit for medical advancement.

Doctrine of Karma: Generally speaking, Indian medicine was put on a religio-philosophical plane by the doctrine of *Karma,* according to which a man's social position in life and his physical advantages or disadvantages are the result of his action in a previous birth.

The doctrine of transmigration of the soul checked medical progress for many centuries. The concept that the soul wanders about after death until it is incarnated in a newly born body of man or beast became widely spread around the world. The doctrine of transmigration afforded a satisfactory explanation of reward and punishment in this world. Blindness for example was explained as retribution for the lust of one's eye in a previous birth, and unusual power of hearing was the reward for listening to the preaching of the law in a previous existence. All diseases and infirmities were ascribed to sins committed in previous existences. The various diseases known to the believers of this concept were traced to particular sins committed in a previous life. Thus, pulmonary tuberculosis was the punishment for murder, dyspepsia for stealing food, lameness for stealing horses, madness for committing arson, epilepsy for engaging in usury, blindness for stealing lamps, and decayed teeth for being an informer.[14]

It is evident that such concepts precluded any progress in medical science. Religious penance was the only measure that could be used to atone for the heinous sins of a former existence.

PERIOD OF RATIONAL MEDICINE

The period of rational medicine began with the Sanskrit treatises of Atreya and Susruta (about 600 B.C.). Scientific medicine in India, as in Greece, originated in mythology. According to Hindu traditions, medicine and surgery were communicated by the supreme god *Indra* to two different agencies. Medicine was handed down to the sage *Bharadavaga,* who, in turn, transmitted it to Atreya (c. 600 B.C.)

whose work *(Atreya Samhita)* is the oldest existing work on medicine. Bharadavaga may be considered the patron saint of medicine and Atreya (600 B.C.), the father of scientific Hindu medicine. Surgery was revealed by the great god *Indra* to *Dhanvantari* and passed from him to Susruta. Surgery thus was separated from medicine coming as it did from a different source.

The story of the birth of this Hindu Aesculapius is related as follows:

A blight has fallen upon the universe, and the anxious gods came to their father, Vishnu, for advice. He declared that they must obtain the *Amrita*, or drink of immortality, and that for this purpose an ocean of milk must be churned. Gods and demons, forgetting for a time their hostility, united in this stupendous work. The great serpent, Vasuki, twined himself round the mountain Mandara, and the gods and demons, grasping the monster by its head and tail, twirled the mountain around in the milk ocean upon the back of Vishnu himself, who lay in the shape of a huge tortoise at the bottom. Long they labored, and the demons, who were nearest the serpent's head, became permanently blackened by the poisonous fumes from his hood; but at last the work was done, and there rose from the churned ocean the moon, a marvellous tree, a sacred cow, the goddesses of Love, Wine, and Beauty, and finally the white-robed physician, Dhanvantari, with the cup of *Amrita* in his hand. In pity for the ills of mortals, he caused himself to be born on earth as a prince of Benares, and having retired to the woods as a hermit, after the manner of ancient Hindu princes, dictated to Susruta, a son of the famous warrior-sage Visvamitra, his Ayur-Veda." [15]

Universities

Hindu tradition, preserved in Buddhist folklore, speaks of two great universities in India during the Vedic Period, where astronomy, mathematics, philosophy, and medicine were taught. One was at Benares on the Ganges in the East, where the head of the medical section was Susruta (c. 600 B.C.). The other was at Taxila in the West (on the Jhelam River), where medicine was taught under the leadership of Atreya. Susruta was perhaps the younger contemporary, for he was acquainted with Atreya's system of anatomy. In his *Samhita* he points out the differences in the teaching of the school of Atreya and his own.[16]

In the compendium *(Samhita)* on *Ayur-Veda*, Susruta enumerates 1120 diseases which he divides into three classes: those that affect the body, such as wounds; those caused by mental disorders; and those caused by natural conditions (incidental to old age, congenital ailments, and starvation).

Teachers

Atreya: Atreya was the first to whom the god of health, Andra, communicated the *Ayur-Veda* (the science of life). He is said to have had six pupils, each of whom individually committed his teaching to writing in the form of compendiums *(Samhita)*. The works of only two of his pupils, Agnivesa Behla and Harita, are known to have survived. *Atreya Samhita* is the oldest known medical book now extant. It contains 46,500 verses.[17] These works were revised, edited, and supplemented about 800 years later by Charaka of Cashmir, a court physician of King Kaniska (c. second century, B.C.).

Charaka: Charaka was a philosopher, astronomer, and physician, a man of high culture and attainments. His medical work is divided into eight parts, containing 120 chapters. It deals with diseases of the heart, chest, abdomen, genital organs, extremities, and others. It describes the diagnosis, symptoms, and treatment. It mentions the use of syringes and other medical appliances. Chapters are devoted to drugs, diet, and antidotes. The use of emetics, purgatives, and enemas are noted. Charaka gives instructions for erecting hospitals and for the construction and provisioning of lying-in and children's rooms. He describes in detail the bedding, sheets, and coverings, and a method to cleanse them by steam and fumigation. He mentions even such a small detail as providing toys for children.[18] He states:

A hospital should be strong and not exposed to strong winds. Every part of it should have access to plenty of air; it should be freely ventilated and spacious enough for walking about freely with ease, not too near any high building or structures, not exposed to smoke, sun, moisture or dust and not exposed to injurious sounds, tastes or smells. [19]

The nurse he considers one of the four limbs of the whole system: "She should be loving, pure in body, speech, and mind, and capable and enlightened."[20] He held that the Hindu physician should serve humanity, regardless of earthly gain: "Not for self, not for the fulfillment of any desire of gain but solely for the good of suffering humanity, should you treat your patients. Those who sell the treatment of disease as merchandise, gather the dust and neglect the gold."[21]

Remedies

Charaka was familiar with 500 medical plants whose fruits, blossoms, leaves, roots, barks, oils, and juices were used as medicine. The medicaments were classified according to their therapeutic actions, i.e. emetics, purgatives, laxatives, sedatives, tonics, and aphrodisiacs.

The last was especially in demand in a land where sterility was counted as one of the great misfortunes.

Antidotes against poisoning were in great demand. The Indian physician was renowned for his knowledge of treatment of snake bites. Hindu medical literature contains minute descriptions of animal, vegetable, and mineral poisoning. Both rational and magical remedies were employed against poisoning. Prayers and spells were followed by bloodletting, constriction of the tissue above the wound, sucking the wound, cauterization, extirpation of the diseased part, or cold water applications. Among the antidotes administered were aconite, brassica, latifolia, and ferox. Black pepper and ginger were used internally or as a snuff.[22]

Diseases

Fever was called the "king of diseases" and was ascribed to the anger of the god *Shiva*. Twenty-six varieties of fever were distinguished. Tertian and quartan malarial fever were described in detail.[23] Seven forms of pyrexia resulted from humoral imbalance. Fever was considered most dangerous on the seventh, tenth, and twelfth days of the month.

Thirteen varieties of abdominal swelling were described. Twelve kinds of "worm" diseases and twenty forms of urinary complaints were listed. Eight varieties of jaundice were known. Five varieties each of cough, asthma, and hiccoughs, eighteen forms of leprosy, seven kinds of impotence, sixty-seven varieties of eye disease, twenty-eight types of ear ailment, sixty-five varieties of mouth infection, thirty-one kinds of nasal disease, eighteen forms of throat disease, and many types of mental disease were tabulated. Diabetes mellitus was first recognized by observing flies and insects feeding upon sweet urine. Many of these diseases were accurately described. Some were no more than symptoms.

Observations were made on the varied character of feces and urine in such diseases as vertigo, dermatitis, apoplexy, epilepsy, rheumatism, insanity, and venereal ailments. Smallpox was unquestionably observed, although a description of the disease was left for later medical literature. The name for smallpox *(sitala)* was also the name of the goddess who caused it. She was located at Benares. The treatment of smallpox consisted of invoking and propitiating the goddess *Sitala*. There was also a rational treatment for smallpox. Indeed some investigators hold that inoculation against smallpox was practiced in ancient India. Pulmonary tuberculosis was called the "royal disease":

The physician who values his reputation should not undertake to take care of a patient who has the three great symptoms: fever, cough, and bloody sputum. If, however, the patient has a good appetite and digests well the food, and the disease is in its infancy, a cure may be hoped for.

Patients suffering from giddiness, and presenting symptoms, such as pain in the side of the head, cough, diarrhea, hoarseness, loss of appetite, and fever (or even fever, cough, and hemorrhage) were not to be treated by any physician seeking a good reputation, for such cases were considered beyond cure. Insane persons were treated barbarously. Starving, burning, whipping, incarcerating them in a dark room, and terrorizing them with wild animals were the order of the day. Insanity was attributed to possession by a rabid demon, and the crude treatment was intended to expel the demon rather than neutralize the disease.

The Hindus, like the Babylonians and the Egyptians, made "worms" (real or imaginary) responsible for many ailments. They believed them to be the etiological agents in eye, tooth, ear, head, and heart ailments.

Susruta and Surgery

The most striking feature is the high place in Susruta's compendium assigned to surgery (salya), a fact sufficient in itself to disprove the priestly origin of these works. "Surgery," says Susruta, "is the first and highest division of the healing art, least liable to fallacy, pure in itself, perpetual in its applicability, the worthy produce of heaven, the sure source of fame on earth." At the same time he emphasizes the unity of medicine, "He who only knows one branch of his art is like a bird with one wing." Practical and theoretic knowledge must be combined:

He who is versed only in books will be alarmed and confused, like a coward on the battlefield, when confronting active disease; he who rashly engages in practice without previous study of written science is entitled to no respect from mankind, and merits punishment from the king; but he who combines reading with experience proceeds safely and surely like a chariot on two wheels.

He similarly warns his pupils against unintelligent repetition from books: the student who thus obtains his knowledge "is like an ass with a burden of sandalwood, for he knoweth the weight but not the value thereof."

In fact, the original text omits many diseases where surgery was not necessary. Some surgical material, found in the present text, was added by Susruta II many centuries later. Of the surgical subjects added in the present text may be mentioned couching for cataract which was not known in the time of Susruta I.

The twenty-fifth chapter of the *Sutra Stahna* is devoted to surgical operations which he classifies into eight groups: (1) extraction of solid bodies, (2) excising, (3) incising, (4) probing, (5) scarifying, (6) suturing, (7) puncturing, and (8) evacuating fluid.

Susruta describes the operation of laparotomy and tells how to extract the fetal head when it is blocked in the pelvis. In his *Samhita*, he describes the different kinds of version and flexion to be performed when the child is in an abnormal position; he discusses the application of forceps and the operation of craniotomy in difficult labor. An adherent placenta was expelled frequently by exerting pressure on the abdomen and occasionally by administering emetics.

He suggests for the first time a plastic operation on a torn ear lobe, using a flap from the neck. Hindu children had their ears pierced for protection against the evil influence of malignant stars and spirits, or for ornamentation. If the earrings were heavy or the piercing had been done badly, a fissure, splitting the ear lobe into two parts, might result. The surgeon had no less than fifteen methods for ensuring the plastic repair of this cosmetic misfortune. One of these operations is known as *ganda-karna*, "Ganda-karna consists in slicing off a patch of healthy flesh from one of the regions of the cheeks and in adhering it to one of the severed lobes of the ears."

Susruta was perhaps the first surgeon to do a rhinoplasty and the plastic operation on the ear lobe. The need for the former procedure was frequent because the nose was often deformed or excised by the authorities as a legal punishment. With reference to plastic surgery of the nose, Susruta says:

If the nose of any one be cut off, the surgeon shall take a leaf from a tree of the same size, lay it on the cheek and take out a piece of skin and flesh equally big, stitch the cheek with needle and thread, scarify the stump of the nose and quickly but carefully place the piece of cheek over it, attach it with a proper dressing and sew the new nose firmly on. He shall then carefully insert two tubes, in order to make breathing easier and when thus raised he shall sprinkle it with oil and scatter on it red sandalwood and other hemostatic powders, whilst white cotton is laid carefully thereon and it is frequently sprinkled with the same oil. [24]

Documents discovered about 200 years ago show that Susruta (c.

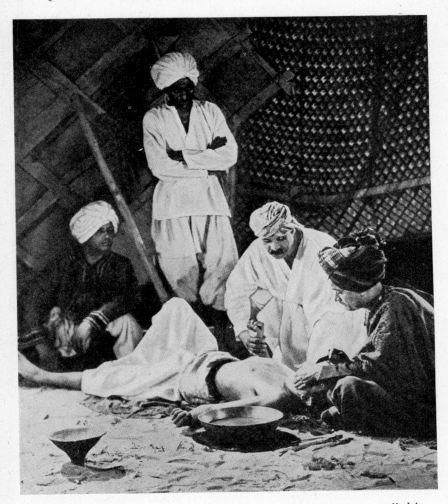

Fig. 85: Surgeons of India. Indian surgeons of the sixth century excelled in plastic operations. Amputation of the nose and ears was a common punishment for adultery. Restoration was effected by bringing down flaps from the forehead and fastening the edges with pure wax or with sutures of linen, plant fiber, hair, or animal tissue. Nostrils were formed over tubes. So vital was skilled suturing held that students were required to practice forms of stitches on thick cloth before being allowed to operate. (Courtesy of Davis and Geck, Inc.; as depicted by an artist.)

1000 B.C.), the father of Indian surgery, was familiar with the clinical picture of cataract. He described a cataract as an opacity of the lens caused by a derangement of intraocular fluids.

Susruta was the first Ayurvedic surgeon to deal systematically, and most exhaustively and elaborately, with the development and the anatomic structure of the eye. He studied the physiological factors and the pathological changes of the ocular apparatus and the symptoms and treatment of ocular diseases. His ophthalmic works have been incorporated in the "Uttara Tantra" of Susruta Samhita, Chapters 1 to 19. He described diseases of the eyelids, conjunctivae, scleras, corneas, uveal tracts, lens, retinas, and vitreous. He presented a good

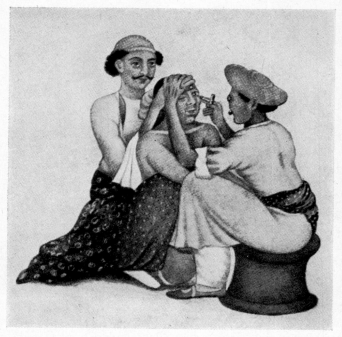

Fig. 86: Couching for cataract. The Eastern (or Indian) operation. (From Brit. J. Ophth.)

account of glaucoma. He was the first ophthalmic surgeon to do the classic couching operation for cataract.

Susruta's description of *arman* (pterygium) was most elaborate. He described five varieties of pterygium, whereas most modern opththalmologists classify only four varieties. His surgical treatment for pterygium was as perfect as, but perhaps more elaborate than, any modern ophthalmic operation. His surgical treatment for *paksma-kopa* (trichiasis) may well be compared with the Jaesche-Arlt operation.

His views regarding the prognosis of the various ocular diseases, for example uveitis *(adhimantha)* and glaucoma *(gambhirika)*, stand fundamentally unaltered today.[25]

Surgery

Tonsillectomies and operations for anal fistula were accomplished with skill. The Hindu operation for vesical calculi, a common disease in India, was performed in Europe up to the sixteenth century. The Hindu surgeon removed tumors of the neck; he tapped the abdomen for dropsy; he repaired prolapse of the rectum and treated hemorrhoids; he made an incision into the bladder to remove stones; and he operated on cases of cataract.

Painstaking care was taken in cases of amputations and dislocations of the long bones. In dislocation of the humerus, for example, the surgeon pulled the arm downward, close to the side of the body, and placed a pillow or similar object in the axilla.

When operating on the temples, cheeks, eyelids, lips, and axillae, the practice was to make a transverse incision; when cutting the palms, a circular incision was effected; when the anus and penis were incised, a semicircular cut was made. The depth of incision for an abscess was two fingers. The pus was evacuated by pressure with the fingers. The abscess cavity was then flushed with a strong solution and packed with a cloth saturated with sesame mixed with honey. Following this it was covered by a poultice and bandaged. The bandage was removed on the third day except when pain was severe, in which case it was removed on the second day. The Hindu physician knew how to ligate blood vessels and use suturing material. The suturing material employed was mostly made from flax, hemp, and bark fiber; occasionally hair was used. Two kinds of needles were employed: straight ones for the fleshy parts and curved ones for the abdomen and scrotum.

Even neural surgery was not unknown. Division of the supraorbital nerve was advised for supraorbital neuralgia which did not respond to medicinal treatment, and there is some evidence that intracranial explorations were undertaken.

Susruta suggests the application of forceps and operations, such as craniotomy and Caesarian section, in otherwise hopeless cases.

Leeching, bleeding, cupping, and actual cautery are recommended. "All the seasons of the year were opportune for cauterization except summer and autumn" . . . "no such distinction (of seasons) shall be observed in cases of impending danger." It is advised that the patient should either fast or take a special diet, according to his or her condition, immediately before the operation. Cautery is thought to benefit glandular inflammation, tumors, fistula in ano, scrofula, elephantiasis, hernia, and warts. Four techniques of cauterization are enumerated. They are, "The ring, the dot, the lateral or slanting lines, and the rubbing modes." Cautery is contraindicated in the weak, the aged, the very young, and the fearful. Preoperative technique and postoperative care are all dealt with.

SURGICAL TECHNIQUE

Surgical procedures attained a high position, and operations were performed at the beginning of the warm season. By way of preoperative preparation, the skin was rubbed with a pledget of cotton saturated with a suitable medicament.

Dressing of wounds was done in a most sanitary manner. The wounded on the battlefield were quickly picked up and carried into a tent. Hemostasis was secured, and then the wound was washed with an anodyne oil. Cautery was frequently used, "The fire cures disease which the knife, physic and herbs do not cure."

Indications of the skill possessed by the early Hindu surgeons is provided in the chapter of the Susruta *Samhita* on incurable diseases, "A case of piles attended with thirst, aversion to food, colic, pain, excessive hemorrhage, local dropsy, and dysentery is soon relieved by death." Cases regarded as extremely hard to cure, and those which usually terminated fatally, were not much more numerous than today.

Susruta enumerates 101 varieties of blunt instruments and twenty kinds of sharp instruments; the latter "should have an edge so fine as to divide the hairs on the skin." The instruments include scalpels, scissors, needles, saws, sounds, lances, hooks, probes, directors, forceps, trocars, catheters, bougies, syringes, and speculums:

The preceptor should see that his disciple attends the practice of surgery even if he has already thoroughly mastered the several branches of the science of medicine, or has pursued it in its entirety. The pupil must be taught in all acts connected with surgical operations, of incision, etc., and injection of oil, etc., the pupil should be fully instructed as regards the channels along or into which the operations or applications are to be made (*Karma-patha*). A pupil, otherwise well read, but uninitiated into the practice (of medicine or surgery) is not competent (to take in hand the medical or surgical treatment of a disease).

Surgical operations were demonstrated to Hindu students on various objects, such as the following: incisions were shown upon fruits;

scarifications upon stretched skins with the hair still on them; punctures on distended skins or bags; venesection on blood vessels of dead animals; extraction of teeth upon dead animals; opening an abscess upon a hump of wax attached to wood; suturing, on thick cloth;

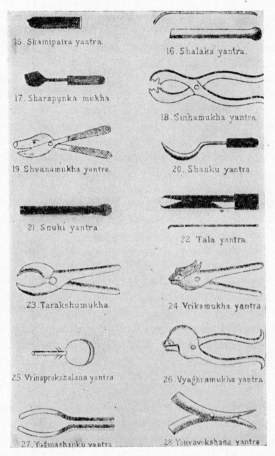

Fig. 87: Surgical instruments of the Hindu surgeon. Susruta (1000 B.C.) enumerated 121 sharp and blunt instruments.

cauterizing, on meats; and bandaging, on fingers. The discipline and the exact training of Hindu students may be best inferred from the following extract from the Susruta *Samhita* which deals with instruction to surgical apprentices:

The art of making specific forms of incision should be taught by making cuts in the body of a *pushpaphala* (a kind of gourd), *alávu*, watermelon, cucumber, or *erváruka*. The art of making cuts either in the upward or downward direction should be similarly taught. The art of making excisions should be practically demonstrated by making openings in the body of a full waterbag, or in the bladder of a dead animal, or in the side of a leather pouch full of slime or water. The art of scraping should be instructed on a piece of skin on which the hair has been allowed to remain. The art of venesection *(vedhya)* should be taught on the vein of a dead animal, or with the help of a lotus stem. The art of probing and stuffing should be taught on worm *(ghuna)*—eaten wood, on the reed of a bamboo, or on the mouth of a dried *alávu* (gourd). The art of extracting should be taught by withdrawing seeds from the kernel of a *vimbi, vilva* or Jack fruit, as well as by extracting teeth from the jaws of a dead animal. The act of secreting or evacuating should be taught on the surface of a *shálmali* plank covered with a coat of bee's wax, and suturing on pieces of cloth, skin, or hide.

Similarly the art of bandaging or ligaturing should be practically learned by tying bandages around the specific limbs and members of a fullsized doll made of stuffed linen. The art of tying up a *karnasandhi* (severed earlobe) should be practically demonstrated on a soft severed muscle, on flesh, or with the stem of a lotus lily. The art of cauterizing or applying alkaline preparations (caustics) should be demonstrated on a piece of soft flesh. Lastly the art of inserting syringes and injecting enemas into the region of the bladder or into an ulcerated channel should be taught by asking the pupil to insert a tube into a lateral fissure of a pitcher, full of water, or into the mouth of a gourd *(alávu)*.

Medicine

The Susruta "Medical Compendium" deals with both medicine and surgery and was intended for students of medicine who were to master both subjects. To cite again, "The physician who lacks knowledge of one of these branches is like a bird without one wing."

In the medical system of Susruta are mentioned the three essential elements supposed to permeate and control the mechanism of the body: air, bile, and phlegm. The air, according to this system, influences the bodily movements and is located below the navel. The bile furnishes the bodily heat and is placed between the navel and the heart. The phlegm is situated higher up and controls the function of the heart. In old age, air is the dominant element. In middle age, bile is the controlling principle. In childhood, phlegm is the governing element. Some Hindu physicians considered the blood as a fourth element.

Health was said to be normal when the three elements were in proper proportion. Disease was the result of a derangement of these three elements. Of course, religious concepts, uncleanliness, poor nourishment, and bad climatic conditions played an important part in both health and disease. Other causes that could upset the equilibrium of the three vital elements that sustained life were heredity, poison, cold, heat, moisture, undernourishment, overwork, psychic disturbance, and contagion.

According to Susruta, there are 1120 diseases which are divided into seven classes in accordance with their etiology: (1) hereditary diseases, (2) congenital diseases, (3) diseases originating from primary elements, (4) diseases due to injury, (5) diseases due to atmospheric influence or to contagion, (6) diseases caused by demonic influence, and (7) diseases due to such causes as hunger or age. The text of Susruta *Samhita* deals, in addition to etiology, with diagnosis, treatment, pathology, surgery, ophthalmology, obstetrics, and elementary medical subjects, such as anatomy, physiology, and chemistry.

It would, however, be a mistake to infer that the conception of the cause of disease was ever separated in India from supernatural influences, such as religion and magic, the wrath of the gods, the envy of the demons, or the *karma*.

DIAGNOSIS

The diagnosis was based upon careful observation of the patient by the use of the special senses. In addition to inspection, palpation, and (direct) auscultation, the senses of taste and smell were brought into service as diagnostic indices. Taste, for example, gave information upon the condition of the urine: sweet urine was indicative of diabetes. The sense of smell was employed in certain diseases to detect the exhalation. Passages in this medical text indicate that the aspects of the tongue and skin were carefully scrutinized. Notice was paid to the crepitus produced by a fractured bone. Tibet physicians were reputed to be able to cure by merely examining the urine.[25] Jumping like a frog, crow, or quail indicated the prominence of bile in the system. A weak pulse, which struck the fingers slowly, like a peacock, a swan, or a dove, indicated the predominance of phlegm. A creeping pulse, like a snake or a leech, suggested derangement of the air element. Different pulses were described in most of the diseases. A woman's pulse was taken on the left wrist, a man's on the right side.

Susruta recognized direct auscultation as a diagnostic method, as may be seen from the statement, "by the ear can be heard the sound of air bubbling in the phlegm of the wind passages."

PROGNOSIS

The desire to predict future events has been the earnest wish of people of all ages, and particularly of persons stricken with disease. All sick people are eager to know how and when their disease will terminate. At present, prognosis is based on clinical history, symptoms, pathology, age, and other factors. But when medicine was looked upon as a result of supernatural forces, prognosis was based upon omens. Among the ancient Hindus, where medicine was a mixture of natural and supernatural concepts, resort was made to omens as well as clinical observations in predicting the outcome of disease.

It was considered a bad omen when the messenger who called for the physician was himself sick, poorly dressed, or of a different caste. If he had seen a snake or blind man while on the road to the physician, if he arrived at midday or midnight, or if he found the physician sleeping upon his arrival, the patient most certainly would take a turn for the worse. It was thought favorable if the messenger met a maiden, a suckling woman, or two persons of the Brahman faith en route to the doctor. There were, however, physicians who based their prognosis on careful clinical observations. It was considered grave if the patient were a diabetic, if the disease was complicated by abscesses or swelling of the mouth, testicles, feet or navel, if the loss of blood was severe, if fever intervened, or if polydipsia or anorexia ensued. Diseases with unfavorable prognoses were the following: dropsy, leprosy, hemorrhoids, fistula, gonorrhea, lithiasis, tetanus, and, in women, abnormal fetal position.[26]

PHYSIOLOGY

The Hindu conception of the workings and machinery of life was similar to that of the Greeks of the same period or later, namely that certain fluids or humors operated in the system. The essence of these elements appeared in the form of an oily, white, cold material. Furthermore, seven secondary substances, that is chyle, blood, flesh, fat, bone, marrow, and semen, contained the vital force which permeated the whole body and regulated the bodily functions independent of the soul. The preponderance of a particular element or secondary substance also influenced character and temperament.[27]

With reference to the soul, variously called *asu* (spirit), *manas* (mind), *atman* (breath), and *prana* (respiration), the Hindus believed that it separated from the body during unconsciousness and continued its existence after the body had been destroyed by cremation or burial; although imperishable, it lived as a mere spirit or shadow, but retained its personal identity in a corporeal state, after the body was purified by the power of the god *Agni* and freed from all imperfections in the other world.

The Hindus believed that respiration was a manifestation of the vital principle. They observed the first gasp of air of the newborn child and the labored breathing at death and attributed these occurrences to the entrance and departure of the soul from the body. They argued that the life-giving breath cannot be of earthly origin but is derived from universal breath. They viewed respiration as a phenomenon of the soul. They noticed the changes from normal breathing in health to the rapid and noisy respirations in sickness and bodily exhaustion, and particularly the irregular respiration preceding death. Their natural conclusion was that the essential differences between health, sickness, and death were due to the respiratory manifestations of the soul. The Biblical statement, "and he breathed into his nostrils the breath of life"[28] appears to be an old tradition among all people of antiquity. In Hebrew, *ruah* (wind) is variously used to designate "breath," "life," and "soul." The same designation is found in other ancient languages.

The Hindus, as far back as in the days of Brahma, concerned themselves with the spiritual aspects of respiration. The regulation of respiration among Hindu ascetics in their ritualistic practices was of paramount importance to their religion.

No people have paid as much attention to the physiology of breathing as the Hindus. They recognized various forms of respiration and assigned to each phase a particular function. They carefully computed the normal respiratory rate per diem and found the average to be 22,636, or about sixteen per minute, which almost agrees with the rate set by modern physiologists. Cultured Hindus still look upon the study of respiration as a science. They maintain that a well-regulated respiration has a vital effect on the mental and physical activities of the person.[29]

MATERIA MEDICA

Medicines were classified according to the disease for which they were thought to be efficacious, such as emetics, purgatives, laxatives, tonics, and aphrodisiacs. Drugs were prescribed in various forms, such as infusions, decoctions, electuaries, mixtures, pills, syrups, pastes, plastics, ointments, suppositories, powders, collyria, and fumigations.

Medicinal plants were gathered by the physician himself, at certain places and at certain seasons of the year. According to Susruta, they had to be prepared free from smoke, rain, wind, and dampness. Incantations and prayers were usually chanted while the plants were collected and prepared for remedies. Medical plants collected by laymen were not considered effective.

The works of Charaka and Susruta embrace an immense number of drugs belonging to the vegetable, mineral, and animal kingdoms. The largest number of drugs were of vegetable origin. Susruta enumerates 760 plants, and Charaka lists 500 medicinal plants. The parts of the plants used included fruits, blossoms, roots, barks, leaves, juices, oils, and resins. Among the vegetable substances used were camphor, cinnamon, sesame, peppers, cardamom, cane sugar, nuts, ginger, and garlic. Of the animal substances, the most important one was milk[30] from humans, cows, elephants, camels, goats, and mares. Butter, honey, meat, bile, blood, and urine were also employed. Of meat, that of fowl and buffaloes was preferred. Ground bones of a goat were used in ointments. Sinews, horn, claws, and nails were used for various purposes. Even sperm had its place in Hindu medicine.

There are special texts of pharmacy and chemistry containing ingenious methods of preparing oxides, sulfates, chlorides, tin, iron, lead, copper, gold, and silver. Mercury was called "king of metals" and was prescribed internally and externally. Oxidized gold was prescribed as a stimulant. Sulfate of iron or copper and oxide of lead were prescribed as aphrodisiacs. Such drugs as arsenic, sulfur, potash, sodium chloride, alum, and ammonium chloride were also employed in the Hindu materia medica.

Many remedies in the modern pharmacopoeia were known to the Hindus. Datura stramonium was used for asthma, nux vomica for dyspepsia and paralysis, arsenic for intermittent fever, and mercury for syphilis. A salt-free diet was employed for nephritis, and flesh and fatty food for tuberculosis.

Both Charaka and Susruta advocated the use of medicinal wine as a sedative, "Wines should be used before operations to produce insensibility." The fumes of burning Indian hemp have been used by Hindus from remote antiquity as an anesthetic.

ANATOMY

Susruta's surgery is based upon a knowledge of anatomy studied on the human cadaver. At the end of the fifth chapter of his compendium, he states, apropos of anatomy:

No accurate account of any part of the body, including even the skin, can be rendered without a knowledge of anatomy. Hence anyone who wishes to acquire a thorough knowledge of anatomy must prepare a dead body, and carefully examine all its parts. For it is only by combining both direct ocular observation and the information of textbooks that thorough knowledge is obtained. For this purpose one should select a body which is complete in all its parts. It should also be the body of a person who is not excessively old, and who has not died of poison or of a protracted disease. Having removed all the excrement from the entrails, the body should be wrapped in rush, bast, grass, or hemp, and placed in a cage. Having firmly secured the latter in a hidden spot, in a river with no strong current, the body should be allowed to decompose. After an interval of seven days, the body should be taken out and very slowly scrubbed with a whisk made of grass roots, hair, bamboo, or bast. At the same time, every part of the body, great or small, external and internal, beginning with the skin, should be examined with the eye, one after the other, as it becomes disclosed in the course of the process of scrubbing. [31]

According to Susruta, the human skeleton is composed of 300 bones: 120 in the four extremities, 117 in the middle part of the body, and 63 above the neck. He includes the teeth and nails among the bones, and also the sclera and trachea. He enumerates 500 muscles, counting each compact mass of flesh which separates into strands as individual muscles; 400 muscles are in the extremities. There are 100 ligaments, 66 in the trunk, and 34 in the head. He enumerates 210 joints, 70 blood vessels, 9 sensory organs, 3 kinds of organs of secretion, and 3 humors which maintain a dynamic equilibrium. The blood vessels, aside from circulating the blood, carry also air, or pneuma. The nerves start from the umbilicus.

Discrepancies in Hindu accounts of human anatomy, as compared with modern knowledge, are probably due, not to lack of observation, but to differences in classification and the fact that dissections were principally made on bodies of children less than two years of age, since older children and adults were cremated.[32]

The osteological system of Susruta is based on the principle of homology, according to which the several organs of the right and left sides and the upper and lower halves of the body correspond to each other.

HINDU OSTEOLOGY, AS VIEWED BY VAGBHATA, SUSRUTA, AND CHARAKA

	I Vagbhata	II Susruta	III Charaka	IV Adopted from Charaka
1. Nails	20	—	20	20
2. Phalanges	60	60	60	
3. Long bones	20	20	20	
4. Bases (sthana)	4	4	4	
5. Clusters (kurea)	8	8	—	
6. Ankle and wrist bones..	8	8	6	
7. Legs and forearms......	8	8	8	
8. Heels	4	4	2	
9. Knees and elbows......	4	4	4	
10. Thighs and arms........	4	4	4	
11. Ribs, sockets, etc.......	72	72	72	
12. Back	30	30	45	
13. Breast	8	8	14	
14. Pubes	1	1	1	
15. a. Sacrum	1	1	—	
b. Anus	—	1	—	
16. Hips	2	2	2	
17. Collarbones	2	2	2	
18. Shoulder-peaks	2	—	2	2
19. Shoulder-blades	2	—	2	2
20. Cheeks	2	2	0	
21. a. Ears	2	2	—	
b. Eyes	—	—	—	
22. Temples	2	2	2	
23. Windpipe (jatru).......	1	—	1	1
24. Palate	1	1	2	
25. Neck (griva)..........	13	9	15	
26. Windpipe (kantha).....	4	4	—	
27. Jaws	2	2	3	
28. Teeth	32	32	32	
29. Sockets of Teeth........	32	—	32	32
30. Nose	3	3	1	
31. Cranium	6	6	4	
TOTALS	360	300	360	57

Other anatomical teachings contend that the body consists of six chief parts, and fifty-six minor members. There are five sensory organs (hands, feet, arms, genitals, and tongue) and seven receptacles where air, bile, phlegm, blood, urine, and digested and undigested food are stored. In women, there is an eighth for the fetus. The human being has nine openings: mouth, two nostrils, two ears, two eyes, the anus, and the urinary opening, and fifteen inner organs. The skin consists of seven layers. There are, in the human body, ten chief seats of life with 107 areas where injuries are dangerous or fatal.

EMBRYOLOGY

Embryology was always associated with mystery and superstition—the Hindus were no exceptions. The sex of a child was thought to be dependent upon the preponderance of the seminal and menstrual fluids.[33] The latter increased in amount on odd days. If conception took place on odd days after menstruation, the child would be female. If conception took place on even days, the offspring would be male. The most favorable time for conception was the twelfth night following the onset of menstruation. Pregnancy was supposed to last an average of ten months. During that period, the mother was kept away from fright and excitement. Violent temper on the part of the mother during pregnancy might result in epilepsy of the child; indulgence in alcoholic drinks might cause the child to have a weak memory. If the mother was dissolute, the child would be depraved or effeminate. When the mother reached the ninth month of pregnancy, she was taken, with religious ceremony, to the place of delivery. Four women assisted in the delivery.

HYGIENE AND PROPHYLAXIS

It is natural that the people under the influence of a religion marked by asceticism and purity of mind and body should practice personal and communal cleanliness. As a matter of fact, the Hindus endeavored to begin this practice when the child was in the embryonic state.

A powdered drug was dusted into the nostrils of a pregnant woman to induce the offspring to become male. Unripe fruits of the *udumbara* tree were attached to a pregnant woman in order to communicate to the child the exuberant maturity which that fruit attains.

By far the most important rite was connected with boyhood, when the lad was introduced to a religious teacher at the ages of seven, eight, and twelve in the case of the first three castes respectively. Standing at the sacred fire, the preceptor invested the boy, whose head had been shaved, with a girdle, which he wound round his waist three times from left to right, at the same time pronouncing certain formulas. He then grasped the boy's hand and, placing his own on the pupil's heart, recited a verse indicating that he had assumed power over the boy's will. On this occasion, the youth also received a garment, a staff, and a sacred cord to be worn over one shoulder and under the other arm. During the whole course of his subsequent apprenticeship, the religious pupil (brahmacārin) was required to practice chastity, to refrain from certain kinds of food, and to tend his preceptor's fire with fuel.

The *Vedic* marriage ceremony was associated with frequent ablution. The ceremony itself was symbolic of the close ties between bride and groom. The act on the part of the bridegroom, of taking the hands of the bride, was intended to place her in the power of her husband. The seven steps which the young couple took and the food which they ate together were meant to establish friendship in the community. Future abundance of male offspring was aimed at when the bride, after being conducted to her husband's house and placed on the hide of a red bull, took upon her lap the son of a woman who had borne only living male children. The husband would then lead his wife three times around the newly kindled nuptial fire, which the couple had to maintain henceforth throughout their lives as their domestic fire.

Death was followed by a period of impurity, varying from three to ten days, according to the degree of kinship. As the return of the soul was feared during this time, the surviving relatives took constant precaution to avoid infection. Thus, only food which was bought or presented by others from outside was eaten to guard against introducing anything tainted into the system.

The ancient law-giver Manu was a sanitarian, biologist, and eugenist. He prohibited the marriage of Hindus to foreigners, because the latter were considered to be inferior in physical, intellectual, and moral qualities. A Vedic sage Vasista, when advising the desirability of marrying a bride from a good family, said, "even a horse is respected on account of his good genealogy; hence a lady of good genealogy should be taken into marriage."[34] The caste system in India is really aimed at the preservation and perfection of race culture, rather than at the division of labor as is commonly believed.[35]

Hindu hygienic rules come under four headings: personal cleanliness, diet, exercise, and prophylaxis. The rules pertaining to bodily hygiene necessitated frequent bathing in cold or warm water, particularly in the sacred baths of the Ganges. Baths were discouraged after meals or after a person had a chill, cold, fever, diarrhea, or disease of the eye or ear. Warm baths were considered wholesome for the lower part of the body. For the upper part, they were thought harmful. Sea water and mineral springs were preferred. Next to frequent bathing, daily evacuation of the rectal and urinary organs was urged. The teeth had to be kept clean by means of toothpicks made of a particular astringent wood. The mouth had to be rinsed after eating with an infusion of camphor, cardamom, betel leaves, or other herbs; the body had to be anointed with an aromatic oil; eyes and ears were treated with a mild salve; the head, ears, and soles with oil; and hair and nails were to be trimmed every five days.

The amount of food to be taken varied with the season of the year, the climatic conditions, and the ability to digest it. Two meals a day, between nine and twelve in the morning and seven and ten in the evening, were prescribed. The meals were preceded by salt and ginger to stimulate the appetite. A moderate amount of water had to be taken. Too much water at the beginning of the meal might cause loss of weight by interfering with digestion, and too much drinking at the end of the meal was thought to cause obesity. After the meal, the mouth had to be rinsed and the person was advised to take a short walk. The best articles of food were cereals, particularly rice. Fruits and vegetables came next. Other wholesome foods were milk, butter, honey, nuts, ginger, sugar cane, and garlic. Of meats, that of fowls and buffaloes were, as noted above, considered the best. Less wholesome were pork, beef, and fish.

In the time of Yuan Chwang, Hindu medical treatment began with a seven-day fast. In this interval the patient often recovered. If the illness continued, drugs were resorted to. Reliance was placed largely upon diet, baths, enemas, inhalation, urethral and vaginal injections, bloodletting, leeches, and cups.

Exercise consisted of daily walks, gymnastics, or massage. Clothing was not to be worn soiled so as not to irritate the skin. Everyone was advised to carry a cane and wear a hat and shoes. Sleep by day was only recommended after too much exertion; by night sleep was indicated until an hour before sunrise. For astrologic reasons, sexual intercourse was forbidden on the eighth, fourteenth, and fifteenth days of the month and in the morning hours. Milk was to be drunk after intercourse. To ward off evil spirits, amulets, in the form of garlands or jewels, were advised.

As a prophylactic measure, an emetic was recommended once a week, a laxative once a month, and venesection twice a year.

Vaccination was known in India as early as 550 A.D., if we are to judge from a text attributed to Dhanvantari, one of the earlier Hindu physicians, "Take the fluid of the pock of the udder of the cow . . . upon the point of a lancet and lance with it the arms (between the shoulders) until blood appears. Then, mixing the fluid with the blood, the fever of the smallpox will be produced."[36] The germ theory was known to the Hindus.[37] Hypnotism originated in India. Braid, who introduced it in England undoubtedly got the idea from the Hindus while he practiced his profession in India.

Strict hygienic rules were ordered during pregnancy, delivery, and the puerperal state. Instructions for the care of babies were definite. To wash the baby with warm water after delivery was mandatory. Instructions were given for the mother and child during lactation. An option was granted between maternal nursing and the employment of a wet nurse.[38] On the tenth postpartum day the mother was permitted to get out of bed. Her diet, however, had to be regulated for a period of six weeks. The child was put to breast on the third day. In the meantime, it was fed on honey and butter. If the child was fed by a wet nurse, she had to undergo a rigid physical examination; and while nursing the child, she was obliged to regulate her diet. The care of a nursing child was under strict regulation as to nourishment, and periods of sleeping, sitting, and lying. Certain charms and amulets were placed in the child's room to drive away evil spirits. After six months, the baby was weaned and fed on rice.

The entire thought of the physician had to be concentrated upon the treatment of his patient. He was warned against divulging what happened in the patient's house and was forbidden to issue a prognosis prejudicial to the patient or the family. Intimacy with women was discouraged. The physician was not to gossip or jest with them. Even the personal appearance of the physician was regulated, "let thy hair and thy nails be cut short; keep thy body clean; wear white clothes; shoes on thy feet; carry a staff in thy hand; let thy appearance be modest and thy spirit pure and without guile." The fees of the physician were in accordance with the social and economic position of the patients.

Medical Education In India

Despite the low castes of Hindus, India has reason to be proud of the many centers of higher education dating from remote antiquity, such as Benares, Taxila, Ujain, and Nalanda, famous for logic, literature, arts, medicine, philosophy, and religion. The University at Benares was famous for theology, that at Ujain for astronomy, that at Taxila for medicine, and that at Nalanda for *Vedic Buddhist* teachings. Students desiring admittance to these schools had to produce evidence of their family background and certificates of their physical, mental, and moral qualifications. Preference was given in the medical schools to the sons of physicians and to those who hailed from medical families.

The moral and ethical aspect of the scholar was emphasized, "The scholar must have a quick tongue, small lips, regular teeth, a noble aspect, well formed nose and ears, a lively spirit, and a graceful bearing. He must be capable of withstanding pain and fatigue." Students entering medical schools were warned to be chaste, to wear a beard, to be moderate, not to eat meat, to speak the truth, to be obedient to their teachers, and faithful to the Brahman religion. On his admission at the opening ceremony, the student took an oath to observe his religious duties and the ethics of his profession, and to treat Brahmans, his teachers, poor friends, neighbors, and orphans gratis. The season of the year for study, the hours of instruction, and the number of students for each instructor were regulated.

Owing to the heat of the Indian summer, the schools opened at the beginning of the cool weather.[39] For astrological reasons, the opening corresponded to the end of the lunar month. The commencement was attended by celebrities of the church and state.

The curriculum extended over a period of six years. No teacher was allowed to instruct more than four students (or at the very most, six students) at a time. The instruction was both theoretical and practical, based upon recognized textbooks. Owing to the scarcity of manuscripts, students had to commit the texts to memory. Great stress was laid on clinical experience.

The practical work consisted of bedside instruction. The physician was urged to broaden his knowledge through intercourse with his professional colleagues "so that the light of wisdom should not be hidden from him."

In contrast to the lay-healers of ancient Babylonia and China, against whom there were rigid laws, the Hindu physician enjoyed privileges and kind consideration from the public at large. During the Brahmanic period (800 B.C. to 100 A.D.), when medicine was a part of priestcraft, there was no question of punishment for malpractice. Both disease and its treatment emanated from the gods; and the priests who only carried out divine wishes, could certainly not be penalized. After the religious concepts with reference to medicine were relaxed, the Hindu physician did not need a legal code to protect him from punishment in the case of injury inflicted on his patient during his medical or surgical practice. The medical regulation to which the physician had to submit was sufficient protection against injustice done to himself or to his patient. The Hindus adopted a code of medical ethics noted for its sagacity and earnestness. The ethical and professional requirements demanded from the medical practitioner were of such a nature that, if they were followed, medical and surgical mishaps would be reduced to a minimum.

INSTRUCTIONS TO THE HINDU PHYSICIAN

General Instructions: Here are some of the instructions given to those who desire to enter upon a medical career:

You must be chaste and abstemious—Speak the truth—Not eat meat—Care for the good of all living beings—Devote yourself to the healing of the sick even if your life be lost by your work—Do the sick no harm; not even in thought—Seek not another's wife or goods—Be simply clothed and drink no intoxicant—Speak clearly, gently, truly, properly—Consider time and place—Always seek to grow in knowledge—Do not treat women except their men be present—Never take a present from a woman without her husband's consent—The physician should enter a house accompanied by a man suitable to introduce him there—He must pay attention to all the rules of behavior in dress, deportment, and attitude—Once with his patient, he must in word and thought attend to nothing but his patient's case and what concerns it—What happens in the house must not be mentioned outside—Nor must he speak of possible death to his patient, if such speech is liable to injure him or anyone else—In face of gods and man, you can take upon yourself these vows—May all the gods aid you if you abide thereby—Otherwise may all the gods and the sacra, before which we stand, be against you—The pupil shall consent to this, saying, "so be it."

Other medical aphorisms are, "A physician, who desires success in his practice, profit, a good name, and finally a place in heaven, must pray daily for all living creatures." "Let his speech be short, clear, pleasant; his transaction in the house should not be bruited abroad."

Importance of Nurse: The relative importance of the nurse to the physician is cited in the following passage:

The physician, the patient, the medicine, and the nurse are the four feet of medicine upon which the cure depends. When three of these are as they should be *(gunavat)*, then by their aid the exertions of the fourth, the physician, are of effect, and he can cure a sore disease in a short time. But without the physician the other three are useless even when they are as they should be, just as the Brahmans who recite the Rig- and Sama-Vedas are useless at a sacrifice without the Brahman who recites the Yagurveda. But a good physician can cure a patient alone, just as a pilot can steer a boat to land without sailors. The physician who has penetrated into the hidden sense of the medical books, who has seen and taken part in operations, who has a ready hand, an honest mind, a bold heart, who has his instruments and books by him, who possesses presence of mind, judgment, resolution, and experience, and who sets the truth above all things, such a physician may be called a true foot *(pada)* of medicine. The patient deserves this name *pada* when he has vital force, and nerve (to resist pain), no incurable disease, no great poverty, self-restraint (to avoid harmful pleasures), faith in the physician, and obedience to his directions. The drug to be called a *pada* must grow on a good soil, and be gathered on a favorable day, be given in proper doses at the right time, and be fresh. Finally the nurse is a *pada* when he is kind-hearted, without false shame, strong, trustworthy, and mindful of the physician's orders. [40]

Attitude towards Patient: Careful attention was paid to the patient's age, mode of life, habits, pulse, body temperature, color of the skin, condition of the eyes, urine, feces, strength of the voice, respiratory sounds, and especially to his intelligence. The last, according to Susruta, was important: "Stupid people are more easily cured than intelligent individuals because the first are more obedient to the instructions of the physician."[41]

If the disease was of an incurable nature, the Hindu physician refused treatment but advised the patient to prepare for the occasion when his soul would be united with God. The physician was advised "to wear his hair short, to keep his nails clean and cut close, and to wear a sweet smelling dress." The superior ethical and practical regulations of the Hindu physician undoubtedly commanded the respect and admiration of his patients and reduced malpractice proceedings to a minimum.

Duties on the Battlefield: The important position occupied by the physician on the battlefield is seen from the following regulations. The duties of the physician to the king on the battlefield are pointed out in Chapter 34 of *Ayur-Veda:*

The physician must see to the food, water, wood, and places of encampment, and examine them carefully for the food may be poisoned by the enemy. If he finds poison he must remove it, and so save the army from death and destruction. He may learn how to do this by reading the chapter on poisons. The pious penitent must, by his prayers keep off evil influences arising from the breath (? incantations) of the powerful, the pains of the oppressed, and the shame of sin (and the astrologer must avert misfortunes indicated by the stars, directing them upon a specially appointed sacrifice). If disease arise in the army the physician must show the greatest diligence, and especially guard the king's person, for he involves the whole people, as saith the proverb: "Were there no king the people would devour one another." His tent shall be near the king's tent, and he shall have his books and drugs always at hand. There shall be a flag over his tent that the sick, poisoned, and wounded may find him quickly.

Hospitals

Hospitals were erected in Ceylon as early as 427 B.C. and in northern India as early as 226 B.C.

Incidentally, it seems that the custom of maintaining hospitals for the poor was practiced in India as early as the second century B.C. It is stated that, when King Dutta Gaman was on his death bed (151 B.C.), he ordered the records of his deeds to be read to him, one of which was that he had established eighteen fully equipped hospitals caring for the poverty-stricken.

King Budhadasa (341 A.D.), was known as a great benefactor. Out of his benevolence he provided hospitals and appointed medical practitioners for all villages.

Having composed a work containing the substance of all medical science, he circulated it among the physicians of the land for their future guidance. He ordained that there should be a physician for every ten villages. He set aside twenty royal villages for the maintenance of these physicians, and appointed medical practitioners to attend members of the army, elephants, and horses. On the main roads he built asylums for the reception of the lame and blind. This man of great compassion was wont to carry his case of surgical instruments in the folds of his loin cloth, and to afford relief to every afflicted person he met.[42]

Development of Hindu Medicine

It is difficult to state with any degree of certainty at what time medicine reached such a remarkable state of development in India. The celebrated Indian physician Mahabharata thought that the works attributed to Atrya and Susruta date at least from the time of Homer (c. 900 B.C.). Others are of the opinion that they flourished about 600 B.C.

If Atrya and Susruta I flourished at about 600 B.C. or about 150 years before Hippocrates, the priority of scientific medicine long credited to the Greeks, becomes a moot question. There is a striking similarity between the Indian and Greek rational medicine; and taking into consideration the independent achievements of the Indians in most branches of science and their aversion to foreign influence, one is inclined to believe that at least some of the Greek medical concepts were borrowed from the Hindus, who preceded them by centuries.

Neuburger seems to support this view when he writes:

On one hand there are shown many parallels to the medical art of the Greeks, corresponding to other great scientific attainments of the Indians (in Philosophy, Astronomy, Mathematics, Geometry and Philology) and to their poetic art. . . on the other hand is seen the determining influence which the East, with the general condition of culture springing from its soil, exercised upon the trend of medical thought.

Recent Sanskrit scholars maintain that, in the language of these medical sages, there are indications that they flourished before Alexander the Great invaded India (327 B.C.). Others place the period as recent as 750 A.D. Perhaps the interval between the last two dates may be correct, as it is contemporaneous with the prevalence of Buddhism in India, which represents the golden days of medicine in India. It was a period when fraternal love and friendly relationship among the various castes was encouraged and the physician was universally held in high regard, in contrast to the Brahmanistic Period when caste prejudice and ritual enslavement prevailed. Dr. Haas ingeniously denies the Hindus' originality. In papers entitled "On the Origin of Hindu Medicine" and "Hippocrates and the Hindu Medicine of the Middle Ages," he asserts that all Hindu medical sciences are of Greek origin, "Nay, Susruta is himself none other than Hippocrates, whose name has been confounded with that of Socrates and misspelled Susruta." He believes his birthplace, which is Benares (or Kasi) stands for Cos (the birthplace of Hippocrates); and to prove his point still further, he finds that Susruta was ruled by his wife as Socrates was henpecked by Xanthippe.

How one clever enough to read Hippocrates in the original and to reproduce it in his own language could mistake the name of Socrates for Hippocrates surpasses one's imagination.

Garrison[43] with his usual penetrating erudition remarks:

Whether the Hindus influenced the Greek medicine before the time of Alexander the Great or were themselves influenced by it, is not known; but it is certain that, at the time of Alexander's Indian expedition (327 B.C.), their physicians and surgeons enjoyed a well-deserved reputation for superior knowledge and skill. Some writers even maintain that Aristotle, who lived about this time, got many of his ideas from the East.

Be that as it may, there is a great similarity in the medical concepts of these two ancient peoples. Both separated superstition from medicine, and both developed a superior code of ethics.

During the reign of Harun-al Rasid (786 A.D.), the great works of Charaka and Susruta were translated into Arabic, under the patronage of Caliph Alamansur. In the same year, Hindu scholars were brought to Bagdad to translate from Sanskrit into the Arabian language works on pharmacology, toxicology, philosophy, and astrology. Indian medical works may be found quoted in the writings of Avicenna (980–1037 A.D.), Razi, Serapion (c. 900 A.D.), and other eminent Arabian physicians.

The works of Charaka and Susruta were translated into Tibetan, again from Tibetan into Mongolian, and into other languages of central and northern Asia, and perhaps into Greek. The last Arabic edition was made in the year 1550 A.D.[44]

Sir William Hunter (1718–1783) declared that Hindu medicine was an independent development. Arab medicine was founded on translations from Sanskrit treatises, and in turn, European medicine down to the seventh century, was based upon the Latin version of the Arabian translations.

References and Notes

1. I Kings 10:22.
2. Professor Max Muller's editions of the text to the Rig-Veda and his eloquent translations of the Vedic hymns into English have opened up new fields of religious thought and philosophical research to English readers.
3. The doctrine of transmigration is not found in the Vedas. Its beginning is met with in the Brahmans, where the information of repeated birth and death appears. It shows itself fully developed even in the oldest Upanishads. It was accepted as early as 600 B.C. before the days of Pythagoras, who is generally credited with having originated this concept.
4. It is a question whether vegetable life was not also included in the transmigrations of the soul.
5. "The man who perceives in his own soul the Supreme Soul present in all creatures, and regards them all with equal benevolence, will be absorbed at last in the highest Essence, even of that of the Almighty Himself." Manu 12:126.
6. Journal Asiatic Society of Bengal, 1875, p. 227.
7. Dinkart: History of Antiquity. Vol. 4, pp. 281, 223.
8. According to Susruta, "Even a Sudra, if of legitimate birth and otherwise qualified, may be taught the art of medicine except the Mantras, i. e. Vedic incantations." Withington, E. T.: Medical History From the Earliest Times, London, 1894.

9. It is to be noted that the term "expelled" suggests that something has entered the patient's body that had to be expelled.

10. Soma is a climbing plant of East India and Burma possessing small greenish-white flowers, and a fragrant smell, which yield a milky juice from which formerly an intoxicating drink was distilled.

11. Vishnu Puramai. Translated by Wilson, 1840.

12. Muthu, D. C.: Antiquity of Hindu Medicine. Paul B. Hoeber, Inc., New York, 1931, p. 87.

13. Hastings, J.J.: Encyclopedia, Vol. 4, p. 754.

14. Ibid.

15. Vishnu-Puramai: Translated by Wilson, 1840. Medical History From the Earliest Times. Withington, E. T.: London, 1894.

16. Hoernle, A. F.: Studies in the Medicine of Ancient India. Oxford, 1907, Part 1, p. 29.

17. "Antiquity of Hindu Medicine", pp. 17-18.

18. Ibid. 23.

19. Ibid. 67.

20. Ibid. 71.

21. Ibid. 49.

22. The writer is indebted to the splendid chapter, Medicine of the Indians in Neuburger, M.: History of Medicine. London 1910.

23. Hastings, J.J.: Encyclopedia, Vol. 4, p. 754.

24. Cited by Neuburger, M.: History of Medicine, p. 58.

25. Bidyādhar, Nabin Kishore: Arch Ophth., 550-574, Oct., 1939.

26. Cited by Neuburger, M.: History of Medicine. p. 52.

27. It may be of interest to note that the Greek teaching of four humors which includes also blood, is found in the Doctrine of Buddha.

28. Genesis 2:7.

29. Erving: Hindu Conception of the Function of Breath. p. 86.

30. Atharva-Veda 9:3-16.

31. Hoernle, A. F.: Studies in the Medicine of Ancient India. Oxford, 1907, Part 1, pp. 210-217.

32. Hoernle is of the opinion that he counts the thirty-two sockets of the teeth, the twenty nails, the windpipe, shoulder blades (two), and the two shoulder peaks as bones.

33. Curious is the following statement of Herodotus: "Intercourse of all these Indians whom I have mentioned takes place openly as with cattle; and all have a complexion closely resembling the Ethiopians." Incidentally Herodotus shows that at his time there was a general belief that "the seed Indians emit is not white as that of other men, but black as their skin; the Ethiopians also emit similar seed." Herodotus 100.

34. Sarkar, B. K.: Hindu Achievements in Exact Science.

35. There were many castes in India that were not influenced by the Vedic wisdom. The Hindu people were divided into many castes and not all of them were Brahmans. According to Herodotus, there were certain barbarous tribes in his time altogether out of the pale of Indian civilization. There were primitive communities, the so-called "aborigines of India," among whom were many cannibals. "Others, Indians, neither kill anything that has life nor show

anything, nor do they have houses, but they live upon herbs . . . when anyone of them falls into any disorder he goes and lies down in the desert and no one takes any thought about him, whether dead or sick." Herodotus 3.98.

36. Hastings, J. J.: Encyclopedia, Vol. 4, p. 754.
37. Ibid.
38. Hindu medical text translated by Hessler into Latin in 1844 and rendered into English by Hoernle in 1897.
39. Neuburger, M.: History of Medicine. p. 53.
40. Cited by Edward T. Withington, E. T.: Medical History From the Earliest Times. pp. 28-29. Ayur-Veda 34.
41. Allen, T. H.: Science-History of the Universe, Medicine. The Current Literature Publishing Co., New York 1901, p. 115.
42. Withington, E. T.: Medical History From the Earliest Times. p. 31.
43. Garrison, F. H.: An Introduction to the History of Medicine. Second ed.
44. Hastings, J. J.: Encyclopedia, Vol. 4, p. 755.

12

Medical Concepts in China

LIKE old Jericho, China was shut up ("none went out and none came in") behind an impenetrable wall; she isolated herself politically, socially, and culturally from the western world. Chinese literature contains no record which might justify the assumption that she was racially or culturally related to her ancient contemporaries in India, Persia, Babylonia, and Egypt. Anthropological studies further contradict the idea that China had any racial connections with these nations. The Chinese themselves assume that their ancestors occupied their present land from time immemorial.

While it is true that there may be certain similarities of practices between the Chinese and other peoples, these may be ascribed to prehistoric connections or to the human common denominator which has led men in different parts of the world to similar goals without ethnic, cultural, or commercial intercourse.

Chinese civilization still seems to be largely independent of other peoples. Great reliance is still placed on tradition and what might be called a disproportionate respect for authority and an exaggerated reverence for the past.

The Chinese have developed their own theory of their prehistoric life. The scene of action has been laid in a part of the world which, from the dawn of history, has never been anything but Chinese territory. According to Chinese genealogy, the first man known was P'an-Ku. His epoch, millions of years ago,[1] was followed by ten distinct periods of sovereigns, including the "heavenly emperors," the "terrestrial emperors," the "human emperors," the Yu-ch'au, or "nest-builders," and Sui-jon, the "Fire Producer." Several of the characteristic phases of cultural progress and social organization have been ascribed to these mythological periods. Authors of less fertile imagination refer these largely mythical characters to later times, when the heroes of their accounts appear in shapes somewhat resembling human beings rather than as gods and demigods.

The Chinese look upon Fu-hi as their first historical emperor, and they place his lifetime in the years 2852–2738 B.C. Some accounts represent him as a supernatural being. He is depicted as possessing a human trunk with a fishtail, something like a mermaid. He is

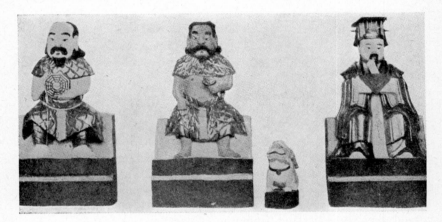

Fig. 88: Chinese gods of medicine. From left to right: Fu Hsi, Shên Nung, and Chang Chung Ching.

credited with having established social order among his people, who, before him, had lived like animals in the wilds. The social chaos out of which Chinese society arose is described as being characterized by the absence of family life; for "children knew only their mothers and not their fathers." Fu-hi introduced matrimony; and in so doing, placed man as the husband at the head of the family and abolished the original matriarchate. This quite corresponds with his dualistic views on natural philosophy.

It is noteworthy that the same ruler who assigned to man his position as the head of the family is also credited with the invention of the concept of "male and female principles," according to which all good things and qualities are held to be male, while their less sympathetic opposites are female (i.e. heaven and earth, sun and moon, day and night).[2]

THE PHILOSOPHY OF YANG AND YIN

For millenniums, Chinese cosmic philosophy held the intellectual life of the nation in bondage. The philosophy was based on the concept that, from the time of creation, there arose the dualistic forces of *yang* and *yin*, the positive and the negative principles from which all phenomena of nature proceed. *Yang* represented the perfect essence of heaven, the sun, the day, heat, and manhood, and was designated by the mark "—"; *yin* stood for the imperfect, the essence of the moon, earth, night, and cold, and was represented by the sign "— —". These two forces that controlled the phenomena of nature were heterogeneous powers, or polarities. Both of these had mutual affinities for each other, and at the same time they were antagonistic to one another. They were present in animate and inanimate substances and were, therefore, the fundamental principle in any discussion of arts, crafts, religion, astronomy, or medicine. There was nothing in heaven or earth which was not governed by *yang* and *yin* forces.[3] The philosopher Haai Nan[4] says:

The cosmic Spirit embraces Heaven and supports Earth. It stretches to the four corners of the universe and generates the eight points of the firmament . . . it endows heaven and earth with the primary element. . . . Expanding, the Cosmic Spirit overspread every part of the firmament, earth, time and space. . . it holds, as in a net, the four poles and comprehends the active and passive forces of creation. . . In the beginning the two forces, *Yang* and *Yin*, having obtained the essence of the Cosmic Spirit became the central organizing powers. . . Without apparent doing, things came into existence under the inspiration of the Cosmic Spirit. . . Its energy is imparted to the minutest thing. . . its virtue gave flexibility to nature and harmonized into unity the operations of the *Yang* and *Yin*. . . It produces all phenomena.

The male principle *yang* was active and positive. The female principle *yin* was inactive and passive. By means of the varying influences of the male upon the female forces, a great variety of things in nature took place. Variations of sex, features, character, and form were fundamentally the result of the preponderance of one principle over the other. Proper balance produced harmony of action. The forces were respectively creative and destructive, contracting and expanding. Their sexual interaction created, and their separation destroyed, all objects in nature.

Five Elements: In addition to the natural forces of *yang* and *yin*, animate and inanimate things were composed of five elements: wood, earth, fire, metal, and water. In the early process of creation, these elements were derived from a single element—water[5]—as follows:

wood (plant) was derived from water; fire (by friction) was derived from wood; earth (ashes), from fire; and metals, from earth. Thus water was the basic or primary element[6] of matter, which is composed of the five elements in various proportions under control of the *yang* and *yin* forces. Transmutation of matter followed the same pattern, beginning with water and ending with metal.

Microcosmic Concept: Chinese philosophy considered man a replica of the cosmos. He was a microcosm, "a miniature of heaven and earth," and a union of the animal and spiritual soul. The animal soul influenced the coarser part of his being; the spiritual soul, the finer

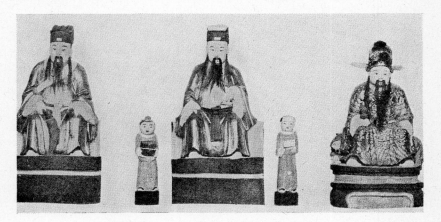

Fig. 89: Other Chinese gods of medicine. From left to right: Hua T'o, Pien Ch'iao, and Sun Ssu Miao (Yoh Wang).

and subtler part of his existence. Man arose from the vital essence, the cosmic soul of *yang* and *yin* that permeated all things in different proportions.[7]

This concept applied also to food, drugs, and herbs. The more invigorating and healing substances were assumed to possess more *yang*, and the less sustaining, more *yin*. The former were life-giving, the latter, life-destroying substances.

Health: Health depended upon the dynamic equilibrium between the male and female principles of the *yang* and *yin*, and on the proper quantitative relationship of the five elements. The male principle, which was vital and warm, ruled, in accordance with its tendency to expansion, over the contracting hollow viscera, such as the stomach, intestines, and bladder. The female principle, which was cold and moist, had, as its seat, the solid organs, such as the lungs, liver, kidneys, spleen, and heart. At death the physical and spiritual souls separated. The spiritual soul of the *yang* went to heaven, and the animal soul of the *yin* returned to earth; thus the souls of the departed ancestors were ever present in heaven and on earth. The great reverence given to the dead not only became a burden to the living, but retarded the study of anatomy.[8]

Medical Skill: With a philosophy of universal sexual dualism in nature as the basis of all sciences, it is not surprising that few major medical inventions and discoveries were made by the Chinese over a period of 4,000 years of experience. The Chinese have had few, if any, medical schools for training. They derived their medical skill from their elders. The art of medicine was passed on from father to son, from master to apprentice. To them, everything ancient was good and everything new was bad. One thing, however, must be credited to this people: they developed a considerable body of practical knowledge.

MEDICAL TEXTS

The oldest of the innumerable medical works of all description with which China has been flooded from time immemorial is a treatise which has been credited to the Yellow Emperor (2698–2598 B.C.). It is entitled "Plain Questions of the Yellow Emperor," or *Su Wên* for short, and takes the form of questions put by the emperor and answered by Earl Ch'i, a minister, who was himself author of the *Nei Ching*, a medical work no longer in existence, which contained traditional lore of a still more remote period. There are treatises on cautery and acupuncture, both of which are still practiced by Chinese doctors, and on the pulse, the variations of which have been classified and allocated with a minuteness that appears incredible. Special treatises on fevers, skin diseases, diseases of the feet, eyes, and heart, are found in great quantities, as well as veterinary treatises on diseases of the horse and the domestic buffalo.

But, in the whole range of Chinese medical literature, there is nothing which can approach the *Pên Ts'ao,* or "Materia Medica," better known in English as the "Herbal," many sources of which hark back to prehistoric times. The work was compiled by Li Shih-chên, who completed his task in 1578 A.D. after twenty-six years of labor. No fewer than 1892 species of drugs (animal, vegetable, and mineral) are dealt with, arranged under 62 classes in 16 divisions; and 8160 prescriptions are given in connection with the various entries. The author professes to quote from the original aforementioned *Pên Ts'ao.*

Prior to this work, the number of recognized drugs known was 365 in all, corresponding to the days of the year; 120 of these were called "sovereigns" and were regarded as entirely beneficial to health,, taken in any quantity, at any time. Another similar number were called "ministers"; some of these were poisonous, and had to be used with discretion. The remaining 125 were agents; all very poisonous, but able to cure diseases if not taken in overdose. The modern *Pên Ts'ao*, in its sixteen divisions, deals with remedies classed under

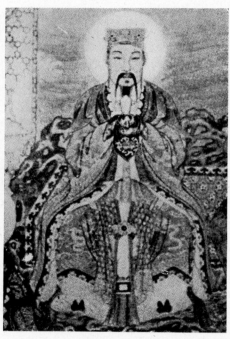

Fig. 90: Portrait of the Yellow Emperor Huang Ti (2698–2598 B.C.), who wrote about whitening the teeth. (From Hume, E. H.: The Chinese Way of Medicine. Baltimore, 1940.)

the following headings: water, fire, earth, minerals, herbs, grain, vegetables, fruit, trees, clothes and utensils, insects, fishes, crustacea, birds, beasts, and man. In each case the proper name of the drug is first given, followed by its explanation. A solution of doubtful points and a correction of errors is then appended. Information as to identification by taste and use in prescriptions is included. The work is fully illustrated, and there is an index to the various medicines, classed according to the complaints for which they are used.

TAOISM

Another fallacy that hindered the progress of medicine in ancient China for many centuries was the concept known as "Taoism" (signifying "a way of life"). Taoism was a form of nature worship which had for its purpose the drawing away of adherents from the cares of the world to worship nature. It substituted the idea of an anthropomorphic deity for an impersonal primal force identified with nature. It was supposed to teach religious, alchemical, and practical methods on how to attain long life and immortality.

Methods of Prolonging Life: The followers of Lao-Tzu (the founder of Taoism, c. 600 B.C.) suggested various methods to prolong life and to attain immortality.

Manipulation of Breath: One of these was the manipulation of the breath, for life and breathing were observed to be dependent upon each other: both ceased together at death. The Taoists practiced holding their breath as long as possible, exhaling very slowly, inhaling very deeply, and breathing imperceptibly. Such practices were believed to conserve the vital spark and in time transform an old person into a young one. Thus declared Lu Pu-Wei (c. third century B.C.), "If the vital breath is renewed every day and the bad breath entirely leaves the body then man may reach the age of heaven itself. Such a man is a saint."

Food Regulation: Frugality and regulation of food were additional means of prolonging life. Abstinence from the five varieties of grains, namely hemp, millet, wheat, rice, and pulse, was urged. "The inhabitants of the Isles of Immortality do not eat the five grains but inhale air and drink dew." On Yng-Chau Island there was reputed to be a spring producing a sweet liquid called "jade-wine," which conferred immortality on human beings.

Vitalizing Substances: Certain substances were thought to be particularly vitalizing, containing a high proportion of *yang*, which was invigorating to the masculine element. The vitalizing substances, especially infused with *tao*, included: pine and peach trees from the vegetable kingdom; the hen, crane, and tortoise from the animal kingdom; and cinnabar, jade, silver, and gold from the mineral kingdom. The most potent substance, having great alchemical properties to influence immortality, was a medicine containing gold as its chief ingredient.

The less important preparations, contributing to long life and immortality, were concoctions made of silver, jade, and cinnabar. The last, by virtue of its producing mercury (the living metal) when subjected to heat, was considered a life-giver. Considering the large quantities of metallic substances used by the Taoists to attain immortality, one wonders that there were not greater disasters from their use.

Tao: The great Chinese philosopher Lao-Tzu (600 B.C.), in his *Tao Te King,* enthroned *Tao* as the central figure and feature of the universe. "The man whose manner of life and behavior," he said, "are in conformity with Tao, will attain the attributes of Tao. The spirits of the departed will not harm such a man; the material world can do him no evil."[9] *Tao* engineered all things, nourished them, developed them, ripened them, tended them, and protected them.[10] Lao-Tzu is known for his aphorisms which are scattered through early Chinese writings. Some of them are:

> The good would be good to the not good. I would also be good in order to make them good.
> Man is an infant born at midnight, who, when he sees the sun rise, thinks that yesterday never existed.
> Leave all things to take their natural course, and do not interfere.
> He who knows how to shut, uses no bolts, yet you cannot open.
> He who knows how to bind, uses no ropes, yet you cannot untie.[11]

Science of Alchemy: The devotees of the Taoist religion developed the so-called "science of alchemy." They employed alchemy in compounding their "pills of immortality" and concocting their "elixir of life." This is reminiscent of the practices prevailing during the Middle Ages.

Wei Po-Yang (c. 100–150 A.D.), author of the earliest treatise devoted wholly to alchemy, and known as the "father" of this science, stated there were over 10,000 formulas for compounding the medicine of immortality. Wei Po-Yang was disinclined to disclose the correct formulas, "A profound subject like this is fit to be treated only by the wise. It is presumptuous therefore for me to write about it, but I cannot hold my peace either, for it would be a great sin on my part not to transmit the Tao (way) which would otherwise be lost to the world forever."

His gold formula for prolonging life, which he hesitated to disclose, was not, however, a specific in all cases. He was disinclined to prescribe it in any case, before experimenting first on a dog. Although the death of the dog did not necessarily signify that the medicine was no good, it did indicate that it was not compounded right. Here then is one of the earliest cases of the use of a biological control:

The student should be industrious and thoughtful; the wise man will follow strictly the directions and will therefore achieve success. The unworthy ones cannot aspire to this...False methods in alchemical research will cause disease; gases from the food consumed will make noises inside

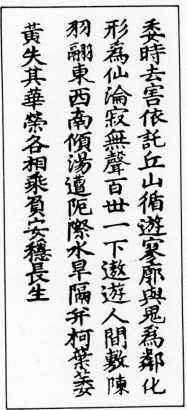

Fig. 91: Cryptogram of Wei Po-Yane, author of the earliest treatise devoted entirely to alchemy (about 142 A.D.). (Courtesy of Professor T. L. Davis.)

the intestines and stomach. The right essence will be exhaled and the evil ones inhaled. Days and nights will pass without sleep...The body will then be tired out giving rise to the appearance of insanity. The hundred pulses will stir and boil so violently as to drive away peace of mind and body.

Alchemy evidently often failed to achieve the desired effect, and the aspirants for long life had to resort to the Taoist religion to realize their aspirations.

Spirit of Tranquility: A more practical plan to attain long life was given by a "sage" to Emperor Huang Ti, the founder of the Chin Dynasty in 249 B.C., "If one embraces the spirit of tranquility, his condition will be good of itself, so if your heart is tranquil and your spirit pure and if you do not strain your body, nor dissipate your essence, you will then attain immortality."

ANATOMY

It is evident that no science could hope to progress when it was impeded by fantastic premises, and least of all the science of anatomy which is based on practical unbiased observation. Anatomy became a mixture of actual and illusionary concepts. It was confined to a few salient facts, hastily observed and incorrectly correlated, on the experience of one or two accidentally killed and crudely dissected bodies.

Dissection: Dissection was strictly prohibited. Confucius (551–479 B.C.) stated:

Whoever enters the realm of death mutilated cannot look forward to a reunion with his ancestors. Hence, the parts of the body, removed in an operation, were kept and placed in the grave after death. Even when a cadaver was secretly obtained and a serious effort at dissection was made, the findings had to be in harmony with the ancient texts and in conformity with the philosophical concepts of tradition. Thus, when the dissection did not agree with traditional concepts, hypothetical and invisible organs and spaces were assumed to exist in the body, such as the "twelve channels," "three burning places," and the "gates of life."

Zo and Fu: According to Chinese anatomy, the body was composed of flesh, bones, and entrails. The latter were differentiated into five *zo* and five *fu*. The *zo* (storehouses) were the principal internal organs, to which belonged the heart, liver, spleen, lungs, and kidneys. Each one of these corresponded to an element and governed a season, color and taste:

The Zo	Element	Season	Color	Taste
Heart	Fire	Summer	Red	Bitter
Lungs	Metal	Autumn	White	Sharp
Kidneys	Water	Winter	Black	Salt
Liver	Wood	Spring	Blue	Sour
Spleen	Earth	The last eighteen days of each season.	Yellow	Sweet

The *fu*, that is to say the "manor houses," assisted the principal entrails. These included the stomach, the large and small intestine, gallbladder, urinary bladder, and *sanstsiao*. The last was a hearing organ containing three parts: the upper part of this organ lies in the heart region and corresponds probably to the ductus thoracicus; the middle part is the pancreas; and the lower part is described as a secretory duct, probably the chyle canal.

Position and Function of Organs: The various organs were bound together by a system of vessels which included those through which the blood flowed and those carrying the pneuma or air.

According to their position, the vessels were divided into fourteen regular and eight irregular ones. Near them lay the so-called *Yu-Ketsu*. This was conceived as a system of holes between the bones and muscles through which the pneuma could wander from the inner to the outer organs.[12]

According to Chinese anatomists there were 365 bones in the male and 5 less in the female skeleton; 190 of these were concealed and could not be seen, and only 265 possessed marrow. The skull, forearms, legs, and pelvis were counted as one bone each. There were 365 articulations, which received air through passages situated at the hips and shoulders. The muscular and nervous systems were not dealt with at all. The brain occupied but a small place in the cranium, not nearly filling the skull.

The vascular system consisted of twelve veins, six of which contained the positive and six the negative elements. They partly began and partly ended in the hands and the feet. The twelve veins were completed by two main collecting channels, one of which, running at the back of the body, contained the positive, and the other, passing in front, contained the negative element. The twelve veins had twenty-three branches, besides a number of smaller vessels. The spinal cord terminated in the testicles.[13]

The writer is indebted to Dr. William R. Morse, Head of the Department of Anatomy in West China Union University, for the following information which is quoted from his handbook "Chinese Medicine."[14]

According to Chinese anatomy there are five organs and six viscera. The organs are the liver, heart, spleen, lungs and kidneys. (The pericardium, brain, and bone marrow are also, sometimes, called "organs".)

The organs store up but do not eliminate. Each has a special pulse. Each organ is supposed to be the habitat of a special animal, for example, a white tiger in the lungs and a dragon in the liver. The organs are solid. They develop the body, control the five senses and all parts of the body and mutually reciprocate in action with the viscera. The *Yin* principle rules organs. The viscera eliminate but do not store up. They are hollow and contractile, and are related to the organs in action and functions. The *Yang* principle rules them. The five organs and six viscera (similar to the five elements), have cognate functions, sympathetic and antipathetic and each exercises a special influence on some distant part. The five organs correspond to the five elements, so through the correlated functions of the organs and viscera the five elements represent both organs and viscera; for example, the element wood corresponds both to liver, an organ, and to its assistant the gallbladder (a viscus). Through these two the juices of the body are filtered.

The five organs and five elements have a telluric manifestation with the constellations, celestial regions, time of year, etc.

The liver is of a rancid odor, sour taste, brown color, and makes the sound *chüeh*. It stores the blood, which contains the soul and is the seat of anger.

The liver produces the ligaments, forms the heart and controls the lungs. It has the eye as its opening, converts the fluids to tears, supplies the ligaments and nourishes the nails. The liver relates to the gallbladder which answers the ligaments. Its duty is that of a general whose function is to meditate carefully. The liver filters out the humors. It has seven lobes and lies on the ninth vertebra.

The heart has an odor of toast, a bitter taste, brownish red color and makes the sound *chih*. It stores the pulse which contains the spirit and is the seat of happiness. The heart produces the blood, forms the spleen and controls the kidneys. It has the tongue as its opening, converts the fluids into perspiration, supplies the pulse and nourishes the complexion.

The heart relates to the small intestines which answer the arteries. It is the king who directs the body. The heart is attached to the fifth vertebra and is conical in shape like a lotus, with openings on the side. It is connected with the tongue, lungs, spleen, liver and kidneys. The larynx opens into it. It has three divisions or chambers.

The spleen has a fragrant odor, sweet taste, yellow color and makes the sound *kung*. It stores the nutrition and is the seat of thought. The spleen is the most important organ because it designates the earth, which is the place of life production and resourcefulness. The spleen produces the flesh, forms the lungs, and controls the liver. It has the mouth as its opening, converts the fluids into saliva, supplies the flesh and nourishes the lips. The spleen relates to the stomach which answers the muscles. It is the officer of granaries, who creates the five tastes. The spleen is sickle-shaped, is attached to the eleventh vertebra and is in the same membrane as the stomach. It moves the voice, grinds on the stomach and aids in digestion.

The lungs have a fishy smell, hot taste, white color, and make the sound *shêng*. They store the energy and are the seat of sorrow. The lungs produce the skin and hair, form the kidneys and control the heart. They have the nose as their opening, convert the fluids into nasal secretion, supply the skin, and nourish the fine hairs. The lungs relate to the large intestine which answers the skin. They are the promulgators who carry out the order of the king (heart). The lungs are attached to the third vertebra and hang down in eight lobes. They are gray in color and are pierced by eighty small holes.

The kidneys have a putrid smell, salty taste, black color, and make the sound *yu*. They store the germinating principle which contains the will and is the seat of fright.

The kidneys produce the bone marrow, form the liver and control the spleen. They have the ears and the genitourinary region as their openings. They convert the fluid into saliva, supply the bones and nourish the hairs. The kidneys relate to the three burning spaces and the bladder which answer the skin and hair. They are the officers of vigor or strength who serve through the intellect. The kidneys rest on the fourteenth vertebra, are two in number, shaped like beans, and are placed one on each side of the spine about 1½ inches apart. They are enveloped in yellow fat and have two pairs of cords which run up and down. The upper pair of cords are attached to the heart, the lower pair pass into the pelvis into a space, and leaving this, pass along with the spinal cord to the brain.

The muscular and nervous and other systems, as such, are not dealt with at all. The brain is a small place in the cranium not nearly filling the skull.

Viscera: The gallbladder is likened to a wine sack, is related to the liver and is the central legal officer who makes judgments.

The stomach is related to the spleen. The stomach is the granary and has five openings, entrances and outlets (of the granary). The food enters the stomach where essence soaks into it and becomes air, which passes to the lower burning space.

The large intestine has sixteen convolutions and serves as the officer of communications who starts all sorts of changes.

The small intestine also has sixteen convolutions and is the receiving officer through whom digestion is carried on. The small intestine and the throat are the post-office system.

The bladder receives the fluids from the three burning spaces. There it is stored and is acted upon by air and passes out.

Two bladders have been described, one for essential fluid, the other for ordinary fluid and urine.

The functions and anatomy of the twelve channels are discussed under acupuncture.

The gate of life "between the kidneys," or sometimes designated as the right kidney, in the male contains the semen, in the female the uterus. The three burning spaces (purely imaginary) constitute the sewage system from which all the canals drain into the bladder. They assist all the organs to function.

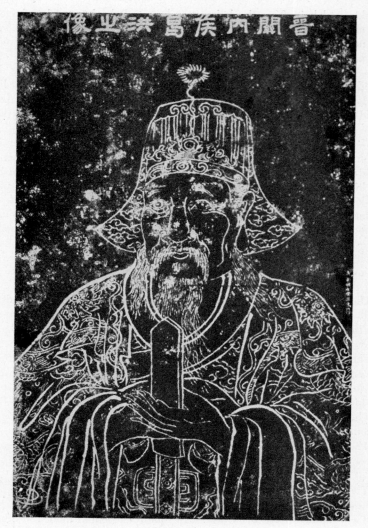

Fig. 92: Portrait of Ko Hung on a stone tablet. (Professor T. L. Davis collection.)

The five organs (i.e. the liver, heart, spleen, lungs, and kidneys), were solid and controlled the five senses. They developed all parts of the body and mutually reciprocated in action with the viscera. These organs were governed by the *yin*. The viscera were hollow organs; they were contractile, related to the solid organs in action and function, and were ruled by the *yang*.

PHYSIOLOGY

Chinese physiology followed the same trend of thought as that of anatomy. It was based largely on a distorted cosmic philosophy. Human life was invested in the blood and air in various proportions, and was carried by the blood vessels.

Blood Circulation: The influence of the blood vessels was manifested in the pulse. The *yang* and *yin* circulated through twelve channels and exercised control over the blood vessels and their contents. The twelve channels were imaginary anatomical units, but were accepted as real by Chinese philosophers, in order to draw conclusions regarding the action of the *yang* and *yin*.

Chinese physicians advanced various theories of the circulation of the blood. The *Nei Ching* (a celebrated ancient medical classic) says:

> All the blood is under control of the heart;....the heart regulates all the blood of the body . . . the blood current flows continuously in a circle and never stops. It may be compared to a circle without beginning or end. The blood flows a distance of six inches with one respiration, making a complete circulation of the body about fifty times in twenty-four hours.

Others assumed that there was a vital principle in the heart, bright like the flame of a lamp, "the burning place." A pile of blood in the center of the heart was devoted exclusively to nourishing the vital force and occupied a "nest." At night the vital force withdrew behind the pile of blood and sleep ensued, while the blood recuperated its vital forces to provide nourishment for the morrow.

The formation and function of the blood was thus elucidated by a physiologist as follows:

> The blood is the fluid tissue of the body. It is formed from the solid and liquid foods which are eaten and enter the belly, where the food is mysteriously transformed. In the abdomen, the formed blood becomes red, passes to the various vessels, nourishes the whole body and transports the vital principles. The fluid part of the blood goes to the *Yin* areas, and the solid part to the *Yang* areas.

According to Wang Ch'ung (27–97 A.D.), man was endowed at birth with either a good or evil nature. He was similarly provided with a vital fluid, or a spirit, which resided in the blood, and was nourished by eating and drinking; this vital fluid had two functions: to animate the body and keep the mind in order. The vital fluid was the source of all sensations, which passed through the blood like a wave. When it reached the eyes, ears, and mouth, the result was sight, hearing, and speech respectively. Disturbance of the vital fluid led to insanity. Without the fluid, the body could not be maintained; without the body, the fluid lost its vitality, since body and fluid were interdependent. Wang Ch'ung argued that when the body perished, the fluid lost its vitality. There remained nothing for immortality in a life beyond the grave. Ghosts, he holds, "are a hallucination of a disordered mind." This materialistic philosopher Wang Ch'ung was a follower of Confucius (551–419 B.C.) who, in his canon, cherished a belief in God but not in the future state of reward and punishment for good or evil action in this world.

Other Doctrines: Other Chinese physiological doctrines were as follows: The formation of semen was dependent on a proper supply of blood and gas. The changes in the blood to form semen took place at the "gate of life" (situated between the kidneys). The blood was purified in the kidneys. The kidneys, according to *Lan Ching* (a medical classic), controlled the secretions: urination, lacrimation and nasal secretion. They also ramified into the heart to produce perspiration and went directly to the mouth to form thick saliva.[15]

Wang Ping says that "the testes generate the marrow and the brain is the ocean into which the marrow runs via the spinal cord. The testes control the bones and the teeth, the latter being an outgrowth of bone tissue." There was complete ignorance regarding the nervous system.

Secretion was also formed by emotions: Sadness caused tears; shame caused perspiration; sexual desire caused secretions of semen; and appetite caused salivation. (This was one of the few correct observations.)

In addition to their direct functions, Chinese physiology as we have seen, endowed each of the five organs with an influence upon some distant part of the body. Dysfunctions of any of the organs always resulted in alteration of the pulses.

The hair was an outgrowth of the brain. When there was lack of brain tissue, the hair was deficient. Hair was the product of a full-blooded system, and blood was a fluid substance which circulated down to the testes.

It is evident from the various citations that, for centuries, medical science had been at a virtual standstill. Chinese physicians did not strive for facts. They were rather unwilling to commit the sacrilege of discarding ancient tradition. The highest ambition of a scholar was to comment on the texts of an ancient authority.

PROVERBS
Confucius' Aphorisms

It is a great disappointment that so clear thinking a man as Confucius (Kung-Futze, 551–479 B.C.) was not interested in medicine. He was primarily a moral philosopher and did not apply his philosophical ideas to the art and science of healing. His ethical teachings, however, applied to medicine as to other trades and professions. Some of his aphorisms are as follows:

Learning without thinking is labor lost; thinking without learning is perilous.

The study of strange doctrine is injurious.

What you do not want done to yourself, do not do to others.

What the superior man seeks is in himself; what the small man seeks is in others.

The superior man is dignified but does not wrangle; social but not partisan. He does not promote a man simply because of his words nor does he put good words aside because of the man.

A man can enlarge his principles; principles cannot enlarge the man; (that is, man is greater than any system of thought).

To serve the dead as though they were living; to serve the departed as though they were still in our midst, that is the acme of filial piety.

A poor man who does not flatter and a rich man who is not proud are passable in character but they are not equal to the poor who yet are cheerful and the rich who yet love the rule of propriety.

In style all that is required is that it convey the meaning.

If you visit a foreign state, ask what the prohibitions are; if you go into a strange neighborhood, inquire what the manners and customs are.

To a question of a disciple as to whether the duty of a man can be expressed in one word, he answered, "Does not 'retribution' do this?"

To a question of a disciple to define death, he replied, "You don't know life yet; how can you know death?"

When one of his disciples asked him as to the future of life, he answered indirectly, "Were I to say that the departed were possessed of consciousness, pious sons might dissipate their fortunes in festivals of the dead, and were I to deny the consciousness, heartless sons might leave their fathers unburied." [16]

Chinese Medicine Proverbs Collected by Wong

Immoderation in food causes illness; immoderation in thought undermines the body.

The blood has its changes like the phases of the moon and the tides of the ocean.

The blood cannot but flow continuously like the current of a river, or the sun and moon in their orbits. It may be compared to a circle without beginning or end.

All the blood is under the control of the heart.

The heart regulates all the blood of the body.

The harmful effects of wind and rain enter the system first through the skin.

The "Difficult Classic" says, "to know by observation is sublime, by auscultation wonderful, by interrogation skillful, by palpation, art."

The "Thousand Remedies" states, "the skillful doctor knows by observing alone, the average doctor by listening, and the inferior doctor by feeling the pulse."

When you treat disease, first treat the mind.

The happy mind is medicine; there is no better prescription.

Keep the mouth shut, close the gateways of sense, and as long as you live you will have no trouble.

A doctor's character should be square, his knowledge round, his gallbladder large, and his heart small. (A large gallbladder signifies bravery; a small heart indicates carefulness.)

Other Chinese Proverbs

Man's body is the same as that of all creatures, but his heart is above all creation.

The blood current flows continuously in a circle and never stops.

If the intellect is not exercised dullness follows; if the circulation is impeded sickness comes.

Prolonged inactiveness causes flabbiness of the muscles as well as weakness of the heart.

If you want eternal life your bowels should be constantly clean; if you want immortality your bowels should be free of residue.

To understand the present, one should examine antiquity; but for antiquity, things would not be as they are now.

By the side of a dead man's body there is a living demon.

The fly though a small insect has its viscera complete.

External complaints are easy to heal; internal ailments are hard to cure.

Heaven is father, Earth is mother.

Heaven and Earth are the parents of all creatures; man is the most highly endowed.

All things come from Heaven; man comes from his ancestors.

One can heal disease, but he cannot cure fate.

The ancients saw not the modern moon, but the modern moon shone on the ancients.

Serving the dead as if they were alive, is the highest form of filial piety.

If there is a custom do not seek to diminish it; if there is no custom do not seek to add to it.

Wide reading increases knowledge of disease; more clinics give experience in diagnosis; repeated tests make properties of drugs better known.

If you would know the whole world's affairs, read the book of the ancients.

OBSTETRICS AND EMBRYOLOGY

The knowledge of female physiology, obstetrics, and embryology of the ancient Chinese was fragmentary and superficial. There are, however, a few salient facts worth mentioning: The blood had its changes like the phases of the moon and the tides of the ocean; therefore every month there was a menstrual flow. Milk was formed from female blood in the spleen and stomach, and was limited to two arteries (the *chung* and *jen*). In the nonpregnant female, the milk formed the menstrual blood; during pregnancy it was retained in the body to nourish the fetus, and as soon as the child was born the red fluid changed to white, to form milk. During the first month of pregnancy, the fetus resembled a drop of water; during the second, a peach leaf; during the third, the sexes were differentiated; during the fourth, the embyro took on human shape; during the fifth, bones and joints could be distinguished; during the sixth, hair. If it was a boy, the right hand moved on the left side of the mother's body at the end of the seventh month; if a girl, the left fetal hand moved on the right maternal side at the end of the eighth. At the end of the ninth month, changes could be made out in the position of the fetus by external palpation; at the end of the tenth month, development was complete. The duration of pregnancy was 270 days. The sex of the child could be determined by the maternal pulse; if the right one was augmented it signified a boy; if the left, it indicated a girl.

Marco Polo, a thirteenth century traveler, related a curious custom among the inhabitants of Yunnan (a mountainous region of China), "When one of their wives has been delivered of a child, the infant is washed and swathed, and then the woman gets up and goes about her household affairs, whilst the husband takes to bed with the child by his side and so keeps to bed for forty days; and all the kith and kin come to visit him and keep up a great festivity."[17]

DIAGNOSIS AND PROGNOSIS

The diagnosis was determined largely objectively. Little of the patient's past history was taken into consideration. The subjective information received by the physician was more in the nature of prognostic omens than signs indicating the presence of disease. The patient was asked about the nature of his dreams, about the kinds of animals he had encountered, about the changes in his hair or nails. The most important diagnostic methods of examination were inspection of the face and tongue and palpation; the last was almost entirely confined to the pulse. The appearance of the face and tongue was a barometer as to the appearance of the internal organs. The color of the tissues in the human body was believed to originate from the air which penetrated into the entrails. Thus, if redness first appeared on the left cheek, this indicated that the fever was in the liver. If on the right cheek, the seat of the disease was thought to be in the lungs. If on the forehead, the heart was diseased. If redness appeared on the nose, the spleen was implicated. A red and dry tongue signified hyperactivity of the *yang*. A white moist one signified overaction of the *yin*. If the tongue, which was normally red, appeared black, it signified that the kidneys, the "heart's enemies," had gained mastery over the heart, and the prognosis indicated the destruction of the heart and death. In diseases of children, the changing color of the index finger was an important prognostic sign. In boys, the left index finger was examined, in girls, the right.

The Pulse: By far, the most important diagnostic sign was the pulse. The sympathy or the antipathy of the pulse upon the dominating organs determined the diagnosis and the prognosis of the case. If sympathetic, the prognosis was considered favorable. If antipathetic, it was unfavorable.

According to Chinese medical authorities, the human body resembled a stringed instrument whose individual parts (organs) possessed their own tone color (pulses of organs): the tone pulses of each organ were the expression of harmony in health and disharmony in disease.

It is not known when and where the system of pulse diagnosis was first originated. Pulse-taking was already known in the third century B.C. A famous Chinese philosopher Pien Chio (225 B.C.) is said to have been a great exponent of pulse-taking. The importance of pulse-taking perhaps arose from the fact that it was considered the objective sign of the actions of *yang* and *yin*, in the system controlling the five elements of which matter is composed. About 156 volumes were written about the pulse.

The pulses were believed to indicate the respective differences in the amount of blood and air in the various organs. When all was in harmony and the flow of the *yang* and *yin* principle was not disturbed, the pulses were said to be in harmony and the person was said to be in a state of health. On the other hand, when these principles were disturbed, there was disharmony in the system and the pulses expressed themselves in the form of disease. There were eleven pulses routinely taken: the radial, cubital, temporal, posterior auricular, pedal, posterior tibial, external plantar, precordial, and three aortic pulses. The most important pulse was the radial. Each pulse was classified as slow, medium, or rapid.

According to Chinese authorities, the best time to take the pulse was the morning. The correctness of pulse diagnosis was not dependent upon the patient only, but upon the sensitiveness of the healer's finger. The latter was warned to be cool in order to have perfect control over his emotions; his respiration had to be calm. A pulse was considered normal when it pulsated four times during the act of one expiration and inspiration. If the radial pulse was taken, the physician used his right hand in the examination of the left pulse and his left hand in palpating the right pulse. The method of taking the pulse was as follows: The examiner laid his middle finger on top of the radial artery, added his index finger, and followed it by the ring finger, while his thumb rested upon the dorsum of the carpus. Three places were palpated on the radial artery of each side. Each was considered a different pulse. The first was felt under the ring finger, the second under the middle, and the third under the index finger. Each pulse was examined three times: first with light pressure, then with medium pressure, and last with firm pressure. The quality and rate of the intermissions (skipped beats) were noted. A single intermission after fifty beats was considered normal. An intermission after forty, thirty, twenty, and ten beats indicated that one, two, three, and four organs were deprived of the vital air and that death would follow within four, three, two, and one years. Absence of the pulses in the male and female, and in the young and aged, were fully discussed in Chinese medical literature. As has been intimated, each of the pulses was correlated with some organ. For example, the pulse on the right side was connected with the stomach and the spleen; on the left side, with the liver and gallbladder. According to the ancient Chinese conception, each organ, in addition to its proper pulse, possessed also an opposite pulse varying with the seasons of the year. The pulse, even in the normal condition, varied in accordance with the influence of the accompanying constellation, the time of the day, and the age, sex, and constitution of the patient. The organs under pathologic conditions reacted unfavorably upon one another and upon the pulses.

ETIOLOGY AND PATHOLOGY

It has been shown that the Chinese attributed disease primarily to a disturbance of the equilibrium between the *yang* and *yin* forces. The predominance of one of these elements over the other was taken as the cause of disease. This disturbance first made itself evident in the circulation of the vital air and blood. Contributing causes were: atmospheric changes, such as wind, draught, and moisture; religious and demonic causes; overeating and drinking; excessive sexual indulgence; partaking of poison; and emotional causes, such as passion and jealousy.

The number of diseases described in the *Ishin-hō* is astonishingly large. Here often a single disease was placed in a number of different categories, according to the symptoms. There were, for example, various kinds of fever termed *shō-kan*. Those caused by cold were the most important. All diseases with fever were designated by this name; smallpox was therefore regarded as a subspecies of *shō-kan*. Six kinds of malarial fever were differentiated: *on-gyaku*, the hot form; *kan-gyaku*, the cold form; *in-gyaku*, with disorders of the stomach; *ro-gyaku*, with a chronic course; *shō-gyaku*, blamed on the influence of miasma; and *kan-kitsu-gyaku*, in which the fever recurred every second or third day.[18]

The physicians of this period were familiar with diabetes and probably also with albuminuria. Numerous skin diseases were described. Of interest is the fact that leprosy was considered a communicable disease transmitted directly from man to man.

With regard to gynecology, the Chinese physician distinguished a large variety of menstrual disorders.

The *Ishin-hō* ascribed the cause of disease to changes in the elements: this was probably taken from the Buddhist *Sutra*.

ETHICS

What China lacked in the scientific principles of medicine, it made up in ethics as may be seen from the following aphorism: Chang Chung Ching, the Hippocrates of China in the "Golden Chamber" remarked, "the skillful doctor knows by observation, the mediocre doctor by interrogation, the ordinary doctor, by palpation."[19]

Other aphorisms are as follows:

You cannot remove trouble if you don't know the cause.

Immoderation in food causes illness; immoderation in thought under-mines the mind.

A phoenix is not to be gotten from a hen's nest.

When you treat diseases, first treat the mind.

When the poor are sick they seek charms and carry idols (they are too poor to buy medicine).

What heaven has ordained cannot be circumvented.

Man's body is the same as that of all creatures but his heart is above all creation.

To complete a thing, one hundred years is not sufficient, but to destroy, one day is more than enough.

No man is a good doctor who has never been sick himself.

It is verily true that good medicine always tastes bitter.

Whenever in danger, one must realize that one doctor heals, two doctors kill.

In ancient times, man learned without a view to his own improvement; nowadays one learns with a view to the approbation of others.

No one takes time to rest before he dies.

You cannot get effective treatment if you conceal your disease.

Do not conceal your symptoms to test a doctor's ability.

The prescription is good, but the medicine, bad.

The superior man, if disinclined for official life, will practice medicine.

To become a good doctor requires breaking three arms three times. [20]

MATERIA MEDICA AND THERAPEUTICS

Chinese therapeutics was based upon the principle that nature tended to create harmony between the two opposing forces which caused disease, and upon the conviction that in nature there existed a remedy for every sickness, which was potent as long as it did not work in opposition to religious faith. The last conviction led to the trial of every imaginable substance: vegetable, animal, and to a smaller extent, mineral. It was the duty of the physician to dis-cover these healing substances and to determine their efficiency. As curative agents, the internal administration of drugs was most important. External remedies were acupuncture and the use of the moxa. Theurgical treatment of disease consisted of amulets, prayers, and pictures of the gods.[21]

Food and all other substances taken into the body were thought to liberate the *yang* and *yin* virtues, some of which produced harmony, others, disharmony. If the remedy was rightly chosen, it tended to correct the physical disturbance and resulted in the restoration of health. On the other hand, if it was ill-chosen it brought on disease and suffering. Certain substances were believed to be more heavily charged with *yang* and *yin* than others. It was the function of the physician to ascertain the proportions of *yang* and *yin* in order to balance the vital economy and to obtain the proper equilibrium.

To compensate for deficiencies and increases of the *yang* and *yin* properties, materia medica and therapeutics were thoroughly studied and a vast number of plant, animal, and mineral materials were experimented upon by ancient Chinese to a degree not exceeded by any other nation.

The Chinese regarded red as the color of fire and light in their philosophy; they identified red with *yang*, the chief principle of life.[22] Red was expected to expel pernicious influences and symbolized good luck, happiness, and delight. Red coffins were favored. The red gate on the south side of the cemetery was never opened except for the passage of the emperor.[23] The Chinese put a red powdered stone in the food or drink called *hun-hong* to destroy the evil spirit which had taken possession of one.

Almost every plant and animal substance was used as a remedy. Many of them were found to possess real medical virtues. Most of the drugs used in China were indigenous. A large number, however, came from countries of the West. The first herbal is reported to have been compiled by Chin Nong, an ancient emperor who reigned c. 2699 B.C. This was devoted chiefly to poisons.

Herbals: Emperor Shen Hung (27 B.C.), known as the patrongod of medicine, as well as the presiding deity of druggists and dentists, was reputed to have been the author of the herbal known as *Pan't'sari-king*, dealing with materia medica. It contained many prescriptions, the ingredients of which he collected himself. He mentioned 358 drugs, 40 of which were derived from mineral sources and 68 from animal sources. In 1596 A.D. Li-hsi Chan collected 1580 prescriptions from various authors, adding 374 of his own. The collection embraced 40 volumes and was accepted as a standard works on therapeutics. The *Pan't'sari-king* listed 1100 species of plants and their parts, and many animal substances, He specified those of 6 domestic animals, the horse, cow, sheep, dog, pig, and hen as most effective. Of human substances, he mentioned hair as a remedy. Others enumerated 13 human items used as remedies.

Ginseng and Shan-luh: Of all the herbs used in China from ancient times, the *ginseng* root was the most highly esteemed for its reputed life-giving properties. It is still believed to prolong life and to have the virtues of an "elixir vitae," and the genuine root still commands a very high price.

Another plant, *shang-luh (Phytolacca acinosa)*, is credited with similar properties. Associated with each, are legends similar to those connected with mandrake in Europe. Both roots have a resemblance to the human form, and are believed to have the power of shrieking when gathered.

Shang-luh was said by the Chinese to grow on the ground beneath which a dead man lies. From early times it was used in China as an ingredient in love-philters. It enjoyed a reputation in the Far East for curing sterility. The black, ripe fruit of the plant was greatly valued by country people, who took it to induce fecundity. It was also employed as a purgative and applied outwardly to scrofulous tumors and glandular swellings.

The Chinese shaped the root into a mannikin which they used in magic, and Chang Urh-ki, a writer of the seventeenth century A.D., stated that "a sorcerer carves the root of shang-luh into a human effigy which he makes through his spells capable of telling fortunes." Similarly German *alraunes*, during the fifteenth and sixteenth centuries, were consulted as oracles and were believed to possess occult powers and the ability to bring good fortune to their owners.

The red variety of *shang-luh*, mentioned in the *Pan't'sari-king*, was said to be a powerful poison: it produced delirium, and was stated to have the power of killing demons. Its use as an anesthetic was here indicated, and it is probable that it was this drug to which the famous Chinese surgeon Hua T'o, who lived in the third century, resorted, when, according to tradition, "he cut his patients' bellies, to cleanse the viscera without harm."

Ginseng has ever had a wonderful reputation in China and was believed to possess marvelous properties. The best kind of *ginseng* was formerly regarded as a royal possession. Within recent years, in the days of the Empire, the Empress Dowager Tze-hsi-hiant-yo, issued an imperial edict granting to one of the viceroys "four ounces of the very best ginseng from the imperial treasury" as a special mark of favor to him.

It is stated by Lieutenant G. C. Foulk, late of the United States Navy, that "mandrake or ginseng formed a chief means of paying the Korean tribute to China, and its value varies in ratio to its resemblance to the male figure." He further states that it is used as a panacea by the Chinese. Numerous purgatives, emetics, expecto-

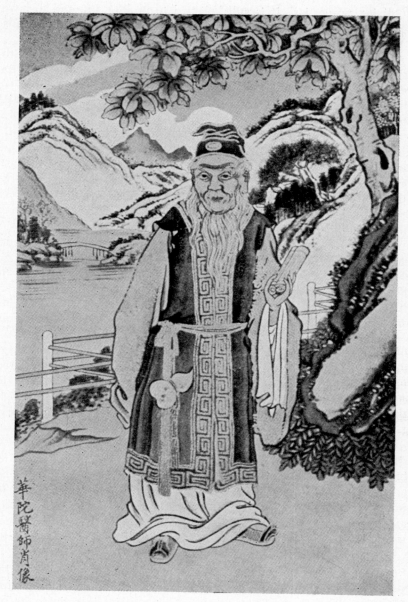

Fig. 93: Hua T'o, a Chinese surgeon (c. 200 A.D.). Hua T'o was famed for his skill in acupuncture and moxibustion, and he was credited with the ability of foretelling the sex of unborn children.

rants, diaphoretics, diuretics, alteratives, and hematinics were employed. Chinese medicine was rich in abortifacients, emmenagogues, aphrodisiacs, and galactogogues.

Other Popular Drugs: Other popular drugs were the root of pomegranate (for worms), camphor and rhubarb (for constipation), aconite, cannabis, iron (for anemia), sulfur (for skin diseases), copper (as an emetic) and alum, musk, opium, asafetida, nutmeg, cinnamon, and pepper for various ailments.

The favorite emetic was betonia. Purgatives were plums, tamarind, rhubarb, pig's gall, and croton. For dysentery, a disease frequently occurring in epidemic form, bat dung, snake skins, and other substances, in addition to drugs, such as aloes, rhubarb, and pomegranate roots, were employed. A favorite remedy for migraine was oil of peppermint. For headache, the brain and marrow of a stag were indicated. For weakness caused by sexual excesses, powdered stag horn was efficient. Epilepsy was treated with silkworm root, and lameness with maple root, cinnabar, tiger's bone, and musk. The black soya bean was supposed to give strength and to act as an antidote for vegetable poisons. Garlic *(allium sativum)* was also widely employed for medicinal purposes. China root was used for rheumatism and syphilis.

Celery, ginger, gentia, cinnamon, poppy (opium), violet, bamboo, and burnt tortoise shell were used for bronchial catarrah. Pig's lungs and licorice, mixed with ammonia, were used for chronic bronchitis and pneumonia. Small doses of red lead, infusion of elamtis, and powdered antelope's horns were prescribed for heart disease. Gentia, ginger, gypsum, borax, burnt hair, garlic, and "dragon bones" were given for hemorrhage.

Uterine hemorrhage was treated with an irrigation of a decoction of stinging nettles. Congestion of the liver was treated with elephant hides, bamboo, and extract of pig liver, ox gall, or bear's gall with arack. There was a long list of remedies for stomach diseases. Among them were peppers, green orange peel, coriander, cloves, magnolia, and chicken crops. Powdered jade and powdered tortoise shell were probably used for their magical properties.

The ancient Chinese physicians were perhaps the first to use animal substances in disease. They may, therefore, be styled as pioneers in the science of organotherapy. Preparations of liver, lung, kidney, and spleen were employed for diseases affecting these organs. Hen gizzards were prescribed for stomach diseases, animal testicles for impotence, the semen of young adults and various animal tissues for weakness, and placental tissue to assist and facilitate childbirth. All kinds of shell fish were employed, and animals' excreta and secreta, repulsive and disgusting, were frequently administered.

Geologists working in China have learned to their disappointment that fossil crabs are rarely found, largely because of the high esteem placed on their medical properties by the natives. Innumerable virtues were credited to these petrified crabs. They were considered an excellent antidote for neutralizing all kinds of mineral, metallic, and vegetable poisons, and were particularly used as a vermifuge. Fossil crabs are still believed efficacious in corneal opacity and other affections of the eyes.

Pliny stated that the ancients had great uses for river crabs. When burned to ashes, they were considered an antidote for all poisons, especially when taken in ass's milk. In Jamaica, there existed a superstition that fiddler crab could cure deafness and earache; it was called the "deaf-ear crab." The treatment consisted of crushing the live crab and pouring the juice thus obtained into the affected ear.

Doctrine of Signature: Medicaments were often classified according to their relationship in color, appearance, and other resemblances to certain organs. Green and sour-tasting drugs were prescribed for diseases of the liver; red and bitter substances were supposed to influence the heart; yellow and sweet, the spleen; white and sharp, the lungs; and black and salty, the kidneys. Ailments of the upper part of the body yielded to remedies derived from the upper parts of plants where *yang* predominated. Diseases of the lower half responded to the roots of plants where *yin* was assumed to dominate. The root of *ginseng,* because of its resemblance to the lower part of a human being, was used in paraplegia. Curative agents were chosen with reference to the season of the year, i.e. spring plants were employed for those undernourished and underweight.

The doctrine of signature was in evidence in China from early times. Drugs and animal organs were used because their color or shapes resembled the patient's diseased tissues. For example, kidney was used for backache, lungs for tuberculosis, necks of animals for cretinism, and goiter and testes for sterility.

It has been authentically recorded that certain organs of children were cut off for the purpose of giving medical aid to other children who were sick in these organs. Kidney-shaped beans were used for kidney diseases and saffron for jaundice.

All warming or cooling substances that possessed a strengthening action were supposed to have the characteristic of the male principle *yang.* Sour, bitter, spicy, or salty flavored preparations had the characteristic of *yin.* Preparations pleasing to the eye, possessing attractive names, or invented by prominent men, were considered efficacious.

Winemaking: It is recorded that the art of winemaking was introduced in China by I-Te as early as 2200 B.C. Its action on the system was tested by Emperor Yu upon himself. The effect of it was very favorable. He enjoyed the beverage very much; but considering the grave consequence which might result if his subjects took to this drink and become addicted to its use, he banished the inventor I-Te from the country. The secret, however, became known, and winemaking became an important Chinese industry. The sweet wine of Shucking was produced from fermented rice with the addition of a leaven of wheat. It does not appear that it was used as often as a medicine in China as in other countries.

Medical Mixtures: Medical mixtures usually combined a number of ingredients, seldom less than nine or ten. Numbers played a prominent part in preparing the mixture. The number of ingredients used in the preparation was frequently a multiple of five, and five doses were generally ordered. Five was considered a holy number: there were five elements, five organs, five colors, five tastes, five smells, and five planets.

Acupuncture and Moxibustion

The invention and technique of acupuncture were supposed to be of Chinese origin. This method consisted of the introduction of hot or cold metal needles into the body as a remedy for certain diseases. The object of the operation was to penetrate certain definite points of the body, presumed to possess channels, in order to allow harmful humors to escape by removing the obstruction, and permitting fresh vital spirits to be introduced into the body. These channels were supposed to exert a profound influence on the circulation of the blood, and on every organ and tissue of the body. The origin of this procedure goes back to ancient times. During the Tang dynasty (c. 618–692 A.D.), Sun Shu Miao, one of the recognized gods of Chinese medicine, collected the writings on the subject in his book "Acupuncture and Cautery." He specified some 650 needling points in the body and listed some 345 special points by name. He pointed out the number of needles used and the depth to which they were inserted. He stated that the length of time they were left in depended upon the nature of the individual case and upon the conception of the healer who was trained in the Chinese theory of disease. He also stated that extraordinary care should be taken in the choice of the spot for the puncture. After the withdrawal of the needles, pressure was exercised upon the seat of the puncture. Other physicians calculated that the body had 388 spots where acupuncture could be performed. Knowing their location was the task of the Chinese physician.

Cauterization by means of moxibustion was another Chinese invention. The procedure consisted of burning powdered leaves of mugwort on the skin. The moxa was rolled into small pellets

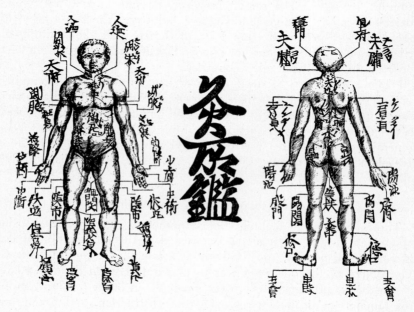

Fig. 94: Indications of the places for applying the moxa. (From Kemfero, 1712.)

mixed with saliva, and lighted with a taper or burning incense stick. When it burned to the skin, the burning mass was crushed into the blister formed. Frequently acupuncture was followed by moxibustion. In China, acupuncture was considered a cure for many diseases. It was used most frequently in fractures, stone in the bladder, sprain, swollen joints, leprosy, rheumatism, lameness, and in deep-seated pain from any cause and in any part of the body.

A Chinese philosopher, named "Nei Ching" gave the following explanation for the efficiency of acupuncture, "the wind scatters through the muscles and comes into conflict with the defensive forces, the channels being choked, the flesh becomes nodular and ulcerates, all because of the stagnant movements and from this offensive force numbness results."[24] Acupuncture relieved the stagnation.

Physical Therapy

Massage was carried out with great skill in China from remote times. At present, it is practiced by the blind or by old women.

Medical gymnastics were supposed to have been first used by the mythical Tschi Sung Tin about 2500 B.C. This practice consisted of rhythmical and systematic inspiration and expiration at different positions of the body, friction of the abdomen, and muscular movements. A complete cure extended over several months. It was associated with dieting and was intended to regulate the circulation of the vital juices.

Hydrotherapy was practiced in China at a very early period as a means of preservation of health. At present, it is associated with religious ritual.

Plasters were used for many ailments, including fractures, dislocations, eyestrain, cancer, headache, carbuncle, and rheumatism. Frequently they were applied at a site distant from the diseased part.

Surgery

Surgery was practiced in China as early as 4000 B.C. Emperor Huang Ti is said to have "employed manipulations," making radical incisions when necessary. "He made incisions through the skin, loosened the muscles, identified blood vessels, sutured tendons, frequently exposed the spinal cord and brain, and cleaned the vessels."[25]

Chou Hong classified medicine into "internal" (medical) and "external" (surgical) diseases. The medicine of wounds he divided under four headings: swellings, ulceration, wounds produced by instruments, and fractures.

Pien Chiao (c. 300 B.C.) used general anesthesia for surgical procedures. It is recorded that he gave two men, named "Lu" and "Chao," a toxic drink which rendered them unconscious for three days, during which time he performed a gastrotomy upon them. A legend tells that he explored their hearts, after removing and interchanging their organs; he gave them a wonderful drug, and the two men went home recovered.[26]

Chang Chung Ching has been called the "Hippocrates of China." He was a contemporary of Hua-T'o, and the author of a treatise on

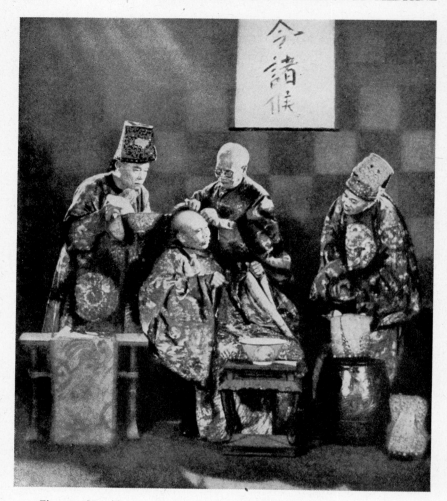

Fig. 95: Hua T'o (c. 115–205 A.D.) court physician of Chao Tsao, King of Wei. He was an exponent of simplicity. However, if medication or acupuncture failed, he did not hesitate to operate. He performed a wide range of abdominal operations, in all major cases rendering his patients insensible to pain by the administration of an anesthetic mixture known as *Ma Fu Shuan*. The wounds were closed with medically treated sutures. (Courtesy of Davis and Geck, Inc.; artist's representation.)

fever and dietetics which remained a textbook for many centuries after his demise. In 170 A.D., he was at the zenith of his fame.

Hua-T'o (115–205 A.D.) has been accepted as the god of surgery. He was skilled in external and internal disease. He performed operations, under anesthesia, on the brain, abdomen, and other parts of the body. "He then withdrew accumulated material. If this material was in the stomach or intestines, they were opened, irrigated, and cauterized, employing suturing materials, and plasters, and in four or five days the patient was well."27 Hua-T'o, who wrote a code on medical ethics, was known as the most ethical physician who ever lived. He lived during the Hau dynasty.

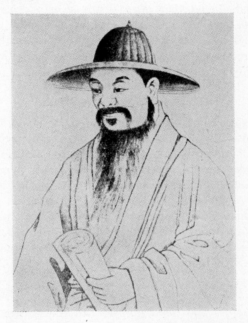

Fig. 96: Portrait of Ko Hung (c. 281–361 A.D.). Ko Hung was the greatest of Chinese alchemical writers. (Courtesy of Professor T. L. Davis.)

Pien Chiao, a contemporary of Hua-To, was famous as an internist, but he was also a surgeon of note. He is credited with having performed the first operation under general anesthesia.

Plastic surgery for harelip was performed in China as early as 229 to 317 A.D. Castration has been performed since 1000 B.C., either by strangulation or a simple stroke of a knife, after which styptics and pressure were applied and the urethra plugged up temporarily. Other surgical works were operations for imperforate anus and cesarian section.

Various eye diseases, including cataract, conjunctivitis, amblyopia, amaurosis, and corneal ulcer are described. It is interesting to learn that the livers of wild pigs were used internally for night blindness. Cataracts were treated with a needle. Apart from this, the therapy in diseases of the eye was meager.

Chinese surgery deteriorated later. It was incompatible with the Chinese religion to sacrifice any part of the body to cure disease. According to Confucius, the human body was the sacred inheritance from one's ancestors and it had to be returned to its ancestors intact. Most Chinese believed that after death a man existed very much as he did in his physical body during life. If a spirit was minus any portion of its body, that spirit would return to earth and revenge itself upon its relatives for failure to protect the body; thus, all kinds of ill luck would come to the surviving relatives.

Responsibility of Physician

When a person died from an overdose of medicine, the healer was not held responsible for his death; but if death occurred after an operation, the surgeon was held for murder, because it was wrong to operate under any circumstances. The death penalty, however, could be ransomed for money, if this was satisfactory to the relatives of the dead. A Chinese physician who lost a royal patient in the course of treatment was buried alive with his dead patient, a practice that continued until 1650. The failure of a physician to save a royal life was thus punished with death until comparatively recent years, regardless of blame.

Fees

Chinese emperors and head ministers of the government engaged in the practice of medicine as an avocation or hobby. Royal physicians as a rule did not charge fees. Grateful patients, however, donated gifts to the state for their generous actions. A considerable amount of healing is still carried on in China by the elders of a clan (i.e. grandfathers and grandmothers) who use home remedies that have been accumulated through the ages.

Upon the subject of medical ethics, a work published in the time of the Ming dynasty is of much interest and will be quoted here:

When a patient is severely ill, treat him as thou wouldst wish to be treated thyself. If thou art called to a consultation, go at once and do not delay. If he ask thee for medicine, give it to him at once and do not ask if he be rich or poor. Use thy heart always to save life and to please all, so will thine own happiness be exalted. In the midst of the darkness of the world be sure there is someone who is protecting thee. When thou art called to an acute illness and thinkest with all thy might of nothing but making money out of the patient, if thy heart be not filled with love of thy neighbor be sure that in the darkness of the world there is some one who will punish thee.

MEDICAL EDUCATION

Already under the Chou dynasty, (c. 900 B.C.), the state held yearly examinations for licensure to practice medicine, and the salaries were fixed according to the showing made in the test.

Most confidence was placed in those who had received their medical education from their parents and especially in those who could point to the greatest number of professional ancestors.

From the data available it is evident that the Chinese were a self-sufficient people, and that their knowledge of medicine was almost completely self-evolved.

PRECURSORS OF MODERN REMEDIES

Much as one may scoff at the Chinese for putting useless and disgusting drugs in their pharmacopoeia, they must be given credit for many remedies which are in accord with the modern pharmacopoeial drugs. According to native writers, seaweed, with its valuable iodide content, has long been used by the Chinese as a remedy for goiter. The best-known remedy of vegetable origin, ephedra, from which the medicinally valuable alkaloid ephedrine is obtained, was known to the Chinese under the name of *ma huang*, and has been employed in China for more than 5,000 years in the treatment of hay fever.

Cinnabar, the chief ore of mercury, was used in China in the production of mercurial preparations and for fumigations. A roll of paper filled with cinnabar was placed in one nostril and the mercurial fumes inhaled. A mercurial inunction of red oxide of mercury and ointments made of sulfur, alum, or arsenic was used for various skin diseases.

The Chinese claim to be the inventors of inoculation against smallpox. It is recorded that they used a cotton-wool pad, saturated with the contents of a fresh smallpox pustule, in the nostrils as inoculation against the disease. Boys were treated this way in the left nostril and girls in the right. One must not judge ancient China by modern standards but by contemporary scales. They made their own contributions to civilization in general. To mention only two basic inventions: The mechanism of a free-swinging magnetic needle had been known to the Chinese since 121 A.D., and the manufacture of spectacles was known to them long before the Europeans had ever heard of them. Indeed, until the conquest of Peiking, the Chinese looked down upon the Europeans as barbarians and devils.

As late as the fourteenth century A.D., Marco Polo, describing the wonderful society of Eastern Asia stated, "There was much for which Europe might envy the Chinese people and little for which the Chinese might envy the Europeans."

References and Notes

1. It is to be noted that the Chinese story of the age of man agrees more with the evolutionary theory than with the Biblical story.
2. Giles, H. A.: Encyclopedia Britannica, Ed. 11, Vol. 6, pp. 226-227.
3. DeGroot, J. J. M.: Religion in China. Putnam, New York, 1912.
4. Cited by Morgan, E.: The Cosmic Spirit. Royal Asiatic Soc., Vol. 62:1920.
5. "Religion in China."
6. Wieger, L.: Taoism. I. Ho-Kien-Fou, 1911, pp. 49-50; 62-65; 172-17, etc.
7. "Out of nothingness was born the Great Extreme; this produced the Yang and Yin; these then produced the four symbols; and they the sixty-four hexagrams." —Chinese Saying (Plopper).
8. "Religion in China." 1:165.
9. Wilson, W. J.: Ciba Symposia, Oct., 1940. Background of Chinese Alchemy. Shanghai, 1928.
10. Ibid.
11. Giles, L.: The Sayings of Lao Tzu. The Wisdom of the East Series, London, 1906.
12. See also Osawa, G.: Zur Geschichte der Anatomie in Japan. No. 16, 1896. Cited by Fujikawa, Y., M. D.: Japanese Medicine. Paul B. Hoeber Inc., New York, 1934, pp. 12-13.
13. Morse, W. R.: Chinese Medicine. Paul B. Hoeber Inc., New York, 1934, pp. 76-77.
14. Ibid. pp. 64-68.
15. Cited by Morse, W. R.: Chinese Medicine. pp. 74-77.
16. Legge, J.: Life of Confucius, p. 101. Giles, L.: The Sayings of Confucius. The Wisdom of the East Series, London, 1907.
17. Polo, Marco: Vol 2, p. 52 (ed. Yule). Cited by Gordon, B. L.: Romance of Medicine. F. A. Davis Co., Phila., 1945, p. 25.
18. "Chinese Medicine."
19. Wong, K. C.: Chinese Contributions to the Science of Medicine. China, M. J., 43:1193, 1929.
20. Foster, A. A.: A collection of Chinese Proverbs.
21. Cited by Fujikawa, Y., M. D.: Japanese Medicine. pp. 14-16.
22. "Religion in China." (Book I), pp. 216-217.
23. Ibid.
24. "Religion in China."
25. Giles, H. A.: A Chinese Biographical Dictionary, 1889. A History of China's Literature, 1901. Chuang Tz, 1889.
26. Translated by Wong, K. C.: China Medical Journal, 44:737, 1930. Cited by Morse, W. R.
27. Rhys, E. (Ed.): Travels of Marco Polo. Every Man's Library, Dutton, New York.

13

Medicine in Ancient Japan

CUSTOMS AND HABITS

THE antiquity of Japanese medicine does not go so far back as that of her neighboring peoples. Japanese civilization is comparatively new. Its prehistoric period is calculated to have been about 1160 years, from 660 B.C. to 400 A.D. Japan derived its culture from China by way of Korea. China was the fountain-head of Japan's civilization: China was to Japan, in medicine, as Greece was to Rome. Even the name "Japan" is Chinese etymologically.

Ancient Japan was peopled with an interesting race of bearded hunters, the Ainu. The Japanese are Mongolians, but of a type distinct from their neighbors in China. Rather they are kin to the Tatar rulers of China, who in the thirteenth century overran the Chinese Empire and have possessed it ever since.[1]

Mythology: Japanese mythology relates that the beautiful islands were made by the gods themselves, two of whom came down to live there, becoming the progenitors of the present inhabitants who are thus the true "sons of heaven." Another mythological tale refers to the god Izanagi and the goddess Izanami, who took a walk around the borders of the newly created realm, going in opposite directions. At length they met. Instantly Izanami exclaimed, "Oh, what a beautiful man!" But Izanagi was displeased that a woman should precede him in anything, even in the matter of flattering speech; so this literal lord of creation commanded that they walk around the island again and that the goddess keep silent upon their meeting, thus giving him his divine right of precedence. Izanami meekly obeyed him, and when next they met, she held her nimble tongue, while her liege lord sluggishly ejaculated, "Oh, what a beautiful woman!"

391

Beginning of Reliable History: Reliable Japanese history does not begin until the fifth century of the Christian era, although native tradition fixes the founding of the empire in the year 660 B.C. According to this tradition, the father of his country was the first emperor Jimmu, evidently a descendant of those Tatar tribes that had secured a foothold in the southernmost island of Kyushu.[2]

Barbaric Skills: The Japanese of the mythical period, preserved by the Hans and Wei records, were a race that had long emerged from the savage stage and had attained a high level of barbaric skill. The Stone Age was forgotten by them, or nearly so, but knowledge of bronze was to be introduced at a later period from the neighboring continent. As a matter of fact, the evidence points to the fact that the Japanese never passed through a genuine Bronze Age. They used iron for manufacturing spears, swords, and knives of various shapes, and likewise for the more peaceful purpose of making fishing hooks and door locks. Their other warlike and hunting implements were bows, arrows, and spears. Bows, arrows, swords, and knives are frequently mentioned, but there is no trace of tools and domestic implements, such as the saw and the axe.

Food, Clothing, and Physique: The Hans and Wei records (25–265 A.D.) furnish a graphic description of ancient Japan and its people. The Japanese are spoken of as "dwarfs" *(wa)*, and their islands are described as mountainous; the climate was mild and vegetables could be grown in winter and summer. The men tatooed their faces and bodies in patterns indicating differences of rank; male attire consisted of a single piece of cloth; females wore a gown passed over the head, and tied their hair with a bow. Food was taken with the fingers but was served on bamboo trays and wooden dishes. Footgear was not worn. When men of the lower classes met a man of rank, they left the road and retired to the grass. They squatted or knelt with both hands on the ground when they addressed a superior. Intoxicating liquor was widely used. The people were long-lived, many reaching the age of 100. Women were more numerous than men. There was no theft, and litigation was infrequent. The women were faithful and not jealous. Many men of high rank had four or five wives; some men of less rank had two or three. Wives and children of lawbreakers were confiscated; and, for grave crimes, the offender's family was extirpated. Divination was practiced by burning bones. After a funeral the whole family performed ablutions.

The food of the early Japanese consisted of fish and wild game. Rice was the only cereal mentioned: its cultivation dates back to time immemorial. Beans, millet, and barley are named. Silkworms are mentioned. A few vegetables and fruits are also listed. An intoxicating liquor called *sak* was known in Japan during the mythical period. No mention is made of the use of fire for warming or cooking.

A high level was reached by the early Japanese in the use of clothing. Combs are mentioned, and much attention was devoted to hair dressing: men seem to have bound up their hair in two bunches, one on each side of the head; young boys tied theirs in a topknot; girls let their locks hang down over their necks; and married women dressed theirs after a fashion which apparently combined the two last-named methods. There is no mention in any of the old books of cutting the hair or beard except in token of disgrace; aside from the headdress, the sexes were not distinguished by apparel or ornamentation.

Nature and Value of Women: From the time Buddhism and its philosophy spread to Japan, a low estimate was put upon the inherent nature and value of women. The notions presented by Buddhism in regard to women were degrading: she was the source of temptation and sin; she was essentially inferior to man in every respect; and before she could hope to enter Nevara, she had to be born again as man. Her social position was low; it was to serve her husband (her lord). She was subject to three obeyances: to parents, to husband, and to her own son—the future lord of the house. The young son was the master of the house in the absence of the husband, and he enjoyed sexual liberties, with the domestics or others, without any embarrassment.

Women had no legal standing in Japan. They were created to perform two functions—begetting children and attending to domestic duties.

A peculiar sort of one-roomed hut, without windows, was called a "parturition house" and was employed for the purpose of delivering parturient women in privacy.

Sexual Relationships: Sexual relationship in Japan has always been characterized by a certain degree of looseness and lack of moral restraint, the prevailing ethical and religious opinion not emphasizing sexual relationship. The naïve openness of speech and conduct in these matters have always astonished and shocked European visitors. Well down to the modern era, phallic worship was popular. Concubines, licensed prostitution, promiscuous bathing, and free exposure of the person were in evidence; little value was placed on sexual purity and personal virtues.

Strange as it may seem, the Japanese never have looked upon bathing with nude women in one tub as immoral or irreligious. Men, women, and children still bathe together undressed without the slightest hesitancy or embarrassment.

Hygiene: Much that was done by the early Japanese for preservation of health may be classified as hygiene, and regarded in the nature of religious duties. For example, the forbidden foods, the cleansing injunctions after touching a corpse, the isolation of the sick, and the burning of the body were regarded as religious duties. They were, however, of hygienic significance.

Ceremonial purification was an old rite in Japan. The *chazu-bache*, which was found before Shinto shrines, containing the holy water with which they rinsed their mouths and washed their hands, was a very old practice. Pilgrims and worshippers invariably made use of these waters. Wiping the hands on the towels which was provided by the faithful, was always a cause of spreading disease and infection. Skin diseases, which have always been so prevalent in Japan, were probably caused by these religious purifications.

The habits of personal cleanliness, which distinguish the modern Japanese from their neighbors in continental Asia, seem to have begun early. One reads frequently of bathing in rivers. To the mind of the ancient Japanese, cleanliness was next to godliness. Any defilement—sanitary, moral, or ritual—received the utmost care. Latrines appear to have been situated away from the houses and generally placed next to a running stream.

JAPANESE MEDICINE

The medicine of ancient Japan, like that of her general culture, has been entirely imported from China, particularly in consequence of the Korean invasion under the Empress Jingo, when the cultural forces of China, as modified by Buddhism, began to pour like a flood. It was a transformation almost as complete and as rapid as the one that took place 100 years ago when Japan came in touch with western civilization through Commodore Perry of the United States Navy. The medicine of Japan, therefore, is a replica of that of China, and little can be added to that of Chinese medicine as described in the previous chapter.

Buddhist Creed: The teaching of Buddha, which was incorporated in the sacred books, first in the doctrine of *suttas* and again in the rules of the society or order he founded referred to disease that could be avoided by personal conduct and to the promise that every person could be his own doctor. The doctrine of *suttas* is found in the following paragraphs:

Now this is the noble truth as to suffering. Birth is attended with pain. decay is painful, disease is painful, death is painful, union with unpleasant is painful, painful is separation from the pleasant, and any craving unsatisfied, that too, is painful.

Now this is the noble truth as to the origin of suffering. Verily; it is the craving thirst that causes the renewal of becomings, that is accompanied by sensual delight and seeks satisfaction now here, now there, that is to say, the craving of satisfaction of the senses or the craving for a future life or the craving for prosperity.

Now this is the noble truth as to the passing away of pain. Verily; it is the passing away so that no passion remains. The giving up, the getting rid of, the being emancipated from, the harboring no longer of this craving thirst.

Now this is the noble truth as to the way that leads to the passing away of pain. Verily; it is the noble eightfold path that is to say right views, right aspiration, right speech, conduct and mode of livelihood, right efforts, right mindfulness, and right rapture.[3]

This Buddhist creed meant to the Japanese much more than the acquisition of a practical religion, with the code of a clearly defined morality in place of the amorphous and jejune cult of Shinto. It meant the introduction of Chinese civilization with all that it stood for: its arts, sciences, crafts, religion, and customs. Priests and scholars crossed in great numbers from China to Japan, and many Japanese came to China to study the *suttas*, which were regarded as the fountainhead of Buddhism.

According to Kukai, a follower of Buddha (774–835 A.D.), every substance was composed of two principles, mental and material, which were inseparably blended: matter contained mind; and mind incorporated itself in matter; and every particle of matter was permeated by the divine personality of Buddahood.

Ancient Japanese medical art was founded upon primitive observations and was free from speculation. It differentiated a considerable number of diseases and had at its command an abundant therapeutic store brought over from China, consisting mostly of endogenous medical plants.

Medical Texts: The oldest existing medical work of Japan is the *Ishinho,* written during the fifth year of the Tengen era (982 A.D.). The author depended chiefly on the Chinese work *Ping-Yuan-hou-Lun* by Chao-yuan-fang, and to a lesser extent on other Chinese medical works. The work deals with acupuncture, diseases of the pneuma, diseases of the intestines, skin disorders, eye, ear, and tooth diseases,

diseases of the hand and foot, tumors, wounds, laryngeal diseases, midwifery, diseases of children, sexual hygiene, dietetics, and drugs.

Anatomy: The status of medicine during the early period may be briefly outlined as follows: Anatomic knowledge was limited to the most superficial parts of the body. Owing to the inviolable reverence for the dead, dissection in Japan, as in China, was not permitted. Anatomy was therefore a highly speculative subject. The body was divided anatomically into flesh, bones, and entrails. The anatomy of the five organs and the six viscera were mentioned and the blood vessels were given brief notation.

Physiology: The physiology of this period was just as obscure as the anatomy. It was based on the concept that there existed in the body a double principle: masculine (positive) and feminine (negative). The working machinery of the body was controlled by these two opposing forces that circulated in the blood and in the pneuma. Accounts of two gods, Onamuj-no-Mikoto and Sukunabikona-no-Mikoto, are found in early writings. These deities, by combining their efforts, discovered the means of curing disease. The brain and spinal cord were regarded as a kind of marrow. The nervous system was not known. Every organ possessed a seat for the spirit.[4]

Etiology: During normal life, the spirit or pneuma pervaded all matter and was found in the five elements that compose the body: wood, fire, earth, air, and water. In the event the pneuma was absorbed through the skin, it penetrated the organs; therefore heat, cold, moisture, and wind played a prominent part in the causation of disease. Sex, age, and constitution were important factors in the pathogenesis of disease. The *Ishinho* attributed diseases to changes in the elements, to the work of gods, to malign spirits, and to the spirits of dead persons which returned to earth to avenge themselves on the living. Other factors were unchastity and carelessness.

Diagnosis: Fever caused by cold was considered the most frequent form of pyrexia and was thought to differ from all other kinds of fever. All diseases accompanied by fever were designated by different names. There was a cold form of fever and a hot form. Six kinds of malarial cases were recognized, including those with disordered stomachs, those running a chronic course, those ascribed to miasma, and those associated with a fever recurring every second or third day. Frequently a single disease was divided into many different varieties, in accordance with the different symptoms presented. Diabetes and a number of skin diseases were diagnosed. Leprosy was considered a communicable disease transmitted from person to person. Smallpox was recognized to be a form of fever bearing a contagious character. The diagnosis of a given disease was reached by interrogation, inspection, and palpation. The last was largely limited to the pulse. Four varieties of pulses were recognized.

Prognosis: Prognosis played an important part in the treatment of disease. The smallest incidents, as for example the growing of two lotus leaves on one stem, the condition of the water in a pond, or rain without clouds, were all regarded as omens.

Materia Medica: The famous book of materia medica known as *Yakkei-Taiso* gave an account of 254 different medicines, vegetable, animal, and mineral, with notes on preparation, preservation, employment, and action. This work was based upon an earlier Chinese work. In the *Hohzo Wamyo* were found 81 remedies derived from minerals, 509 from plants, and 181 from animals. The most favorite remedies were *sak* (a rice wine), licorice root, ginseng, magnolia, rhubarb, and croton oil.

Surgery: Surgery of early Japan was limited to wounds, ulcers, and abscesses. The treatment consisted of superficial incisions, bandages, and salves. Cauterization was practiced on ulcers and on wounds caused by the bites of mad dogs. Hemorrhage was checked by ground oyster shells, chalk, and sawdust. When this did not stop it, it was controlled by applying compresses. Bloodletting appears to have been employed early. Mineral baths and douches were frequently used. Decayed teeth were first loosened with a piece of wood and a hammer and then extracted with a finger. Acupuncture and moxibustion were favorite methods of counterirritation. There were specialists of acupuncture.

Acupuncture: One of the chief therapeutic measures of ancient Japan, brought over from China, was acupuncture, one of the three great nostrums still popular in Japan: the other two are massage and moxa. The operation consisted of perforating the skin and underlying tissue, to a depth ranging from ½ to ¾ inch, with a fine needle of gold, silver, or steel. The form and construction of the needles varied; but generally speaking, they were several inches long and of an average diameter, $\frac{1}{48}$ inch. The needles were usually fastened into a handle which was spirally grooved from end to end.

To perform the operation, the handle of the needle was held tightly between the thumb and the first finger of the left hand, the point resting upon the spot to be punctured. A slight blow was then given the head of the instrument with a small mallet held in the right hand, and the needle was gently twisted until its point had penetrated to the desired depth, where it was left for a few moments. It was then slowly withdrawn and the skin in the vicinity punctured rubbed for a few minutes. The number of perforations ranged from one to twenty and they were usually on the skin of the abdomen, although other portions of the body were not infrequently punctured.[5]

Moxibustion and Massage: The art of moxibustion was practiced by low castes. Massage was the profession of blind persons. Corresponding to the conception that diseases were produced by spiritual forces, prayers, sacrifices, exorcisms, incantations, and the like were used as remedies.

Eye Diseases: Certain eye diseases were recognized, including cataract, conjunctivitis, amaurosis, amblyopia, and corneal ulcer. Cataracts were cured by gouging, operation, or needling. The liver of a wild pig was prescribed internally for amaurosis. The puerperal woman was regarded as unclean and was confined in a separate room or house during parturition. Incantations and magic were employed to facilitate paturition.

The Insane: The insane were badly treated, as they are in a measure to this day. Gulic[6] observed an insane person kept in a cage. He was given but little food and had few clothes on him. He was treated like a wild animal, not even being provided with bedding.

Lepers: The same treatment was accorded to lepers. They were carried out from their homes and compelled to wander as outcasts, living in the outskirts of the villages in rude huts of their own construction, and depending on begging until merciful death gave them relief.

Theurgical Concept: The diseases of this period were purely theurgical in origin. Some diseases were the works of the gods and were designated as *kami-no-ke* (the spirit of the gods). Others were regarded as the work of malign spirits, such as those caused by the influence of demons. The spirit of a dead person was believed to be capable of making his erstwhile fellowmen ill, and there were a number of other causative factors, such as unchastity and carelessness.

Corresponding to the conception they had at that time of the causation of disease were the means used to ward off the disease-making influences, such as sacrifices, prayers, exorcisms, and magical incantations. The use of internal medicine belonged to a later period in which *sak* (rice wine) was the principal medicament. Of the medicines of botanical origin, the most important may be mentioned: *amaki* (Glycerrhiza glabra, L.), *nikota* (Panax quinque-folium), *hohokashiwa* (Magnolia hyolenka, S. and Z.), *ohoshi* (Rheum undulatum, L.), and *inumame* (Croton tiglium, L.).[7]

Outside Influences: The prehistoric era drew to its end toward the close of the fourth century A.D. The historical period began with Emperor Richu (c. 400 A.D.). It is related that during the reign of Emperor Ojin various Chinese books, including the "Confucian Analects" *(Lunyu),* were introduced into Japan from Pekche, China, a small state in the southwestern part of the peninsula. At a later period, a certain physician named Oyu-Ryoda came with two apothecaries to Japan, bringing with them various medicines from Korea. After that it is recorded that Korean medicine spread throughout Japan. In the northern part of Korea, a colony of Chinese medicinal plant cultivators existed who produced the most highly prized ginseng root found at that time.

According to one Japanese source, the Chinaman Jofuku of Tsing, under the Emperor Korei, came to Japan in search of the medicine that would prevent death. Among his traveling companions, there ought to have been a physician, but a foreign physician was called for the first time during the Inkyo dynasty on the occasion of the illness of the Emperor. At the Emperor's wish, the king of Silla sent the skilled physician Kon-Bu to the Imperial Court, and he arrived at Yamato in the eighth month of the third year of the Emperor's reign (414 A.D.) and quickly cured him of his illness. In the third year of the reign of the Emperor Yuryaku (458 A.D.), a Korean physician named Tokurai came out of Koryo (or Koma), a state in the northwestern part of the Korean peninsula, and with his family settled in Naniwa. He busied himself exclusively with the practice of medicine, and after his death his family from generation to generation continued to follow in his footsteps.

A New System: In the fifteenth year of the Emperor Kimmei (552 A.D.), the physician Oyu-Ryoda and the apothecaries Han-Ryoho and Tei-Yuda of Pekche came to Japan. They brought with them various medicines from Korea, and after that Korean medicine began to flourish and to spread throughout Japan.[8]

New Drugs: The new religion promised immortality and stimulated the devotees to search for drugs that could impart eternal life. Death was known as "disappearing," "going away," or "concealing one's person." As a pastime Japan's nobility gathered in groups to collect herbs, hoping to discover some possessing medical virtues. During the search, many valuable remedies were discovered. Ginseng root has been used in Japan from ancient times and was highly esteemed for its reputed life-giving properties. It was believed to prolong life and to have the virtues of an "elixir of life," and it commanded a high price. It came first from Korea, which China colonized because of the reputed marvelous medical plants that thrived there.

Other Modes of Treatment: Of course, divination and augury of various kinds were also practiced, and magic and charms were employed to avert evil. The followers of the Buddhist religion established, in addition to temples and pagodas, hospitals, dispensaries, and asylums for the sick, aged, and helpless. Students were sent directly to China to study the Buddhist doctrine, and they brought back the Chinese culture which included medical learning. Chinese medicine received state recognition when native medicine lost its hold on the general public.

Schools of Medicine: At the end of the seventh century, schools of medicine were founded in the capitals of the various provinces under the guidance of a Korean physician. The schools were made up of the following departments: medicine, acupuncture, massage, exorcism, and pharmacology. The medical department was further subdivided as follows: *tai-ryō*, or internal medicine; *sō-shu*, or wounds and tumors; *shō-sō*, or pediatrics; and *ji-moku-kō-shi*, or ear, eye, mouth, and tooth diseases. Acupuncture comprised the introduction of needles and small operations. In the massage department, they taught massage, the treatment of fractures, and bandaging. The exorcism department was instituted for the purpose of teaching the formulas of exorcism, but later this was entirely abandoned. The teachers of every branch comprised only those who exclusively devoted themselves to their teaching. The number of years of each course was as follows: internal medicine, seven; pediatrics and surgery, five; ear, eye, mouth and teeth, four; acupuncture, four; massage, three; and exorcism, three. The students were educated at the expense of the government. The examinations were held monthly by the teachers of the faculty and yearly by the chief of the medical department of the court. The final examination was held before the court minister himself; and after the examination, he bestowed the title *ishi* (physician). In addition, yearly, thirty women between the ages of fifteen and twenty-five years were chosen and educated in midwifery, the treatment of wounds, bandaging, and in administering acupuncture.[7]

The influence of Chinese and Korean teachers was strong until the sixteenth century, when some medical practitioners had the temerity to oppose Chinese doctrine, and they were successful in securing recognition for their individual experience.

Fees: For a long time, the Japanese physician was at the mercy of the charity of his own patients who determined his fees on the principle that "when the disciple of medicine successfully cures a potentially fatal illness, he must not be accorded too great an income, lest he begin to neglect his duties." The average fee allowed the physician was two to four times the value of his home-made medicine. To secure his position and his rights, the physician had only one weapon at his command—flattery. The young apprentice accompanying his master had ample opportunity to learn this method of insuring adequate fee collection.

Respected Status of Physicians: The art of healing, however, was highly respected in old Japan. Physicians were employed as court doctors and as central and local government medical officers. The modern art of healing which helped to save Japan from oriental stagnation did not emerge until 1771 A.D., when a few able physicians in Yedo began to study the Dutch language and Dutch medicine. This eventually opened the eyes of the intelligent class to the importance of science: "Be a prime minister or become a physician for they are both benevolent arts." This was a common saying in China and continues in Japan to this day.

Japan's Contribution to Modern Medicine: Japanese medicine made great progress in the last two centuries, when the Japanese began to mingle with Europeans. Takamine's discovery of adrenalin and his studies on vitamins are well known. The most famous Japanese medical investigator, Neguchi, produced the first pure culture of the syphilitic germ. He also isolated the yellow-fever parasite.

References and Notes

1. Scherer, J.: Young Japan. J. B. Lippincott Co., Philadelphia and London, 1905, p. 18.
2. Ibid., pp. 21-24.
3. There is not a word about God or the soul, not a word about Buddha or Buddhism. It seems almost empty, so thin and weak that one wonders how can it have formed the foundation of a system so mighty in its historical results; but the simple words were pregnant with meaning, and their implications were clear enough to the hearers to whom they were addressed.
4. Cited by Fujikawa, Y.: Japanese Medicine. Paul B. Hoeber, Inc., New York, 1934, pp. 1-2.
5. Whitney, W. N.: On the History of Medical Progress in Japan. Asiatic Transactions. 12: Part 4, p. 35.
6. Gulic, E. L.: Evolution of the Japanese. New York, 1903.
7. "Japanese Medicine," p. 2.
8. Ibid., pp. 3-4.
9. Ibid., pp. 6-7.

14

Medicine Among the Prehistoric Amerinds

DOCUMENTARY EVIDENCE

Few documentary evidences pertaining to medicine among the aboriginal American Indians from the pre-Columbian era are available. In fact, our knowledge of disease among the American Indians before the arrival of the white man is not satisfactory even for the semicivilized natives of Central America and Peru. Whatever knowledge we possess of prehistoric Amerind medicine is largely deduced from the practices and folklore of the modern Indian, from the records of the early Spanish travelers, from inscriptions carved on stones, and particularly from skeletal remains found in various parts of America.

The inscriptions are little more than mnemonic signs marked on clothing, mats, tents, and especially on rocks. In Mexico, the inscriptions are in the form of ideographic writing, where signs of animals and things represent ideas. In some localities, as for example, in the Yucatán, the Mayas had a well-devised alphabet of twenty-seven different elementary sounds. The letters of this alphabet vary from those of all other nations and evidently were original with this group.

PRIMITIVE CULTURE

The primitive culture of the aborigines of North America was fundamently indigenous—an almost direct environmental reaction. The Indian inherited his rude equipment and primitive mind from his remote ancestors, who, it is believed by most authorities, reached the new world from the old at an early date. According to Ameglimo, who based his studies on anthropoid and human fossils found in southern South America, America was the scene of the origin of man. Cooper states the following:

Few men exhibit such diversity, or if we may so express it, greater antithesis of character, than the native warrior of North America. In war, he is daring, boastful, cunning, ruthless, self-denying, and self-devoted; in peace, just, generous, hospitable, revengeful, superstitious, modest, and commonly chaste. These are qualities, it is true, which do not distinguish all alike; but they are so far the predominating traits of these remarkable people as to be characteristic.

Folklore: The culture of the aboriginal American is expressed in his practical knowledge and in his folklore. One of his favorite pastimes was the telling of tales and legends; each tribe and family had its own particular myth, told and retold, rivaling in interest the myths of the Greeks and the Vikings. The tale of Hiawatha by Longfellow may be taken as one example of the Amerind appreciation of the beauties of nature.

Practical Knowledge: The fascination which folklore held for the redskins almost obscured their practical knowledge. As is so often the case, theory is one thing and practice another. Some tribes were at least on the road to civilization. The Mayas had a calendar of 360 days with intercalendary days. The Indian knowledge of the atmospheric air and its properties was profound. Heat and cold, rain and drought, and the winds, in relation to the points of the compass, were never out of their thoughts. In each province, they found the best springs, flints, rocks, clay, beds, and stones for their tools, weapons, and dwellings.

They were familiar with the vegetable kingdom; edible plants and those used for medicine were on their list. They recognized poisonous plants and knew in many instances how to eliminate the poisonous properties from such plants. Their reliance on animal food to sustain life prompted them to observe animals. They knew well their nature and habits and could imitate their vocal noises with perfection. They knew a large number by name. Animal substances were the basis of their industries and fine arts. Their devotion to hunting enabled them to learn at least some anatomic parts of animals.

DISEASES

The condition of the skeletal remains of the prehistoric Indian, the testimony of early observers, and the folklore of many of the present tribes warrant the conclusion that, on the whole, the ancient Indian was a comparatively healthy person. If he was not immune to many epidemics and diseases of the old world, he was essentially free from local ailments by virtue of his environment and mode of life.

John Josselyn, who visited America twice (1674), says, speaking of disease among the Indians:

The great pox is proper to them, by reason (as some do deem) that they are Man-eaters . . . . In New England the Indians are afflicted with pestilent Feavers, Plague, Black-pox, Consumption of the Lungs, Falling-sickness, Kings-evil, and a Disease in the back, with us Empyema. Their physicians are the Powaws or Indian Priests who cure sometimes by charms or medicines, but in a general infection they seldom come amongst them, therefore they use their own remedies, which is sweating, etc. Their manner is when they have plague or small pox amongst them to cover their wigwams with Bark so close that no Air can enter in lining them (as I said before) within, and making a great fire till they are in a top sweat, and then run out in the Sea or River, and presently after they come into their Huts again they either recover or give up the Ghost.[1]

Immunity to Diseases: Many diseases common in urban Europe were not known to the prehistoric Indian who lived a free life by hunting and fishing in healthy surroundings. Such diseases as yellow fever, scarlet fever, and diphtheria were strange to him. They were brought over by the white man. The Indians were not immune to white man's diseases. On the contrary, during colonial days, when epidemics broke out in their midst, they were literally decimated, for they were not prepared hereditarily or medically to grapple with them. There are cases on record where parties of Spaniards or other white Europeans, apparently in good health, camped overnight near an Indian village not seeing the redskins. None the less they introduced fatal epidemics to the natives, so that when other European groups passed later, they found the entire community wiped out with only corpses populating the area.[2] During the Black Hawk war, a troop ship near a Chippewa camp, landed a soldier stricken with smallpox. Within six weeks, more than two thirds of the tribe in that region had succumbed to the disease. The epidemic among the Indians of New England in 1616 to 1620 was accompanied by a great mortality although the English seem to have been immune. This epidemic was perhaps the bubonic plague which raged in London earlier and was transmitted to America by English sailors.

Prevalent Diseases: Twitchel has collected the testimony of several explorers and has found record of numerous deserted Indian villages with a great number of unburied corpses lying in their ruins. Warner records a trip through the central part of California in 1832:

On no part of the continent over which I have been or have since traveled was so numerous an Indian population as in the villages of the Sacramento and San Joaquin Rivers . . . On our return late in the summer of 1833, we found the valleys depopulated. From the head of the Sacramento to the great bend and slough of the San Joaquin, we did not see more than six or eight live Indians. The disease appeared, as far as I could judge, to be a most acute and violent type of *remittent fever*.[3]

There is a popular belief among the Indians that diseases were unknown in America before the advent of the white man, that their great decrease of numbers was due to the introduction of diseases and to the changes of their habits of life introduced by the European intruders. That there is a basis for this belief has been attested by the records of many early European travelers which show that epidemics and outbreaks of diseases took place among the Amerinds contemporaneously with the new settlements in the various parts of the continents by the Europeans. This theory, however, is questioned by many observers who point out that bone diseases among the prehistoric American existed in the same form as prevails at present; this fact is evident from fossilized remains found in the various parts of the new continent. Bacterial diseases of the soft tissues must also have existed, for bacteria were known earlier than pre-Columbian days.

Skeletal remains, found in many parts of the American continent, reveal that *arthritis deformans* of the hip and spine was common among the aboriginals. Ritchie reports that 15 per cent of the natives in the New York area were inflicted with this disease.[4] *Mastoid infection* appears to have been frequent among the prehistoric Indians. Hrdlica reports five Peruvian and two Southwestern skulls of North American Indians with abscess of the external auditory meatus.[5]

MacCurdy[6] records a case of *osteosarcoma* of the cranium in Peru. Hrdlica is of the opinion that the prehistoric aborigines of America were not affected by rickets, tuberculosis, microcephaly, hydrocephaly, typhus, cholera, smallpox, plague, leprosy, syphilis, and flattened arches. He thinks that cancer and skin diseases were rare and that mental disease was infrequent.

It is not certain whether malaria, yellow fever, typhoid fever, scarletina, and diphtheria existed.[7]

With reference to the prevalence of *syphilis* among the prehistoric Amerinds, there is considerable divergence of opinion. Williams and Denninger are confident of its existence in prehistoric America. They first identified it in three skulls found in Pecos, New Mexico. Grana identified syphilis among the Peruvian Kuanti, and Iwan Bloch demonstrated, from historical and osteological evidence, the presence of syphilis among Indian Tribes of prehistoric times.[8] On the other hand, Hrdlica and others are not convinced that syphilis existed among the prehistoric Americans. The existence of tuberculosis among early Indians is also questionable.

Tumors, arteriosclerosis, heart disease, and endocrine disturbances rarely occurred.

Diseases common among the prehistoric Amerinds were chiefly of a *gastrointestinal nature*. Their custom of abstaining from food, often for days, followed by a period of overindulgence, brought on various gastrointestinal disorders. It was customary during tribal wars and hunting expeditions to abstain from food for several days at a time; but after these were over, the redskins engaged in an orgy of feasting. This fast-and-feast routine resulted in abdominal pain, colic, flatulence, nausea, vomiting, and diarrhea.

Other diseases, common particularly in the Great Lakes area, were *rheumatism, bronchitis, pleurisy,* and *pneumonia*. Living in tents filled with tobacco smoke, the Indians were troubled with various forms of *opthalmia*. *Deficiency diseases,* such as *scurvy* or *hemolytic anemia,* were found, according to Krogman, in 3.27 per cent of adult craniums in Pecos, New Mexico. *Urinary calculi* and *goiter* were not infrequent among the indigenous Americans.

Williams identified in the effigy pottery *(huacos)* of Peru, the possibility of *leprosy, lupus, syphilis,* and *verruca peruviana*. He concludes: "The diagnosis of syphilis of the skull is as certain as is possible in any dry bones without clinical history." Denninger diagnosed luetic periostitis in the long bones of adults found in Illinois mounds, as well as in the facial bones in a skull from Arizona, dating back to 1000 to 1350 A.D.

According to Krogman, the percentages of *caries, alveolar abscesses, periodonitis,* and *calculus deposit* were quite large among the American Indians. He states:

If we were to summarize the essentially indigenous disorders of the American Indians, we would have to include *deficiency diseases* (rickets [denied by Hrdlica], osteomalacia, and osteoporosis), *arthritis, rheumatism, neuralgia, stomach disorders* (especially in infancy and old age), *osseous tumors* of the external auditory meatus, and, in certain areas, *endemic goiter* and *urinary calculi*. In more restricted areas we would note the *infectious verrucae* of the Andean area of Peru, and in the same area the endemic facial ulceration known as *"uto";* in the Great Lakes area, *pleurisy* and *pneumonia* were common; and among the tipi-dwellers of the Plains area, *conjunctival disorders* were traceable to smoke-filled lodges. The subject of malarias and fevers must be held in abeyance. Dental disease was far more common than is generally accepted.[9]

A peculiar affection characterized by an *eruption of the skin,* somewhat resembling smallpox, was observed by Lawson (1700) in North Carolina.[10] Among other things he states:

The struma is not uncommon amongst these savages, and another distemper which is in some respects like the pox, but is not attended with gonorrhoea. This not seldom bereaves them of their noses. I have seen three or four of them rendered most miserable spectacles by this distemper. Yet when they have been so negligent as to let it run on so far without curbing of it, at last they shift to patch themselves up, and live for many years after; and such men commonly turn doctors. I have known two or three of these no-nose doctors in great esteem among these savages.

In his account of the original tribes of Massachusetts, Daniel Gooking[11] refers to a disease of high mortality among the tribes of Massachusetts:

This people were a potent nation in former times . . . . A very great number of them were swept away by an epidemical and unwanted sickness (1612 and 1613) . . . about seven or eight years before the English first arrived in those parts to settle the colony of New Plymouth . . . What this disease was, that so generally and mortally swept away, not only these but other Indians, their neighbors, I cannot well learn. Doubtless it was some pestilential disease. I have discoursed with some old Indians, that were then youths, who say that the bodies all over were exceeding yellow, describing it by a yellow garment they showed me, both before they died and afterwards.

Span of Life: The average longevity of the aboriginal American was about thirty-seven years. The struggle for survival, the rigorous life of war and chase, and the long periods of fasting followed by periods of gourmandism cut down their span of life. Their women, who carried the main burden of their existence, matured young and died early. Child mortality was very high. In Peru a number of young females were found buried, evidently full-term stillbirths.

Indian Concepts of Etiology of Disease: With reference to the causation of disease, the prehistoric American attributed all illness without apparent causation to supernatural agencies, such as the entrance into the body of malevolent or offended supernatural beings, witchcraft, enchantment, the ill will of certain persons, ghosts of the dead, and shadows of the living. Among some tribes of British Columbia, widows and widowers who observed mourning regulations had to avoid letting their shadow fall upon a person, lest the latter fall sick at once.

Animals: Animals were believed to cause diseases in man. Mooney relates that, among the Cherokees, it was held that animals became so offended and outraged at the carelessness of men and the invasion of their rights on the part of mankind that they held council and determined to obtain revenge on each of them, inflicting disease upon their human oppressors. All animals, large and small, shared in this vengeance. The incantations and rites of the Cherokee medicine men, pertaining to disease, refer often to animals as being the cause of disease. The legend goes on to state that, as a result of the action of the animals, all plants held a council and resolved to save man from the evil conspiracy of the animals. They devised remedies for him to combat all diseases caused by animals. "Thus it happens that for every disease brought about by animals, there is a remedy to be found in the plant world." This legend, that animals large and small are the cause of disease, may be considered a premonition of the modern scientific doctrine of the microbic origin of human diseases.[12]

Menstruation: Ploss states that, among many Indian tribes a menstruating woman was isolated because she was regarded as the cause of disease. According to Boas,[13] menstruating women, among Indian tribes of Vancouver Island, were not allowed to come near sick persons lest their presence further debilitate the ailing. The same author states that, among some tribes of British Columbia, "women during their monthly periods are forbidden to cook for their families for fear that the food will become poisonous." He further states that the *shamans* of the Shushwap were convinced that the proximity of a menstruating woman caused sickness and that the shadow of a mourner produced disease in whomever it fell upon. To combat such ailments, the *shaman* "shot" at the disease directly from his eyes.

Plurality of Souls: Many American tribes thought that diseases were dependent upon the existence of a plurality of souls. Some tribes of the Northern Pacific regions and of the Fraser River in British Columbia believed in this doctrine. When a man was sick, it was because the principal soul had left his body, and recovery was only assured when the *shaman* or medicine man had caught the soul and returned it to him. The loss of all souls entailed death. According to Boas, the Amerinds believed that the soul was a physical being, having the shape of a tiny man, and located at the crown of the head. As long as it stood erect, the person to whom it belonged was in good health, but when it lost its upright position for one reason or another, its owner lost his consciousness.

Winds: Diseases were attributed by some Indian tribes to the winds, not in the rational sense, but in the supernatural conception. They believed that the winds themselves were evil spirits. When one contracted a cold, the wind spirits were the cause of it. Disease, they believed, was a punishment for known or unknown sins, committed by themselves, by the family, or even by the community, for breaking a taboo or for disregarding religious regulations. Father Gerste[14] states that in cases of severe illness, the medicine man told the patient that he must have committed some sins, and kept questioning him until he confessed his guilt. The remedy for such disease was purely spiritual.

Deities or Demons: The conception of disease as caused by the deity or by a demon, is still entertained by many Indian tribes. The Iroquoian believed that the evil demon, known as *Hondi*, caused disease and misfortune among man, but when he was appeased by dances and other ceremonies, or by offerings of food or tobacco, he became friendly and protected them from sickness and disease as well as from witchcraft. During the dances, women masked themselves as disease demons with distorted human faces. The Sacs and Foxes believed that the spirit of sickness, *Apenaveni*, hovered about seeking entrance into the huts. Among some tribes of Brazil, when recovery from illness was not expected and when all the arts of the *shaman* had been exercised in vain, last minute appeal was made to "the great water snake," a prominent figure in Indian mythology.

Personification of Disease: Disease was personified by many Indian tribes. It assumed the form and was recognized as having the shape of some object or creature which could only be expelled by a *shaman* who was learned in secret healing methods. The Sioux Indians personified disease as a worm, the Californians as a frog, and the Dakotas as a tortoise.

THE MEDICINE MAN

The medicine man long held sway over the life of the indigenous Americans. At all times he held an important position in the communal life of his tribe and frequently was the chief of his tribe. His office was not obtained by heredity but by choice of the tribe. His position was usually achieved by performing an allegedly miraculous deed, by living a pious or eccentric life, by explaining a dream the interpretation of which later became a reality, or by foretelling successfully events during a state of ecstasy. Women as well as men were eligible for the position of *shaman*. An Apache woman became a *shaman* by escaping death after she was mangled by a mountain lion and struck by lightning. Among the Hopis and the Navahos, boys became medicine men after being trained for many years by older *shamans* in the ritual dances, mysteries, and ceremonies, as well as in the physical therapeutics of their calling. They were, as a rule, permitted to enter the profession after serving as an apprentice to an established practitioner. Of course, those reputed to possess occult powers were preferred.

Medicine men were usually organized into guilds, each having its distinctive secrets, and each practitioner following the accepted secrets of his organization. There was, however, general unanimity of opinion with reference to the administration of medicine.

Despite all the chicanery and deception involved in their practices, the medicine men had complete faith in their own practices and took great pride in their profession. They were respected by the community and were consulted on all matters concerning their tribe. They officiated at births, weddings, and funerals. Their remuneration depended upon the wealth of the patient and was paid in kind, that is with horses, buffaloes, sacks of corn, skins, or utensils. Among some of the Algonquian tribes, wampum was used as a medium of exchange, and was used as his fee.

Lawson gives a graphic description of the methods used by the medicine man:

As soon as the doctor comes into the cabin, the sick person is set on a mat or skin stark naked . . . . . Then the doctor begins and utters some few words very softly; afterwards he smells of the patient's navel and belly; and sometimes scarifies him a little with a flint, or an instrument made of rattlesnake teeth for this purpose; then he sucks the patient and gets out a mouthful of blood and serum, but serum chiefly, which perhaps may be a better method in many cases than to take away great quantities of blood, as is commonly practiced, which he spits in the bowl of water. Then he begins to mutter and talk apace, and at last to cut capers and clap his hands on his breech and sides, till he gets into a sweat, so that a stranger would think that he was running mad, now and then sucking the patient, and so at times keeps sucking till he has got a great quantity of very ill-colored matter out of the belly, arms, breast, forehead, temples, neck and moist parts, still continuing his grimaces and antic postures, which are not to be matched in Bedlam. At last you will see the doctor all over of a dropping sweat, and scarce able to utter one word, having quite spent himself; then he will cease for awhile, and so begin again till he comes in the same pitch of raving and seeming madness as before; all this time the sick body never so much as moves . . . . . At last the conjurer makes an end, and tells the patient's friends whether the patient will live or die; and then one that waits at this ceremony takes the blood away, which remains in a lump in the middle of the water, and buries it in the ground in a place unknown to any one but he that inters it.[15]

HYGIENE AND PROPHYLAXIS

Boas' remarks concerning the Tisimshian Indians of British Columbia may well be applied to other tribes of the redskin. "The Tisimshians," Boas says, "make themselves agreeable to the deity by cleanliness; therefore they must bathe and wash their whole bodies before praying. For the same reason they take a vomitive when they wish to please the deity well. They fast and abstain from touching their wives if they desire their prayer to be successful."

The idea that "cleanliness is next to godliness" was widely spread among the aborigines of America. Bathing and other cleansing practices were commonly employed. Even the most primitive tribesmen were very careful to bathe frequently. This practice began with birth; the newborn infant was plunged into cold water even in the coldest northern weather. The mother also underwent ablution as soon as possible after the birth of a child. The sudatoriums, or sweathouses, were used after menstruation, after coitus, and after coming in contact with the dead. The use of the bath was often accompanied by religious and mystical ceremonies.

Bathing, fasting, and sprinkling the body with water were common practices in connection with games, which often assumed a religious character. Among the Dakotas, Creeks, Ojibways, and Klamaths, hot baths were followed immediately by cold, the person rushing at once from the sweat-house to plunge into the nearest cold stream. The sudatoriums were more than mere cleansing places. They were gathering places of the cultured and the storage houses of the cultural achievements of the indigenous American.

According to Henshaw, sweating was practiced for three different purposes: (1) as a purely religious rite for purifying the body and propitiating the spirits, (2) as a therapeutic measure to combat disease, and (3) as an institution for social and hygienic purposes. In the last case, a number of persons entered the sweat-house influenced by social instinct and appreciation of the luxury of a steam bath.

The sudatoriums were used by boys and girls at the age of puberty for performing the religious rite of initiation into the tribe. They were used before undertaking a special exploit and at time of danger to the tribe. Only the males used the public steam-houses; the females had their own baths.

The sudatorium consisted of a temporary hut, made airtight by animal skins and blankets. The steam was produced by bringing hot stones into the hut and pouring water on them. As a rule not more than four persons occupied the sweat-house at one time. In Mexico pueblo regions and Central America, these structures were dome-shaped and made of stone. The primitive structures were entered by crawling through a hole at a level with the floor. A cap made of bird skin was worn during the procedure.

The Alaskan Eskimo invented a device to protect his lungs from inhaling the fumes of the sudatorium. It was a sort of small gas mask through which air was filtered through layers of grass. This apparatus had a wooden mouthpiece which was placed between the teeth.

Those who found it hard to bear the fumes of the bath-house lay flatly on the floor. The bathers themselves were usually passive. They were often attended by two masked dancers, equipped with horns of a mountain sheep and wearing leather clothing, who brushed them, anointed them with fish oil, and sprinkled them with helebore water. The Navahos concluded the ritualistic bath with a massage.

The baths were considered a panacea for all external and internal diseases and particularly for ailments such as gout, rheumatism, typhoid fever, pneumonia, skin diseases, constipation, and blood poisoning. Bassu ascribes to these steam baths the absence among Indians of gout, kidney gravel, goiter, and obesity. The Cherokees used these sweat baths during a smallpox epidemic in 1865 during which over 300 persons died. In Guatemala, during the grippe epidemic of 1918, the government felt compelled to prohibit the use of steam-houses.

PROGNOSTICATION

Indians, like all ancient peoples, believed in the prognostication of disease. The Central Mexican natives, according to Bartels,[16] believed that if the leaf of a certain plant, when placed on a sore part of the body, stayed, it was a good omen; if it dropped off, death was a certainty. The Mayas of Yucatan used a crystal for the purpose of prognosticating the favorable or unfavorable termination of an ailment.

THERAPEUTICS

Indian therapeutics may be divided into two categories: natural and supernatural. The natural method was practiced when the cause of the ailment or symptoms (with few exceptions they did not identify the disease as a whole, but treated the symptoms), was evident. On the other hand, when the cause was obscured or when natural remedies were of no help and the case appeared hopeless, occult treatment was resorted to. But even when natural remedies were used, they were accompanied by mystic formulas. The plants or herbs were collected at night or before sunrise when the tribe was asleep. The nature of medicines used for severe diseases was kept secret. Drugs were administered in a single large dose, usually in the form of a decoction or infusion, but occasionally as a powder or inhalation. Religious rites were always observed.[17]

Isolation

The Aztecs, according to Gerste, treated severe diseases where death might be expected in a very strange way. The family of the patient carried him to the highest point of a nearby mountain; they gave him food and a vessel of water and left him to die or to recover, as the case might be, forbidding all persons to see him. The isolation of the sick was intended to keep away evil spirits. It was the custom of the Winnebagos of Wisconsin and the Mosquitos of Honduras to surround the sick bed with poles, on which various animals were hung, or to hedge the patient in with painted sticks, allowing no one but the medicine man to approach the spot.[18]

Scapegoats

The idea of surrounding the sick with animals and other objects was perhaps to use them as a scapegoat and transfer the disease to them. Many Indian tribes believed that an ailment could be transferred from one person to another or from a person to an animal. The Aztecs of ancient Mexico, according to Gerste,[19] tried to relieve fever by transferring it to a figure of a dog made of maize flour, which was then placed in a maguey plant on the public highway. It was believed that the first passerby would take over the fever, thus enabling the patient to recover. The natives of Peru were in the habit of exposing the clothes of the sick on the public highway in the belief that a passerby would take the disease upon himself and so relieve the patient.

The idea of unloading disease on others was, and still is, a common practice in the east. The Hindus in Vedic times used a blue jay as a scapegoat to whom they transferred consumption by whispering, "Consumption fly away, fly away with the blue jay."

The Romans allegedly cured fever by paring the patient's nails and sticking them on a neighbor's door with wax before sunrise. The fever then was supposed to pass from the sick person to the neighbor. In Bavaria, the healer wrote upon a piece of paper, "Fever, stay away, I'm not at home," and placed the paper in the pocket of the first passerby. The fever then passed, it was thought, from the patient to the stranger.

The natives of the Orkney Islands bathed the sick person and spilled the water near the gate of the village in the belief that the disease would be transferred to the first person who stepped on it.

In Oldenburg, one contracting a fever placed a bowl of sweet milk before a dog and murmured, "Good luck, ye hound, may ye be sick and I be sound." The Australian magician agreed to take over the disease into himself by sucking out the evil witchcraft.

Scapegoats were used particularly for transferring of warts. One method was to have the patient touch the wart with a pebble, place the pebble in a bag, and drop it in the street. The first one who picked up the pebble was said to get the wart. Another method was to steal a piece of bacon, rub it on the wart, and slip the bacon under the bark of a tree. In this case the wart was said to disappear from the skin and appear on the bark of the tree. Still another remedy was to tie as many knots in a hair as there were warts on the body and throw the hair away; if a person could be found foolish enough to pick up the hair and count the knots, he would surely take over the warts.[20]

In Germany, the healer who attended to wounds placed the removed plasters and dressings at a crossway in order to transfer the disease to a passerby. Tyler[21] states that the bunches of flowers offered by children to travelers in Southern Europe are sometimes intended for an ungracious purpose, the transferring of disease. Persons in Eastern Europe hesitate to pick up an article found on the highway for fear that someone has left it for malevolent purposes. Perschel remembers being warned never to pick up a flower lying in the road; for one cannot tell the motive of the person who threw it away.[22]

Ehrenreich reports that the Caraya Indians of Brazil inquire of every stranger, "Have you a catarrh?" They permit the stranger to enter their cabins only after being assured that there is no danger of consumption. These Indians evidently well recognize the infectious character of this disease.[23]

Medical Guilds

The Amerind treatment of disease varied from the procedures of the medicine man, who used incantations, dancing, noises made with rattles and drums, and the practice of laying the hands on the affected part and pretending to extract the principle causing the disease from the body by sucking the injured part, to more elaborate and highly developed ritual activities practiced by the medical leagues for the benefit of the family or the community.

Hrdlica[24] states that certain stocks of Indians were organized in guilds and on special occasions performed curative or life-giving ceremonies, which consisted of songs, prayers, rituals, and drum rhythms. The ceremony extended over a period of from a few hours to nine days. The healing ceremonies were exceedingly elaborate both in ritual and in paraphernalia. According to Dorsey,[25] the principal purpose of such ceremonies was to heal the ailing person, but the aim as well was to implore the gods for various blessings, not only for the sick but for all who participated in the ceremony, and their friends and relations. In most instances, the patient defrayed the expense of the ceremony.

Among the Navahos, the *shaman* employed a large number of fetishes and amulets, on the principle of *similia similibus curantur*. The fetishes used were made from peculiarly shaped stones or wooden objects, feathers, claws, hair, fingers, or mystic animals, which were fashioned to resemble the diseased part of the body. They were supposed to embody mysterious powers capable of preventing and counteracting the ailments. Sympathetic magic was also resorted to.[26]

The *shaman*, while officiating for the sick, frequently disguised himself in the skin of an animal in order to inspire fear and confidence in the patient. At all times, the *shaman* wore a distinctive form of dress while carrying out the healing ritual. The dress varied, in accordance with the disease he was about to cure, from the most ridiculous to the finest examples of Indian art. Members belonging to "medical societies" wore the costumes of the society. Some tribes conducted ceremonies for the purpose of rendering the medicine man more powerful through intimate communion with supernatural agents. These ceremonies entailed public performances to impress the people with his magical skill.

Treatment of Specific Diseases

Malaria: Malarial fever was commonly encountered by the ancients and was one of the few diseases identified by antiquity. They recognized its symptoms, which consisted of chills, fever, moist and dry skin, muscular pain, thirst, and prostration, but did not know its true cause. The sudden onset of chills and fever prompted ancient man to view it as the work of an avenging spirit; consequently, heroic treatment was indicated. As in all cases of possession, occult measures were first resorted to. When these were exhausted, natural remedies, such as, rest, purgation, diuretics, and a liquid diet were employed. Some tribes practiced phlebotomy to combat fever. Other remedies employed were watermelon and decoctions of the leaves of wild sage and the leaves and bark of the willow and dogwood trees.

Diseases of Lungs and Chest: Diseases of the lungs and chest were fairly well understood by the American Indians. They did not differentiate between the various types of bronchitis or between pneumonia and pleurisy, treating all as one disease. Because of the climatic changes in the rigorous climate of the north and in the neighborhood of the Great Lakes, the natives in these regions were subject to respiratory diseases. They used the same remedies for all chest affections associated with cough or painful respiration.[27]

For the relief of pain in the chest, cupping over a wide area of the chest was practiced, followed by oral suction. They used as a cup the horn of a buffalo from which the pointed end was removed; a negative pressure was effected by sucking through the small end. The Chinese method of applying *moxas* was known to the indigenous Americans. They used certain crushed plant's stems, moistened them with saliva, lighted them, and allowed them to burn down to the skin. They also used animal dung, various seeds, and punkwood for this purpose.

Among drugs used for chest affections were decoctions of sassafras and infusion of leaves of flax. Some of these remedies are still considered helpful in bronchial diseases. They employed decoctions of the nuts and leaves of red cedar and also inhaled its burning twigs. Holly plants were used in the form of decoctions as an expectorant. The head of a sunflower in the form of a decoction was used for the same purpose. Hot decoctions of basil were used as an expectorant.

Rheumatism, Arthritis, and Neuritis: The exposure to the inclement weather and the dampness of the caves, tents, and huts where they dwelled exposed the indigenous Americans to attacks of rheumatism, arthritis, and neuritis. As in the case of respiratory diseases, they did not classify these ailments but considered them as one. The remedies for the relief of these diseases were many. The most important therapeutic agent was the steam-house, described previously in the present chapter. Perhaps these painful affections influenced the Amerinds to establish steam-houses in every village.

The Dakotas and the Ponchas from Omaha applied the crushed leaves of pasque flowers to the skin over the affected parts, which acted as a counterirritant, producing a blister. Other remedies employed locally were the balm of Gilead, hot applications of jalap slit root, hot poultices of sheep dung, and sprigs of cactus plant ground and powdered on the surface. Internally, decoctions of bugbain and many others were used.

An early traveler describes a decoction of a certain mushroom, which was used in Mexico as an intoxicant and an anodyne. The peyote bean (also known as devil's food) was used by the Apache for the same purpose. One bean is said to produce loss of muscular co-ordination and exhilaration followed by visual hallucinations of swirling colors.

Jimson weed *(Datura stramonium)* was another plant that produced delirium, which state, the Indians believed, enabled the *shaman* to communicate with the spirits. In large doses it was thought to act as an aphrodisiac. It was known to many of the tribesmen and was given to youths during the ceremony of their initiation into manhood.

Gastrointestinal Disorders: By far the most frequent ailment of the American Indian was gastrointestinal malfunction. Realizing the cause to be indiscretions of diet, he resorted largely to natural remedies in treating gastroenterological ailments. He treated such symptoms as gastric distress, colicky pains, flatulence, nausea, vomiting, diarrhea, and constipation. He employed emetics daily. He produced emesis by inserting a feather at the back of the palate. His pharmacopeia was rich in roots and herbs that would produce emesis. Some of the remedies were decoctions of holly leaves, bloodwort, and butterfly weed. Decoctions of wild verbena were taken internally for gastralgia. Infusion of wild mint acted as a carminative. Pounded ragweed was applied locally, after the abdomen was scarified; it acted as a counter-irritant. Salines in the form of magnesia salt found in the mineral springs were used as a purgative. As a remedy for constipation the leaves and husks of cereal and grass pulp were employed. Decoctions of aloes, the bark of the sycamore tree, or powdered jalap root were used in obstinate constipation. Some used a syringe to induce bowel evacuation. The syringe was made of an animal bladder attached to a hollow long bone of a turkey.

Cardiovascular Diseases: Few primitives understood the mechanism of the heart and circulation; they commonly confused cardiac disease with chest affections. Consequently, few remedies were listed for cardiovascular diseases.

Edema: An ailment which the indigenous Americans could not help recognizing was dropsy. The causes of this condition were not known to him, and he attributed it to the entrance of an evil spirit into the patient. In this case, as in other diseases which he suspected were of a spiritual nature, the medicine man resorted to natural drugs after his ritualistic measures were exhausted. External medicaments consisted of tobacco leaves and scarification. Internal medication consisted of infusions and decoctions of wintergreen, yarrow, sarsaparilla, juniper, and magnolia.

Neurological Disorders: Neurological disorders were not common among the Indians. Insanity was comparatively rare. Mild forms of nervous depression and hysteria responded satisfactorily to the medicine man's theatrical performance and to his clever ritual. In this branch of medicine he was a master.

First-Aid Treatment: The prehistoric Indian frequently was bitten by snakes and scorpions, and for these, remedies were naturally plentiful. First-aid treatment consisted of suction applied to the bitten area or excision of the tissues around the wound. This was followed by various local applications.

Among the southwestern tribes, snakebite was treated by applying to the wound a portion of the ventral surface of the snake that had done the damage. Crickets, lizards, spiders, and spider eggs were used by some tribes.

The Navahos used red ochre combined with fat to prevent sunburn. The Hopis blew charcoal ashes or other products of fire on an inflamed surface to counteract the supposed fire which caused the ailment. The oil and grease of certain animals were used externally and internally as antidotes. Scorpion oil was used in Central Mexico for scorpion bites. Among Brazilians, infected areas were plastered with feathers.

Drugs

The greatest mass of primitive remedies was derived from the vegetable kingdom. Roots, twigs, limbs, bark, flowers, and seeds were employed, usually as decoctions made either from fresh or dry plants, but sometimes as powder.

Signature: The concept of "signature" largely influenced the use of plants in medicine. This doctrine was probably the earliest therapeutic system in the history of medicine. It was based on the belief that the Creator stamped all objects medically beneficial to mankind, and on the assumption that there was a connection of every part of the human body with a corresponding part in the world of nature. This hypothesis originated in the ancient idea that man was a microcosm (little world), and each anatomical part of man had a counterpart in the macrocosm (larger world). Accordingly, disease readily responded to remedies bearing some real, symbolical, or fanciful resemblance to the diseased part, either in appearance or structure. The doctrine of signature presupposed that there were specifics for all pathologic conditions, if man could only recognize them. Color and shape were the two principal factors in selecting remedies. Persons troubled with jaundice were treated with yellow drugs. Disease characterized by redness of the skin was treated by covering the patient with scarlet blankets. Red color was considered an acceptable substitute for blood. Liverwort was employed in combating liver ailments because its leaf was shaped like a liver. Lungwort, the leaves of which bore a fancied resemblance to the surface of the lungs, was considered good for pulmonary complaints. Heart-shaped leaves were placed over the sore breasts of a nursing woman.[28]

Number of Remedies: The number of herb remedies was quite large. The Ojibways, according to Hoffman, counted eighty-nine different medicinal plants.[29] The Hopi Indians, according to Hough,[30] counted forty-five different therapeutic plants. Several North American tribes used as many as 160 indigenous species. Fifty-nine of them are found in our pharmacopeia. The Indians possessed a large number of plant remedies for cuts, burns, bruises, wounds, bites, stings, and gastrointestinal disorders.[31]

The planting and gathering of medicinal plants were associated with certain ceremonies. Both priests and laymen smoked plants which were strongly narcotic and caused them to become ecstatic and to see strange visions.

Tobacco: Few herbs have occupied as important a position in religious and medical folklore as tobacco. It was known as the "holy herb" and, among many Indian tribes, it was reserved exclusively for the use of priests, sorcerers, and medicine men who employed it for religious and magical purposes. They chewed tobacco often in conjunction with coca before they were ready to communicate with the "Great Spirit." The use of it made them see strange phantoms and induced in them exhilaration accompanied by shouting and dancing.

To the Ottawas, tobacco was a sacred plant. They used it to quiet the waves of the Great Lakes that threatened their safety. There, while the waves crashed and foamed at their feet, they lifted their eyes to the sky, addressed an invocation to the "Great Spirit," and scattered over the troubled waters large pieces of tobacco.

Tobacco played a prominent part during all solemn occasions in peace and in war. The calumet (peace pipe) had a great symbolic value. An herb capable of possessing such power was destined to make a strong impression on native medical folklore. The idea prevailed that all plants coming from the New World possessed healing virtues. The favorable reports of tobacco's medical potency received from the colonies soon gave this plant a therapeutic prestige in the mother countries of Europe.[32]

John Josselyn, an Englishman who lived in the early settlement of Massachusetts, left an interesting account regarding the use of tobacco among the Indians:

> The vertues of Tobbacco are these, it helps digestion, the Gout, the Tooth-ache, prevents infection by scents, it heats the cold and cools them that sweat, feedeth the hungry, spent spirits restoreth, purgeth the stomach. killeth nits and lice; the juice of the green leaf healeth green wounds, although poysoned; the Syrup for many diseases, the smoak for the Phythisick, cough of the lungs, distillation of Rheume, and all diseases of a cold and moist cause, good for all bodies cold and moist taken upon an emptie stomach, taken upon a full stomach it precipitates digestion, immoderately taken it dryeth the body; enflameth the blood, hurteth the brain, weakens the eyes and sinews.[33]

Intoxicating Drinks: In South America, a number of intoxicating or stupefying drinks from plant juices were employed by the Indians on ceremonial occasions. Getting drunk was not an uncommon practice on festive occasions among certain tribes of Brazil and Paraguay. According to Hrdlicka,[34] a species of *Datura* (poisonous plant) was added to the liquor to make it stronger and increase its medical virtues. Certain Californians made drinks from *manzanita* berries. *Peytol* and a certain variety of cactus plant were extensively used in the north of Mexico for ceremonial and medicinal purposes.

Surgery

Trephination: The knowledge of surgery of the prehistoric American was limited to setting of fractured bones, reducing dislocations, treating wounds, stopping hemorrhages, and performing one major surgical operation—trephination. This operation was practiced by the Peruvians and the Pueblos and especially by the Andean Indians. The original purpose of its performance has not been made clear. It might have been done to relieve pressure on the brain produced by a fracture of the skull or, as some supposed, in order to permit the evil spirit causing persistent headache to pass through the opening in the skull. The operation might also have been performed just before death for the purpose of permitting the soul to escape the dying body.

In most of the trephined skulls found in Peru, the perforation was made in the right parietal bone; less often the opening was made through the frontal and occipital bones. One operation was the rule, but as many as five openings have been found in some skulls. Hrdlicka[35]

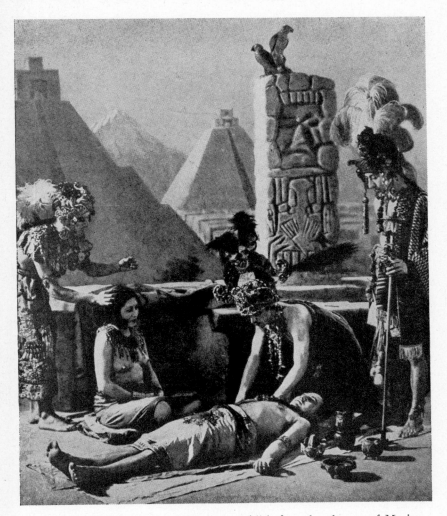

Fig. 97: In the great Aztec Empire, established on the plateaus of Mexico, the physicians played an important role, though their practice contained some mysticism. The Spanish conquerors wrote of the high standards of surgery and the excellent wound hygiene. Sutures were made from human hair, and effective methods of splinting fractures were developed. (Courtesy of Davis and Geck, Inc.; as depicted by an artist.)

states: "The highest surgical achievement, undoubtedly practiced in part as a curative method, was trephining." This operation was of common occurrence, and is still practiced in Peru where it reached its highest development among the American tribes.

Trephining was also known in quite recent times among the Tara-humare of Chihuahua, but has never been found north of Mexico. It has been estimated that about 2.5 per cent of the Peruvian population were trephined; some survived the operation, as is evident from the healed skulls. Those who succumbed were probably thought to have been hopelessly possessed by the demon. The instruments employed for the operation were largely made of flint, obsidian, and quartz.[36]

Care of Fractures: Fractures were fairly well taken care of by the American Indians. They had for long ages used bark splints which were bandaged around a broken limb with great care. Unfortunately, they usually did not attempt to set the fractured bone before applying the splint; the results, therefore, were often not satisfactory. Some tribes fashioned splints from raw hide; when the leather dried, the splints became immobile.[37] Karl Jaeger found 53.8 per cent of neolithic bones, which had been broken during life, to have healed with good union as compared with 46.2 per cent which had united badly.

Bone setting was accomplished quite cleverly by a number of tribes all over the continent, particularly the Sioux Indians, the Winnebagos, the Creeks of the southeastern United States, some of the groups of the North Pacific Coast, and certain Brazilian tribes.[38]

With reference to dislocations, the results appear to have been satisfactory. Stone cites a case of an Indian hunter who reduced his own hip dislocation. He was alone in the woods when his leg caught in a tree and his hip joint became dislocated. He managed to reduce it himself.

Amputation: Amputation of the limbs does not seem to have been practiced among the American Indians, even among the tribes which were skillful in bone setting. Amputation of the digits was frequently practiced, not as a surgical measure to relieve an abnormal condition, but more as a religious rite. Frequently digital amputation was meted out as a punishment for violating a taboo.

Certain Amazon tribes carried the theory of localized demoniacal possession to its logical conclusion. If the pain, swelling, or whatever the symptoms were, did not respond to the ritual procedure, the surgeon amputated the affected area and thus made quite sure to dispose of the demon responsible. There is no evidence that the prehistoric American directed his attention to muscle surgery. Nothing has remained of the soft tissues to warrant an opinion. One can only turn the spotlight on the modern Indian to see how he treats wounds in order to infer how his prehistoric ancestors treated them.

Bloodletting: John Lawson, who traveled in the Carolinas in 1700, recorded an incident among the Tuscaroras which he witnessed. He saw an Indian medicine man administering to a young woman suffering from "fits." He placed her "on her belly and made a small incision with rattlesnake teeth; then laying his mouth to the place he sucked out nearly a quart of black, coagulated blood and serum."

On another occasion, Lawson states that one of his companions became lame in one knee. The chief, at whose abode they were staying, after looking at the injured member, proceeded as follows:

. . . pulled out an instrument something like a comb, which was made of split reed with fifteen teeth of rattlesnakes, set at much the same distance as in a large horn comb. With these he scratched the place where the lameness chiefly lay till the blood came, bathing it both before and after the incision with warm water spurted out of his mouth; this done, he ran into his plantation and got some sassafras root, which grows there in great plenty, dried it in the embers, scraped off the outward rind, and having beat it between two stones, applied it to the part afflicted, binding it up well. Thus in a day or two the patient became sound.[39]

Treatment of Wounds: As a local application on wounds, certain Indian tribes applied leaves of plants or cobwebs in association with incantations. The last were calculated to impress the patient and his anxious relatives. In a few instances, attempts were made at minor wound surgery.

It is likely that several methods were employed in the treatment of wounds among the neolithic Indians. The Dakotas, for example, were accustomed to flush a wound with water squirted from a syringe, using the bladder of a sheep attached to a quill of a turkey.

Another primitive technique was that of closing a wound by means of the powerful jaws of a leaf-cutter ant. After the edges of the wound were approximated and the ant's jaws were set, the body of the ant was cut off. This method of closing wounds anticipated the device of Michel, whose metal clips are widely used at the present time.

Foreign Bodies: Most tribes recognized the obvious necessity of removing foreign substances from the body. They used not only their fingers but also their teeth to extract them.

Judging from the surgery of the head performed by the neolithic men, one carries away the impression that the prehistoric Indian had more surgical boldness than the modern Indian.

Resistance to Pain and Healing Power: It is the opinion of many observers that Indians are better able to resist pain and surgical shock than white men and that their wounds heal easier and more quickly.

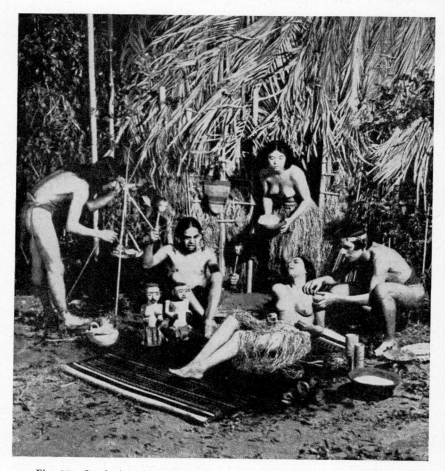

Fig. 98: South American natives have, for generations, used the large, leaf-cutting, Sauba ant in closing wounds. The ant is permitted to bite through the approximated edges; and since its tenaculum-like jaws retain their grip after death, the body is then pinched off. A row of these ant heads and lo!—they have Nature's challenge to the modern skin clip. (Courtesy of Davis and Geck, Inc.; as depicted by an artist.)

The reasons are not clear. Stone mentions the case, reported by Bourke, of two wounded Indians who were discharged from a military hospital as hopeless cases. Both were permitted to leave the hospital so that they could die among their own people, and both recovered after treatment by their medicine man. Could the redskin's healing herbs be a factor in such cases, or is their resistance to infection naturally better?

Some writers attribute such remarkable occurrences among Indians to hygienic regulations. Indians, they say, understood the value of cleanliness when treating external injuries and kept their sick scrupulously clean. They used many types of dressings and dressed wounds frequently. To treat large wounds, the Dakotas and the Winnebagos used stitches of thread made of sinews, needles made of bone, and drainage wicks made of pieces of cloth or twists of fiber. In cases of contusion, they used helebore or tobacco poultices. Water-lily roots were applied to granulations, and pitch was used as a salve.

Hemorrhage: The Amerinds had many methods to stop bleeding in the various parts of the body. The North American tribes filled a bleeding wound with some dry powder used as a styptic and then applied firm pressure, bandaging tightly with strips of bark. The Miscarleros packed oozing wounds with eagles' down or with scrapings from the inside of a freshly tanned hide. The Haidas packed bleeding wounds with spider webs. The Dakotas used hot ashes for epistaxis. The Brazilian Carayas used a binder on the limbs in case of severe bleeding. All tribes knew the use of the tourniquet.

Obstetrics

Labor and Delivery: Obstetrics was practiced by women. Labor was connected with little pain and rarely lasted more than three hours. The Navaho and Apache women assumed a semirecumbent position during delivery. The parturient Crow knelt during labor and rested her head against a support, while the midwife pressed her hand on the back of the woman during her labor pains. The Sioux women and the squaws of the Warm Spring were delivered while standing. The Creeks reclined on their stomachs with pillows strapped to the epigastrium; as labor progressed, the strap was tightened. In most cases, where the squaws were delivered in a kneeling position, they stood upright after the fetus passed to deliver the placenta.

Indian women were often delivered in their huts while the members of the family were sent away. The tribes of the Plains erected huts in bushes away from the village and near a stream, where they placed their pregnant women during confinement. Among some tribes (for example the Sioux and the Umquas), friends and relatives were invited to witness the birth. Among most tribes, however, the confinement was witnessed by two women friends or midwives.

In prolonged labor, the midwives performed abdominal manipulations to correct the fetal position; if this failed, a number of novel techniques were employed. In one of these, the midwife knelt behind the laboring woman locking her fingers over the patient's abdomen and exerting downward pressure. In another, the Sioux warrior walked about, carrying his woman on his back with her abdomen pressing on his back. The Dakotas placed a wide strap around the abdomen and tightened it. The Nez Perces turned the woman upside down and shook her. If these devices were not effective, the midwife inserted her hand in the vagina and attempted to pull on any part that was presented.[40]

Some tribes used psychotherapeutic measures to induce labor. They posted a man with a gun, and at a signal he fired a shot. The fright sometimes seemed to bring on delivery.

In spite of all this rude management on the part of the midwife, the mortalities of mother and child were low. Stone quotes Dr. Feed of the United States Army, who was for many years in intimate contact with one tribe, to the effect that he knew of no maternal deaths and only one death of a child during labor. Another observer tells of one maternal death in 800 deliveries, and this was due to transverse position.

Complications: Diseases like eclampsia, puerperal sepsis, and postpartum hemorrhage, which are responsible for much of the obstetrical mortality among white women, were rare among the Indians.

Abortion: Abortion was resorted to rarely and only on occasions where the pregnancy of the Indian woman was caused by contact with a white man. Indians did not tolerate half-breed babies. Abortion was induced by some tribes by trodding on the pregnant woman's abdomen; others placed a board across the abdomen with women on both ends of it who seesawed up and down. Frequently, slippery-elm sticks were inserted in the cervical canal. As abortifacients for internal use, decoctions of scrapings of bear claws, of ground cedar, of the inner bark of pine, or of powdered rattlesnake were used.[41]

Phlebotomy

Bloodletting was practiced in ancient Peru and Mexico and also by the Brazilian Carayas, Central Californians, and certain tribes of the Isthmian region of Central America. The place of venesection differed according to the location of the disease.[42] The Carayas incised a vein of the forehead for headache, and the ancient Peruvians cut into the veins at the root of the nose for the same condition. The Indians of Honduras opened the veins of the leg or shoulder in diseases of the lower parts of the body. Certain tribes of the Isthmian region are said to have practiced bloodletting by shooting a small arrow from a special bow into a vein of the part of the body affected.

Implements used for scarification were sharp pieces of stone, bits of shell, pieces of flint and obsidian, thorns, fish spines, or teeth of animals. Some tribes developed special instruments for this purpose.

Cauterization was accomplished with smoldering cedar bark, and this method is still in use by several tribes in the North Pacific Coast. California tribes cauterized a chancre with hot coal. They considered this condition to be of a local nature. Many North American Indians practiced cauterization for all obstinate soreness.

As mentioned above, cupping was used among many tribes. The horn of a buffalo with the narrow end cut off was frequently used as a cup.[43]

AMERIND CONTRIBUTIONS TO MODERN MEDICINE

While most Indian medicine was of an empiric nature, there were some remedies discovered by the Amerinds that have made a distinct contribution to the modern art of healing. One of these was quinine, extracted from the bark of the cinchona tree. It was used by the Indians to combat malarial fever. Another was cocaine, prepared from the leaves of the coca bush, and used as a narcotic. The Spaniards rationed it to their workers to relieve pain and to stop the monotony of endless labors which they imposed upon the natives. This drug, in many instances, gave the invaders a more complete control over the Indians than any other effort to subdue them.[44]

Dr. Lyman mentions that the *hechiceras* (Indian medicine man) used Eriodictyon glutinosum, which grows profusely on our foothills, in afflictions of the respiratory tract. So efficacious and valuable did it prove to the missionaries that they called it *yerba santa,* or "holy plant." The Rhamnus purshiana, which grows luxuriantly in the timbered mountains of Southern California, was used extensively as a cathartic. So highly esteemed was it by the followers of the Cross that they christened it *cascara sagrada,* or "sacred bark." Grindelia robusta was used in pulmonary diseases and as external applications following exposure to Rhus toxicodendron, or poison oak.[45]

PSYCHOSOMATIC AND BACTERIAL ORIGINS OF DISEASE

The etiology of disease was viewed rationally among some tribes. According to the "Jesuit Relations," the Iroquois considered ailments to be the result of unsatisfied craving. Among the main sources of disease was the fact that the mind of the patient himself, who desired something, would vex his body until he possessed the thing required. Their concept was that there are in every man certain inborn desires often unknown to himself upon which his happiness depends. For the purpose of ascertaining the desire and innate appetite, they summoned soothsayers who, as they thought, had divinely imparted power to look into the innermost recesses of the head. The Myettas had an idea that sickness was brought about by insects flying in the air.[46] The first idea of disease anticipated the psychotherapy of Freud; the second, the bacterial origin of disease.

References and Notes

1. Packard, F. R.: History of Medicine in the United States, 1:19.
2. Chamberlain, A. F.: Hastings Encyclopedia, 4:731-741.
3. "History of Medicine in the United States," 2:910.
4. Ritchie, W. A.: Prehistoric Fortified Village Site at Canandaigua, Ontario County, New York.
5. Hrdlica, A.: Seven Prehistorical Skulls with Complete Absence of the External Auditory Meatus. Am. J. Phys. Anthropol., 17:355, 1933.
6. MacCurdy, G. G.: Human Skeletal Remains From the Highlands of Peru. Ibid., 6:217.
7. Ashmead: Am. J. Dermatol., pp. 226-228, 1908.
8. "Hastings Encyclopedia," 4:731-741.
9. Krogman, W. M.: Ciba Symposia, pp. 111-117, April, 1939.
10. Lawson, J.: History of North Carolina, 1709. Cited by Packard, F. R.: 1:23.
11. Gooking, D.: Historical Collections of the Proceedings of the Plantation at Plymouth (1612-1613), reprinted in the Mass. Historical Society Collections, Series 1, 1:148. Cited by Packard, F. R.: p. 66.
12. Ploss: "Das Weib" in der Natur und Volkskunde. Leipzig, 1891.
13. Boas, F.: The Doctrine of Souls and of Disease among the Chenook Indian. I.A.F.L., 1893, pp. 39-43.
14. Gerste: Sur la medicina et la botanique des anciens Mexicaines. Paris, 1910, p. 19.
15. Cited by Packard, F. R.: p. 21.
16. Bartels: Die Medezin der Naturvoelker. Leipzig, 1893, p. 168.
17. "Sur la medicina et la botonique des anciens Mexicaines," p. 242.
18. "Die Medezin der Naturvoelker," p. 244.
19. "Sur la medicina et la botanique des anciens Mexicaines," p. 47.
20. Strack, J. L.: Aberglaube und Sagen aus dem Herzogthum Oldenburg, 1867, p. 71.
21. Tyler: Primitive Culture, 2:150.
22. Perschel, O.: The Races of Man. D. Appleton-Century Co., New York, p. 342.
23. Cited by Bartels: p. 238.
24. Hrdlica, A.: Bull. 30, Bur. Ethno., Smithsonian Institute, Part I, p. 838.

25. Dorsey, G. A.: Anth. Pub. Field Columbia Museum, IX, 1905. Cited by
    Hrdlica, A.: Note 24, p. 229.
26. Hrdlica, A.: p. 837.
27. Much of the Amerind's healing measures in this chapter were drawn from
    Stone, E.: Medicine Among the American Indians, Paul B. Hoeber, Inc.,
    New York, to which work I am greatly indebted.
28. For a fuller description on the subject of "Signature" see Gordon, B. L.: Ro-
    mance of Medicine, F. A. Davis Co., Philadelphia, p. 367.
29. Hoffman, W. J.: Grand Medicine. Society of the Ojibway, 7, R.B.E.W., 1891,
    pp. 143-300.
30. Hough: American Anthropology, 1898.
31. "Die Medezin der Naturvoelker," p. 209.
32. "Romance of Medicine," pp. 417-449.
33. "History of Medicine in the United States," pp. 19-20.
34. Hrdlica, A.: p. 837.
35. Ibid., p. 838.
36. Von Storch, T. C.: American Medical History, 1930, 2:614.
37. Morice, Father, A. G.: T. Roy. Canad. Inst., 7:15-27, 1901.
38. "Medicine Among the American Indians," p. 82.
39. "History of North Carolina," p. 26. Cited by Packard.
40. "Medicine Among the American Indians," pp. 71-76.
41. Ibid.
42. "Die Medezin der Naturvoelker," p. 269.
43. Chamberlain, A. F.: Proc. American Antiquitics Soc., 16:91, 1905. See also
    Hastings Encyclopedia, 4:731-741.
44. Brown, M. J.: America's Yesterday. J. B. Lippincott Co., 1937, p. 228.
45. Cited by Packard, 2:910.
46. Palmer, R. A.: The North American Indian. Smithsonian Institute Series, 1929,
    4:8.

Part II

THE GRECO-ROMAN PERIOD

15

Dawn of Greek Medicine

THE most interesting and significant records on medicine of antiquity are furnished by ancient Hellas. These may be divided into three periods: (1) Aesculapian, (2) Homeric, and (3) Hippocratic. In the first period, preceding the Trojan wars, Greek medicine was a mixture of empirical remedies, theurgic rites, and priestly magic.

AESCULAPIAN MEDICINE

The first period of Greek medicine is veiled in mystery. The greater part of their erudition was borrowed from the priests and magicians of Egypt and perhaps also from the Brahman priests of India. It is a question whether the Greeks of this period acquired any substantial stock of medical formulas not known to the Egyptians. But, however disguised, early Greek medicine is, by its nomenclature, clinical description, medical divinities, and mythology, the successor and disciple of Egypt in much the same fashion as Rome at a later date followed Greece. The medical divinities of Egypt, Apis, Serapis, Isis, Osiris, and Thoth, are related to the Greek Apollo, Minerva, Hermes, Orpheus, and Aesculapius.

Early Greek Physicians

Orpheus: Orpheus, the son of Apollo and Calliope, according to a mythological account, inherited from his mother the power of producing melodies, and from his father, skill in the healing art. Orpheus, according to tradition, was a pupil of Melampus, the reputed son of Amytheon and Drippe, and the counterpart of the Egyptian Hiero-Ietero, who demonstrated his skill in the healing art and his fam-

433

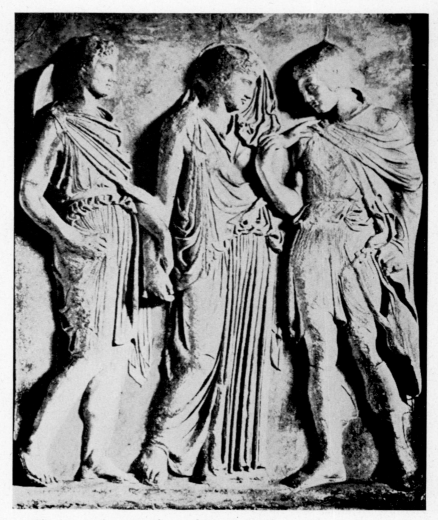

Fig. 99: Orpheus, Eurydice, and Hermes. Orpheus (on the *right*) was permitted to regain his mate Eurydice from Hades on condition that he would not
look behind him on the journey. When he violated this agreement, Hermes (on
the *left*) had to take her back to the underworld. (Greek marble relief of the
fifth century B.C., now in the National Museum in Naples.)

iliarity with healing plants. The name "Melampus" has been preserved in the plant, melampodium, a genus of hellebore, with which
Melampus successfully cured the daughters of Proetus, King of Argos,
from attacks of insanity.

Melampus: Melampus was the founder of the "family of seers" who, according to Herodotus,[1] acquired the art of divination from the Egyptians. A popular legend tells how, in consequence of his having his ears cleansed by a snake, he became proficient in prophecy and magic and, by magical means, enabled Iphiklos to regain his lost virility. Another legend relates that he cured the celibate women of Argos who, in numbers, became obsessed with the thought that they had been transformed into cows and roamed the fields and wild forests aimlessly. Melampus ordered them to bathe in the fountain of the Anigridian nymphs. The water from this font was considered highly efficacious also in combating skin eruptions and herpes.

According to another version, Melampus, having observed the purgative effect of helebore upon goats, treated the women with the milk in which white hellebore had been steeped. While these remedies, of course, were not particularly effective against monomania, the treatment might be regarded as natural (if not quite rational) and therefore contrary to the occult practices of the day. It is further related that King Proetus, in appreciation of the excellent remedies administered to his daughters, presented Melampus with half of his kingdom as an honorarium.

Chiron: Another of the early Greek physicians was the fabulous Chiron. According to a Greek mythological tale, he was the fifth son of Cronus and Philyra, whose equestrian skill gave him the reputation of having been a centaur—a compound of man and horse. The mighty Apollo was indebted to him for instruction in music and medicine. Chiron supervised the expedition of the siege of Troy in 1192 B.C., on all matters pertaining to medicine and surgery. Chiron dwelt on Mt. Pelion and was famous for his great wisdom. Many of the celebrated heroes of Greece were brought up and instructed by him.[2] Tradition speaks of Chiron's pharmaceutical skill rather than of his surgical achievements. He was known for the "hand applied to the skin with magic effect."

According to Xenophon, Chiron had a number of famous disciples: Achilles, remembered in anatomy for a tendon he discovered (*tendo achillis*); Amphiarus, who died on the way to Thebes, where he was taken against his will; Castor, who was said to be the first to employ pepperwort in epilepsy; Hippolyte, the son of the famous physician Theseus, who was restored to life by Aesculapius at the intercession of Diana; and last, but not least, Aesculapius.

Chiron lived in a period of transition from occult to empirical therapeutics. Incantation was not used by itself, as it was among the

Babylonians and Egyptians, but in conjunction with physical remedies.[3] According to the fourth and tenth books of the Iliad, Aesculapius and Achilles received efficacious drugs from Chiron. The first received the remedy for relieving pain and the second, for assuring

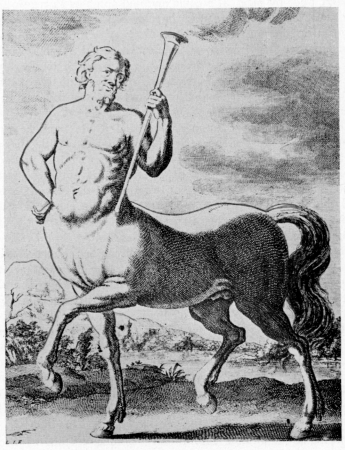

Fig. 100: Chiron Centaurus. Chiron Centaurus, a legendary figure, was a compound of man and horse. According to legend, Chiron supervised the expedition of the siege of Troy in 1192 B.C. on matters pertaining to medicine and surgery. Apollo was indebted to him for instruction in medicine and music, and Aesculapius for his knowledge of medicine. (From an old print.)

hemostasis. The art of military surgery, which was free from magic, is traced back to Chiron.

For centuries down to modern times, there was a tribe near Mt. Pelion, claiming descent from Chiron. They had a tradition that a

certain sacred herblore was handed down to them from father to
son from their early progenitor Chiron. The Magnesians sacrificed
the first-fruits of the herbs and plants to this divine physician. In
another district, near Mt. Pelion, a certain plant grew which had the
reputation of possessing miraculous virtues. The extent of Chiron's
medical skill, as handed down by tradition, is summarized by Pindar
in the curriculum of his pupil, Aesculapius.

Chiron, according to another mythologic tale, was accidentally
pierced by a poison arrow dispatched by Hercules. He renounced
his immortality in favor of Prometheus and was placed by Zeus among
the stars in the constellation of Sagittarius.[4]

On a wall painting in Pompeii, Chiron is shown teaching Achilles
to play the lyre.[5]

Discounting much of the mythologic significance attached to his
name, it cannot be denied that his talents were of the very first order
and that his knowledge must have appeared supernatural in the days
of superstition in which he lived. He is credited with the invention
of a probe, of employing bandages when treating wounds, of using
purgatives, and of extracting teeth. His superstitious contemporaries
elevated him to the dignity of godhood after he died. From the
fragments of the history of his life that remained, his real worth cannot be accurately estimated.

Aesculapius: The most famous pupil of Chiron was Aesculapius
(the patron god of Greek medicine), the son of Ischys and Korônis,
daughter of Phlegyas of Thessaly. Homer mentions him as a "blameless physician." His sons, Machaon and Podalirius, according to
Homer, were surgeons in the Greek camp before the siege of Troy.[6]

Legends: Numerous fabulous legends have been woven about him.
The most persistent one is that his mother, who was beloved by
Apollo and became impregnated by him, cultivated an immoral intimacy with a young Arcadian named Ischys, son of Elatus, and consented to wed him. A raven brought Apollo the news of her infidelity.
The great god became so incensed that he changed the color of the
bird from white, as it previously had been, to black.[7] Artemis, to
avenge the wounded dignity of her brother Apollo, put Korônis to
death; but Apollo preserved the male child of which she was about
to be delivered, and consigned it to the care of the Centaur Chiron.
The child was named Asclepius or Aesculapius, and acquired partly
from the teaching of Chiron and partly from inborn and superhuman
aptitude, a knowledge of the virtues of herbs and a mastery of medicine and surgery, such as had never before been witnessed. He not

only cured the sick, the wounded, and the dying, "but even restored the dead to life." Zeus, however, now found himself forced to take precautions lest mankind, unexpectedly protected against sickness and death, should no longer stand in need of the immortal gods.[8] He consequently smote Aesculapius with a thunder bolt and killed

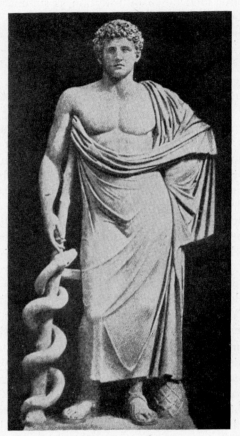

Fig. 101: Aesculapius. (Greek marble in the Vatican Museum.)

him. Apollo was so enraged by the slaughter of his highly gifted son that he killed the Cyclones who had fabricated the thunder bolt. When Zeus was about to condemn him to Tartarus for doing this, Latona interceded on his behalf, and the king of the gods relented and was satisfied with imposing upon Apollo a temporary servitude in the house of Admetus at Pherae.

Temples and Hymns: Among the Homeric hymns belonging to the time of Hesiod, there is a part of a hymn to Aesculapius which reads:

> I began to sing of Aesculapius
> Son of Apollo and healer of sickness,
> In Dotion plain fair Korônis
> Daughter of King Phlegyas bore him a great joy to man
> A shooter of cruel pangs.

Aesculapius was worshipped with very great solemnity at Trikka, at Cos, at Cnidus, and in many different parts of Greece, but especially

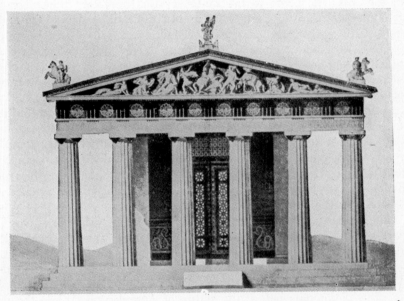

Fig. 102: Façade of Temple of Aesculapius. (Restored [Delfrasse]. Courtesy of Burroughs Wellcome & Co., Inc.)

at Epidaurus. The temples of Aesculapius were erected on high places, often surrounded by gardens and forests, adjacent to baths and mineral springs. Catton found among the ruins of Epidaurus a central shrine dedicated to Aesculapius and another one to his daughter Hygeia—a great abaton, a hostel, mineral baths, and what was probably a library. The springs that the patients were bathed in contained sulfur and other minerals. Some of these edifices date from the seventh century B.C.[9]

About 300 temples were constructed in different parts of the world in honor of Aesculapius, where distant hierarchial guilds of priestly physicians (Asclepiades) were trained to minister to the sick. Epidaurus was perhaps the greatest medical center of antiquity. A theater with a seating capacity of 20,000 and a stadium seating 12,000 people were discovered there. A probable library was also found, which was a part of the accommodation for students and patients who came to that center.

Tablets: The Greek archaeologist, Cavidas, discovered at Epidaurus inscriptions on tablets dating from ancient times; forty-four of these tablets go back to the fourth century B.C. These tablets are records of patients who came to the sanctuary for treatment; they give details of the nature of the disease and of the famous cures. On arriving at the shrine, the patient received instructions from the priest on how to conduct himself. He was urged to perform certain rites, to offer sacrifices to the healing god, and to adhere to such other sacred observations as to put him in a thoroughly recipient frame of mind.

Admission of Patients to Resorts: Before the patient was admitted to the divine healing resorts, he underwent a preliminary examination; if he appeared to be too sick, he was not admitted to the temples at all. The preliminary treatment consisted of abstinence from certain foods and drinks (wines) and other bodily wants; purgatives and baths were ordered; then the doors of the temples were opened to the pilgrim patient.

The patient was taken to the abaton of the sanctuary. One of the essential methods of treatment at the temple was the "incubation sleep" (which denotes sleeping in the shrine with the object of receiving divine revelations or aid with reference to the particular disease), for which the sick were placed on the floor of the temple on skins of animals before the statue of Aesculapius. While the patient was in a lethargic state, he received oracular messages from Aesculapius which were interpreted by the priestly physicians.[10, 11] Perhaps the sleep was induced by the use of poppy seed or hemlock. The soul, which was believed to depart from the body during sleep, was in a better position to communicate with the divine powers than when imprisoned in the sinful body.[12]

Serpents: During the temple sleep, the gods often manifested themselves in the form of serpents, which visited the patients and licked the diseased portions of their bodies. According to some ancient authors, the serpents were trained to act at the sound of music or whistling and to respond to special contrivances. Excessive heat may have been used to arouse the snakes and force them from their retreat. Coming into the open, they would appear to the visitors and profoundly impress them.

Another mythological tale attributed the medical skill of Aesculapius to a sacred serpent, which presented him with an herb possessing miraculous powers for cure. This herb healed all diseases and even resuscitated the dead. It is of interest to note that a certain species of serpent found on the north side of the Alps near the location of an ancient health resort has been identified with these ancient snakes of Aesculapius. The idea of cunning serpents was familiar among all ancient peoples; in the Biblical narrative, the serpent was the tempter connected with Mother Eve in the Garden of Eden.[13]

The serpent coming out of the earth became a symbol of the underworld power it was believed to possess. Particularly was this true with regard to the early Greeks, who worshipped the earth as a major deity and benefactor of all creatures and the serpent as the most representative creature of the underworld. The caduceus, two snakes twined on a staff, has come to be the symbol of Aesculapius and is still the most commonly used medical emblem.

Treatment Methods of the Asclepiade: From an inscription on a stele discovered in 1891 at Epidaurus, it may be gathered that the system of Aesculapius was based on miracles and not upon medical arts. Hypnosis and suggestion are, however, closely akin in their effects to modern hypnotism, which has proved efficacious in many painful diseases of a mental character.

Some of the patients unquestionably realized that the natural methods used, such as the open air baths, gymnasiums, and medical regulations contributed to their recovery. But the priests had to live up to their miraculous tradition, and they brought in an atmosphere of secrecy.

Pindar aptly describes Aesculapian medicine in the following poem:

> On some the force of charmed strains be tried,
> To some the medical draught applied
> Some limbs he placed the amulets around
> Some from the trunk he cut and made the patient sound.
>
> Pindar (Translated by Wheelwright)

The followers of Aesculapius were known as "Asclepiade." The name was first applied to priests who served in the healing temples. Subsequently, it also included lay-healers who were not of the priestly caste. The methods of treatment employed by the Asclepiade included both natural and supernatural elements.

The rite of incubation for the cure of disease is still widely employed in churches of the Greek and, to a lesser extent, Latin countries. Some of the cures resulting from incubation have been acknowledged by even prejudiced writers, and there can be no doubt that faith is a potent agency in the amelioration and even complete cure of certain bodily ills. The patient abstained from food, drink, and the pleasures of life, and the mystical environment of the temples readily contributed to the psychic factor in the treatment employed by the priestly healers. A large number of the cures reported probably also resulted from the natural measures administered.

Galen appears to be uncertain whether Aesculapius was a god or a deified mortal. It is certain that in Homer's time, Aesculapius was only considered a mortal. He is described in the second book of the Iliad as a minor chieftain from Thessaly; and although he is said to have lived about 1300 years b.c., he was elevated to godhood in post-Homeric times, possibly around 950 b.c. Aesculapius is usually represented as standing in a long cloak, with bare breast, and holding a clublike staff with a serpent coiled around it. He is frequently accompanied by Telesphorus, the boy genius of healing.

There is no doubt that the Asclepiade exploited human weakness to suit their purpose. They had to live up to the truly godlike tradition that had impressed itself upon the public. Not one of the thousands of patients treated at the temple died there. At the first sign of approaching death, patients were dumped in the woods nearby, lest their death should suggest that the healing god was fallible.

Fees: The healing practice of the Asclepiade was not motivated by altruistic principles. The person healed was required to pay a fee; nonpayment was punished by recurrence of the disease. Votive offerings were also made and, in some instances, were commanded by the god. Costly votive offerings were the earlier mode of showing gratitude. An actual fee was introduced only when the shrine had become comparatively elaborate and expensive in upkeep; this naturally varied according to the means of the patient who had been cured. Phalysius of Naupactus gave 2000 gold staters (£ 1900) when healed of blindness;[14] a boy offering the gods ten dice for a cure was healed without charge. Even the patron god Aesculapius, himself, on one occasion is said to have demanded silver or gold for his medical services. He told the patient, "Thou art healed; now pay the fee."

It is easy to understand how these demands were gladly accepted. Those suffering from illnesses were prone to believe that their suffering arose from the displeasure of the gods; and since they found that personal sacrifices and worship were insufficient for their protection and cure, they were ready to offer any of their possessions as a ransom to escape eternal punishment. To relieve the troubled conscience and to reconcile the sick or suffering with the offended gods required mighty influence. Only the priests could impart the rites of confirmation and purification to the troubled minds and bodies.

In many cases, these rites fell into the hands of mountebanks who volunteered their services to healthy men as prophylaxis against disease. These imposters degraded their profession by extravagant promises, although occasionally the price of the promises was lowered to bring them within the reach of the poor and even of the slaves.

Miraculous Cures: The votive tablets discovered in the ruins of the temples describe the nature of the miraculous cures. Some of the cures recorded on these tablets were the work of unscrupulous priests to attract the credulous public. The motive of personal gain characterizes these medical and surgical records.

The following are some of the cures credited to Aesculapius:

Julian, being in a hopeless state on account of spilling blood, was directed by the god to take pine seeds from the altar, mix them with honey, and eat them during three days. He recovered and returned thanks openly before the people.

A man who had only one eye was visited by the gods in the abaton (an airy sleeping chamber). The god applied an ointment to his empty orbit. On his awakening, the man found he had two sound eyes.

A certain Cleo, whose abdomen grew unusually large, consulted the Asclepiade who diagnosed a five-year-old fetus in her abdomen and placed her in the abaton where she slept one night. The next morning she gave birth to a grown-up child who washed himself at the fountain, took his mother's arm, and strolled back home. A Spartan girl, Arete, was dying from dropsy. She was cured by Aesculapius who simply cut her head off and drained the dropsical fluid while holding the decapitated body upside down; then he skillfully replaced the head.

A certain Hermo of Pasos was cured by the god from blindness. He, however, made the mistake of refusing to pay the honorarium to the sanctuary. The god promptly smote him again with blindness as a punitive measure for the oversight. When he returned again and paid, he slept once more in the temple, and the financially satisfied god once again healed him.

A certain woman was told that she had a worm in her belly. She was taken to the temple of Traixenes, and the god appeared to her in a dream. She dreamt that the son of the god, in the absence of his father, cut off her head. She, not being able to attach it again to the body, sent a messenger to Traixenes, to summon Aesculapius. The next morning, the attending priest found that her head was actually separated from her body. When night came again, the patient had a second dream during which the god arrived from Epidaurus, put the head back on her body, and operated on her belly and took out the worm.

The long-bearded Heramus of Mytilene was ridiculed by his neighbors because of his bald pate. During incubation sleep, the god anointed his head with a drug. In the morning, Heramus sported a crop of luxurious black hair.

A boy stole the staff from the lame Nicator. Nicator pursued the thief and, by the grace of Aesculapius, was cured of his lameness.

Hermadius consulted the god for general debility. He was so sick that he could not move. He was told by the god to go outside of the temple and bring back the largest stone he could find. Sure enough, he carried back a boulder. According to the inscription this mammoth rock still lies upon the ground.

Aesculapius' Sons: There is no record that the sons of Aesculapius resorted to miraculous cures. They were prominent leeches of the Greek army commanding the contingent at Trikka in the northwestern region of Thessaly at the siege of Troy by Agamemnon. The eldest son Machaon is represented as unrivaled in surgical operations. The other, Podalirius, who first noticed the glaring eyes and the disturbed behavior which preceded the suicide of Ajax, was sagacious in detecting and appreciating morbid symptoms. He is said to have been the first to introduce phlebotomy. Mythology credits the third son Telesphorus with having been associated with convalescence. If his statue does him justice, Telesphorus was a diminutive, dwarfish youth with short legs and perky face, wrapped in a mantle and barefooted. He is pictured generally by the side of his father. Mythology credits him with medical genius; if so, his appearance makes him a poor competitor of his divine father.

Aesculapius' Daughters: Of the daughters of Aesculapius, the most prominent was Panakeia (Panacea). She was popularly personified as the healing goddess of all diseases. She used herbs which she received from her father. She was omnipotent as a healing goddess. Her sister Hygeia (the goddess of hygiene) was not known as a healer but as a guardian of health—the stewardess of the supreme blessing of life. This blessing was to be acquired not by healing but by safeguarding the health and strength of those that were well, through rational conduct. Hygeia was worshipped by those who instituted the athletic contests and the Olympic games in Greece.

Thus, the family of Aesculapius presided over everything pertaining to health. This was emphasized by the physician Eryximachos, who was quoted by Plato as saying, "Aesculapius took over the whole art of medicine on one hand and gymnastics and agriculture on the

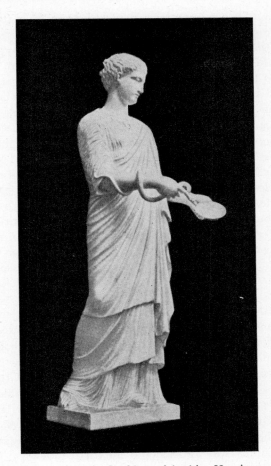

Fig. 103: Hygeia, the Greek goddess of health. Hygeia was worshipped, together with Aesculapius, first at Titane in the territory of Sicyon. Her cult was founded in Epidaurus at a later date. Hygeia was probably introduced into Athens to ward off a plague which raged in 420 B.C. Gradually, she came to be regarded as the daughter of Aesculapius. The cult Hygeia was introduced in Rome after she was admitted into the Epidaurian family of gods in the year 293 B. C. In art, as this picture shows, Hygeia is depicted as a maiden of benevolent appearance, giving food and drink to a serpent out of a bowl.

other hand." The followers of Aesculapius formed a special caste, transmitting the healing art from generation to generation as a family heritage.

In Grecian art, Hygeia appears as a radiant maiden. In the Athenian, she appears as the only other partner in the sanctuary with her divine father. She is sometimes depicted as waiting for the sacred snake to whom she offers food or, more frequently, a bowl.

Towards the end of the thirteenth century B.C., Hygeia and her sister Panacea migrated with their divine father from Thessaly to Trikkala, and to Cos, the birthplace of Hippocrates. There is a widely disseminated belief that the latter was a direct descendant of Aesculapius. From Cos, they came to Epidaurus and thence to Athens, where they spread the new medical doctrine.

Influence of the Aesculapian Cult: The diffusion of the cult of the hero of Thessaly rapidly influenced the Hellenic mind and his doctrine spread all over Greece. According to a well-founded tradition, the poet Sophocles (fifth century B.C.) was one of his apostles. In the next generation, the Athenians still worshipped the hero of Thessaly, and from Athens the Aesculapians penetrated the entire Hellenistic world. The Aesculapian cult must be reckoned as one of the strongest religious forces of later Hellenism. Aesculapian medicine was in striking contrast to Babylonian medicine, which never dissociated itself from magic.

Deities

From earliest times, belief in gods was connected with their power over health and disease. In all kinds of trouble, especially where illness was involved, appeals were made for divine help.

Originally there were no special healing deities in Greece. Every deity could properly exercise the healing power. The sufferer applied to his tribal or family god in case of sickness. Later, certain gods came to be regarded as specialists in healing diseases. Apollo, for example, was the god of pestilence though he also governed other diseases. Aesculapius was appealed to for all pathological conditions.

Leclerc enumerates some thirty Greek divinities, heroes, and heroines who were supposed to govern or cultivate some branch of medicine. First in importance among the Grecian divinities that held sway over medicine was *Zeus*, the sovereign of the Greek pantheon. He was known as a sender of disease. He seldom appears as a healer. *Athena*, his daughter, is shown with him in some vague relation to the healing god.

Next in importance is *Apollo* "who chases away evils." At the time of Homer, he was not yet connected with healing faculties. He is mentioned in the Iliad as the disseminator of plague and the stayer of pestilence. He is particularly known as the god of pestilence. His sister *Artemis* was known as the mistress of women and children.

Gruppe describes her as having been the source of psychic and nervous ailments as well as the restorer of health to those who were afflicted with these diseases. Her special concern was females.

Demeter was proficient in the art of nursing and of fire baptism, which imparted eternal youth. She did not prescribe remedies for general use. Her main power was limited to prognosis, and she revealed whether the patient would die or recover. Her specialty was also the healing of ophthalmia.

Dionysos conveyed his power of healing by touch. The priests of his sanctuary specialized in incubation and dream reading.

Pan's specialty was prophylaxis and hygiene. His power to stop pestilence was by means of oracles. He also represented the hygiene of nature.

Paieon was mainly interested in surgery. In the Iliad, he is described as the physician of the gods. He healed the wounds of Hades and Aris. The Odyssey speaks of him as the ancestor of the Egyptian physicians.

Hades, or *Pluto,* was of great importance in Greek religious medicine. He incubated patients in a cave filled with earthly vapor and directed curative dreams while the sick person was in an ecstatic trance. The task of interpreting dreams developed entirely upon the priests and their temples. Hellius was known as the restorer of sight to the blind. He restored sight to Orion.

Therapeutics

While the medical treatment of the early Greeks was directed by oracles, natural remedies were also administered. The therapeutic value of such treatment, however, is not possible to determine; for investigations of that period have so far yielded no original votive tablets dedicated by restored patients containing records of the prescribed remedies. It may, however, be reasonably supposed that the Aesculapian curative methods kept better pace with the higher state of medical knowledge than the debased character of religion. It may also be supposed that cures during incubation and in the waking state were wrought quite apart from oracular suggestion, although such were extolled as divine miracles.

Homer does not attach any supernatural powers to Aesculapius, but he refers to him as the "blameless physician." His two sons, Machaon and Podalirius, were soldiers as well as doctors. They fought before the walls of Troy. Machaon was highly praised for his heroism and for his surgical skill, as shown by the following lines of Homer:

Of two great surgeons, Podalirius stands
This hour surrounded by the Trojan bands,
And great Machaon, wounded, in his tent,
Now wants the succor which so oft he lent.

(Pope's translation)

HOMERIC MEDICINE
Treatment of Wounds

Occult medicine is placed in a minor position in Homeric writings. It is interesting to note that in Homer's "Iliad" the effects of different wounds are accurately described and the treatment is simple, straight-

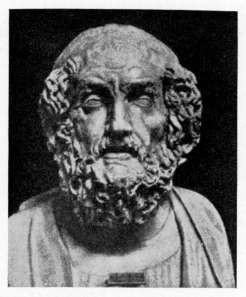

Fig. 104: Homer (c. 1000 B.C.). Seven cities claimed the honor of being Homer's native city, and many busts represent the blind bard of the Iliad and Odyssey. None is authentic, but all show how the Greeks envisaged the creator of their heroic epics. (This marble bust is in the National Museum in Naples.)

forward, and rational. In Homer's time (c. 1000 B.C.), medicine appears to have been a well-established profession. There was considerable knowledge of first aid at that period, at least among the warriors who were of great aid to themselves and to their comrades when wounded; their field work was systematic and based upon recognized principles of surgery which came only as a result of considerable thought and practice. There were no cases of imflammatory or traumatic fever, and no one died from secondary hemorrhage. The wounded either died at once or after simple treatment returned to the battle-field.

In his "Iliad," Homer, while describing the wounded heroes and heroines, exhibits a considerable knowledge of anatomy, physiology, and traumatic surgery. He describes how Ulysses struck Priam with a spear in the temple and "the brazen point penetrated to the other temple and darkness veiled his eye"; also, how Pirus struck Diores "with a hard stone at the ankle of the right leg. The reckless stone crushed both tendons and bones." To kill him, "he struck a spear in his navel and thereupon all his entrails poured forth upon the ground."

Reference is made to 149 different wounds in his poems. Some of these were superficial, others deep. The average mortality, as figured out by Frohlich, was 77.6 per cent. The highest mortality was among those whose wounds were inflicted by the sword and spear; the lowest mortality among those injured by the arrow. In the fourth book of the "Iliad," Homer describes the technique of the treatment of a wound sustained by an arrow: The surgeon sucked out the blood from the wound caused by the poisoned arrow and then sprinkled it with a remedy. It relates how the hero Menelaus, sustained a wound by a "bitter arrow which fell on the well-fitted belt, and through the deftly wrought belt was it driven, and it stuck in the variegated corselet and the brazen plated belt which he wore—the main defense of the body, a guard against weapons which protected him. Instead it grazed the surface of the hero's skin and straightway black gore flowed from the wound." King Agamemnon dispatched the divine herald Talthybius to summon with all speed:

. . . the hero Machaon, the son of the blameless physician, Aesculapius, that he may see Marshal Menelaus, the chief of the Greeks, whom some skillful archer of the Trojans wounded with a shaft . . . Machaon, in the presence of the King and with the brave ranks of the shield-bearing hosts around him, extracted the arrow from the belt, but when he perceived the wound where the bitter shaft had fallen, having sucked out the blood, he skillfully sprinkled in it shooting remedies which the benevolent Chiron had frequently given to the father.

In the eleventh book of the "Iliad," Eurypylus, wounded with an arrow in his thigh, calls upon Patroclus to remove it:

Thereupon Patroclus bore him to his tent, laying him at length, cut with a knife the bitter sharp arrow from the thigh and washed the black blood with warm water, which art he is said to have learned from Achilles, who himself had it from the centaur Chiron. Then he applied a bitter pain-assuaging root, rubbing it in his hand, which checked all his pangs. The wound indeed was dried up and the bleeding ceased.

Knowledge of Anatomy

In the following poems, Homer reveals considerable knowledge of regional anatomy. Minerva "directed the weapon to his nose near the eye and it passed quite through his white teeth and then the unswaried brass cut the root of the tongue, and the point came out at the bottom of the chin."

A compound fracture of the femur at the hip joint is described in the fifth book of the "Iliad" with reference to the injury of Aeneas:

> With this stone he smote Aeneas on the hip
> Where the thigh joins its socket. By the blow,
> He broke the socket
> And the tendon twain
> And tore the skin with the rough jagged stone.[15]

In the same book, a fracture of the skull causing death to a Trojan warrior is described, "The brazen point of his arrow fixed itself in his forehead, then forced the bone and darkness veiled his eyes."

The relation of the heart, liver, and diaphragm is described in the eleventh book of the "Iliad," "Eurypylus . . . pressed hard with many darts, advancing he stood beside him, and took aim with his shining spear, and smote Apisaon, son of Phausias, in the liver under the diaphragm." Another passage reads, "Patroclus smote his foe where the diaphragm is set close about the throbbing heart and he fell with a thud and the spear was fixed in his heart."

The high esteem in which the surgeon was held may be seen from the eleventh book of the Iliad. Paris, the husband of fair Helen, disabled Machaon, the shepherd of the people, wounding him in the right shoulder. Machaon was hurried by Nestor toward the ship. The injury of Machaon caused great consternation among the Greeks, for Idomeneus said to Nestor, "a doctor is equivalent to many other men, both to cut out arrows and to apply mild remedies."[16]

> A surgeon's skill our wounds to heal
> Is worth more than armies to the Public weal.
>
> (Pope's translation)

Machaon was surgeon to Menelaus. He fought in the army of Nestor. Fearing for the surgeon's safety, King Domeneus placed him under the charge of Nestor, who was instructed to take the doctor into his chariot. The medicine or food which Nestor gave to the wounded Machaon, adding honey to the mixture, formed a mass which Circe gave to the sailors of Ulysses in which she placed her baleful *pharmakon*.[17]

In the same book, the following are mentioned: severance of both tendons of the neck; injury of the arm below the elbow; and injury to the breast "near the right pap passing through the shoulder on the opposite side."

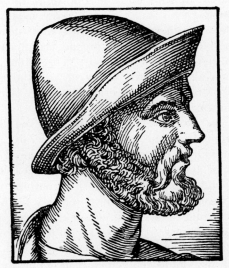

Fig. 105: Machaon, son of Aesculapius. Machaon was the elder brother of Podalirius. They are mentioned as leaders commanding thirty vessels in Homer's "Catalogue of Ships." In the "Iliad," Homer mentions the skill of these men in extracting weapons, binding up wounds, and applying soothing drugs. (Courtesy of William R. Warner & Co., Inc.)

Incidentally, the Greeks, like the ancient Egyptians, Babylonians, and Hebrews, believed that the mind was situated in the heart or breast, "Hear me, ye Trojans! . . . I speak what the mind in my breast commands me."[18] In the ninth book of the "Iliad," the same idea is expressed, "In thy breast, the gods have put an unyielding and evil mind."[19]

The gods and goddesses in the "Iliad" were as susceptible to injury as the mortals. The fifth book of the "Iliad" states, "Immortal blood flowed from the goddess Ichor such to wit as flowed from the blessed gods, for they eat not bread, nor drink dark wine; therefore they are bloodless and they are called immortal." The physician of the gods in Homer was Paioen. It may be interesting to note that the Iliad mentions the aid given to the war heroes by nurses.[20]

Magic and Theurgy

In the absence of occult elements in the surgical practice of the "Iliad," some medical historians venture to assert that, in Homer's time, medicine in general was free from magic and theurgy. This is erroneous. Homer dealt with surgical conditions, the causes of which were apparent to the eyes and devoid of any mystery. In cases of such obvious etiology, where skilled hands were needed to practice natural measures, even the Babylonians and Egyptians that preceded the Greeks employed rational methods. The Code of Hammurabi places the surgeon alongside the architect and the artisan, and the Edwin Smith Papyrus, which concerns itself only with surgery, prescribes practical measures.

This however, was not the case with internal medicine, where the etiology was hidden from the eye. Internal diseases, marked by insidious onset and violent symptoms, were considered by all ancients as a punishment of the gods or caused by magical influence of ill-disposed forces, and were treated by supernatural means. Homer himself refers to the sons who were happy to see their father recovering from a longstanding illness with which an angry god assailed him. Their pleasure was compared to the joy of Ulysses at the sight of land.[21] The blinded and howling Cyclops was told by his friends that, if he was ill, he should remember that sickness came from Zeus and was unavoidable, indicating that internal disease was attributed to supernatural causes.[22]

In the epics of Homer, the healers who treated their surgical cases by natural means were at a loss when confronted with pestilence sent by Apollo. There they had recourse to supernatural measures of healing administered by priests, seers, and dream readers.[23]

In the "Odyssey," where Homer dealt with internal medication, divine influence was evident:

She (Helen) cast into the wine of which they were drinking (pramian cheese and barley meal)—drugs to quiet all pain and strife and bring forgetfulness of every ill; whoever should drink it down when it is mingled in the bowl, would not in the course of that day let a tear fall down over his cheeks, no, not though his mother and father should lie there dead, or though before his fall, men should slay with the sword his brother or dear son, and his own eyes beheld it; such cunning drugs the daughter of Zeus, drugs of healing which Polydamina, the wife of Thou, had given her by a woman of Egypt, for there the earth, the giver of grain bears greatest store of drugs. Many that are healing when mixed and many that are baneful; there every man is a physician, wise, human, kind; for they are of the race of Paioen.

Status of Medicine and Surgery

It appears that, as early as 770 B.C., medicine was separated from surgery. Aretimus of Lebos (770 B.C.), in his "Sac of Iteum," referring to the sons of Aesculapius, states:

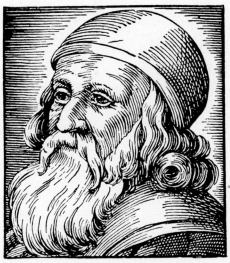

Fig. 106: Podalirius, son of Aesculapius. According to Diodorus of Sicily, Podalirius and his brother Machaon lived and worked harmoniously. Their reputation was such that they were exempt from fighting. However, they declined this privilege, taking a leading part in attacks against the Trojans. (Courtesy of William R. Warner & Co., Inc.)

For their father the famous "earthshaker" gave both of them gifts, making each more glorious than the other.[24] To the one (Machaon) he gave skillful hands, more light to draw or cut out missiles from the flesh and to heal all kinds of wounds; but in the heart of the other (Podalirius) he put full and perfect knowledge to kill hidden disease and cure desperate sickness. It was he who first noticed Ajax's flashing eyes and clouded mind when he was enraged.

It is related that Podalirius, returning from Troy, was wrecked on the coast of Caria. He was rescued by a herdsman who took him to the palace. He found everyone there concerned about the king's daughter, Syrna, who had fallen from the roof in a fit and was still

unconscious. Podalirius restored her to health by drawing blood from
both arms and received her hand and a fortune as a fee.

It is apparent that in the state of society pictured by Homer, medicine was already a distinct and organized profession, and war surgery
was advanced. According to Daremberg, the anatomical nomenclature
was already substantially the same as that employed long afterwards
in the Corpus Hippocraticum. The description given of wounds betrayed a knowledge of the relationship of the organs of the human

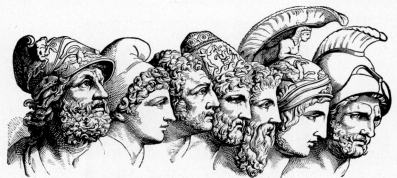

Fig. 107: Heroes of the Trojan War. (From Grote: History of Greece. Vol. 10.)

body. In short the art and science of medicine, however imperfect
as compared with later times, were far from being in their infancy.

The Homeric heroes were represented as skilled in administering
first aid to ordinary wounds and injuries; but there was also a professional class, as represented by Achilles, Patrocles and especially by the
cunning leeches, Machaon and Podalirius. These professional physicians were treated with great respect. There is no record in the
Homeric poems of the subordination of medicine to religion, as was
the case during the 300 years that intervened between Homer and
Hippocrates, or in ancient Egypt, Babylonia, and India; nor are priests
charged, as they were in those countries, with medical functions.
These facts throw grave doubts on the commonly held opinion that
medicine derived its origin in all countries from religious observances.

During the 500 or 600 years that elapsed between the siege of Troy
and the rise of the Ionian School of Philosophy, medicine was controlled chiefly by the priests, among whom the spirit of rivalry existed
on behalf of their respective divinities. This, however, was not without its advantage in promoting medical art and science, since the
priests had to take advantage of the aid of observers and investigators
to accomplish their cures, although credit was given to their gods.

Votive Tablets

In order to add to the celebrity of the temples, it was considered a solemn duty for every patient, on recovery, to leave in the temple a representation of the part of the body affected, accompanied by a tablet which described the symptoms and recorded the cure. Such tablets were attached to the walls of the temples.

Aristophanes (388 B.C.), in his "Plutus," indicates that in his time temples were erected to the gods of medicine. The sick were laid down in the temples after they had offered their sacrifices and undergone purification. The priest disguised himself as a deity. The mode of treatment was revealed to the patient directly or through a dream. Before leaving the temple, the cured patient presented offerings of thanks and medals representing the affected parts in gold, silver, or wax. The temple at Athens possessed, among other things, a silver heart, golden legs, and gilded or golden eyes. A tablet was put up describing the illness and the treatment.

Grueter, a German investigator, preserved a number of these votive tablets. Large collections of medical trophies have been collected by others which attest to the successful cures of the temples and provide important facts and observations. Gradually, these temples were converted into medical schools, varying in excellence as they did in reputation. Thus, the foundation was laid for the great revolution in medicine which was first effected by the Ionian School of Philosophy and which emancipated medicine from the trammels of superstition and elevated it to the dignity of a rational science. According to Pliny and Strabo, these tablets found in the Aesculapian temples of Cos, the birthplace of Hippocrates, were used by the father of medicine to form some of his medical ideas. Later writers even made him a "priest of Aesculapius," but not enough is known of these tablets to attach so much importance to them. The few that have been discovered in Epidaurus and Rome, as shown earlier in the chapter, mentioned miraculous cures which Hippocrates opposed. If he had seen them, the only use he would have made of them would be to oppose them as a means of therapy.

Medical Schools

In later years, schools independent of temples were opened, as for example the school of Cnidus in Asia Minor, which produced such men as Euryphon, Ctesias (fragments of whose history have been preserved in Persia), and Photius. Hippocrates received his training in the art of healing at the school in Cos. At this school, medical instruction was first confined to lineal descendants of Aesculapius. In the course of time, other students were granted admission. In these schools, sages, conspicuous for their talents and eminence, directed their attention to medical research and labored to enhance the medical art.

Theopompus, the analyst (350 B.C.), is of the opinion that the physicians of Cos and Cnidus were descendants of Podalirius; they were called "Asclepiade." The early Asclepiade might have hailed from the priestly family, but it is generally agreed that later laymen were also admitted in the temples. The idea that the Asclepiade were priests is now generally abandoned, as is the idea that Greek medicine originated in the temples of Aesculapius.

In the middle of the seventh century B.C., the school that was founded in Cnidus largely discarded magical and superstitious concepts. The causes and symptoms of diseases were based upon facts and not upon omens, stars, and other superstitions, and the treatment was based upon experience. The events contributing to such revolutionary changes will be described in the next chapter.

References and Notes

1. Calliope 9:34.
2. Apollodorus 3:10, 13.
3. Odyssey 19.
4. Apollodorus 2:5; Ovid (Fasti) 5:14.
5. Encyclopedia Britannica, Vol. 6, p. 239.
6. Iliad 2:131.
7. The change of the color of the crow is noted in Ovid, (Metamorphoses) 2:632.
8. This legend is analogous to the story that Adam and Eve were driven out of the Garden of Eden lest they eat of the tree of life. Genesis 3:5.
9. Catton, R.: The Temple and the Ritual of Asklepios. Clay and Son, London, 1900.
10. Grote, G.; Greece: R. F. Collier and Son, 1900, Vol. 1, p. 178.
11. Genesis 28:12; 37:5; 41:1-36. I Kings 3:5-15. The entire basis of incubation could not be better expressed than in the words of Job 33:15: "In a dream in a vision of the night when deep sleep followed upon me in slumberings upon the bed; then he (God) openeth the ears of man and sealeth their instruction."
12. Hastings, J. (Editor): Encyclopedia of Religion and Ethics. Article by Gray, L. H. Charles Scribner and Sons, New York, 1928, Vol. 7, pp. 206-207.
13. Genesis 3:1.
14. Pausanias 10; 38:7.
15. Rendered into English by William Cullen Bryant.
16. Iliad 2:197.

17. The word *"pharmakon,"* from which "pharmacy" is derived, denotes an outward application in the Iliad, and in the Odyssey it signifies "poison," or "charm."
18. Iliad 7.
19. Ibid., 9.
20. Ibid., 14.
21. Odyssey 5:395.
22. Ibid., 9:411.
23. Iliad 1:63.
24. Among the early Greeks, the medical art passed from father to son. The sons of Hippocrates, Draco and Thessalus, were physicians and were the founders of the medical cult known as "dogmatism."

16

Influence of Philosophy on Medicine

THE RISE of rational medicine in Greece may be traced to the year 670 B.C. when Psammetichus, king of Egypt, opened the land of the Nile to the inhabitants of the Mediterranean and European countries. Before that time, the Valley of the Nile was a land of mystery. All that was known about Egypt was vague reports that leaked out through political refugees who fled Egypt to escape punishment or from adventurous Greek pirates. These men stealthily visited the Valley of the Nile and brought back prodigious and miraculous reports of great pyramids covering acres of land, their tops rising to the heavens; of obelisks of enormous height, erected by superhuman skill from a single block of stone on everlasting pedestals, the surfaces of that stone being inscribed with mysterious hieroglyphics, unknown to the uninitiated; of great temples; and of sphinxes, grim and silent, guarding the portals of palaces and temples.

Because Greek aid helped Psammetichus in attaining supreme power over Egypt in a civil war against the Pharaohs, this monarch made Egypt accessible to the Greeks and other neighboring peoples who flocked there to obtain valuable products from the Egyptians. Psammetichus also opened the schools, for which Egypt was famous, to young Greeks who were thirsty for the "wisdom of the Egyptians."

It has been pointed out in a previous chapter how the hieroglyphic script furnished interesting medical evidence; how it underwent a two-fold ideographic and phonetic development (one expressing ideas and the other, sounds); and how these enigmatic characters have revealed the existence of an extensive literature, embracing music, astronomy, medicine, anatomy, geography, cosmogony, and other subjects that have attracted the curiosity of men.

458

To the Greeks, who were blessed with lively intellectual curiosity, Egypt appeared truly a great spiritual and intellectual center. The Greeks imbibed the wisdom of the Egyptians, made additions to it and, at times, sharp diversions from it, and finally embarked on a new route—on a scientific course unknown to the Egyptions. They discovered a path which led to a mechanical explanation of the universal phenomena.

IONIAN SCHOOL OF PHILOSOPHY

It must be borne in mind that Greek thought first took root, not on the mainland of Greece, but on the eastern shore of the Aegean Sea, known as "Ionia." Ionian philosophers attempted for the first time to replace the anthropomorphic gods by natural causes and to explain the universe in terms of natural laws. They promulgated a rule that "nought can come from nought or return to nought" which excluded the intervention of the gods in the affairs of nature. True, the gods were not altogether eliminated. An open avowal of agnosticism or atheism was avoided out of respect to the popular religion, but religious forces became impotent.

The Ionian philosophers (excepting the Pythagoreans and the Eleatic followers) sought, in matter, motion, and force, an explanation of the universal phenomena, and they established the principle that all matter was composed of elements. The atomist carried further the thought of the Ionian school, postulating that every occurrence is the product of cause and necessity and visualizing matter, in a variety of forms and substances, as composed of atoms.

Thales

Thales of Miletus (c. 650–580 B.C.) was the founder of the Ionian School of Philosophy. He was the first to break away from the mythological tradition and to adopt a program for investigating natural phenomena. Thales was the first to enunciate the principle that all matter was created from water[1] ("the semen of nature").[2] The importance of this declaration lies in the fact that it assumed for the first time that all phenomena of the universe are based on natural principles and must be explained through rational inquiry and knowledge.

This idea is said to have dawned on Thales when he visited the schools of Egypt and observed that, with little care on the part of man, the fertilizing Nile water yielded abundant crops, making Egypt the granary of the world and the source of life of animals and plants. He observed how necessary water was to growth, "that without moisture, even his own body would not have been what it was, but a dry husk falling to pieces."[3]

Aristotle attributed to Thales the saying, "All things are full of gods," a pantheistic idea promulgated about 2000 years later by Spinoza. Aristotle suggested that Thales conceived the view that water was the first principle by observing that the seed of all living things existed

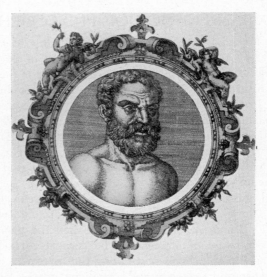

Fig. 108: Thales (640–546 B.C.). Thales, Greek sage and philosopher, and one of the seven wise men of Greece, was born at Miletus, Asia Minor. He was noted especially as an astronomer and geometer and was the earliest of the Ionian natural philosophers. He regarded water as the principal ingredient of all things. He is said to have been the first one to predict an eclipse of the sun, which was alleged to have occurred on May 25, 588 B.C.

in a moist medium and were kept alive by it.[4] "Dominant in the Ionian school," said Aristotle, "was the recognition of matter, motion, and physical causation, that is of objects extended in space and orderly movements and changes in space as being themselves the manifestators of absolute reality."[5]

In Egypt, the doctrine that "water is the origin of all living things" had existed for millenniums and, being protected by antiquity and venerable tradition, it did not create any controversy or even examination. But in young Greece it was challenged. The very idea of a primary element tended to reduce all possible agencies to one, to substitute monotheism for polytheism, and to encourage philosophical skepticism. Thales met with strong opposition. The main argument was, "if plants and metals are essentially the same as water, then the evidence of the senses is not trustworthy." Thales was opposed, not only by those who believed in the Orphic mysteries, but even by open-minded philosophers like himself. The challenge, however, yielded good results. Thales was perhaps the first Greek philosopher to explain the working of the universe on materialistic and mechanical principles and this was the first instance on record where scientific inquiry was attacked.

Anaximander

Thales was followed by Anaximander (610–545 B.C.), his younger contemporary and townsman, who postulated that, in some sort of sequence, heat, cold, water, earth, air, fire, plants, animals, and human beings developed from a primordial cause. He was in accord with Thales that the basic principle of all structural and functional morphology was one element or principle, but he thought a corporal substance was the primal source of life. His opinion was based upon the fact that, when an animal or any other form of matter was destroyed, dust was the only thing that was left. Primary matter he believed to be eternal, but all created things, even the heavenly bodies, were doomed to destruction and to return to the undivided unity of the universal being. The infinite principle has been, is, and always will be immutable. Growth and decay he explained on the principle of mechanical compensation.

Some of the other theories presented by Anaximander were as follows: Living creatures arose from the moist element as it was evaporated by the sun. Man was like another animal, namely a fish, in the beginning. The first animals were produced in moisture, each enclosed in a prickly bark; as they advanced in age, they came out upon the drier part; and when the bark broke off, they survived for a short time.

Anaximander regarded primordial substance as eternal. He considered all generated substances as doomed to destruction, although they were derived by a transformation of an indestructible substance.

Anaximander was probably the first to enunciate the theory that man evolved from animals of a lower species. He argued that, while other animals quickly matured and found food by themselves, man alone required a lengthy period of suckling. Hence, had he been originally as he was then, he would never have survived. His theory of the evolution of man differed, however, from the modern doctrine of "Origin of Species."

He declared that the first animal arose from sea slime and that the first human beings evolved from the inside of fishes; and having been reared like sharks and become capable of protecting themselves, they finally were cast ashore where they took to the land.[6]

Anaximander's investigations represented conclusions drawn from the study of nature. His biological conclusions, like his cosmological physics, which appear to be an integral part of his philosophy, were free from superstition. He had little religious awe, admitted no magic, and recognized no supernatural phenomena. Such unprejudiced observations of nature were unique in the ancient world and tended to build up a systematic body of natural knowledge.

Anaximenes

Anaximenes (611–546 B.C.) rebelled against the extreme materialism of his master Anaximander. He ventured to advance the doctrine that the primary element from which everything was created was atmospheric air. Common observation supported his theory; for water itself appeared to be generated from atmospheric air, clouds were formed in the air, and from them springs and fountains were formed. Anaximenes attributed infiniteness to air, a dogma that did not require much imagination in that early period, for who could discern the boundary of the atmosphere when looking upward? Indeed, life itself, depended upon inhaling and exhaling atmospheric air. Anaximenes believed that the soul was nothing but air and ceased to exist as soon as the process of respiration stopped. As proof that the origin of all things was air, he offered the erroneous observation that, when one breathed with the lips closed, the air was cold, but became warm when breathing through the open mouth. Hence, he argued that, with sufficient rarefaction, air might turn into heat; and if by chance it should undergo condensation, it would turn into clouds and water. Since air was a life-giving principle to man, he inferred that the infinite air was the first principle of creation.[7] This primordial matter was endowed with generative or transmutive force by virtue of which it passed into a succession of forms. Thus, he regarded the world with its infinite forms as having been issued from a single substance.

Diogenes

The theory of Anaximenes was later elaborated by Diogenes of Apollonia (460 B.C.), who emphasized the importance of breath, or pneuma, and held that air was distributed throughout the body by the arteries arising from the heart and the aorta. Diogenes applied the philosophy of the elements to the human economy. His doctrine contributed to the erroneous concept that the arteries contained air, and this principle checked medical progress for ages.[8]

Diogenes regarded the universe as a living being, spontaneously evolving and transforming itself. He agreed with Anaximenes that the soul of man was nothing but air as was also the soul of the world.

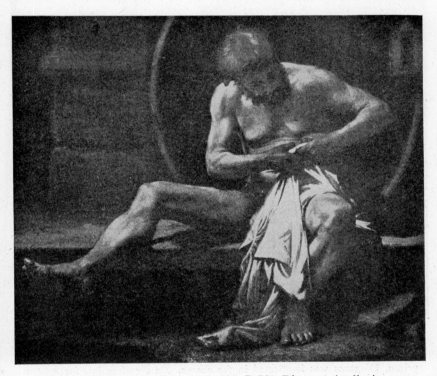

Fig. 109: Diogenes Apolloniates (c. 460 B.C.). Diogenes Apolloniates was an Ionian philosopher, who lived for a time in Greece. He came from Dorian stock, although he wrote in the Ionian dialect. While sojourning in Athens, his liberal views on religion made him so unpopular with the Athenian population that his life was threatened. His "De Natura" is not complete; only some fragments are extant.

From this it followed that the air had to be eternal, imperishable, and endowed with consciousness:

It knows much; for without reason, it would be impossible for all to be arranged so duly and proportionately as that all should maintain its fitting measure, winter and summer, night and day, rain, wind and weather; and whatever object considered will be found to have been ordered in the best

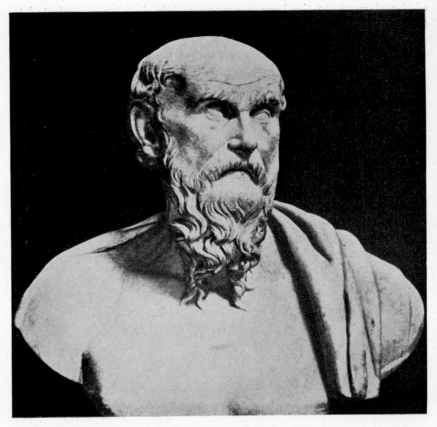

Fig. 110: Diogenes, "The cynic" (412–323 B.C.). This Greek philosopher, "the cynic," should not be confused with Diogenes Apolloniates. The former was born at Sinope. When his father was accused of counterfeiting and put in prison, Diogenes was implicated in the charge. He therefore left for Athens where he became the pupil of the ascetic Antisthenes. All of his life, Diogenes taught the doctrine of self-control. On a voyage to Aegina, he was captured by pirates and sold as a slave in Crete. At one of the Isthmian games, he is reported to have requested that Alexander the Great "not stand between him and the sun," to which Alexander replied, "If I were not Alexander, I would be Diogenes."

and most beautiful manner possible . . . but that which has knowledge is that which man calls air; it is that which regulates and governs all and hence it is the use of air to pervade all, and to dispose all and to be in all, for there is nothing that has not part in it.[9]

His conclusion that the air was actually a spiritual being converted the theory of Anaximenes from a physical into a psychological system and marked the beginning of the special philosophy of Greece. It led to the principle that the thinking power of man arose from the flowing of air through the body and blood.

Diogenes explained the formation of the world by the hypothesis of condensation of the earth from air by cold, the warmth rising upward and forming the sun. In the stars he recognized the respiratory organs of the world. He attributed the difference of mentality between men and beasts to the air in its various condition of moisture and warmth: "The variation in the souls of brutes, which differ from men and from one another in intelligence, is only due to the air in its various conditions of moisture and warmth." From the preponderance of moist air in the constitution of animals, he inferred they were like the insane, incapable of thought, for thickness of the air impeded respiration, and therefore quick comprehension. Plants having no cavities wherein to receive the air were altogether unintelligent. He also explained the different character of the air in humans and in brutes by the fact that brutes carried their nostrils near the ground and men carried their breathing organ high above the ground. Anaximenes believed air to be possessed with intelligence, and Diogenes' chief advance was beyond this doctrine. The air which was the origin of all things was necessarily eternal and imperishable and endowed with consciousness.[10]

Heraclitus

One who contributed greatly to both metaphysical and scientific speculations was the Ionian philosopher and poet, Heraclitus of Ephesus (540 to 475 B.C.). Heraclitus expressed a contempt for the materialistic tendencies of Anaximander and Anaximenes. He maintained that ethereal fire was the predominant cause of all life. His system was based on the axiom, "All is convertible into fire and fire into all." In the term "fire," he included dry and warm conditions.

He considered the element of fire to be in a state of perpetual activity, forming and absorbing every individual thing. The motion of this primordial principle moved in the upward and downward direction and in the higher and lower region. The chief accumulation was above, the chief deficiency below. He regarded the soul of man as a portion of fire migrating from heaven.

His moral system was based altogether upon the physical, the fundamental dogma being, "the excellence of fire in the system." He ascribed the stupidity of the drunkard to the fact that he possessed a moist soul and drew the inference that a warm or dry soul was of the highest quality. He declared that the noblest souls had to belong to a climate

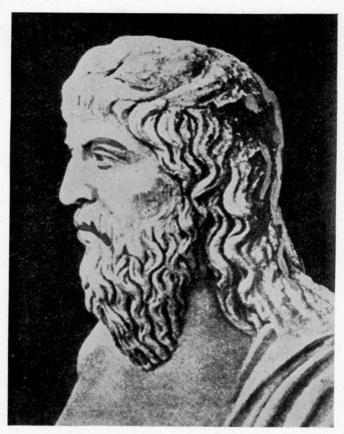

Fig. 111: Heraclitus of Ephesus (540–475 B.C.). Heraclitus of Ephesus was known as the "dark, or weeping, philosopher." He had a contempt for mankind and spent a lonely life in isolation. He denied the reality of "being." Contrary to the views of his contemporaries of the Ionian school of philosophy, he was not a thoroughgoing materialist, although he frequently held materialistic views. He is considered to be the founder of metaphysics.

that was dry, intending thereby to indicate that Greece was man's fittest and truest country.

"Fire," he maintained, "is the kind of stuff of which all is made, to which all returns." The perpetual alteration of opposites in this world, such as sleeping and waking, life and death, health and disease, made the ceaseless rhythm of the ever-living fire. His idea was that all which appeared to us to be permanent was only a regulated and self-renewing occurrence of similar and opposite motions, and that there was a constant destruction and renewal.[11]

Heraclitus' notion that conflict was the father of all things and that harmony was the result of a dynamic equilibrium of discords—an endeavor of individual things to maintain themselves, in permanence against the universal process of destruction and renovation—reminds one of the theory of survival of the fittest.

"Truth," he said, "can only be found within the reflection of the universal logus or reason." The last remark shows that Heraclitus believed in the doctrine of a soul of the world. In Heraclitus, the Ionian school reached its highest peak of learning.

Some of his teachings were as follows: The element of fire in itself was a divine rational process, the harmony of which constituted the law of nature. Knowledge consisted in comprehending this all-pervading harmony as embodied in the manifold processes of perception. The senses were "bad witnesses" because they comprehended phenomena, not as a manifestation, but as "stuff" and "dead." Real value consisted in the subordination of the individual to the laws of disharmony and the universal reason, wherein alone universal freedom was to be found. Moral failure was proportional to the degree in which the individual declined to recognize his personal transience in relation to the eternal mind.

Heraclitus regarded the organs of sense as the channels through which the outer life of the world, and therewith truth, entered the mind, and he believed that in sleep, when the organs of sense were closed, all communion with the surrounding universal spirit was shut out.

The individual, like the phenomenon of sense, came out of the infinite and again was merged with the infinite. Hence man was not a true separate entity but existed in the infinite and had to continue to exist. The soul approached most nearly its perfection when it was least akin to the fiery vapor. According to his philosophy, while one was alive, the soul was dead within him; but when he died, the soul was restored to life. This belief was a step further than the philosophy of Pythagoras who believed that, while one lived the soul was incarcerated in the body, as punishment for sin committed in a previous existence.

Some of Heraclitus' aphorisms are as follows:

All is and is not; for though it does in truth come into being yet it forthwith ceases to be.

No one has ever been twice on the same stream for different waters are constantly following down it.

It disappears its waters and gathers them anew. It approaches and it recedes, overflows and fails.

On the same stream he embarks and embarks not.
Being and not being are related.

Of the early life of Heraclitus and his education, nothing is known. From the contempt with which he spoke of his colleagues, one may gather that he regarded himself as a pioneer of wisdom. In contradistinction to Democritus (the laughing philosopher), he was known as "the dark philosopher" and "the weeping philosopher," because of the lonely life he led and because of the extreme profundity of his philosophy and his contempt of mankind. The school of disciples founded by Heraclitus flourished long after his death. Cratylus was the chief exponent of his teaching. Heraclitus had great respect for Pythagoras, "Of all men the son of Mansachus was the most assiduous inquirer."

Aims of Ionian Philosophers

The Ionian philosophers sought to explain the natural universe as given in the sensible perception. Their explanation was in terms of matter, movement, and force. In this they differed from the Eleatics and the Pythagoreans, who thought in the abstract sense and explained knowledge and existence in metaphysical terms.

In tracing the development of their ideas, the following differences may be distinguished: The earlier thinkers down to Heraclitus endeavored to find a material substance of which all things were composed. Heraclitus, by his principle of universal flux, took a new line of thought: He explained everything in terms of force, movement, and dynamic energy. In other words, the early philosophers sought to solve the problem, "What is the status of the things we see?" and Heraclitus sought to explain, "Of what nature is the motive force?"

ELEATIC SCHOOL OF PHILOSOPHY

Xenophanes

Another type of critical philosophy was the school founded by the philosopher and poet, Xenophanes of Colophon (c. 530 B.C.). Xenophanes was a native of Ionia, from which he was exiled. After leading for many years the life of a wandering rhapsodist, he settled in Elea (a Greek colonial city of Italy), where he founded (at the end of the sixth century B.C.) the Eleatic School of Philosophy. He became conspicuous for his opposition to Homer, Hesiod, and other Greek popular poets whom he denounced for promoting the base polytheism of the times, and for degrading the idea of the divine by the immoralities they attributed to the gods. He proclaimed God as an all-powerful being, existing from eternity, and without any likeness to man.

In his natural philosophy, he believed that the phenomena of nature originated in combinations of the primary four elements—earth, air, fire, and water. He regarded the earth as possessing a flat surface, the interior region of which extended indefinitely downward, and so gave a solid foundation. His physical views almost bordered on skepticism.

He was a strict monotheist; he asserted that "of the all-powerful and all-perfect there could not, in the nature of things, be more than one; for if there were even two, those attributes could not apply to one of them; much less then, if there were many." This one principle or power was to him the same as the universe, the substance of which, having existed from all eternity, must necessarily be identical with God; since it was impossible that there should be two Omnipresents, so also it was impossible that there should be two Eternals.[12] The vulgar belief which imputed to the Deity sentiments, passions, and crimes of man, was blasphemous and accursed. Xenophanes[13] assailed popular anthropomorphism, "The Ethiopians make their gods black-haired and flat-nosed. The Tracians make theirs red-headed and blue-eyed. Men think their gods are begotten as they are, dress as they do and look and speak as they do. If horses or oxen had hands to carve and paint, they would represent them in the equine and bovine shape."

He exposed the impiety of those who would figure the Great Supreme in the form of a man, "He has no resemblance to the bodily form of man, nor are his thoughts like ours. . . No mortal man ever did, or ever shall know God and the universe thoroughly, for since error is so spread over all things, it is impossible for us to be certain even when we utter the true and the perfect." To Xenophanes, the discovery of the invisible was to be made by the intellect of man, not by the senses.

Parmenides

The chief exponent of this school was Parmenides, who flourished about the year 480 B.C. Parmenides pushed to an extreme the characteristic Greek assumption that what was inconceivable was impossible, even if the senses told them that it had in fact happened. He argued thus: Creation was impossible because something could not be conceived to arise from nothing; a being could not originate from a non-being. Conversely, destruction was impossible because something could not vanish into nothing. Even change was impossible, because a thing could not arise from another thing which was in essence unlike itself. Sense perceptions were unreal, nonbeing; thought alone was real, true-being. In the apparent world of phenomena, the unreal but still observed universe was a series of concentric shells of fire and earth, though all this was but "opinion" and not necessarily "truth."

Thus the appearances of changes, of diversity and multipliciy, of time and space, which were thought to be seen in nature, were but false impressions of the senses, which thought proved to be self-contradictory. By thought alone could one arrive at the fundamental truth that "the all is one."

Zeno

Some of these ideas were carried further by Zeno of Elea, a younger contemporary of Parmenides, who opposed the Pythagorean doctrine that all things were made of integral numbers. He discredited multiplicity by his famous series of paradoxes, "A manifold must be divisible to infinity and therefore must itself be infinite, but, in trying to build it up again, no number of infinitely small parts can make a finite whole."

Zeno proved that the idea of division without limit into infinitesimal units as then understood, was inconsistent with experience.

The Eleatic philosophy, by discrediting the senses, helped the atomists to seek reality in things imperceptible to the senses. It explained what afterwards came to be called the "secondary or separable qualities of bodies" (such as heat or color) as mere sense perceptions.

Anaxagoras

Among the early contributors to Greek philosophy, the name of Anaxagoras of Glazomanae (born at Smyrna c. 500 B.C.) stands out prominently. He went in his boyhood from his birthplace in Asia Minor to Ionia, from there to Athens, which was rapidly becoming the headquarters of Greek culture, and he remained in that city for thirty years. He visited Egypt in quest of knowledge. Returning to Athens, he met the orator Pericles and the poet Euripides with whom he became closely connected by cultural and friendly ties. Both derived from him an enthusiasm for science and humanity. It is asserted that Socrates was among his disciples to whom he taught the spirit of scientific inquiry and philosophical knowledge, which he had brought from Ionia to Athens.

He was accused by the superstitious Athenian populace of atheism and impiety to the gods. He allegorized Zeus and other personal gods and advanced materialistic ideas with reference to cosmogony. His observation of the planets led him to form new theories of the universal order. He asserted that the sun and moon consisted of a mass of ignited stone and were not animate beings as was even later taught by Plato. He emphatically declared that the so-called "divine miracles" of his time were nothing more than common, natural phenomena. He also taught the dualism of mind and matter, a dogma promulgated by the Persians.

He was thrown into prison and condemned to death, from which he barely escaped through the influence and eloquence of his disciple Pericles; and he fled to Lampsacus, where he ended his days in exile. His countrymen conveyed exaggerated honor upon his memory, claim-

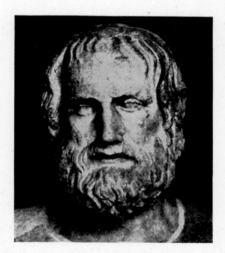

Fig. 112: Euripides (480–406 B.C.). Euripides, youngest of the three great dramatists, was the most tragic of the tragedians.

ing that he was the first to explain the phases of the moon and the nature of solar and lunar eclipses, and that he had the power of foretelling future events. Born in affluence, he devoted all his means to philosophy; and in his old age, he encountered poverty and want.

The basic principle of his philosophy was the recognition of the unchangeability of the universe as a whole, that the variety of forms seen was produced by new arrangements of their constituent parts. His doctrine included the idea of the eternity of matter. "Wrongly do the Greeks suppose," he stated, "that aught begins or ceases to be, for nothing comes into being or is destroyed, but all is an aggregation or secretion of preexisting things, so that all becoming might more cor-

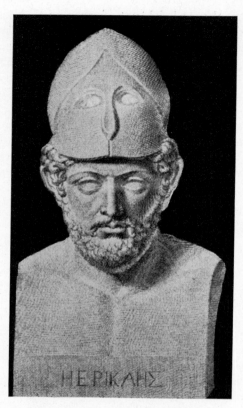

Fig. 113: Pericles (490–431 B.C.). Pericles was a pupil of the great philosophers Anaxagoras and Zeno. The latter revealed to him the power of dialectics.
Another teacher of his, Daman, instructed him in music. He was a great statesman, and all through his life he conducted himself with dignity and sagacity.
He was noted as a great orator, soldier, and patriot. He died during the plague
that ravaged Athens in 431 B.C.

rectly be called becoming-mixed, and all corruption becoming-
separate."[14]

His philosophy was somewhat similar to that of Anaximander:

Things have existed from the beginning but originally they existed as
infinitesimally small fragments of particles endless in number, inextricably
combined throughout the universe. All things existed in a confused and
indistinguishable form. There were, however, the seeds or miniatures of
everything in the primitive mixture, but these had to be eliminated from
the complex mass before they could receive characters and names.[15]

Anaxagoras was among the first in Greece to advance the knowledge of the anatomy of the brain by dissection of animals. He explained mental perception upon the hypothesis that one had naturally within him the contraries of all the qualities of external things and that, when one considered an object, he became aware of the preponderance of those qualities in his mind which were deficient in it. Hence, all sensation was attended with pain. As to the nature of human knowledge, Anaxagoras asserted that, by the intellect alone, one became acquainted with the truth, the senses being altogether unreliable. This he illustrated by letting a drop of colored liquid fall into a quantity of clear water; the eyes were unable to perceive any change in the aqueous vehicle. He also asserted that snow was not really white, but black, since it was composed of water which he considered to be black in color. Hence he drew the conclusion that things were to each man, not what they were, but merely how they appeared to him.[16]

The concept of unreliability of senses brought forth from him the following statement, "Nothing can be known; nothing can be learned; nothing can be certain; sense is limited; intellect is weak; life is short; and motion is not real." Matter, he argued, was composed of many different entities, with qualities as the sense suggested, regardless of size. The individual parts of matter contained things like the whole, although differences could arise from different proportions of the ingredients.

In addition to the elements composing matter, he mentioned many subordinate agents in the government of things (such as color). This doctrine implied that, in compound things, there was not only formation but an arrangement that required many elements instead of a single one, that is flesh was made of fleshly particles and bone of bony particles. Anaxagoras held that all the parts of an animal's body preexisted in the food and were merely collected therefrom. Plants he regarded as rooted animals, motionless, but having sensation and desires. He ascribed the superiority of man to the mere fact that he possessed hands. His doctrine of the origin of animals was founded on the observation of the apparent action of sunlight on moist earth. Anaxagoras believed that the mind or soul (nous) was the prime controlling force over all bodily activities.

Reasoning of Eleatic Philosophers

It is evident that the philosophers of the Eleatic school reasoned from the general knowledge of their time in the light of the prevailing metaphysical concepts and on the basis of the four elements. But granting that matter was composed of the four elements, the question arose as to how they were held together and how particles could move in a fully packed space, or plenum (air was now known to be corporeal; thus an empty space could only be a vacuum). Did the properties of matter change? Was water always water? Was earth always earth, even if divided into infinitesimal parts? Were the special senses to be trusted? How could one be sure that matter was composed of the elements?

Democritus

Such were the trains of thought which agitated the mind of Democritus (460-356 B.C.), and as a solution to all these perplexing problems, he suggested the theory that matter consisted of ultimate particles scattered in a void, a theory with which he explained all the relevant facts then known—evaporation, condensation, motion, and the growth of new material. The atomist held that atoms were physically indivisible because there was no void within them.

Atomic Theory: Democritus adopted the principle of atomism which he received from his preceptor and townsman Leucippus, who wholeheartedly believed that "nothing happens without a cause, but everything with a cause and by necessity." Democritus elaborated the theory of his master in his attempt to furnish a rational explanation of the phenomena of the universe. While agreeing with Thales, Anaxagoras, and the Eleatic school in the basic principle that "nothing can arise out of nothing and nothing can be reduced to nothing," Democritus denied the oneness and immobility of matter which they taught.

According to Democritus, plurality, movement, and space were essential to explain the workings of the physical universe. "Space" had an equal right with "being" to be considered existent. "Being" was the full (plenum). "Not being" was the void (vacuum). An infinite number of atoms moved in the infinite space. These atoms were eternal and so small that they could not be divided any more; they were indivisible, incomprehensible, invisible, and poreless; they filled completely the spaces they occupied; they were homogenous, differing only in figure as "A" differs from "N," in arrangement as "AN" differs from "NA," and in position as when the letter "N" is laid on its side to form a "Z." The atoms differed in quantity, not in quality. The apparent difference in quality was due to the impression caused to the senses by the combination and configuration of the atoms.

According to the philosophy of Democritus, "Nothing is true, or if so, such truth is not certain to us." The sweet, the bitter, the hot, and the cold, were simply creations of the mind. Atoms and space alone existed, and the opinions of the properties of such objects were founded upon images inflicted by them upon the senses. He included "reflexion" as necessary for true knowledge, since "sensation" by itself was untrustworthy. Thus, although "sensation" may have indicated that sweet, bitter, hot, and cold occurred in bodies, "reflexion" taught that this was altogether an illusion and that, in reality, atoms and space alone existed.

The atoms composing stone or iron could only throb or oscillate. Those forming air and fire rebounded at great distances. They moved in all directions through infinite space. They struck against each other, producing lateral movements and vortices. The atoms of water, being smooth and round, were unable to hook onto one another and therefore rolled about, whereas the atoms of stone or iron, being rough, jagged, and uneven, clung together and formed a solid body.

Since all matter was composed of atoms of the same character, it could be concluded that nothing came into being or perished; hence matter was indestructible, although the atoms were liable to attach or detach themselves one from another and so change the appearance of matter.

Motion, according to Democritus, was equally eternal. It had its origin in a preceding motion, and so on *ad infinitum.*

Democritus substituted fixed natural laws for the combination of matter, disagreeing with the concept of love and discord conceived by Empedocles and in the idea of *nous* (mind or soul) taught by Anaxagoras. He explained the creation of the world on the basis that a definite number of atoms were carried downward through space. The larger and heavier, falling with a greater velocity, overtook and collided with the smaller which were thereby forced upward. This caused various lateral and contrary movements which resulted in a whirling movement, whereby smaller atoms were brought together and united to form larger bodies. As atoms and voids have always existed, there always had to be an infinite number of whirls in various stages of growth and decay, corresponding with the position of the atoms.[17]

Anatomy and Physiology: Democritus devoted considerable attention to the structure of the human body. Diogenes Laertius referred to a treatise by Democritus, "The Nature of Man," which treated of the anatomy of the human organism. It is related that Hippocrates was once sent to examine Democritus and to cure him from what the common people of his town thought was madness. Hippocrates found him engaged in dissecting animals to determine if disease was influenced by the bile. After having a lengthy discussion with his patient, Hippocrates addressed the people of Addaras. He expressed great veneration and respect for his patient. He rebuked those who had sent him on his mission with the remark that they themselves were mad, but stated that Democritus "is not only in full possession of his senses but he is the wisest man living."

THE SOUL: Democritus ascribed the physiology and psychology of the human organism to the soul. The soul, which pervaded the entire body, he thought was composed of fine invisible atoms, finer even than those of wind and heat; hence the exquisite fluency of the soul to govern thought, sensation, and motion, and its ability to bestow life on the coarser materials of the visible body. Sensation, thought, and all other functions were in reality movements of soul atoms produced by mechanical laws of pressure and impact.

The infinite particles of which the soul was composed he believed to be fiery, ethereal, and vaporous in character; they could not hold together when released from the body. While accepting the idea that the soul governed the body, he considered the soul not a separate entity, but rather a material automaton. After death, the atoms of the soul were blown away like smoke and perished together with the body. The soul reverted to the primeval matter from which it originated. While it was true that the individual atoms of the soul were indestructible, the soul, as such, lost its identity at the moment of death when it was liberated from the body. Thus he was opposed to Pythagoras who held that transmigration of the soul into another body took place after death.

Regarding the problem of perception of things, Democritus was of the opinion that objects constantly threw off images of themselves which were assimilated by the air through which they had to pass and entered the soul by pores of the sensitive organs. The all-pervading soul atoms exercised different functions in the different organs. In the head, they produced reasoning; in the heart, anger; and in the liver, desire. Life was maintained by the inhalation of fresh atoms to replace those lost by exhalation. Consequently, when the supply of atoms ceased, life ceased. Thus Democritus explained perception by external impressions to be the result of contact of the bodily atoms with the atoms from without. These external contacts consisted of subtle atoms thrown off from the surface of an object that penetrated the body through the pores and effected changes in the soul.

Atoms of the Senses: The atoms of the senses were particularly affected by those which resembled them. One saw atoms by means of the eye and heard atoms by means of the ear. These were best adapted to receive the images or sound currents. The sense organs, he held, were passages through which the atoms penetrated the soul. The eye, for example, was damp and porous, and the act of seeing consisted of the reflection of images mirrored on the smooth and moist surface of the pupil. He evidently believed, as did most ancient physiologists, that the pupil was the chief structure involved in the act of vision.

Because air was interposed between the eye and the object, visual images were blurred to some extent. Democritus distinguished between obscure cognition resting on sensation alone and genuine vision which was the result of inquiry by reason.

Color: Democritus was the first to explain color. He regarded white, black, red, and green as primary. The other colors resulted fom various mixtures of these four and were infinite in number. Color, itself, was not objective. It was found not in the ultimate *plenum* and *vacuum*, but in accordance with physical qualities and relations.[18]

Mechansim of Disease: The atomic concept was elaborated still further by Epicurus (342–270 B.C.) and later by Asclepiades, who explained the mechanism of disease as follows: The body was composed of minute particles, or atoms, and interspaces, or pores. These particles in the state of health were in perpetual motion. They kept circulating in the pores of the body, especially in the intestines where they were most active, in order to maintain the normal physiologic functions. According to this concept, disease was occasioned by clogging of the pores and by the stagnation of small particles caused by contraction of the tissues *(status strictus)* or by relaxation of the tissues *(status laxus)* due to an insufficient number of atoms in the pores.

According to the atomists, all things, even the elements, were composed of atoms. The character of all substances was determined by the shape, order, and position of its component atoms; and while the element of atmospheric air played an important part in human psychology, fire or heat was the most important element. Its atoms were the moving principle of all organic bodies. The soul itself was composed of fire or heat atoms. Mental activity was affected by the motion of such atoms.

Psychology: It is apparent that the system of psychology of Democritus differed from that of Heraclitus and Anaxagoras. The latter also explained human psychology on a materialistic basis, but he believed mental activity was produced by invisible particles exhaled from the vapor of warm blood, similar to the evaporation of water and diffusion of scent. The *nous* (soul or intelligence) of Anaxagoras was supposed to come from outside of the system from the universal mind and spread throughout the human body via the nerves.

The system of Democritus, however, was based upon mathematical considerations. He took as his starting point a vacuum and atom. The former was motionless; the latter moved in all directions through infinite spaces. The atoms struck against each other, producing lateral movements and vortices, bringing similar atoms together to form elements, and starting the formation of worlds which grew, decayed, and ultimately perished. Only those systems which were fitted to their environment survived. The last remark may be considered a premonition of Darwin's theory of natural selection.

Modern Atomic and Molecular Theories: The modern atomic and molecular theories, formulated by Dalton, Avagadaro, and Cannizzaro, have no relation to the atomic theory of Democritus. The discoverers of the modern chemical theory had before them exact quantitative measures of the properties in which chemical elements combined by weight and volume. Their concepts were not deduced from philosophical concepts nor even bound up with any philosophical theory of the universe.

Democritus' Family Education, and Influence: Democritus had the great advantage of being born in a wealthy family. His father was a prominent statesman of Thrace. It is related that his father had once entertained the Persian King Xerxes; and in evidence of friendship, the King sent several Magi from Persia to educate his son Democritus. His father died when he was quite young. After his death, Democritus asked for his part of the inheritance in money in order to be able to devote himself better to travel in the quest of knowledge. The land and other possessions he left to the rest of the family. Democritus visited Persia, Ethiopia, India, and other eastern countries. He resided in Egypt for seven years, during which time he studied mathematics and physics at the ancient schools. It is stated that when he returned to his native land he was penniless.

It is a matter of conjecture as to what extent he was influenced by his Magi teachers of the eastern schools. He wrote in the Ionic dialect. His works, according to Diogenes Laertius, numbered seventy-two. His purity of style compares favorably with that of Plato.

His views on the physical universe came down to posterity through the works of later writers, such as Aristotle, and particularly through his follower and admirer Epicurus (341-270 B.C.), who adopted and elaborated his atomic theory at Athens as a basis of physics, philosophy, ethics, and psychology.[19]

The teachings of Democritus are also derived from the criticism of his opponents, especially Aristotle and Theophrastus. According to Aristotle, Democritus regarded the primitive atoms as the seeds out of which individual things were developed. He traced the progressive genesis of vegetable and animal forces out of the earth. He said that many races might have survived by craft, courage, or speed. Thus he again vaguely anticipated the modern idea of survival of the fittest. Aristotle, although frequently disagreeing with the conclusions of Democritus, spoke of him with admiration.

The atomic theory was never popular in antiquity, since Democritus avoided dialectical discussions so dear to the Greeks of the time of the Sophists. Like Pythagoras, he became a legendary figure. One of the legends passed down from antiquity is that he put his own eyes out with a burning glass so that he might no longer be deluded with false indications, thus enabling himself to exercise his reason with tranquility.

References and Notes

1. Burnett, F.: Early Greek Philosophy. 1892.
2. Aristotle stated that Thales attributed to water divine intelligence which he opposed. De Anima 1:5.
3. Cornford, A. M.: Before and After Socrates. Cambridge, 1932.
4. Metaphysics 3:383–418.
5. De Anima 411, 8. Aristotle states, "Thales believed that the magnet has a soul because it makes iron move."
6. Heath, Sir T.: Greek Astronomy. London, 1932. Fairbanks, A.: First Philosophy of Greece. London, 1898.
7. "First Philosophy of Greece."
8. Sarton: History of Science. Baltimore, 1927, Vol. 1, p. 75.
9. Grote: History of Greece. Chap. 8.
10. Mulach, F. J.: Fragmenta Philos. d. Graec. 1860. "Early Greek Phil." 1892.
11. "Fragmenta Philos. d. Graec."
12. Freudenthal: Ueber d. Thelogie d. Xenophanes. Breslau, 1886.
13. Diels: Fragmente der Vorsocratiken. P. 59.
14. Gamperz: Griech Denkers. Leipzig, 1897. Zeller: Phil. der Griech. Leipzig, 1893.
15. A description similar to that of Genesis 1:2, "Now the earth was unformed and void."
16. Neuburger, M.: History of Medicine. Oxford University Press, London, 1910, p. 109.
17. Marion, Jr.: The Atom Theory of Lucretius. London, 1884.
18. Lange, F. A.: Gesch. d. Materialismus, 1866-1878. English trans., London and New York, 1925.
19. Baily, C.: Greek Atomists and Epicures. Oxford University Press, 1925.

17

Medical Philosophers and Practitioners

PHILOSOPHERS

THE contribution of the Ionic and Eleatic schools of philosophy to medicine was of inestimable value. The structure and function of the human body ceased to be merely an object of creation. It became a substance composed of basic elements subject to natural laws, and a change in the quantitive or qualitive proportion of those elements or in the surrounding nature could effect a change in the bodily substance and result in disease. The discussion and conclusion of these schools of learning, however, were of an abstract nature and largely academic, relating to the mind, the special senses, and the phenomena of birth, death, sleep, dreams, and memory. It is not known that any of the sages mentioned adopted the art of medicine as a profession. There might have been some who treated their sick disciples or friends. Several of the sages have been reported to have rendered medical aid during the prevalence of epidemics, but these were isolated cases.

Pythagoras

The first Ionic philosopher, recorded to have written on medical subjects and practiced medicine as a craft, was Pythagoras of Samos (580–510 B.C.). It is related that he traveled to Syras to render medical aid to his master Phereeydes (sixth century B.C.), one of the seven wise men of Athens and founder of the Orphic community, who is said to have been sick with phthisis. Pythagoras was especially known for his system of dietetics.

Concept of Four Elements: Pythagoras seems to be the first who applied the concept of the four elements to explain the processes of health

480

and disease. He was first to add four proximate qualities to the elements: hot and dry, hot and moist, cold and dry, and cold and moist.

Health he regarded as a proper tuning of the body, so that the right proportion of hot and cold, and moist and dry was preserved. Disease was the disproportionate expansion of one or the other. The pre-

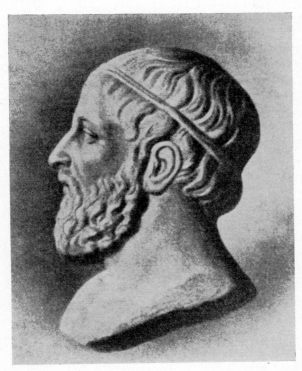

Fig. 114: Pythagoras (580–510 B.C.). Pythagoras was a Greek philosopher and a native of Samos. While still a youth, he was expelled from his native town by the tyranny of Polycrates. For a time, he belonged to the Ionian school of philosophers. His great search for knowledge took him to the Far East, the wisdom of which he introduced into his native land. He is said to have been the first Ionian philosopher to have taken a deep interest in medicine. Heraclitus, who was not given to compliments, said of him, "Of all men, Pythagoras, the son of Menesarchus, was the most assiduous inquirer."

occupation of Pythagoras with medicine led him to regard the soul more and more as the function of the body. Philolaus, who was an inspired pupil of this great master, explained the cause of disease to be due to a disturbance of the elements that made up the bile, blood, and phlegm, as for example an excess or lack of warmth (fire), or nourishment.[1]

Concept of Three Functions: Pythagoras thought that there were three functions in man: human, animal, and vegetable. The human function was located in the brain; the animal element, in the heart; and the vegetable, in the region of the naval.

Musical Relationships: The Pythagoreans experimented with sound and proved certain numerical musical relationships. Aristaxinus states that the Pythagoreans used medicine to purge the body and music to purge the soul. They advocated the use of music in diseases of the mind and in ailments prevailing in the spring. If high and low pitch, they argued, could be brought together in perfect attunement, it was natural to suppose that all other opposites could similarly be treated and all stable reality was a blend of opposites in proportions which could be numerically expressed.

Mystical Approach to Problems: Pythagoras opposed the purely materialistic tendencies of the Ionic school. He promulgated a mystical approach to the problems of man and his universe, seeking to find its solution in abstract mathematical concepts. He and the school which he founded exhibited a mystic attitude toward the universe, accompanied by a readiness to observe and experiment. Pythagoras objected to the idea that all matter was composed of one single element and he substituted the theory that the universe and all that it contained was composed of four elements. It is said that he arrived at this conclusion from the observation of the burning of a green stick. When green wood was burned, all the four elements of which wood was composed could be analyzed. The fire was seen by its own light. The smoke vanished into the air whence it originated. The water boiled off; and only the ashes which were the element of the earth, were left to join its own element.

According to the Pythagoreans, all matter was composed of pairs of the four underlying qualities: hot and cold, wet and dry. Water for example, was cold and wet; fire was hot and dry. Blood, according to the Pythagoreans, was composed of four equal elements, whereas bones contained one half fire (heat) and one quarter each of water and earth. During the process of solution of matter, the liberated elements united with their like in space, that is air to air and earth to earth.

The fundamental dogma of the Pythagoreans was that "number is the essence or first principle of all things." This led them at once to the study of the mysteries of figures and of numerical relations. It plunged them into the wildest fantasies, even to the point of believing that numbers were actually things. Aristotle states that "the Pythagoreans seem to have looked upon numbers as the principle of which

all that exists consists of." The Pythagoreans also believed in the fundamental importance of opposing principles, such as love and hatred,
good and evil, light and darkness[2]—an idea which often recurred in
Greek thought.

The Pythagorean system dealt with the philosophy of form as contrasted with the Ionic philosophy of matter. The Pythagoreans held
that the soul of man was merely an emanation of the universal soul,
and that it came into the body from without. They believed in a disembodied soul. They supposed that souls could exist without a body,
leading a kind of dream life. Their heroes and demons were souls not
yet embodied, or which had become disembodied. The doctrine of
metempsychosis (transmigration of the soul) which they had adopted,
perhaps from India, was in harmony with such views; and if it did
not imply the absolute immortality of the soul, at least it signified its
existence after the death of the body, when the disembodied spirit became incarnated again as soon as it found a suitable body. To life after
death, the Pythagoreans added a doctrine of reward and punishment.

The Pythagoreans, according to Philolaus (who wrote during the
fifth century B.C.), recognized the earth as a sphere, an idea opposed
by the Ionian school. Even Anaxagoras and Democritus maintained
that the earth was flat. The Pythagoreans realized that the apparent
rotation of the heavens could be explained more simply, by supposing
a moving earth. The earth was thought to revolve, not on its own axis,
but balanced by the counterearth, around a point fixed in space; it hung
free in space in the center of the universe, and it kept its place because
there was no reason why it should fall in one direction rather than in
another; it rotated like a stone at the end of a string.

Writings: Of the writings ascribed to Pythagoras, little is known
which is definitely authentic. Which material is his and which is the
work of his disciples or others who used his name to attract readers
is not known.

Doctrines: The scientific doctrines of the Pythagorean school had
no apparent connection with the religious mysticism of the society or
their rules of living. They had their origin in the same disinterested
desire of knowledge which gave rise to the other philosophical schools
of Greece, and in the idea of "philosophy" or the "theoretic life" as a
method of emancipation from the evils of ancient dogmas.

Aristotle, in his accounts of Pythagorean doctrines, never referred
to Pythagoras but always, with a studied vagueness, to "the Pythagoreans." Nevertheless, certain doctrines may be traced to the founder's
teaching. Foremost among these was the theory of immortality and

transmigration of the soul. Pythagoras' teaching on this point was connected, by one of the most trustworthy authorities, with the doctrine of the kinship of all living beings. The Pythagorean rule of abstinence from flesh was thus, in its origin, a taboo resting upon the blood-brotherhood of men and beasts, and the same line of thought appeared in a number of the Pythagorean rules of life which we find embedded in different traditions.

The moral and religious applications which Pythagoras gave to the doctrine of "transmigration" continued to be the teaching of his school. The view that the body was the tomb of the soul, besides being in the philosophy of immortality in the "Phaedo," was expressly connected by Plato with the teaching of Philolaus, disciple of Pythagoras. The strain of asceticism and self-denial of worldly pleasure which we meet here and elsewhere in Plato is usually traced to Pythagorean influence. Plato's mythical descriptions of a future life of retribution and purificatory wandering can be traced to Pythagorean teaching, though the substance of them may have been drawn from a common source in the mysteries.[3]

Foreign Influence: Pythagoras spent the first part of his life in Ionia. His accumulated wisdom was attributed to his wide travels which brought him into contact with the Egyptians, the Pheonicians, the Chaldeans, the Indians, the Jews, and the Arabians, as well as with the Persian Magi and the Brahmans. According to tradition, he was driven from Samos by the tyranny of Polycrates. He found refuge first in Egypt where he resided twenty-two years. In his philosophy may be detected many Egyptian concepts. His admission into the land of the Pharaohs was not without difficulty. The laws of the Egyptian priesthood rendered it impossible for a foreigner to become initiated without being circumcised, and Pythagoras had to submit to this operation.

From Egypt, he went to India. It is not known how long he resided there; but on his return, he brought back the doctrine of metempsychosis (transmigration of the soul) and the doctrine prohibiting the partaking of meat and other fanciful and visionary tenets. He settled in Crotona, a Greek colonial city in Italy, where he established a school.[4] Among many other branches of knowledge which he imparted to his pupils was the study of animal economy. He introduced a system of dietetics and taught his pupils the theory and practice of medicine. His visionary attempt to account for everything on the basis of the power of numbers exposed him to ridicule. His system of therapeutics hardly rose above the level taught in the temples. It does not appear that Pythagoras had the courage to brave the prejudice of his age by dissection of human bodies. Comparative anatomy and dissection of animals seems to have been the usual practice among the Pythagoreans.

Political Organization: The philosophers of the Pythagorean brotherhood were not, however, timid. Nor was this group merely a religious or mystical cult. The Pythagoreans formed an aggressively active political organization. Their master Pythagoras was of a restless and revolutionary nature. He organized the youths (who availed themselves of his instructions) into a secret political fraternity to combat oppression and fanaticism. His disciples, to join the Pythagorean brotherhood, had to undergo a period of probation and submit to examinations. At least on one occasion they constituted a ready instrument of intrigue against the state, which ended in successfully supplanting the senate of Crotona and the elevation of Pythagoras and his followers to the administration of the government. This, however, was not of long duration. Soon an overwhelming reaction set in. While his friends exalted Pythagoras above mankind, his opponents denounced him as a charlatan or, at best, a visionary mystic, who had turned the weak-minded into shallow enthusiasts and grim ascetics. He was openly accused of having conspired against and brought disorder and bloodshed upon a state which had given him an honorable refuge. Perhaps at the bottom of these political movements lay the hope of establishing a central point of union for the numerous Greek colonies in Italy, which, although they were rich and highy civilized, were by reason of their isolation and antagonism essentially weak.

One of Pythagoras' works begins, "Of the gods I cannot know what they are or are what they are not." Tradition adds that the book was burned and the author exiled. His institution was destroyed and the founder fell victim to his enemies. The Pythagorean brotherhood had its share in the wave of religious revival which swept over Hellas in the sixth century B.C. and had much in common with the Orphic community which sought by rites and abstinence to purify the believer's soul and enable him to escape from "the wheel of rebirth." A religious organization of this description, however, had no place in the tradition of Greek life and could only maintain itself by establishing the rule of Samos on a political basis.

The Pythagorean brotherhood remained an aggressively active political organization; and even after it was subdued, it still remained a subversive political force to be reckoned with.

Ethics: Aside from their political activities, however, the Pythagoreans formed a highly ethical community. They taught the principles of moderation in all things, the cultivation of friendship, the observance of faith, and the practice of self-denial. It was a maxim with them that a right education was not only of importance to the individual, but also to the interest of the state. Pythagoras directed his disciples, in their secret worship, to engage in gymnastics and dancing to the accompaniment of music. In accordance with his principle of imparting to men only such knowledge as they were fit to receive, he communicated to those who were less perfectly prepared exoteric doctrines, reserving the esoteric for the privileged few who had passed five years in silence, endured humiliation, and undergone purging by self-denial and sacrifice.

Alcameon

One of the most distinguished Pythagoreans was the philosopher Alcameon of Crotona (c. 500 B.C.). While most Ionian philosophers occupied themselves incidentally with medicine, Alcameon made medicine the chief object of his philosophy. He was the founder of the Sicilian dogmatic school of medicine and is said by some to have been the first Greek investigator to study anatomy by dissecting animals. According to Aristotle, Diogenes, and Plutarch, Alcameon was the first Greek investigator who possessed considerable knowledge of anatomy. Calcidus asserted that he was the first who dissected animals in order to learn the internal structure of the body. It is said that he dissected monkeys because they closely approximated the human form.

Anatomical Studies: Alcameon is said to have discovered the optic nerve and the eustachian tubes. Some of his teachings were as follows: The brain was a gland that generated thought as the salivary glands produced saliva and the lacrimal glands gave rise to tears. The brain was the central organ that governed thought, motion, and sensation; it was the seat of the soul. The sense of hearing was mainly the result of the concave form of the interior of the ear, just as all hollow places resounded when any noise entered them. The sense of odor was effected by the passing of odoriferous elements through the nose to the brain. Because of its humidity, moderate heat, and softness, the tongue was enabled to discriminate taste.

According to Plutarch, Alcameon originated the theory that sleep was caused by the storage of blood in the larger vessels; if this process proceeded to the extent of complete congestion, death resulted. Waking followed the redistribution of the blood throughout the system. The head of the fetus was the first part to be formed so that it could take nourishment in the uterus. He disproved, by experiments on animals, the old belief that seminal fluid passed from the brain to the spinal cord.

He taught that health depended on the equilibrium (attraction and repulsion) of the four elements and the adjustment of heat, coldness, dryness, humidity, and the sweet and bitter qualities of the tissues of the body. He attributed disease to changes in the secretions, especially

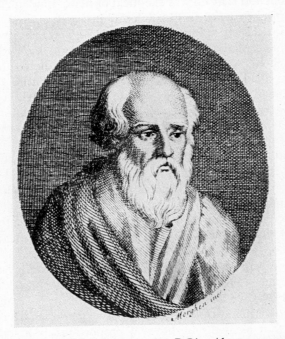

Fig. 115: Alcameon of Crotona (c. 500 B.C.). Alcameon was one of the most distinguished Pythagorean philosophers. He was perhaps the first on record who made medicine the chief subject of his philosophy. He was the founder of the Sicilian dogmatic school of medicine and the originator of animal dissection for the purpose of demonstrating the internal organs of the body. He should not be confused with Alcameon of Agros of an earlier date, whose name is associated with many Greek legends. He was deified after his tragic death. His tomb was on Cypress at Esaphis.

to the altered condition of the bile (black or yellow) and to changes in the blood and mucus (phlegm). Thus, he anticipated the humoral theory, later promulgated by Hippocrates. Alcameon taught the old concept, that the human microcosm was a miniature of the universe (macrocosm) and reflected the structure of the world. To cure disease, he determined, by study, what elements were lacking and then restored balance by adding the missing qualities.

Empedocles

Another disciple of Pythagoras, who rivaled him in his mystical philosophy, was the poet and philosopher Empedocles (c. 490–430 B.C.) of Agrigentum, a town in Sicily. From the scattered fragments of ancient writers, it may be inferred that he did not belong to any particular school and that he was skeptical of many fundamental theories.

Philosophical System: In his philosophical system, he seems to have been paradoxical—the physical, metaphysical, and moral were all combined. He accepted much that had been taught by Pythagoras and the Ionic school. On the one hand, he supported the Orphic mysteries and, on the other hand, he presented germs of scientific truths which were developed a century later by Plato and particularly Aristotle. For example, he accepted Pythagoras' dogma of transmigration of the soul as interpreted by the Orphics, that is the soul was a wanderer and a fugitive from God; it was yoked to the body and buried in it, as in a tomb. Empedocles considered this dogma as a kind of condemnation of the soul for sins committed in previous existences; and in the same breath, he taught that matter was composed of four elements: fire, earth, air, and water.

With reference to the elements, he taught that they were divine and eternal and that they were united and separated from each other by divine powers, love and discord (attraction and repulsion). According to him, these could be seen by the ordinary eye working among men in the phenomena of love and hate, but they really pervaded the whole world. Just as a painter made all shades and tints by combining four pigments, so matter was composed in many shapes and forms by combining the four elements in different proportions. For example, flesh and blood were made of equal parts by weight (not volume) of all four elements, whereas bones were one half fire and one fourth each earth and water.

Concept of Evolution: Empedocles took an important step in the direction of the modern conception of physical evolution by teaching that all things arose, not by transformation of some primitive form of matter, but by various combinations of a number of permanent elements. The elements were continually being combined and separated by two forces, "love and hatred" (attraction and repulsion). Empedocles may be said to have had a considerably advanced idea of evolution as a strictly mechanical process.

The four qualities, heat, cold, dryness, and moisture, were used by Empedocles to explain the construction of matter. These elements were also active in the human organism and had to be considered a part of "nature." The following is from a fragment of his poem "On Nature," "Listen first while I sing the fourfold root of Creation, fire and water and earth and the boundless aether, for therefrom is begotten what is, what was and what shall be." If "air" is substituted for "aether," there is the doctrine of the four elements which Empedocles introduced into philosophy and which, with the corresponding four qualities, heat, cold, moisture, and dryness, and the four humors, blood, phlegm, and black and yellow bile, lies at the base of Greek medical theories. He classified the elements, and their qualities and humors as follows:

Elements	Qualities	Humors
Fire	Hot and dry	Blood
Earth	Cold and moist	Phlegm
Water	Hot and moist	Black bile
Aether	Cold and dry	Yellow bile

Empedocles, like the atomists, explained the growth of an organism (increase and decrease) by the aggregation and segregation of the elements, "Nothing new comes or can come into being; the only changes that can occur are a change in juxtaposition of elements with elements."

His views that the early developments of animal life were derived from the union of incomplete structures and separate members were strange, as the following quotation shows:

As the elements entered into combination, there appeared strange results —heads without necks, arms without shoulders. Then as this fragmentary structure met, there were seen horned heads on human bodies, bodies of oxen with men's heads and figures of double sex but most of these products of natural forces disappeared as suddenly as they arose; only in these rare cases where the several parts were found adapted to each other and casual members fitted into casual members did the complex structure thus formed, last. Thus from spontaneous aggregations of casual aggregates which suited each other as these have been intended, did the organic universe originally spring. Soon, various influences reduced the characters of double sex to a male and female and the world was replenished with organic life.[5]

One may readily see in this strange concept, a crude prediction of the survival of the fittest. The animal characteristics, often seen in man, he explained on the basis of the principle that plants, animals, and man were composed of the same elements in different proportions. Thus there had to be some identity of nature in them all. They all had sense and understanding. Men, however, had a mind situated in the blood and the heart. The mind was dependent upon the body and varied with its changing constitution.

Concept of Knowledge: He explained knowledge on the basis that several elements in the things outside were perceived by the corresponding elements inside the body. One knew only in so far as he had within him a nature cognate with the object of knowledge, "Like is known to like." In the organs of sense there were pores, especially adopted to receive effluxes, which continually rose from bodies around men. In this way, perception was somewhat obscurely explained.

Concept of Vision: He explained vision on the principle that certain particles went forth from the eye to meet similar particles coming forth from the object; the resulting contact constituted vision. This concept conveyed the idea that perception was not merely a passive reflection of external objects. It was indeed difficult to harmonize his semi-scientific theories with the concept of transmigration of the soul which he expounded. Perhaps in this concept there was a germ of the doctrine that divinity passed from element to element, nowhere finding a home, which was a mystical way of teaching that continued identity was at the bottom of every phase of development from inorganic nature to man.

Other Concepts: Among his other concepts were the following: The law and identity of elements pervaded all nature. Plants and animals were links in a chain where man was a link too, and even the distinction between male and female was transcended. He anticipated the origin of species elaborated by the Darwinian school of the nineteenth century, "Beasts are akin to man; he who eats their flesh is not much better than a cannibal."

"We see," said Empedocles, "but a part and fancy that we have grasped the whole, but the senses cannot lead to truth; thought and reflection must look at a thing on every side. It is the business of a philosopher, while he lays bare the fundamental differences of elements, to display the identity that subsists between what is seen in the unconnected parts of the universe."[6]

Empedocles was perhaps the first among Greek philosophers to present a rational theory of fecundation:

The embryo is born jointly from male and female elements; the preponderance of the male or female semen, and the temperature and moisture of food determines the sex of the child. If the female sustains herself on cold and moist food, a daughter will be born. Twins are the result of a large amount of semen in the horns of the uterus. The embryo is completely formed on the fourth day; the resemblance of the child to the parent depends upon the one who contributes most towards its formation.

Empedocles, according to Galen, entertained a paradoxical opinion concerning the structure and function of the various parts of the body He explained respiration as follows:

As soon as that humidity of which there is a great stage in the first formation of the fetus begins to be diminished, the air insinuating through the pores of the body succeeds it; after this, the natural heat, by its tendency to make its escape, drives the air out and when the natural heat enters the body again, the air follows it afresh. The first part of this action is called inspiration and the latter, expiration.

Empedocles was of the opinion that respiration began before birth. He claimed that hearing was occasioned by impulses of air striking against the interior of the ear, which he fancied to be convoluted like a shell and fixed to the most elevated part of the body like a small bell, sensitive to every undulation of the air entering from without. Flesh was formed of equal portions of the four elements. Nerves were manufactured from two parts of water, one of fire, and one of earth. Bones consisted of equal parts of earth and water. He viewed sweat and tears as being merely the thinner parts of the blood. He wrote a book in Greek on the nature of things in which he compared the seeds of plants to the eggs of animals, both of them dropping when they attained maturity.

This puerile system of physiology was such that it betrayed an ignorance of the structure of the body and the analysis of the solids. But the philosophies of Alcameon and Empedocles were of the age when wild intuition and imagination were permitted to usurp the place of observation. Yet their theories and absurd speculations show that they possessed the keenest minds of their age.

Empedocles did not belong to any definite school of thought. He combined much that had been suggested by Pythagoras, Parmenides, and the Ionic school. At the same time he was a firm believer in Orphic mysteries.

Practical Application of His Theories: Empedocles was credited with having prevented an epidemic in his native city of Agrigentum by sealing an opening in the adjoining mountains through which the miasma was about to enter the city.

On another occasion, when the inhabitants of Selinus were afflicted with a plague in consequence of the stagnant water of the river which

surrounded its walls, he ordered that two neighboring streams be made
to flow into the channel. This feat of sanitary engineering carried away
the putrefaction and restored health to the town. Thus the wisdom of
his practice compensated for his mistaken theories.

Status in the Community: Empedocles belonged to a distinguished
family of statesmen and merchants. He himself was a statesman,
prophet, physicist, physician, and reformer. To his contemporaries and
the general public, he seemed more than a mere man. The Sicilians
greatly honored him and looked upon him with reverence as he moved
about them with his purple robes and golden girdle. Surrounded
by a retinue of followers, he made a conspicuous appearance with
his long hair bound by a Delphic garland and brazen sandals on his
feet.

Numerous legends were woven about him. One was that he restored
the life of a woman who was in a deathlike trance. Another was to
the effect that he had miraculously rendered salubrious the marshes
around Selinus. The manner of his death was also surrounded with
legends. According to one story, Empedocles, after a midnight feast
held in his honor, was called away in a blaze of glory to the gods. According to another, he threw himself into the crater of Etna in the hope
that man, finding no trace of him, would suppose him to have entered
heaven. This legend goes on to say that his hopes were in vain, because
the volcano cast forth his brazen sandals and betrayed his secret.[7]
Empedocles dedicated his poem "On Nature" to Pausanias. This poem
made first mention of the Asclepiades, to which Hippocrates himself
belonged.

The people of Agrigentum never ceased to honor him, and even
in modern times he has been celebrated by the followers of Mazzini
as the democrat *par excellence* of antiquity.

Neuburger has this to say of Empedocles:

He was physician, seer, priest, and poet in one. Honored as a god by
his contemporaries, his influence made itself felt throughout Hellas; his life,
his deeds and his death were surrounded by a halo of myth. "In a purple
robe, gold encircled, long hair framing his gloomy countenance, crowned
with the priestly laurel, he travelled through the country districts of Sicily,
surrounded by a host of worshippers of both sexes. Thousands, even tens
of thousands, acclaimed him, prostrated themselves before him, and demanded of him favorable forecasts for the future no less than healing for
all manner of disease." He freed the town of Selinus from a devastating
scourge by reclaiming the swampy land, and he assured his native town of
Agrigentum, favorable climatic conditions by blocking up a rift in a hill.[8]

Acron

A contemporary of Empedocles was his townsman Acron of Agrigentum (fifth century B.C.). Süidas gives the titles of several medical books written by him in the Doric dialect. According to Plutarch, during the great plague of the year 473 B.C. which depopulated Athens, Acron was instrumental in arresting the progress of the contagion and diminishing the mortality by recommending large fires to be kindled in the street and the practice of fumigation in the houses.

Archelaus

Another Ionian medical philosopher was Archelaus of Miletus (c. fifth century B.C.),[9] a pupil of Anaxagoras and teacher of Socrates. Archelaus identified primitive matter with air and ascribed to this element all mental activities, thus disagreeing with the doctrine of dualism or the principle of disembodied soul taught by his master Anaxagoras. "Out of this conscious air by the process of thickening and thinning arose cold and warmth or water or fire; one is passive—the other, active. The earth and heavenly bodies are formed from mud, the product of water and fire, from which springs also man first in his lower forms. Man differs from lower animals by the possession of moral and artistic faculties." His philosophy was frequently met with in the works of contemporary physiology and pathology. Nothing of his literary remains is extant. Extracts from the works of Diogenes, Laertius, Plutarch, and Hippolytus[10] contain what is known of his doctrine.

Hippo

Another physician, a contemporary of Archelaus and classed among the scientists of Ionia of that period, was Hippo of Miletus. He held that the principle of all things was moisture, and that fire developed from water, and from fire the material universe. He denied all existences save that of material things as known through the senses. He was classed among the "atheists." "The gods," he said, "are merely great men canonized by popular tradition." It is said that he composed his own epitaph wherein he claimed for himself a place in this company. He explained sickness as dependent upon an excess or a lack of humidity and upon the viscidity and thinness of the air. "Moisture was the fundamental status of nature from which heat and cold are derived." He described the soul as "a humor derived from the semen."

PRACTITIONERS

Aside from medical theorists there were practical physicians. Some of them enjoyed an international reputation.

Democedes

Herodotus[11] spoke highly of a certain Democedes (c. 520 B.C.) of Crotona and a contemporary of Empedocles. Democedes was a famous physician of international reputation whose professional services were solicited by King Darius of Persia when he dislocated his ankle while leaping from a horse:

He was without sleep for seven days for which his court physicians found no remedy until Democedes was sent for by the advice of one of his ministers . . . Fearing if his skill was discovered he would never be allowed to return to Greece, (Democedes) first denied that he knew his art; but Darius recognizing that he was unwilling to attend to him threatened him with corporal punishment, whereupon he changed his story by saying he did not know his art perfectly; he had some knowledge of it because of his connection with a physician. Darius placed himself under his care and by using Grecian medicine and applying lenitives after violent remedies, he caused him to sleep and in a little time he restored him to health, though he (Darius) had despaired of ever recovering the use of his foot.

Democedes returned to Crotona but did not remain there long because he was harshly treated by his father who had a severe temper. He left for Aegina. In the first year after he settled there, though he had none of the instruments necessary for his art, he surpassed the most skillful of the local physicians and, because of his skill, was engaged as chief physician on the yearly salary of one talent ($1200) out of the state treasury; on the third year he was called by the Athenians at a salary of one hundred minae ($2024); and the year after, he was summoned to Samos to be court physician of Polycrat, on a salary of two talents ($2400). From this time on, Democedes reflected great credit upon the physicians of Crotona. (Herodotus relates that owing to the treacherous murder of Polycrates by the Persians, Democedes was made a slave by Darius.)

Not long after, Atossa, daughter of King Cyrus of Persia and wife of Darius, had an abscess on her breast. After some time, it burst and spread considerably. As long as it was small, she concealed it and from delicacy she informed no one of it. When it became dangerous, she sent for Democedes . . . who cured her from the breast abscess . . . He exacted from her a promise that she, in return for the cure, would do for him whatever he should require from her, adding that he would ask nothing that would bring disgrace upon her. When she recovered, the king presented him with much wealth, but he wanted the liberty to return to Greece, and to obtain it he offered to act as a guide to the Persian spies that were sent to Greece. On reaching Crotona, he refused to accompany his escorts any further.[12]

The story of Democedes, as related by Herodotus, is of interest not only because of his distinction as a surgeon but also because this is the first case on record of public medical service.

In estimating the fees he received, it must be taken into consideration that money then had many times its present purchasing power; that the salary of an Athenian ambassador in the time of Aristophanes was less than one twelfth the amount paid to Democedes.

It is not known to which school Democedes belonged; but judging from his great popularity in his native land and in the East, it may be assumed that he was a *coan*. The school of Cnidus was at that period not so popular in Greece as that of Cos. The school of Cnidus undoubtedly received much of its erudition from the East as shown by its leaning toward dream interpretation and by the symbolic designation of its scientific terminology. Physicians of this school visited Persia, which was then a world empire, to learn the wisdom of the East.

Ctesias

One of these distinguished Cnidian visitors who went to Persia was Ctesias. Upon his arrival, war broke out between Cyrus the Younger and Artaxerxes Mnemon, and he was taken prisoner and inducted into the army as a military surgeon. When the war was over, Artaxerxes Mnemon, recognizing in Ctesias great professional ability, appointed him as court physician but prohibited him to leave Persia. For seventeen years, he was retained in the emperor's palace where he was held in high esteem. He did not spend his time, however, in leisure. He collected a large number of historical and geographical notes, many fragments of which are still extant.

In one of his historical notes, he described the tragic fate of his colleague, Asclepiad Apollonius of Cos, who having given immoral medical service to Princess Amytis, was tortured for two months and finally buried alive. His history "Persica" unfortunately exists only in fragments. It contains another interesting story as to how the Queen Pary Satis poisoned her rival Statira. After dividing a bird with a knife smeared with poison on one side, she gave the poisoned half to Statira while she ate the other half in order to show there was no deception.

He wrote a book on hip articulation, denying the possibility of reducing dislocation of the hip joint. He gained much publicity when he returned to Greece in the polemic with Hippocrates regarding his idea of dislocation of the hip joint. He also wrote books on medical plants, including one on the use of hellebore in medicine.

Euryphon

Among the most distinguished physicians of the school of Cnidus was Euryphon. According to Le Clerc, Euryphon was the author of the "Cnidian Sentences." He is credited with the introduction of percussion as a means of distinguishing tympanitis from dropsy, and he advised the use of milk (from an ass) for the treatment of phthisis. This does not tally with the statement of Coelius Aurelianus who reports that Euryphon was of the opinion that pleurisy was an affection of the lung; if he was skilled in percussion, he would not have made this mistake.

Eurypon did not always use the cautery iron judiciously. Galen preserved a fragment of Plato in which is described a certain Cinesias who was "thin as a skeleton, his legs like reeds, his chest still full of pus, and his ribs covered with scars from the cautery iron of Euryphon."

This is a fair example of the practices of the Cnidian school, whose motto was "accurate diagnosis and vigorous treatment." Their diagnosis was far from accurate and the treatment was vigorous, but not rational. It often produced very disastrous results. One is not surprised that the rival school of Cos quickly outshone the medical college of Cnidus.

Two quotations from the Hippocratic collection show that Euryphon practiced anatomy, and that he wrote a book on "Livid Liver." Euryphon ascribed the causes of disease to insufficient evacuation of waste products from the digestive tract. He was one of the few physicians of his period who knew that the arteries contained blood; he taught that hemorrhage could come from the arteries as well as from the veins.

Contributions of Physicians to Society

Physicians in Greece since the days of Homer held honorable positions in society. Herodotus attributed to them two of the most important events of antiquity—the conquest of Egypt by Cambyses and the invasion of Greece by the Persians. An inscription, dating from the fourth century B.C., found in the Acropolis at Athens reads:

Since Evenor the physician had sometimes shown goodwill to the city and people, and made himself useful by his art of healing to many, both citizens and strangers, and now having been chosen inspector of drugs

had spent a talent (240 pounds) in that office, it seemed good to Demus
to praise Evenor, son of Evepios the argive, to crown him with a crown
of green olive for his goodwill to the people of Athens, and that he be an
Athenian and his descendants, and that it be lawful for him to enter his
name on the list of whatever tribe he pleases, and this decree be engraved
on stone and preserved on the Acropolis.

Many inscriptions of a similar character are found in Greece dedicated
to physicians for their good and faithful services.

Argaeus

Another prominent physician was Argaeus, the Athenian physician,
who cured Batakis of rheumatism; and aside from getting a liberal fee
he got an inscription in his honor, dated in the first century B.C., which
reads:

> If ever mortals by wisdom discovered ought worthy of honor
> Surely Argaeus 'tis thou, O man of marvelous mind:
> Thou who hast gathered from books the learning and love of physicians,
> Wherefor the fame of thy art shall live through the ages to follow.
> Passing in brightness the stars shinging far over on high.[13]

Argaeus appears to have belonged to the sect of "wine doctors"
who flourished at that period.

Satyrus

The island of Cos, the birthplace of Hippocrates, was famous for its
great physician Satyrus. "The people of Istnus honored with triple
honors, Satyrus, son of Themistocles the physican and bestowed on him
a crown valued at fifty gold pieces." A bronze statue was also given,
because of his skill in art and his good will toward the Demus.[14]

References and Notes

1. Burnett, J.: Hasting's Encyclopedia, Vol. 10. pp. 520–530.
2. Ibid.
3. Allman, G. J.: Encyclopedia Britannica, Ed. 11, University Press, Cambridge,
England, 1911, Vol. 22, p. 699.
4. Pythagoras spent the latter part of his life at Crotona; this colony in south
Italy was famous for its healthy climate. According to Herodotus, the most
famous physicians of his day came from this city. Most of them were said
to be Pythagoreans.
5. Windelband: History of Philosophy. English translation.
6. Stein, H.: Empedocles Agrigenti Fragments. Bohn, 1882.

7. Fairbanks, A.: The First Philosophers of Greece. 1898. Gamperz, T.: Greek Thinkers. 1901, Vol. I. Eng. trans., L. Magnus.
8. Neuberger, M.: History of Medicine. London, 1910, p. 108.
9. Diogenes Laertius 2:16.
10. "Greek Thinkers." P. 402.
11. Herodotus 3:129–131.
12. Ibid. 3:127–137.
13. Cited by Withington: P. 67.
14. Patton and Hicks: Inscriptions of Cos. No. 408.

18

Hippocrates, the Great Teacher

IT is related that two sages expressed opposing views. One vehemently declared, "The time is adopted to the leader." The other just as forcefully proclaimed, "The leader is adopted to the time."[1] As is often the case when views diverge, both are expressions of eternal truths. This is particularly true in the case of Hippocrates. He was adopted to the time. Seldom, if ever, has there been a period within the memory of man in which history recorded so many literary giants within such a short period of two centuries. It was an age of transition from simple faith to enlightenment, a time when old mythology gave way to science. Beginning with Thales of Miletus, there were the philosophers Anaximander, Heraclitus, Anaxagoras, Pericles, Alcameon, Empedocles, Pythagoras, Diogenes, and a host of others. Among Hippocrates' own contemporaries, were Herodotus and Thucydides, the two greatest historians of all times, Aeschylus, Sophocles, and Euripides, the great writers of tragedy, Aristophanes, the author of comedies, Phidias, the eminent sculptor, and, of course, his younger contemporaries, Socrates and Plato.

The time was adopted to him beyond doubt. "His capacious mind and his penetrating judgment clearly discerned and carefully directed the removal of the obstacles which the bigotry and superstition of the vulgar, the impudence of the vain, the pretense of the quack, and the pride and vanity of the Sophists imposed."[2] He combated the dangerous and deceptive doctrine of the supernatural origin of disease inculcated by the priests—a doctrine which had been detrimental to the progress of medicine for ages. Hippocrates was not against the gods *per se*. He was against the idea of divine agencies. In his "De Morbo Sacro,"[3] he attacked those who masked their ignorance beneath a veil

499

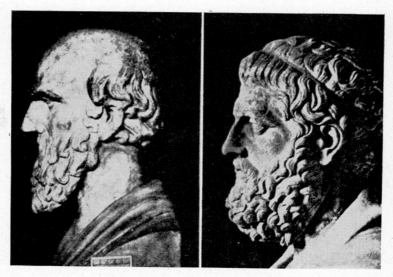

Fig. 116: *Left:* The oldest of the three great dramatists was Aeschylus, the creator of great tragedies. *Right:* Sophocles distinguished himself by nobility and loftiness both in portrayal of character and in language. (The portraits are now in the Capitoline Museum in Rome.)

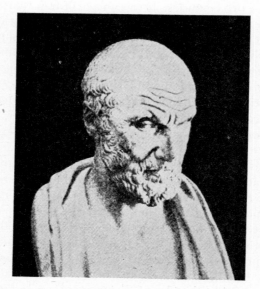

Fig. 117: Hippocrates (460–357 B.C.). (Courtesy of Yale University Press.)

of piety, and who pretended to subdue by charm and incantation those complaints which they had not the skill to encounter with rational means. He stated that our chief study should be how to learn the true properties of a thing, not by vain theories and delusive reasoning, but by actual experiments, patient investigation, and careful deductions.

HIPPOCRATIC SYSTEM OF MEDICINE

Hippocrates applied to medicine the same principle used by the Ionian philosophers in all matters pertaining to universal phenomena. He shared the opinion of Anaxagoras who modified his idea of divine agency so as to suit his thirst for scientific research. He sought the cause of disease in nature, in the earthy surroundings of man, and in the mechanism of his body. His great medical investigations were not in themselves a means of curing or preventing disease but represented a new approach to the study of disease. He disclosed where this human foe called "disease" was to be detected and how it could be subdued. He said that the purpose of medicine was to assist nature's recuperative power to throw off disease. The tendency of a wound was to heal and of sickness to give way to recovery.

Celsus, in the preface of his "De Medicina," states that Hippocrates was the first to emancipate medicine from the trammels of superstition and the delusions of philosophy.

Hippocrates freed medicine from philosophy, religion, and magic. What he said of these subjects is so interesting that a lengthy reproduction is pertinent for the proper evaluation of the life and work of the "father of medicine." With reference to the relationship of philosophy to medicine, Hippocrates questioned the usefulness of philosophic theories for medical practitioners:

Certain physicians and philosophers assert that one cannot know medicine without knowing what man is, how he originally came into existence and of what substances he was compounded in the beginning . . . Now the contention of these men really looks to philosophy, as do Empedocles and others who have written concerning nature. As for me, I consider that what a philosopher or physician has said or written of Nature has less relevancy to medicine than to painting; and I am of the opinion that, so far as concerns knowledge of Nature, one can know nothing definite about it except from medicine; but this may be thoroughly learned, when men go about it rightly. Hitherto, it seems to me, we have been far from it: far, that is to say, from having scientific knowledge of what man is (that is to say, what his constitution is) and to what cause he owes his origin and the rest, in any exact sense. Now, so much at least, it is indispensable that the physician should know concerning Nature and should greatly concern himself to know, if he is to do any part of his duty; to wit, what a man is (that is what his constitution is), relative to meat and drink, and what he is, relative to the rest of his mode of life, and what results follow for the individual from particular things, and all this not merely in general terms, as for example "cheese is unwholesome food, for it distresses one who eats plentifully of it"; but what particular distress it causes, and for what reason, and to what ingredient of the man's constitution it is unsuitable.[4]

The most exemplary arguments for freeing medicine from religion and magic and anxieties and irrelevant considerations is found in the Hippocratic text "On the Sacred Disease." Epilepsy, which was commonly regarded as a visitation of a god or demon, appeared to Hippocrates as follows:

. . . to be no wise more divine nor more sacred than other diseases, but has a natural cause from which it originates like other affections. Men regard its nature and cause as divine, from ignorance and wonder because it is not at all like other diseases. And this notion of divinity is kept up by their inability to comprehend it, and the simplicity of the mode by which it is treated, for men are freed from it by purifications and incantations. But if it is reckoned divine because it is wonderful, instead of one there are many diseases which would be sacred; for, as I will show, there are others no less wonderful and prodigious, which nobody imagines to be sacred. The quotidian, tertian, and quartan fevers seem to me no less sacred and divine in their origin than this disease, although they are not reckoned so wonderful. And I see men become mad and demented from no manifest cause . . . They who first referred this disease (epilepsy) to the gods, appear to me to have been just such persons as the conjurers, purificators, mountebanks, and charlatans now are, who give themselves out for being excessively religious, and as knowing more than other people. Such persons, then, using divinity as a pretext and screen of their own inability to afford any assistance, have given out that the disease is sacred, adding suitable reasons for this opinion; they have instituted a mode of treatment which is safe for themselves, namely by applying purifications and incantations, and enforcing abstinence from baths and many articles of food which are unwholesome to sick men . . . [5]

Hippocrates, for the first time, based the science of medicine on investigation and experience. He examined all the sick carefully and recorded the history and the symptoms of disease. He attempted to find out how one diseased man differed from another. He gathered facts and systematized them. He recorded his failures as well as his successes.

Experience and not hypothesis was the foundation upon which he built his medical structure. He demonstrated that, through observing the needs and diseases of men, medicine had developed through the ages, and not because of the acceptance or rejection of some particular hypothesis as to the reason for cure.

Healing by Nature: He laid down as his cardinal doctrine the adage *"vis medicatrix naturae"* which may be paraphrased, "Nature heals; the physician is only nature's assistant."

The fact that some forms of food will make a healthy person sick speaks against those who imagine that diseases, being produced by an excess of warmth or cold, dryness or moisture, may be cured by remedies believed to have the opposite properties. For if hot, or cold, or moist, or dry, be that which proves injurious to man, and if the person who would treat him properly must apply cold to the hot, hot to the cold, moist to the dry, and dry to the moist—then let a man eat wheat raw from the threshing floor, and raw meat, and drink water with it. By using such a diet I know that he will suffer severely; for he will experience pains, his body will become weak and his bowels deranged, and he will not live long. The surest and most obvious way is to change his diet, give bread instead of wheat, boiled flesh in the place of raw, and a little wine.[6]

Hippocrates confessed he could not tell which drugs possessed specific curative qualities and felt that other physicians resorted to their imaginations in selecting such drugs. In his own method of treatment, he relied upon nature, which he considered the great healer, and he believed in following the policy that would assist nature. This he did by measures founded on common sense, consisting in supervision of the patient's surroundings as to light, air, and cleanliness, and by encouragement and advice as to diet and exercise.

Traditional Medicine: Hippocrates was a believer in tradition since he felt that it is impossible for medicine to progress in any other way than as a result of experience. "The art of medicine," says this author of ancient medicine, "has from the earliest ages contained everything in itself, a principle as well as a method, by means of which, in more spacious times, many beautiful discoveries have been made; the rest will yet be found out, if capable investigators, knowing what has already been achieved, commence their research from that point."

Hippocrates' methods were far removed from the crude casual empiricism of his Asclepiadic predecessors. His opposition came, not because traditional medicine was old and out of date, but because, as he said, "I do not say that the old art of healing should be abandoned as of no account or as though its investigations were wrongly conducted; on the contrary, I maintain that its way of thinking came so near to truth that one should take it more into consideration and wonder at the discoveries made in spite of so great a lack of knowledge."

There is hardly a statement in his writing that has failed to leave its impression upon medicine. For example, the following may be cited:

He who would know correctly beforehand those that will recover and those that will die and in what cases a disease will be protracted or shortened must be able to judge from a thorough acquaintance with all the symptoms and a comparison of their weightiness, not omitting a consideration of the season of the year, yet being sure that at every season bad symptoms prognosticate ill and favorable symptoms good . . . You should not complain because the name of any disease may not be mentioned here, for you may know all such as come to a crisis in the above-mentioned times by the same symptoms.

The Hippocratic decision to abide by clinical experience in acute diseases and the significance of constantly recurring symptoms reflected the master's medical genius. His refusal to distinguish between diseases which were beyond any physician's knowledge, also showed his medical wisdom.

Natural History of Disease: What Hippocrates appears to have studied with particular attention was the natural history of diseases; that is to say, their tendencies to a favorable or fatal issue. "Without this knowledge, what can all medical practice be but blind empiricism? —a haphazard experiment, which perchance may turn out to cure or to kill the patient? The physician who cannot inform his patient what would be the probable issue of his complaint, if allowed to follow its natural course, is not qualified to prescribe any rational plan of treatment for its cure."

Prognosis: One of the most distinguishing characteristics, then, of the Hippocratic system of medicine was the importance attached to prognosis, under which was comprehended a complete acquaintance with the previous and present condition of the patient, and the tendency of the disease. Hippocrates was opposed to the overstrained system of diagnosis practiced in the school of Cnidus, according to which diseases were divided and subdivided arbitrarily into endless varieties. His common sense and high intellect led him to the discovery that to accidental varieties of diseased action there was no limit, and that what was indefinite could not be reduced to science.

STATUS OF MEDICAL ART

The reader may be interested in ascertaining what the status of the art of medicine of Greece and its colonies was at the time of Hippocrates. It has been shown that, as early as the time of Homer, Greek medicine was already at a fairly high level, and that the 500 years elapsing between the Greek poet and Hippocrates witnessed the transformation of many Aesculapian temples into medical schools where lay Asclepiade were trained in the art of medicine. It is logical, therefore, to conclude that, before Hippocrates arrived on the scene, medicine was fairly well advanced, and even the germ of rational medicine had already been planted in the schools. The Sicilian school, founded by Empedocles a century before Hippocrates, had already attempted to convert the medical art into a science by means of philosophical conclusions. The medical school of Cyrene received the praise of the philosopher Heraclitus, for its good physicians. (This school was not the Aesculapian temple which was erected in Cyrene in the year 429 B.C.)

In Hippocrates' own time, two famous schools flourished in the Greek colonies; the older one was that of Cnidus and the newer one with which Hippocrates was affiliated was Cos. The first school was mentioned by Hippocrates in his works and was praised by the rival college of Cos for its accurate descriptions of disease. It was censored only for too much emphasis on subjective symptoms and too little on objective signs. Because of this frailty, the members of the older school, like the Egyptians and Mesopotamians, distinguished a large number of diseases which were in reality only symptoms. This fault, according to Neuburger,[7] was corrected in a revised edition of the "Cnidian Sentences." The members of this school made use of the method of direct auscultation in the examination of the chest. The school attained considerable prominence in gynecology and possessed a comprehensive pharmaceutical formulary. Its therapeutic methods were in accordance with its topical diagnostic methods.

The Cnidians did not hesitate to perform excision of a rib in the case of empyema or nephrotomy for renal abscess. The cautery was frequently used. Excessive purgation, the injection of fluid in the air passages to produce cough, and the expulsion of mucus and pus from the lungs were frequently resorted to. The school of Cnidus was much influenced by the East, and learned the use of the medicinal plants from the East. Some Cnidian remedies were analogous to those mentioned in the Ebers Papyrus, including the use of human milk from a

mother who gave birth to a son and the use of whey and barley prepared in various ways. In later years, the Cnidians applied the principle of the nature philosophers to the art of medicine. The Cnidians
followed the trend of experience which led them often to sacrifice
truth for pseudoscientific precision.

The members of the school of Cos paid more attention to objective
symptoms and did not rely too heavily upon the statements of the patient. They employed their special senses to the limit when examining
a patient. They did not concern themselves with philosophical theories
and were not interested so much in a differential diagnosis as in the
patient. They recognized the systemic nature of disease; they held that
disease was generally not limited to a certain organ, although it could
manifest itself locally. They particularly studied acute diseases presenting precise symptoms.

According to Gamperz,[8] the members of the school of Cos worked
inductively. This group attempted, as far as possible, to start with
individual observation, although it was not able to completely without the support of the concepts of natural philosophy and physics.
The Cnidian school, on the other hand, was concerned chiefly with
knowledge derived from the mysteries. It developed directly in continuous tradition from archaic Greek, Babylonian, and Egyptian healing, and the school worked largely in a deductive manner. The influence of both the schools of Cos and Cnidus may be found in the
Hippocratic writings.

HIPPOCRATIC ANATOMY

Hippocratic anatomy is probably a collection of the anatomists that
preceded him; the respect for the dead, which was religiously observed
in all of Greece, prevented dissection of the human body. Knowledge
of human anatomy was superficially obtained through the treatment
of wounds, by external examination of clinical patients, and from the
observation of bodies found in tombs and from bodies of executed criminals. This knowledge of anatomy, as far as can be learned from the
Hippocratic writings, ranked far behind that of Alexandria a century
or so later. There is a difference of opinion as to whether Hippocrates
did original work in the anatomic field.

Rufus Epheseus and Galen[9] refer to Hippocrates with great deference
as one of the ancient authorities on the subject. Others say that he
organized a complete system of anatomy. His thorough acquaintance
with the bones, they assert, is evident from the brazen model of a

skeleton which was hung up in the temple of the Delphian Apollo as a testimony of his diligence and skill in this department. He is credited in one of his treatises, "The Heart," with having bestowed the name "aorta" on the great artery that arises from the left ventricle of the heart. This last claim, however, is denied by Galen who credits the discovery to Aristotle. It is by no means certain that Hippocrates dissected human bodies. If he did, he would not have confounded the nerves with the tendons and ligaments. With all these defects, Hippocrates was unquestionably the most gifted man of his age, and his opinion upon all medical subjects retains authority even to the present day.

The Hippocratics counted 91 bones in the body and, with the addition of the nails, the total rose to 111. The bones were fairly well observed as is evident from their bone surgery. The head consisted of one frontal, 2 temporal, 2 parietal, and one occipital bones. The frontal was the thinnest and weakest; the occipital, the strongest and thickest. They also made note of the sagittal sutures and certain abnormalities connected with them. They spoke of a *lamina externa* and a *lamina interna* and *diploe* (the cellular bony tissue between the cranial tablets).

Under the skull, there were two meninges covering the brain. The upper one was thick, and the lower one was thin. In the face, they described the nasal and cribriform bones and the spongy cartilage, and the superior and inferior maxillary bones and their apophyses. In the oral cavity, they named the teeth, gums, tongue, hard and soft palate, uvula, tonsils, sublingual glands, and esophagus.

The chest had seven ribs on each side, most of them false and connecting only with the vertebrae. Some were connected also to the sternum. The lungs had five lobes, spongy in texture. The heart was located between the lobes. Many tubes (bronchi) passed through the lungs. The stomach was on the left side of the liver in the abdominal cavity. The liver was connected to the gallbladder. From the stomach proceeded a serpentine-shaped, 12-cubit-long intestine "which some call the colon," and which ended at the rectum. The Hippocratics also noted the jejunum, the mesentery, and the mesocolon through which the intestines, with the exception of the lower part, passed. The mesocolon was attached to the lower part of the vertebrae. The plexuses were mentioned. The peritoneum was listed in one place.

The liver was situated right under the diaphragm with which it was connected. It was divided into two parts *(quadratus* and *spiglii)* which formed the porta. The gallbladder was described in its relation to the liver. The spleen resembled the sole of a foot. The pancreas was not mentioned. Of the urinary organs, the Hippocratics spoke of the heart-shaped kidneys, the ureters, and the bladder. The bladder was suspended from ligaments. They noted also the abdominal aorta and the vena cava.

There were ten vertebrae which were described as containing certain processes; the vertebrae were held together by intervertebral ligaments. There were anterior and posterior cords and the spinal processes. The spinal cord arose from the brain and was provided with little depressions or cavities. There were four curvatures to the spinal column.

Other anatomic descriptions were the acromion process, which was considered a special bone connecting the scapula with the clavicles. The bones were connected by tendons. The joints were lined with synovial membranes which facilitated their movements. Few muscles were mentioned: the deltoid, the pectoralis major, the flexors of the hands and fingers, the psoas, the gluteus, the biceps femoris, and the gastrocnemius. Other muscles were mentioned collectively as, for example, "the flesh above the bone." No distinction was made between tendons, nerves, arteries, and veins, although some veins must have been known to the practitioners of "blood-letting."

The word *phlebes* was applied to vessels containing blood. "Artery" was simply applied to tubes carrying air, such as the trachea and bronchi, and to the vessels found empty after death which were believed to contain air.

HIPPOCRATIC PHYSIOLOGY

The defective knowledge of anatomy at times gave rise to fanciful views of physiology. The brain was regarded as a gland and was the center of thought, will, and sensation, whose function was also to collect the excess fluid from the body. The chief organ of sight was the pupil. Vision was explained as the result of images thrown on the pupil. The bones of the ear carried the auditory sensation to the brain. The uterus was described as bicornate. In the right cornus, the male was believed to be conceived; in the left, the female. Fertilization was produced by both male and female seeds. This, in brief, was the knowledge of anatomy and physiology scattered in the Hippocratic literature.

HIPPOCRATIC PATHOLOGY

Humoral Theory: While Hippocratic therapeutic practices were not always aimed at counteracting the cause of disease, the Father of Medicine was always interested in the causation of abnormal phenomena. He followed the doctrine of Empedocles that the essence of matter was to be found in the four primary elements, fire, water, air, and earth. He also advocated the theory of the four proximal qualities, hot, cold, wet, and dry, a doctrine that finally culminated in the humoral theory of disease, which he elaborated and which became known as the humoral theory of Hippocrates.[10] His picture of the physical world is built on the following:

Elements	Humors	Qualities
Fire	Yellow bile	Hot and dry
Earth	Black bile	Cold and dry
Water	Phlegm	Cold and moist
Air	Blood	Hot and moist

The body of man (declared Hippocrates) has in itself blood, phlegm, yellow bile, and black bile; these make up the nature of his body, and through these he feels pain or enjoys health. Now he enjoys the most perfect health when these elements are duly proportioned to one another in respect to compounding, power, and bulk and when they are perfectly mingled. Pain is felt when one of these elements is in defect or excess, or is isolated in the body without being compounded with all the others. For when an element is isolated and stands by itself, not only must the place which it has left become diseased, but the place where it stands in a flood must, because of the excess, cause pain and distress. In fact, when more of an element flows out of the body than is necessary to get rid of superfluity, the emptying causes pain. If, on the other hand, it be to an inward part that there takes place the emptying, the shifting and the separation from other elements, the man certainly must, according to what has been said, suffer from a double pain, one in the place left, and another in the place flooded.[11]

The humoral theory of disease was supported 400 years later by Galen and remained the leading theory of disease until comparatively recent times. To the Hippocratics, life was bound up with the four primary fluids, blood, phlegm, and yellow and black bile. The blood, originating from the heart, represented the warm-moist quality; the yellow bile, secreted in the liver, represented the warm-dry properties; the black bile, arising from the spleen, had cold and dry characteristics; and the phlegm, formed in the brain, the cold-moist quality. The humors were formed and renewed by the daily supply of food, and were influenced by the season of the year, the wind, warmth, cold, sunshine, shadow, manner of life, and age.

Health depended upon the equilibrium and the normal blending of the humors. When their proportions were disturbed or unbalanced, when the humors had changed in quality, when they were not properly mixed, or when there was an abnormal accumulation of a given fluid in one part, health was impaired because of the production of sanguine, phlegmatic, melancholic, or choleric temperaments. Humoral disharmony in one part of the body could affect the entire system, or could cause abnormality in an organ located in a distant part of the body.

Hippocrates went on to explain how various diseases were caused by humoral pathology. Abnormal phlegm, for example, arising in the head could be the cause of pneumonia, pleurisy, dropsy, diarrhea, dysentery, vertigo, or sciatica. If phlegm penetrated the blood (or was suppressed, whereby cooling and excretion were hindered), fever or chill resulted. If bile was mixed with the blood, it produced fever-heat; impoverishment of the blood caused suppuration.

"Coction," or thickening of the humors of the body, was supposed to be necessary to cure disease. Coction was supposed to follow the combination of morbific matter in the economy. It was believed that a disease could not be properly expelled until the morbific humors were so prepared as to form excrementitious material. These physical changes were supposed to be brought about by the vital principle variously called "nature" (physis), "soul" (psyche), "breath" (pneuma), or "heat" (thermos).

Dyscrasia of the four principle fluids which determined, according to the Hippocratic view, the nature of disease, was often to be found under unfavorable external influences, such as the seasons of the year, climatic conditions, faulty habits of life, and morbid inheritance. In the spring, blood predominated; in the summer, yellow bile; in autumn, black bile; and in the winter, phlegm was in the ascendant.

The system of humors had a morphological basis: yellow bile arose from the liver; black bile, from the spleen. When the blood coagulated, it separated into its humoral components: the bottom, black part of the clot was black bile; the upper, red part was the blood; serum was the yellow bile; and fibrin was the phlegm.

Qualities were used by Empedocles to explain such things as sex, growth, and senility. Males were of warmer temperament and evolved in a northerly climate. Growth was an increase in bodily warmth. Senility occurred because of a loss of warmth. In much the same way, such physiological processes as respiration, sight, and hearing were interpreted.

Three Stages of Disease: Every disease had to undergo three stages: acridity (crude state, or irritation), coction (ripening, or crisis), and solution (or elimination). The last terminated in cure or death. The day on which coction took place was known as the crisis. It was usually accompanied by signs which received the designation "critical signs." It was for this crisis that the physician anxiously watched. On the critical day, nature (or rather *vis medicatrix naturae)* was supposed to remove the morbific material spontaneously. The crisis was accompanied by sweats, urination, or defecation. Sometimes the physician had to assist nature by the administration of purgatives, diuretics, or other measures. The term "critical period" has left an indelible mark on medicine which lingers still among physicians of various countries.[12]

The critical day was originally held to be the fourth day of the disease *(quarternary).* Some reckoned with the seventh day *(septenary).* The Pythagoreans, who were accustomed to juggle with figures, added many complicated numbers to the critical days. Thus, the thirty-fourth, fortieth, and sixtieth days of disease were figured by them as the most critical days.

The crisis was supposed to be local when one organ was affected and general when more than one organ was implicated. The term "crisis" was applied when the disease terminated rapidly with diaphoresis, diuresis, secretion, or excretion. When the diseased products were disposed of slowly or when one form of fever changed to another, the term "lysis" was applied. Fever was thought to rise on even days. The crisis, therefore, was also supposed to be on even days, such as the fourth, sixth, eighth, tenth, fourteenth, twentieth, twenty-fourth, thirtieth, fortieth, sixtieth, eightieth, and one hundred and twentieth days. Where the exacerbation occurred on odd days, the crisis was to be looked for on the third, fifth, seventh, ninth, eleventh, seventeenth, twenty-first, twenty-seventh, or thirty-first day. Any deviation from these days was considered a grave sign. It signified relapse or death. According to medieval writers a physician had to beware of all days, but especially the fourteenth, twenty-eighth, and forty-second days of the disease.

Celsus and Galen subscribed to the doctrine of critical days. Critical days were recognized in the seventeenth, eighteenth, and nineteenth centuries by such men as Sydenham, Stahl, Van Swieten, and many others. Some physicians still wait for certain days for a change in the disease. This might be explained by the fact that there are actually self-limited diseases of nearly regular periods and that the critical doctrines might have been founded upon the observation of such diseases.

Theory of Fluxions: Another prominent theory in the system of Hippocrates was the theory of fluxions (gathering of fluid, or catarrh). Fluxions were ordinarily considered to be caused by cold, although certain fluxions were supposed to be caused by heat, because the tissues thereby became attenuated so that the fluxions flowed easily when compressed. The theory of fluxions was founded on the ignorance of the histology of tissues and the laws of physics. The body of man in the Hippocratic works was sometimes likened to a sponge and sometimes to a sieve. The treatment recommended for fluxion was as vague as the theory. Certain other theories have complicated or disfigured the Hippocratic writings.

Hippocratic Opinion on Theories: Hippocrates did not follow his theories blindly as may be seen from the beginning of his medical tract:

There are those who have essayed to speak or write concerning medicine, basing their argument on the hot or cold, on the moist or the dry or anything else they choose, reducing the causes of human diseases and death to a minimum, one and the same for all, basing their argument on one or two (such causes); but in many of the novelties they utter they are clearly in the wrong. This is the more blameworthy, because they are touching an actual art which all men employ in the greatest emergencies and in which they honor most the skillful practitioners. Now there are practitioners, some bad, some excellent; which would not be true if medicine were not actually an art, and no observations or discoveries had been made in it. All would be equally unskilled and ignorant of it, and the cure of diseases would be wholly subject to chance. As a matter of fact, it is not so; but, as artisans in all other arts excel one the other in handicraft and knowledge, so also in medicine. Therefore I maintained that it had no need of vain hypothesis, as is the case in matters inaccessible to sense and open to doubt. Concerning these, if one essay to speak, one must resort to hypothesis. So, if one should speak and entertain an opinion touching things in the heavens or under the earth, it would be clear neither to the speaker nor to those who heard him whether his opinion was true or false; for there is no appeal to aught that can establish the truth.[13]

HIPPOCRATIC PROPHYLAXIS AND HYGIENE

In the Section "On Airs, Waters, and Places," Hippocrates conveyed the idea that it was not enough for a physician to study diagnosis and materia medica; he should also be learned in geography, meteorology, climatology, and sanitation. He begins the subject with the following:

Whoever wishes to investigate medicine properly, should proceed thus: in the first place to consider the seasons of the year, and what effects each of them produces (for they are not at all alike, but differ much from themselves in regard to their changes). Then the winds, the hot and the cold, especially such as are common to all countries, and then such as are peculiar to each locality. He must also consider the qualities of the waters, for as they differ from one another in taste and weight, so also do they differ much in their qualities. In the same manner, when one comes into a city to which he is a stranger, he ought to consider its situation, how it lies as to the winds and the rising of the sun; for its influence is not the same whether it lies to the north or the south, to the rising of the sun or to the setting sun, and concerning the waters which the inhabitants use, whether they be marshy and soft, or hard, and running from elevated and rocky situations, and then is saltish and unfit for cooking; and the ground, whether it be naked and deficient in water, or wooded and well watered, and whether it lies in a hollow, confined situation, or is elevated and cold; and the mode in which the inhabitants live, and what are their pursuits, whether they are fond of drinking and eating to excess, and not given to excess in eating and drinking.

From these things he must proceed to investigate everything else. For, if one knows all these things well, or at least the greater part of them, he cannot miss knowing, when he comes into a strange city, either the disease peculiar to the place, or the particular nature of common diseases, so that he will not be in doubt as to the treatment of the diseases, or commit mistakes, as is likely to be the case provided one had not previously considered these matters.[14]

In the same chapter, Hippocrates gave a general observation on the importance of cultivating a knowledge of the effects which the different seasons, the winds, the various kinds of water, the situation of cities, the nature of soils, and the modes of life, exercised upon the health, and the necessity of a physician's making himself well acquainted with all these matters, if he would wish to practice his profession successfully. The author insisted, with particular earnestness, on the utility of studying the constitution of the year and the nature of the seasons, and refuted the opinions of those persons, in his days, who held that a knowledge of all these things belonged to meteorology rather than to medicine. He treated of climate and the diseases prevalent in localities characterized by their exposure to particular winds. He treated of the various kinds of water and their effects in different states of the human constitution. The remarks contained here were of an eminently practical nature, and evidently must have been the result of patient observation and experiment, so that, even at present, it would be difficult to detect in our author a single error of judgment.[15]

HIPPOCRATIC THERAPY

Bathing was among Hippocrates' favorite remedies in a variety of cases, but he appeared to have employed aqueous affusion instead of immersion. There were contraindications against bathing after exposure to cold, after eating or drinking, when the stools were too loose or too costive, when there was loss of appetite or nausea, and when one was susceptible to nosebleed.[16]

He advised exercise in chronic cases but not in acute diseases; but even in acute diseases, he did not recommend constant confinement, observing, "We must sometime push the timid out of bed and rouse up the lazy." When diet and exercise failed to effect a cure, he had recourse to more active remedies, among which purging was one of the first.[17] He believed that purgation helped to rid the body of morbid humors. He was cautious however, never to administer them to pregnant women, since abortion might result. Purgatives were seldom prescribed for the very young or the very aged. Hippocrates stated that purgatives should not be used in the beginning of a disorder, nor between the first and fourth day. Each humor had its specific purgative which acted upon it alone. He judged the potency of the humor by the feeling of the patient after use of the purge. He used emetics as a prophylactic measure and occasionally for the purpose of cleaning the *primae viae*. He used an active emetic, such as white hellebore, when he wanted to recall the humors from the innermost recesses of the body. He administered it chiefly to insane and melancholy patients.[18]

As the author of "On Purgative Medicine," he emphasized idiosyncrasy in the use of both purgatives and emetics and advised physicians to make inquiry beforehand as to what effect such medicine had formerly produced on the patient. It should not be administered during the height of fever, and during the hot season of the year.

As the author of "On the Places in Man," he declared under certain circumstances a purgative would bind the bowels and astringents would loosen them. He further made the important remark that, although the rule of treatment was *contraria contraris curantur*, the opposite rule also held good in some cases, namely *similia similibus curantur*. It thus appears that the principles of allopathy and homeopathy were recognized by the author of this treatise.

He frequently had recourse to phlebotomy as a method of depletion, evidently as a prophylaxis and cure "to recall the blood when taking a wrong course and to procure free motion of the blood and spirits." He drew off the blood from the arms when the complaint was above the liver and from the foot or ankle or the back part of the thigh when below the liver. He stopped diarrhea before attempting phlebotomy.

He occasionally bled the patient to a great extent, even in chronic diseases. He related the case of a young man who complained of much pain in his belly, attended with rumbling noises while the stomach was empty, but with none when full. His food, however, did him no good. He became further emaciated each day. When none of the remedies benefited him, Hippocrates resorted to venesection, first in the arm, and then in other places, until the patient had scarcely any blood left in his body. By this means a cure was effected.

He bled in cases of dropsy, in enlargement of the spleen, and sometimes even during syncope. The veins that he opened included those of the arms, hands, forehead, occiput, posterior auricular region, under the breast, the ankles, and behind the thigh. He occasionally employed cupping and scarifying.

He resorted occasionally to diaphoretics, when bleeding or purging failed to offer the expected relief. His favorite external applications were fomentations. Fumigations were another method of cure, especially in famale complaints, and as a gargle in tonsillitis or quinsy. Other measures used included oil, ointments, cataplasms, and collyria.

The treatise "On Disease" contained many sound observations which might have been written by a present-day physician, as for example:

. . . having given an emetic to a woman to induce abortion, or applied an ointment for some disease of the eye when acute pain supervenes which ends either in rupture of the eye or amaurosis; the physician, in such a case, gets the blame, and when a physician gives anything to a woman in labor on account of pain in the bowels and the woman gets worse or dies, the physician incurs censure; and in disease and injury when there is a necessary succession of bad symptoms, the physician gets the blame, as man does not perceive that the aggravation of symptoms is a necessary consequence of the nature of the disease; and if a physician visits a patient in fever or who has met with an injury, and if the patient gets worse after the first medicine that is administered, the physician is blamed whereas he does not get the same amount of credit if the patient improves, as the amendment is attributed to nature.[19]

ETHICS OF HIPPOCRATES

One of his most repeated and favorite aphorisms was that life was short, the art long, the occasion fleeting, experience fallacious, and judgment difficult. The physician should not only be prepared to do what was right himself, but also to make the patient and attendants, felicitously cooperate. Hippocrates did not content himself with a general formula for the acquirement of knowledge, but gave explicit directions as to the physician's behavior in particular cases:

Touching his state of mind he must be heedful of the following: He must not only know how to be silent at the right time, but must lead a well-ordered life, for this adds much to his good repute. Let his disposition be that of a man of honor and as such let him behave to all honorable men in a friendly and easy spirit. Precipitation and impetuosity are not liked even though they be of use. As to his bearing, let him wear an expression of sympathy and not show vexation, which would indicate presumption and misanthropy. Who, on the other hand, laughs readily and is at all times merry, becomes a burden whence this is particularly to be avoided.

Medicine is of all the arts the most noble; but owing to the ignorance of those who practice it . . . it is far behind the other arts . . . as the mute figures on the stage have the shape, dress, and appearance of actors, and yet are not, so physicians are many in title, but very few in reality. You must not only do the proper thing, but do it at the right time . . . Whoever is to acquire a competent knowledge of medicine ought to have the following advantages: a natural disposition; instruction; a favorable position for the study; early tuition; love of labor; leisure. First of all, a natural talent is required, for when Nature opposes, everything else is in vain; but when Nature leads the way to what is most excellent, instruction in the art takes place, which the student must appropriate to himself by reflection, early becoming a pupil in a place well adapted for instruction. He must also bring to the task a love of labor and perseverance, so that the instruction, taking root, may bring forth proper and abundant fruits . . .

In the treatise "On Decorum," the author states:

A philosophical physician is equal to a god. In practice of medicine, all virtues relating to wisdom are exercised, namely contempt for money, modesty, simplicity in dress, character, judgment, quietness, accessibility, purity of life, knowledge of purifications which are proper and necessary in life, abstinence from lucre, freedom from superstitions, and divine excellence. The physician should keep himself aloof and not hold much converse with the common people unless when necessary.

Instruction in medicine is like the culture of the productions of the earth. For our natural disposition is, as it were, the soil; the tenets of our teacher are, as it were, the seed; instruction in youth is like the planting of the seed in the ground at the proper season; the place where the instruction is communicated is like the cultivation of the fields; and it is time which imparts strength to all things and brings them to maturity.

Having brought all these requisites to the study of medicine, and having acquired a true knowledge of it, we would thus, in traveling through the cities, be esteemed physicians not only in name but in reality.

In the treatise "On the Physician," he had some good advice for the physician himself. The physician should have a healthy look, for people fancy that a person who does not keep himself in good health is not qualified to take charge of the health of others; he should be of a prudent disposition and a gentleman of morals.[20]

HIPPOCRATIC OATH

The other great legacy left by Hippocrates was the Oath which was administered to physicians before entering upon medical practice, and which is still administered in full or in part in various parts of the world:

I swear by Apollo, the physician, and Aesculapius, and Health, and Panacea, and all the gods and goddesses that, according to my ability and judgment, I will keep this oath and this stipulation—to reckon him who taught me this Art equally dear to me as my parents, to share my substance with him, and relieve his necessities if required; to look upon his off-spring on the same footing as my own brothers, and to teach them this Art, if they shall wish to learn it, without fee or stipulation; and that by precept, lecture, and every other mode of instruction, I will impart a knowledge of the Art to my own sons, and those of my teachers, and to disciples bound by a stipulation and oath according to the law of medicine, but to none other. I will follow that system of regimen which, according to my ability and judgment, I consider for the benefit of my patients, and abstain from whatever is deleterious and mischievous. I will give no deadly medicine to anyone if asked, nor suggest any such counsel; and in like manner I will not give to a woman a pessary to produce abortion. With purity and with holiness I will pass my life and practice my Art. I will not cut persons laboring under the stone, but will leave this to be done by men who are practitioners of this work. Into whatever houses I enter, I will go into them for the benefit of the sick, and will abstain from every voluntary act of mischief and corruption, and further, from the seduction of females, or males, of freedmen and slaves. Whatever, in connection with my professional practice, or not in connection with it, I see or hear, in the life of men, which ought not to be spoken of abroad, I will not divulge as reckoning that all such should be kept secret. While I continue to keep this Oath inviolate, may it be granted to me to enjoy life and the practice of the Art, respected by all men in all time! But should I trespass or violate this Oath, may the reverse be my lot!

References and Notes

In the preparation of the chapters on Hippocrates, some of the quotations and other material are taken from the translation of W. H. S. Jones (Loeb Classical Library). However, for the sake of simplicity, the reader is referred to the appropriate section of Adam's translation.

1. Talmud Airechin 17a.
2. Puschmann, T.: History of Medical Education. 1839.
3. Adams, F.: The Genuine Works of Hippocrates. Wm. Wood & Co., New York, Vol. 2, pp. 334, 335, 336.
4. Ibid., Vol. 1, p. 143. ("On Ancient Medicine.")
5. Ibid., Vol. 2, pp. 334–335.
6. Ibid., Vol. 1, p. 138.
7. Neuburger, M.: History of Medicine. Oxford University Press, London, 1910, Vol. 1, p. 113.
8. Gomperz, T.: Griechische Denker. Leipzig, 1896, Vol. 1.
9. Galen: Politic. Vol. 3, p. 339. (Tauschnitz: De dissect.)
10. "The Genuine Works of Hippocrates," Vol. 1, pp. 85–87. Galen holds that Hippocrates was the author of the theory of humors.
11. Ibid., Vol. 1, p. 51. (On Ancient Medicine.)
12. Ibid., Vol. 1, pp. 208–209. (Air, Waters, and Places.)
13. Ibid., Vol. 1, p. 132. (On Ancient Medicine.)
14. Ibid., Vol. 1, pp. 156–159. (Air, Waters, and Places.)
15. Ibid., Vol. 1, p. 157.
16. Ibid., Vol. 1, pp. 252–253. (On the Regimen in Acute Diseases.)
17. Ibid., Vol. 1, p. 103.
18. Ibid., Vol. 1, pp. 262–276. Also Vol. 2, p. 204.
19. Ibid., Vol. 1, pp. 74–75. (Preliminary Discourse.)
20. Ibid., Vol. 1, p. 99.

19

Hippocrates, the Clinician

It has been noted in the last chapter that Hippocrates viewed the human body as a unit. Accordingly, his therapeutics was of a general nature, in contrast to the Asclepiade of the school of Cnidus who viewed the pathology of each organ separately and treated it locally. The Hippocratics examined not only the affected organ but the patient's entire body. They utilized the impressions of their eyes, and ears, and all sensory and intellectual means to aid them in arriving at a diagnosis.

MEDICAL HISTORIES

In addition to a direct examination, the statement of the patient was carefully recorded. Each symptom was considered a natural phenomenon which was to be studied with all available means. Personal observation, with due regard to individual peculiarities and to nature as a whole, was taken into account before arriving at a diagnosis. They were particularly impressed with the idea that the fate of the patient rather than the study of the symptoms had to be considered, and that, frequently, clinical observation even without deeper insight could furnish clues for his treatment.

Hippocrates was the first physician, and the only one on record from antiquity, to introduce the method of taking medical histories. He has left forty-two clinical histories; and no less than twenty-five of the forty-two cases (59½ per cent) ended fatally, a fact brought out by commentators as scientific honesty. Hippocrates did not give the diagnosis, which allowed many diagnostic attempts for commentators; and with the exception of some cases in which bleeding and enemas were mentioned, no remedies were employed. Perhaps the routine

519

treatment was generally known. Six of these histories, quoted at random, will be presented here:

CASE II: Hermocrates, who lived by the New Wall, was seized with fever. He began to have pain in the head and loins; an empty distention of the hypochondrium; the tongue at first was parched; deafness at the commencement; there was no sleep; not very thirsty; urine thick and red, when allowed to stand it did not subside; alvine discharge very dry, and not scanty. On the fifth, urine thin, had substances floating in it which did not fall to the bottom; at night he was delirious. On the sixth, had jaundice; all the symptoms were exacerbated; had no recollection. On the seventh, in an uncomfortable state; urine thin, as formerly; on the following days the same. About the eleventh day, all the symptoms appeared to be lightened. Coma set in; urine thicker, reddish, thin substance below, had no sediment; by degrees he became collected. On the fourteenth, fever gone; had no sweat; slept, quite collected; urine of the same character. About the seventeenth, had a relapse, became hot. On the following days, acute fever, urine thin, was delirious. Again, on the twentieth, had a crisis; free of fever; had no sweat; no appetite through the whole time; was perfectly collected; could not speak, tongue dry, without thirst; deep sleep. About the twenty-fourth day he became heated; bowels loose, with a thin, watery discharge; on the following days acute fever, tongue parched. On the twenty-seventh he died. In this patient deafness continued throughout; the urine either thick and red, without sediment, or thin, devoid of color, and having substances floating in it; he could taste nothing.[1]

CASE IX: The woman who lodged at the house of Tisamenas had a troublesome attack of ileac passion; much vomiting; could not keep her drink; pains about the hypochondria, and pains also in the lower part of the belly; constant tormina; no thirst; became hot; extremities cold throughout, with nausea and insomnolency; urine scanty and thin; dejections undigested, thin, scanty. Nothing could do her any good. She died.[2]

CASE X: A woman of those who lodged with Pantimides, from a miscarriage, was taken ill of fever. On the first day, tongue dry, thirst, nausea, insomnolency, belly disordered, with thin, copious, undigested dejections. On the second day, had a rigor, acute fever; alvine discharges copious; had no sleep. On the third, pains greater. On the fourth, delirious. On the seventh she died. Belly throughout loose, with copious, thin, undigested evacuations; urine scanty, thin. An ardent fever.[3]

CASE XII: In Larissa, a young unmarried woman was seized with a fever of the acute and ardent type; insomnolency, thirst; tongue sooty and dry; urine of a good color, but thin. On the second, in an uneasy state, did not sleep. On the third, alvine discharges copious, watery, and greenish, and on the following days passed such with relief. On the fourth, passed a small quantity of thin urine, having substances floating towards its surface, whch did not subside; was delirious towards night. On the sixth, a great hemorrhage from the nose; a chill, with a copious and hot sweat all over; apyrexia, had a crisis. In the fever, and when it had passed the crisis, the menses took place for the first time, for she was a young woman. Throughout she was oppressed with nausea, and rigors; redness of the face; pain of the eyes; heaviness of the head; she had no relapse, but the fever came to a crisis. The pains were on the even days.[4]

CASE XIV: In Cyzicus, a woman who had brought forth twin daughters, after a difficult labor, and in whom the lochial discharge was insufficient, at first was seized with an acute fever, attended with chills; heaviness of the head and neck, with pain; insomnolency from the commencement; she was silent, sullen, and disobedient; urine thin, and devoid of color; thirst, nausea for the most part; bowels irregularly disordered, and again constipated. On the sixth, towards night, talked much incoherently; had no sleep. About the eleventh day was seized with wild delirium, and again became collected; urine black, thin, and again deficient, and of an oily appearance; copious, thin, and disordered evacuations from the bowels. On the fourteenth, frequent convulsions; extremities cold; not in anywise collected; suppression of urine. On the sixteenth, loss of speech. On the seventeenth, she died. Phrenitis.[5]

CASE VII: A woman at the house of Ariston with sore throat which began from the tongue; speech indistinct, tongue red, and became parched. First day, she felt chilly and was feverish. Third day, a rigor and acute fever, a reddish, hard edema on both sides of the neck and chest. Extremities cold and livid; respiration labored; fluid returned to the nose, could not drink; constipation and suppression of urine. Fourth day, all the symptoms grew worse. Fifth day, the patient died.[6]

It is evident that Hippocrates strictly followed the principle laid down in the treatise "The Physician's Establishment," namely, "The physician is directed, when he comes to the patient, to seek to recognize similarities; that is to say, he shall, by observation of the patient, discover what manifestations indicate a deviation from the normal. In this connection he is enjoined to pay attention to the most salient phenomena first."

In addition to this, the physician was to examine not only the affected organ, but the condition of the patient's entire body, utilizing impressions from all the senses, and going into the minutest details. But however admirable the observation of such minutiae may be, the essence of "the art" of Hippocratism rested on the fact that the practitioner could, in individual cases, decide which impressions collectively permitted conclusions upon prognosis and indicated the occasion for therapeutic measures and the form they should take.

SYMPTOMS

The Father of Medicine was one of the first to point out that different diseases were to be distinguished by characteristic groupings of symptoms. Greek physicians before his time described cases of illness by the recital of a long list of symptoms. Each and every symptom was set down without emphasis or attempt at correlation.

Some symptoms are common to many diseases. Fever and such concomitant symptoms as headache, thirst, and dry skin, for example, may be present in diseases of the respiratory tract or of the gastrointestinal tract. In diseases of the former, the fever is apt to be accompanied by cough or pain in the chest; in diseases of the latter, the fever is apt to be accompanied by abdominal discomfort, nausea, or diarrhea.

Hippocrates laid stress on individual symptoms; he separated the essential from the nonessential ones. He pointed out that the combination of certain symptoms formed a clinical picture which characterized a specific disease and differentiated one disease from another. His knowledge of symptomatology aroused the admiration of Celsus and caused him to declare that "succeeding physicians, notwithstanding their improvements in the treatment of disease, were indebted to Hippocrates for the whole of their knowledge of signs."

He was especially skilled in bedside observations. He judged the patient's state of health by the facies, posture, voice, and excretions. It was his custom to examine the urine, feces, expectoration, sweat, and pulse of the patient.

It has been pointed out by critics that Hippocrates paid too much attention to the prognosis and not enough to the diagnosis of the disease. Such a criticism of the greatest physician in history is not justified. The fact is that Hippocrates based his prognosis upon a comprehensive study of the symptoms and the causes of the disease, particularly with reference to the acute diseases common in Greece at his period, such as, for example, pleurisy, pneumonia, and various fevers. In order to arrive at an intelligent prognosis, he employed all available diagnostic signs.

DIAGNOSIS

His diagnosis was based upon inspection, palpation, direct auscultation, taste, and smell. He examined the excreta, such as urine, feces, expectoration, and sweat, and paid particular attention to the patient's pulse. By inspection, he observed the so-called *"facies hippocraticus"* which included a sharp nose, hollow eyes, collapsed temples, cold and contracted ears, ear lobes turned out, skin above the forehead rough and distended in parts, and the color of the whole face green, black, livid, or lead-colored. Unless such features could be explained by some special reason, such as want of food or sleep, they represented a grave condition.[7]

Grave prognoses were also indicated by inspection when the patient was found in bed lying upon his back with his hands, neck, and legs extended, and when he was seen waving his hands before his face or moving his fingers aimlessly as if gathering bits of straw or picking the bed clothes (carphologia). ". . . for after I saw him fumble with his sheets and play with flowers and smile upon his finger ends, I knew that there was but one day."[8]

Emphasis was laid upon the appearance of the patient's eyes, particularly such ocular signs as cross-eyes (strabismus), protusion, inequality of the pupils, and ophthalmia. Any prominence of veins, pulsation of arteries, or other such visible evidences of pathology were considered important. Pulses were taken in the temples, arms, cardiac region, over the abdomen, and in the wrist joints. Unlike the Chinese who wrote volumes on the pulse and could distinguish many kinds of pulses, the Greeks did not concern themselves excessively with pulse counting. However, they used the pulse rate in estimating the temperature. The temperature was also ascertained by palpating the chest of the patient with the palms of the hands. Hippocratists were able to map out by palpation, the position, size, and consistency of the kidneys, liver, spleen, and uterus (vaginal exploration was done by the midwife). They were able, by means of palpation, to ascertain whether there was fluid within the abdominal and thoracic cavities.

Direct auscultation was expressly described. The patient's chest was shaken before auscultation was practiced. The so-called "Hippocratic succussion-splash" was observed to establish the presence of pus. The ear was applied to the thorax to listen for a noise which sounded like snoring when there was pus in the thorax. Pleurisy was described as producing a noise similar to that produced by rubbing a leather strap.

The sense of taste furnished many clues of internal diseases. All secretions and excretions were examined. The sweetness of urine gave evidence of diabetes. The taste of sputum, vomit, feces, ear wax, tears, nasal mucus, and the discharge of wounds gave evidence of many pathologic conditions. Such examinations were done by the physician or the patient. The odor of the sweat was ascertained in certain patients. Cold, clammy perspiration was a bad omen, particularly when it occurred on critical days. All in all, the Hippocratic examination was very thorough and excellent, considering the lack of diagnostic equipment.

According to Neuburger, the Hippocratic clinical history included such information as the following: age; temperature; mental state; memory; delirium; picking at the bed clothes; facial expression; condition of tongue; tones of voice; attitude when standing in bed; conditions as to nourishment and strength; power of movements; sensibility to pain; behavior during sleep; sensations of hunger and thirst; exhalation; condition of the skin, hair, and nails; state of the sense organs, particularly the eyes; possible abnormalities of the hypochondrium (enlargement of the liver and spleen); abdominal swelling; tumors or abscesses; the amount, color, taste, smell, and consistency of the blood and excretions; and such symptoms as gnashing of the teeth, shivering, and twitching.[9]

Aphorisms: Hippocrates was so perfect in the observation of external signs of disease that he has never in this respect been excelled. That he paid attention to the smallest details may be seen from his aphorisms, a few of which are presented here at random:[10]

Spontaneous lassitude indicates disease.

Those bodies which have been slowly emaciated should be slowly recruited; and those which have been quickly emaciated should be quickly recruited.

In acute disease it is not quite safe to prognosticate either death or recovery.

It is better that a fever succeed to a convulsion, than a convulsion to a fever.

In every disease it is a good sign when the patient's intellect is sound, and he is disposed to take whatever food is offered to him; but the contrary is bad.

Old people, on the whole, have fewer complaints than young; but those chronic diseases which do befall them generally never leave them.

In autumn, diseases are most acute, and most mortal, on the whole. The spring is most healthy, and least mortal.

In persons who cough up frothy blood, the discharge of it comes from the lungs.

It proves fatal to a woman in a state of pregnancy, if she be seized with any of the acute diseases.

Persons are most subject to apoplexy between the ages of forty and sixty.

Pains of the eyes are removed by drinking undiluted wine, plenteous bathing with hot water, and venesection.

If one gives to a person in fever the same food which is given to a person in good health, what is strength to the one is disease to the other.

Those diseases which medicines do not cure, iron (the knife?) cures;

those which iron cannot cure, fire (cautery) cures; and those which fire cannot cure, are to be reckoned wholly incurable.

Autumn is a bad season for persons in consumption. Winter (is a bad season) for pleurisy, pneumonia, coryza, hoarseness, cough, pains of the chest, pains of the ribs and loins, headache, vertigo, and apoplexy.

At the approach of dentition, (there occurs commonly) pruritus of the gums, fevers, convulsions, diarrhea, especially when cutting the canine teeth, and in those who are particularly fat, and have constipated bowels.

Persons who are naturally very fat are apt to die earlier than those who are slender.

To old people, (there is a predilection for) dyspnea, catarrhs accompanied with cough, dysuria, pains of the joints, nephritis, vertigo, apoplexy, cachexia, pruritus of the whole body, insomnolency, defluxions of the bowels, of the eyes, and of the nose, dimness of sight, cataract (glaucoma), and dullness of hearing.

If, in a person affected with fever, the neck becomes suddenly distorted, and he cannot swallow unless with difficulty, although no swelling be present, it is a mortal symptom.

Cold sweats, occurring along with an acute fever, indicate death; and along with a milder one, a protracted disease.

When in a fever not of the intermittent type, dyspnea and delirium come on, the case is mortal.

Blood or pus in the urine indicates ulceration either of the kidneys or of the bladder.

When small fleshy substances like hairs are discharged along with thick urine, these substances come from the kidneys.

In those cases where there is a spontaneous discharge of bloody urine, it indicates rupture of a small vein in the kidneys.

In those cases where there is a sandy sediment in the urine, there is calculus in the bladder (or kidneys).

Those cases of epilepsy which come on before puberty may undergo a change; but those which come on after twenty-five years of age, for the most part terminate in death.

Phthisis most commonly occurs between the ages of eighteen and thirty-five years.[11]

PROGNOSIS

The object of his careful clinical observation was perhaps not so much to foster and develop the diagnosis as to foretell the outcome of the disease. The wish to know the future was strangely characteristic of the ancient mind, and Hippocrates was no exception. He naturally held that it was better to exert all possible means to cure the patient than to waste energy in order to tell what was going to be, but this was not always possible. Some patients were incurable. It was best therefore, for the physician to be able to establish a prognosis, penetrating and exposing first of all, at the bedside, the present, the past, and the future of his patients, and adding what they omitted in their statements. He gained their confidence and, being convinced of his superiority of knowledge, they did not hesitate to commit themselves entirely into his hands.

He begins the "Book of Prognostics":

It appears to me a most excellent thing for the physician to cultivate prognosis; for by forseeing and foretelling, in the presence of the sick, the present, the past, and the future, and explaining the omissions which patients have been guilty of, he will be the more readily believed to be acquainted with the circumstances of the sick; so that men will have confidence to intrust themselves to such a physician. And he will manage the cure best who has foreseen what is to happen from the present state of matters. For it is impossible to make all the sick well; this, indeed, would have been better than to be able to foretell what is going to happen; but since men die, some even before calling the physician from the violence of the disease, and some die immediately after calling him, having lived, perhaps, only one day or a little longer, and before the physician could bring his art to counteract the disease; it therefore becomes necessary to know the nature of such affections, how far they are above the powers of the constitution; and, moreover, if there be anything divine in the diseases, and to learn a foreknowledge of this also. Thus a man will be the more esteemed to be a good physician, for he will be the better able to treat those aright who can be saved, from having long anticipated everything; and by seeing and announcing beforehand those who will live and those who will die, he will thus escape censure.12

SYNDROMES

Hippocrates was slow to name the disease. He described the syndrome and prescribed the remedy to neutralize it. A consumptive was seen in the following description, "little hair, a feminine skin, a complexion the color of a lentil, yellow eyes, a skin as in anasarca, prominent shoulder blades." Favorable signs of recovery were the observation that the patient's body was not wasted and that he possessed a chest with a plentiful growth of hair. With reference to the prognosis of consumption, he stated, "Many and in fact most of them die and of those confined to bed I do not know of a single individual who survived any considerable time."

The contagious effect of pulmonary consumption was mentioned by Hippocrates. He advised a young man suffering from consumption to leave the city and rest in the sunshine, to eat nutritious food, and to imbibe much milk, until his flesh rounded his frail frame, and until his cough was gone and strength had returned. He believed that phthisis was caused by small foci of pus.

His writings contained classical descriptions of gout, cirrhosis of the liver, arthritis, puerperal sepsis, diphtheria, tuberculosis, mumps, hysteria, epilepsy, different types of malaria (which are still designated by the Hippocratic nomenclature as quotidian, tertian, and quartan), acute inflammation of the throat, pneumonia, tetanus, erysipelas, inflammatory diseases of many organs, paralysis due to cerebral apoplexy, and diseases of the spinal cord now known as transverse myelitis and infantile paralysis. His descriptions, with a few changes, would be appropriate in a modern textbook.

Perhaps the most remarkable description, from the modern viewpoint, was that of pleurisy and the operation for purulent inflammation of the pleura. For this condition he advised the opening of the chest between the ribs. He made his diagnosis by the location of the pain and the presence of a splashing sound in the chest. This evidence of air and fluid in the chest is today a very rare physical sign of the disease, because modern methods of examining the patient yield an earlier diagnosis than was then available. There was no means for the physician of the fifth century B.C. to detect such a lung condition until this sign became manifest. Hippocratic pleurisy included not only empyema or purulent pleurisy but also pleurisy due to perforation of the lung in tuberculosis and lung abscess. Hippocrates described chest sounds when adhesions existed and caused friction between the lung and the chest wall. How much more he knew of the physical examination of the chest can only be surmised, but he could hardly have heard these friction sounds without putting his ear in direct contact with the chest.

The origin of pneumonia was attributed to phlegm, which, when descending from the head, was transformed into pus causing empyema or clots of blood. Undoubtedly, the Hippocratics knew that cavities could be formed in the lungs. Pleurisy was described as a disease following pneumonia, an adhesion of the lung with the costal pleura.

Such conditions as epilepsy, paraplegia, tetanus, apoplexy, and convulsions were considered as due to a loss of phlegm from the brain which had a tendency to deprive it of its humidity. Phrenitis was a disease characterized by hallucination and delirium.

In the first book on "The Epidemics," he recognized that there were diseases which were always present among the population. He coined the term "endemic" for such diseases and "epidemic" for diseases which were not always present, but at certain times became prevalent.

REGIMEN

The tract "On the Regimen in Acute Diseases" is of great interest.[13] This tract opens with a polemic against the Cnidian school for their differential diagnoses of diseases which went beyond their knowledge of the course and nature of disease, and far beyond their restricted remedies.

Diet was one of the most efficient weapons wielded by Hippocrates in combating disease. In acute disorders, especially in fevers, he preferred liquids to solids; and he was particularly partial to the use of *ptisans* (a drink made of peeled barley), which he prescribed to be taken twice a day by those who were accustomed, when in health, to take that number of meals. He disapproved of the sick eating oftener than when they were healthy. During paroxysms of fever as well as during all complaints, which had suffered exacerbations, he prohibited food altogether during the continuance of the paroxysm. Young persons were permitted a larger dietary intake than older people, always, however, bearing in mind the previous habits of the patient. He did not approve of the rigid and indiscriminate system of abstinence with which the practitioners of his day were in the habit of treating every complaint; for, he observed, this practice weakened the patient too much at the beginning of the disease and rendered the subsequent feeding of the patient at the improper stage indispensable. With respect to drinks, he was unfriendly to the use of plain water, substituting for it various refreshing beverages. He did not forbid wine, even in fevers and other acute disorders, provided delirium and pains in the head were not present. In complaints of a chronic nature, he ordered the use of milk and whey.[14] In his treatise "On the Regimen in Acute Diseases," dietary therapeutics was thoroughly discussed; he advised against sudden changes of diet even in disease:

One may derive information from the regimen of persons in good health what things are proper; for if it appear that there is a great difference whether the diet be so and so, in other respects, but more especially in the changes, how can it be otherwise in diseases, and more especially in the most acute? But it is well ascertained that even a faulty diet of food and drink, steadily persevered in, is safer in the main as regards health than if one suddenly change it to another. Wherefore, in the case of persons who take two meals in the day, or of those who take a single meal, sudden changes induce suffering and weakness; and thus persons who have not been accustomed to dine, if they shall take dinner, immediately become weak, have heaviness over their whole body, and become feeble and languid, and if, in addition, they take supper, they will have acid eructations, and some will have diarrhea whose bowels were previously dry, and not having been accustomed to be twice swelled out with food and to digest it twice a day, have been loaded beyond their wont.[15]

Hippocratic therapeutics was governed by the principle that recovery could be best achieved within the bounds of nature, and the duty of the physician was to adjust the condition of the patient to enable nature to function. In view of the limitation of the physician to cure every ailment, the Hippocratic physicians occupied themselves only with those diseases in which a cure could be anticipated. He approached the sickbed inspired by the principle, "Do good, or at least do no harm."

Drugs were used with caution, and drug treatment was conducted upon the principle of aiding the elimination of abnormal materials from the system which were increased, diminished, or diverted from unfavorable regions.

SURGERY

It is impossible in the available space to give an adequate account of Hippocratic surgery. One may form an idea of their surgical pathology from their knowledge of tuberculous bone infection now known as "coxalgia" or "Pott's disease." It seems that the Hippcratics knew of this condition. They described the symptoms of this disease as local and radiating pain coming on spontaneously or with little provocation, stiffness of the joints, restricted movements, stiffness of the back, necrosis of the bone (of the head of the femur), dislocation of the hip joint and abscess formation. The prognosis of this disease, according to the Hippocratics, was grave, particularly when the cartilages grew together; ankylosis set in and the patient became hopelessly lame.

Empyema: Another instance of the advanced stage of Hippocratic surgery may be seen from the description and treatment of empyema.[16] The symptoms were described as cough, purulent sputum, dyspnea, intermittent fever, profuse sweat, anorexia, and in the case of pyopneumothorax also the sign known as "succusio Hippocratica" (which was performed by shaking the patient and listening to a splashing sound). The Hippocratics did not distinguish between empyema and pyopneumothorax, but they knew that the succussion sound was sometimes absent, a condition which they ascribed to the thickness of the secretion. "When the patient suffers from rapid respiration, swelling of the feet, and cough, we take it for granted that the chest is full of pus." Bulging of the intercostal spaces was the guide for locating the pus in the chest. Another diagnostic sign was obtained by spreading over the suspected area a cloth soaked in moist soil. The place where the moist material dried first was taken as the area where the pus cavity was located.

The treatment of empyema was as follows: As soon as the pus area was located by the succussion sound, rales, or by bulging of the intercostal spaces, an incision was made in the skin behind the affected area with a *bistoury*. Then the point of a knife, thrust into the depth of a fingernail, was introduced into the incision in the intercostal space. In order to prevent the knife from going deeper, a cloth was wound above the desired point; the pus was then allowed to escape, and a wick was introduced for drainage. The pus was evacuated every day for ten days. If the pus was found to be thin, a tube was introduced. As soon as the cavity was free of pus, it was filled with an infusion of wine and oil. The idea of using the infusion was to keep the pleural cavity moist and not allow it to dry.

The prognosis depended upon the nature of the pus. If the pus was white and clear, the patient was promised recovery. On the other hand, if it was bloody and discolored or had a foul smell, the prognosis was fatal.[17]

Abscesses: Hippocrates ascribed inflammation to the accumulation of blood. Pus derived when blood did not leave the tissues in due time and particularly when pressure was exerted upon the inflammatory part. Inflammation and suppuration were always accompanied by fever and pain. The fever and pain were most intense during the process of pus formation and became ameliorated when pus had already formed.

He recognized two kinds of abscesses: circumscribed and diffused. He based the diagnosis of the presence of pus or abscess, upon fever, chills, pressure-pain, and swelling. The prognosis of suppuration depended upon the density of the inflamed area. If the area was soft and the surrounding tissue not hard, or if the abscess was pointing, the prognosis was favorable. His treatment of an abscess was medical and consisted of using measures that would tend to open the abcess spontaneously. He was averse to the use of a knife to hasten recovery.

Fractures and Dislocations: The Hippocratic descriptions and management of fractures and dislocations show to what good use they put their limited knowledge of anatomy. The Hippocratics knew that extension was of a vital importance if a broken bone was to be set accurately.[18] In a fracture of the humerus, the two fragments are drawn apart and then manipulated into the correct position. Usually the shoulder is fixed, and the elbow is pulled strongly downwards until the two fragments have been adjusted so as to come accurately together again.

The Hippocratics applied this principle to a break in the upper end of the humerus: A stout piece of wood was suspended by two chains from the ceiling of the room. The patient's broken arm was placed over this in such a way that, to all intents and purposes, he was suspended by the armpit from the wooden crossbar. This effectively fixed the upper fragment of the broken bone. The arm was bent at right angles, the wrist being supported by an assistant. A broad silk scarf was placed loosely over the bent elbow and, to its tied ends, a heavy weight was attached. This weight, pulling on the lower fragment, drew it into line with the fixed upper part of the broken bone, that is weight extension brought down the overriding broken bone and kept the two fragments roughly in a line with each other. It was then easy for the surgeon to manipulate the two broken ends into exact position. The same principle of fixing one end of a broken bone so that traction could effectively be exerted at the other end was applied in setting a broken thigh or a broken leg. A stake was driven firmly into the ground, and the patient was placed with one leg on either side of it, so that his own weight fixed his body against the immovable stake. Pulling on the ankle or knee would then separate the ends of the fractured bone and allow it to be set.

In fractures of bones below the knee, an ingenious use was made of the natural elastic springiness of twigs from the cornel tree. Thickly padded rings, one just above the ankle and the other just below the knee, were placed around the injured leg. Four twigs a little longer than the distance between the padded rings were then cut and forced into position between the rings. The slightly bent twigs, by their tendency to spring into a straight line, constantly forced the padded rings apart, and so transmitted the body-weight from ankle to knee without allowing undue strain on the broken bone. Hippocrates considered it disgraceful on the part of the surgeon to allow a broken bone to be set in a faulty position.[19]

Fractures are divided into (1) simple fractures, (2) fractures with slight exfoliation, (3) fractures with great exfoliation, and (4) compound fractures. According to Vectiarius, the treatment of fractures constituted the most interesting part of Hippocratic surgery. Every fracture, as well as dislocation, was carefully investigated by the Hippocratics. A careful history was taken of the age of the patient, the place of fracture, and how the accident happened. It was noted whether paralysis or atrophy resulted, and whether there was an open wound or any other abnormalities.[20]

Dislocations of the hip, shoulder, and jaw were described to per-

fection in the Hippocratic works and treated almost as we would treat
them today. The reductions of a dislocated shoulder and of a dislocated jaw are shown in a ninth century manuscript of Apollonius
of Kitium, believed to have been copied from the pre-Christian manuscripts of surgeons in the direct line of Hippocratic descent. The patient with a dislocated jaw was seated; an assistant stood behind him
fixing his head. The surgeon was in front, both his thumbs inside the
patient's mouth pressing the jawbone downwards, while his fingers

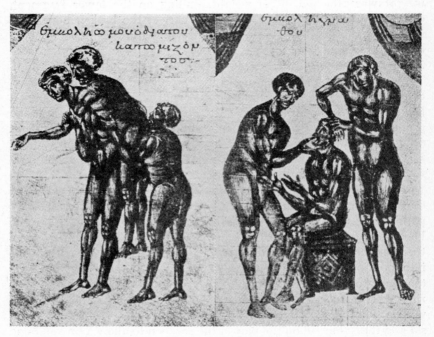

Fig. 118: *Left:* Reducing a dislocated shoulder. *Right:* Reducing a dislocated
jaw. (From a ninth-century manuscript by Apollonius of Kitium, which was
copied from a pre-Christian original.)

were outside, reaching behind the angle of the dislocated bone to
rotate it back into position.

The modern surgeon, faced with the same dislocation, varies the
technique depicted by Apollonius in only two minor particulars. The
patient with a dislocated shoulder is lifted onto the surgeon's back.
An assistant drags his body downwards while the surgeon, whose
shoulder is beneath the patient's armpit, is forcing the dislocated bone
upwards into its natural position. This is an application of the simple

lever principle, but it is important to note the positio... dislocated arm. The surgeon is holding it firmly above the... is bent at right angles with the hand, palm-upwards, and t... rotated outwards. If a dislocated arm is forced into this positi... then abruptly released from it, the dislocation will be reduced. ... Hippocratics dexterously employed a mechanical table to help put dis- located bones into position.

The Hippocratic description of the treatment of a wrestler who had sustained a dislocated hip is excellent.[21] There was "something masterly about it, pleasing to those who like to make some display in such mat- ters." The patient's arms were bound by his sides. A broad, soft strap encircled his legs just above the knee, so tied that the limbs were "four fingers' breadth or even less" apart. These preliminaries com- pleted, the patient was lifted until his feet reached either side of a stout beam, some 6 feet from the ground. Strong but soft bands about the ankles suspended him head downwards from this miniature gal- lows. In this position, the weight of his body tended to reduce the dis- location of the hip. Actually, the reduction was effected by an as- sistant inserting his forearm between the patient's thighs and abruptly suspending his whole weight from the already suspended patient. A dexterous twist of the forearm was then all that was needed. The dislocated bone slipped back into its socket with a sickening crack, and the reduction was completed. Bandages were applied, and at length the patient was lifted down and restored to his bed.[22]

Surgery of the Head: The most remarkable advance was made by the Hippocratics in surgery of the head. Head lesions were divided as follows: (1) fractures with depression and contusion; (2) fractures with impression; (3) simple contusions of the scalp; (4) weapon wounds, with or without fracture and contusion; (5) contracoup frac- tures. The Hippocratics believed that no matter how light a head in- jury seemed, it required most careful investigation and early diagnosis. To establish the diagnosis in a given case, the Hippocratics investigated the following: (1) the location of the injury; (2) the bone affected; and (3) the degree and kind of involvement. The history of the injury was considered important, especially in determining whether the pa- tient lost consciousness at the time of the accident. Probing was recom- mended by some Hippocratic writers only in weapon wounds if the history and careful examination established a definite head injury.

When further investigation was deemed necessary, an incision was made to separate the soft tissues from the bone. If no injury to the bone was found, the exposed part was filled with lint upon which a

cond day, the dressing was removed
examined. If there was any doubt
ne was curetted and searched for a

to discover a fracture was to apply to
that penetrated into fractures but was
ostances like bones. The black line left
vidence of fracture. Still another curious
cient bite on hard rice and instruct him to
he bones in the skull. Lesions in the front
isidered more dangerous than those of the
d by heavy sleep and dreams. The symptoms
of fever, u.. oma indicated that the brain was implicated.

When the lesion s. ined was in the vicinity of the skull sutures,
the prognosis was considered unfavorable. The prognosis was thought
to be fatal in fracture of the skull when the patient was not trepanated
early. In winter, a skull fracture, if not trephined, would be followed
by fever and other distressing symptoms after the fourteenth day; in
the summer, after the seventh day. The first symptom of approaching
danger was discoloration of the wound and a copious watery discharge. The soft part was first to undergo gangrenous degeneration and
was soon followed by necrosis of the bone and loss of consciousness.
In some case, the discharge separated the muscles from the cranial
bones; and in such cases, cure was hardly possible. The prognosis was
considered particularly grave when the opening of the wound was
small and did not permit a free discharge of pus. This caused inflammation of the surrounding tissues followed by chills and fever. When
early fever was complicated by monoplegia and unconsciousness, the
patient would surely die. A favorable prognosis was given when the
brain was not implicated.

As soon as fractures or contusions of the head were diagnosed (at
the latest within three days), trephining was indicated. Simple impression very seldom required trepanation. Impression with laceration of the head, a simple puncture wound, and even a clear penetration
of the bone did not indicate trepanation. The purpose of this operation
was to prevent inflammation of the dura. The earlier the skull was
trepanated, the more favorable was the prognosis. The trephining was
to be done at the place where the pus (if there was any) would most
freely escape. The Hippocratics advised not to trephine over a decayed
and destroyed bone, because such a bone would dissolve and disinte-
grate by itself. On the other hand, when a cranial bone was fractured

and the fissures of the broken bone were exposed, it should be trephined at once. Otherwise the fluid discharged would be absorbed in the dura and would cause putrefaction and decay because it had only a narrow place to escape.[23]

The trepanation should not be done too close to the dura, lest the dura be injured. As soon as the bone began to move, the trepan had to be removed and an effort made to loosen the fragment by other means. The trepan should not be allowed to get too warm. It had to be immersed in cold water during the operation because the heat might injure the healthy part of the bone. If, however, the trephining was being performed on a long-standing case, it could be drilled right to the dura. Care, however, had to be exercised not to push the drill too hard because the bone that had undergone necrosis could give way and the trepan injure the dura. The same cautions were advised when trephining young children whose bones were tender.

The reasons for trepanation were: (1) traumatism of the bone depression; (2) pus or blood below the cranial bones; and (3) water in the cranial cavity.

Three kinds of trepans are mentioned: (1) crown trepans; (2) perforative trepans; and (3) saw trepans. No description is given as to their character. To avoid *caro luxurians*, the wound in the head had to be made dry in order to promote fast healing. The dura had to be cleared of any discharge to prevent it from decaying. Nothing was so striking in Hippocratic surgery as the treatment of head wounds.

Trepanation is a dangerous operative interference which is seldom done in modern times. The fact that the operation was resorted to so frequently shows that the procedure must have met with some success; otherwise people would not have submitted to it.

Trepanation was practiced as far back as the Stone Age, as has been discussed in a previous chapter. Pruniers and Brocca have shown that neolithic skulls, discovered in France, Germany, Bohemia, Portugal, and South and North America, furnish evidence that this operation was performed during life in prehistoric times and not, as some believe, as a postmortem procedure. As a rule, the opening was irregular, mostly elliptic in shape, seldom square, and was made with a rather rough saw.

This operation of skull trephining was probably the earliest major surgical procedure. In remote antiquity, one of the prime objectives for this procedure was magical, that is the production of a hole in the skull permitted the incarcerated demon, causing epilepsy, blindness, or migraine, to pass out of the body of the possessed person. The re-

moved bone was used as an amulet by members of the family to ward
off diabolic diseases.

From excavations conducted some years ago in Peru,[24] it has been
estimated that about 2.5 percent of the population were trephined.
A few epileptics and more particularly victims of skull fractures, such
as those resulting from stone slings and clubs used in battle, were perhaps relieved by this operation. Some operations might have been performed as a punishment for crime or as a method of subduing a foe. Few
survived the operation.[25] Those who succumbed were of course thought
to be hopelessly possessed by the demon. Trepanned skulls have also
been discovered in Sweden, dating from the second or third century A.D.[26]

Other Surgical Diseases: Other surgical diseases dealt with in the
"Corpus Hippocraticum" are the following: fractures of the ribs, malar
bones, nasal bones and ear bones; injuries of the palate; inflammation
of the uvula, tonsils, and salivary glands; the presence of polyps; and
abdominal pathologies, such as hernia, ascites, fistulas, hemorrhoids,
proctitis, abscess of the liver, and stone in the kidneys and bladder.
Excision of tumors was not commonly practiced by the Hippocratics
although the Hindus had performed such operations previously. Amputations are not mentioned but it is reported by later writers that the
Hippocratics removed limbs which were threatened by gangrene.

Diseases of the eye were studied, and certain conditions, such as
cataract, ectropion, and many cases of ophthalmia, were treated surgically and medically.

There is no evidence that arteries were ligated, but the hot cautery
was used to stop bleeding vessels and for other purposes.

Wounds: Wounds were divided into two classes, "incised" and
"lacerated." There is an account in Hippocrates' work "Epidemics" of
a case of an arrow wound. The arrowhead was left in the soft tissues
for six years before it was removed, during which interval the victim
had no discomfort. The following diseases, complicating wounds, are
listed: erysipelas, tetanus, and phlegmon. Mention is made of a depressed
wound and a metastatic wound. Hippocrates understood the pathology
of clubfoot and cured cases of this deformity.

Bloodletting: Certain rules are laid down for bloodletting: the skin
had to be punctured above the exact place of the vein. If the blood,
after the phlebotomy, did not stop by itself, it was necessary to elevate
the limb from which the blood was drawn "in order that the blood
stream shall stop flowing"; following this procedure, a tight bandage
was applied. The bloodletter was admonished not to leave clots in the

wound in order to avoid suppuration. A number of sites are favored in the Hippocratic writings for bloodletting. According to Bouchut, the Hippocratics made a careful study of the veins. It is more likely that they used the superficial veins which were more visible to the eye.

Hemostasis: Measures included to assure hemostasis were various styptics, cold applications, cauterization of the bleeding vessel, and a tight bandage above the wound. The last, while not found in the Hippocratic writings, was employed even by the Homeric physicians.

Dressings and Bandages: Directions are listed as to dressings and bandages. The dressing had to be clean, light in weight, soft, and thin. At the same time it had to be firmly applied. The bandage had to be applied quickly and comfortably, without undue pressure. The dressing should not be dry. It had to be saturated with some moist substance. Sutures are only mentioned once in the Hippocratic writings, with reference to a nasal polyp where the nose was cut.

Techniques: Instructions were given how to bring together the opposing parts of a wound. Minute details are given as to personal cleanliness of the surgeon. His nails had to be cut to medium length; his hands had to be thoroughly cleansed; and the instruments and other equipment necessary to the operation had to be arranged at the proper place. Even the kind of light, natural or artificial, and the position of the operator were carefully regulated.

Hippocrates was as proficient in surgical technique as in medicine. His aversion to major surgery was due to the fact that he did not possess, at that early date, the necessary knowledge of measures to safeguard his patients against intense pain and various surgical complications. He had no knowledge of ligatures and of course no adequate anesthetic. He endeavored to do bloodless surgery whenever possible.

The operating room was built according to a standard plan, with reference to such things as wind and light. The instruments and dressing materials necessary for the operation had to be ready on hand. Water used to wash the patient's wound had to be clean (or boiled?). Wine and oil were most commonly used for washing wounds. Andreas Anagostakis thought that the Hippocratics had an idea of the antiseptic method of treating wounds, since they used such articles as wine, salt, copper solution, tar and asphalt, aromatic substances such as resin, and employed cautery frequently. He believed that the water used by the Hippocratics in surgery was boiled. Hirschberg[27] ventures a similar opinion. The evidence, however, is not conclusive, and the Hippocratics certainly did not know of antiseptics in the modern sense. If they did use them, it was simply for the purpose of cleanliness. Nowhere

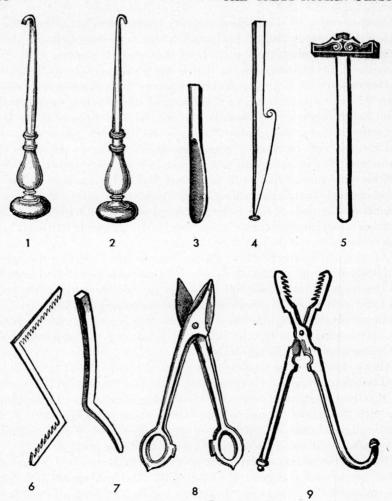

Fig. 119: Surgical instruments used by Hippocrates. *1* and *2:* A scalper, or raspatory, with which the moderns scrape the bone. *3:* Scalper cavus, or scooped raspatory. *4:* A lenticular. *5:* A malleolus, or mallet. *6:* A lever, by which modern surgeons protect the dura mater, and raise a depressed bone. *7:* The ancient meningophylax. *8:* Forfex excisoria, or cutting scissors. *9:* A forceps, used for extracting bones. (Reproduced from Adams: Genuine Works of Hippocrates.)

do the Hippocratic writings definitely say that the water used for surgical purposes was boiled. The Hippocratics had various lotions for promoting the healing of ulcers. Some of these have been used up to recent times.

Instruments: The following surgical instruments are mentioned in the Hippocratic writings: bistoury (broad and pointed); trepans for the head and for empyema; curettes; catheters; cautery instruments; speculums; dental forceps; uvula forceps; probes; syringes; and cups for bloodletting. Hippocrates used the sound for exploring the bladder. He knew the use of the speculum for examination of the rectum and the operation for fistula and piles.

In one of the books credited by some authorities to Hippocrates, he writes of sounds made of wood and of lead. He speaks of dilators and catheters. Vaginal tampons were made by rolling lint or wool into an oblong shape and were made emolient and astringent as needed for local action. Frequently, one half of a pomegranate was used as a mechanical pessary. There are also references to rectal suppositories, sitz baths, and fumigations, the last used in gynecological practice.

OBSTETRICS AND GYNECOLOGY

Hippocrates gave his views on conception, generation, and obstetrical management; and although some of his theories are at present out of date, on the whole the treatment he recommended is sound. The Hippocratic collection includes a monograph on generation, the nature of the infant, the seventh month of pregnancy, the eighth month of pregnancy, and accounts of superfetation, dentition, diseases of women, and extraction of a dead fetus.

The Hippocratics considered only vertex presentations as normal, which they explained as being due to the gravitation of the heavy head. Besides these they knew breech, transverse, and partial and complete foot presentations. In complete foot presentations, they either took no action or practiced shaking of the parturient woman or turning by external, internal, or combined methods. Prolapse of the arm in transverse presentation was thought to indicate death of the child and was an indication for embryotomy, which was carried out by means of a crushing instrument and a hook.

For delivery of the placenta, the woman kept her seat upon a chair with a hole in it, which was at other times used for vaginal fumigations; and the child with the cord still unsevered, was placed upon leather water-bags on the ground. These bags were then pricked so that their contents slowly escaped, by which means the child gradually sank and by its own weight brought away the placenta. The stool of delivery, the forceps, cesarian section, and ligature of the cord are not mentioned. A series of clinical histories deals with puerperal fever, which was supposed to depend upon retention of the lochia.

An important cause of abortion was held to be a disproportion between the development of the child and that of the uterus. Frequently the induction of abortion was attempted by shaking and by means of abortifacients, of which there were a number (as there were also means of preventing conception). In this connection, it was advised by the author of "De Natura Pueri" that the patient repeatedly jump up into the air, and at the same time kick the heels against the buttocks.

In his treatise "On Air, Water, and Places," he touches on the subject of gynecology. Mention is made of ulcers and hypertrophy of the labia, amenorrhea, a variety of discharges, narrowing of the os uteri, hemorrhage, inflammation, prolapse, versions, and carcinoma of the uterus. The methods of treatment, as far as they are directed against the frequently resulting sterility, are distinguished by their variety. The system of fumigation-therapy, as well as many of the means of recognizing fruitfulness and pregnancy, or of prevention of conception, are vividly reminiscent of Egyptian and oriental methods.

OPHTHALMOLOGY

Ophthalmology occupied a considerable place in Hippocratic medicine. It dealt largely with external diseases of the eye; very little was known of diseases of the uvea and fundus before the invention of the ophthalmoscope. External diseases of the eye included styes, blepharitis, conjunctivitis, ectropion, trichiasis, trachoma, pterygium, corneal ulcer, strabismus, nystagmus, nyctalopia, and hemianopia. Amblyopia was ascribed to the flow of phlegm from the brain. Blue color of the pupils indicated future cataract. Amaurosis was attributed to fever, loss of blood, and injury to the adjacent organs of the eye.

Operative measures were used for tumors, hypopion, and chemical and mechanical irritation of the mucus membrane. Cataract was removed by gouging. Surgical means were employed to arrest the flow of phlegm and to get rid of the accumulation of fluid in the brain. The measures consisted of repeated incisions to the skin of the scalp right down to the bone.[28]

HIPPOCRATES' PERSONAL HISTORY

Very little is known of Hippocrates' private life beyond the fact that he was born in the year 460 B.C. in the little island of Cos, in the Agean Sea some distance from Rhodes. This minor island is distinguished as the birthplace of three or four of the most eminent men of antiquity: Hippocrates; Apellas, a great painter of antiquity; Philetas the poet; and, perhaps, Theocritus. Hippocrates was the second of seven sons of a physician named Heracleids. He belonged to the family of Asclepiade, a sect of doctors who resorted to suggestions and prescribed drugs as indicated in dreams. According to tradition, he was a direct descendant on his father's side from Aesculapius. A genealogical table, professing to give a list of the names of his forefathers up to Aesculapius, has been transmitted from remote antiquity. On his mother's side, Hippocrates traced his ancestry to Hercules. His medical education is said to have been received from his father. He was taught rhetoric, philosophy, and literature by the Greek Sophist, Gorgias, and philosophy by Democritus, whom he cured of some mental derangement.

It is certain that he traveled widely, since his writings manifest a knowledge beyond the land of his birth. He commenced the practice of his art in his hometown on the island of Cos. Being dissatisfied with local educational facilities, he visited the principal foreign cities where he collected many of his ideas. His medical reputation spread, and he soon was considered the supreme representative of the Coan school, the teaching of which was included in the medical code known as "*Coaccae Praenotiones*" at Cos. He disapproved of some of the doctrines of the rival school of Cnidus, as included in "the Cnidian Sentences," a work probably consisting of the observations and theories made in the temple of health at Cnidus.[29] That he achieved great renown during his life is evident from the writings of Plato and Aristotle. According to all contemporaneous accounts that have come down to us, it is evident that Hippocrates was the model physician of experience and common sense. Since the basis of his system was rational experience and not blind empiricism, the Empirics in later ages had no bonafide grounds for claiming him as belonging to their sect.

Hippocrates died at Larissa, a town near Thessaly, about the year 361 B.C. at the advanced age of ninety-nine years.[30]

Hippocrates had two sons, Thessalus and Draco: the former became physician to Archelaus, King of Macedonia, and the latter, physician to the wife of Alexander the Great. They, together with their brother-in-law Polybus, were the founders of the School of Dogmatism based on their father's aphorisms, a sect which emphasized the importance of investigating not only the obvious, but the underlying and hidden causes of disease. It was the most prominent medical sect until the founding of the Empirical sect of Alexandria. During the life of his sons and son-in-law, the principles of Hippocrates were preciously guarded. Their writings bore the name of their illustrious father. It was difficult to distinguish his works from theirs. Later, some unscrupulous authors who bore no relation to him at all, signed his name to their own writings. In the course of time, various ideas and concepts detached themselves from the system of Hippocrates and gave rise to new lines of thought and speculation which had nothing in common with the thoughts of the savant of Cos.

HIPPOCRATIC WRITINGS

The following works, according to Renouard, seem to be authentic Hippocratic writings: "The Prognostics," "The Aphorisms," the first and third books "On Epidemics," "The Regimen in Acute Diseases," "On Airs, Waters, and Places," "On Articulations," "Luxations and Fractures," and treatises on "Instruments and Reduction."

Books considered almost certainly genuine are "Ancient Medicine," "Surgery," "The Law," "Fistulae," "Ulcers," "Hemorrhoids," and "On the Sacred Diseases."[31]

EVALUATION OF THE HIPPOCRATICS

Charles Singer, evaluating the Hippocratics, says:

The work of these men may be summed up by saying that without dissection, without any experimental physiology or pathology, and without any instrumental aid, they pushed the knowledge of the course and origin of diseases as far as it is conceivable that men in such circumstances could push it. This was done as a process of pure scientific induction. Their surgery, although hardly based on anatomy, was grounded on the most carefully recorded experience. In therapeutics they allowed themselves neither to be deceived by false hopes nor led aside by vain traditions. Yet in diagnosis, prognosis, surgery, and therapeutics alike, they were in many departments unsurpassed until the nineteenth century, and to some of their methods we have reverted in the twentieth. Persisting throughout the ages as a more or less definite tradition, which attained clearer form during and after the sixteenth century, Hippocratic methods have formed the basis of all departments of modern advance.[32]

References and Notes

1. Adams, F.: The Genuine Works of Hippocrates. Vol. 1, pp. 324–325. Probable diagnosis: Obstruction of the bowels.
2. Ibid., Vol. 1, p. 330. Probable diagnosis: Internal hemorrhage due to tubular gestation.
3. Ibid. Probable diagnosis: peritonitis.
4. Galen ascribes the recovery to copious menstrual discharge.

5. "Genuine Works of Hippocrates," Vol. 1, p. 348. Probable diagnosis: Septicemia.
6. Ibid., Probable diagnosis: Scarlet fever with kidney complications or erysipelas.
7. Ibid., Vol. 1, pp. 195–197.
8. Ibid., Vol. 1, pp. 194–195.
9. Neuburger, M.: History of Medicine. Henry Frowde, London, 1910, Vol. 1, p. 145.
10. "The Genuine Works of Hippocrates," Vol. 2, pp. 184–273.
11. Ibid., Vol. 2, pp. 192–273.
12. Ibid. (On Prognostics), Vol. 1, pp. 194–195.
13. Ibid., Vol. 1, pp. 227–259.
14. Ibid. (On the Regimen in Acute Diseases), Vol. 1, pp. 230–232.
15. Ibid., pp. 242–243.
16. Singer, C.: On the Legacy of Greece. P. 228.
17. For the sources, see Lurje, S. (to whom the writer is indebted): Studien über Chirurgie der Hippocratiker. Dorpat, 1890.
18. "The Genuine Works of Hippocrates," Vol. 2, pp. 35–49.
19. Ibid., pp. 36–37.
20. "Studien über Chirurgie der Hippocratiker," pp. 99–100.
21. "The Genuine Works of Hippocrates," Vol. 2, pp. 37–39.
22. Graham, H.: The Story of Surgery. pp. 57–59,
23. "The Genuine Works of Hippocrates," Vol. 1, pp. 386–388.
24. Wakefield, E. G., and Delinger, M. S.: Possible Reason for Trephining of the Skull in the Past. Ciba Symposia, 166, Sept., 1939.
25. The operation might also have been postmortem surgery for the purpose of permitting the escape of the soul before interment.
26. Broca, P.: Cas singulier de trapane chez les Incas. Bull. Soc. Anthr., 11: 403, 1867. Squier Exploration in the Land of the Incas. New York, 1877, Vol. 8. The operation appears to have been performed in the Talmudic days, where it is noted that a plate (kidduk) was used to replace substance from the cranium.
27. Hirschberg, J.: Die Asepsis bei den alten Griechen. Deutsche med. Wchnschr., 1070, 1889.
28. The writer is indebted to Max Neuburger for much of the information with reference to Hippocratic obstetrics and ophthalmology.
29. It is regrettable that this medical code has been lost. From his commentary, Galen appears to have seen this work.
30. Hamilton, W.: History of Medicine and Surgery. London, 1831.
31. Emile Littre deserved much credit for his splendid translation of the "Corpus Hippocraticum" in ten volumes, with two large introductions containing the Greek text printed opposite the French translation (1839–1853).
32. "On the Legacy of Greece," p. 236.

20

The Drift Towards Dogmatism

AFTER the death of Hippocrates, medicine suffered a setback. The followers of the sage of Cos either failed to comprehend the spirit of his instructions or abandoned themselves to delusions of vanity when deviating from the straight path, which had been so ably and so clearly demarcated by their illustrious preceptor. They returned to philosophic speculation which was denounced by Hippocrates. Their philosophy differed from that taught in the schools of Ionia and Elea. It was the moral philosophy or psychology developed in Athens by Socrates and Plato instead of the natural philosophy taught by the Ionians and Eleatics.

The ancient Greeks loved to talk and to carry on discussions. They preferred discussions on general subjects rather than investigation of a subject in particular. Instead of applying the Hippocratic method of deduction to cases under examination, they depended upon the written work of their master. They searched between the lines of his texts to find an answer to every medical problem; and when this was not possible, they indulged in philosophical speculations. They made commentaries on the text to suit their erroneous views, and as a result spurious texts bearing the name of the great physician appeared that tended to detract from his original works. In time, it became difficult to differentiate between the gold of the leader and the dross of the students.

Those who revered the memory of their great teacher became known as "Dogmatics." Their motto was as follows: "The physician who is also a philosopher is godlike."

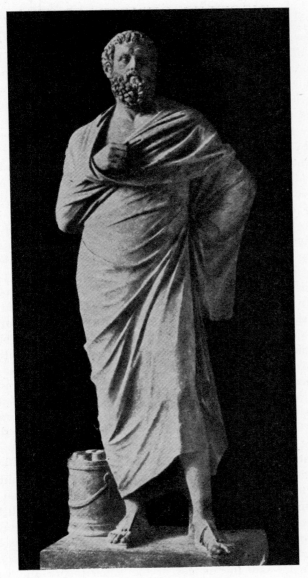

Fig. 120: Sophocles (495–406 B.C.). Sophocles was the greatest tragic poet of Greece. He was a contemporary of Hippocrates. At the age of twenty-eight, he was awarded the prize which was held for many years by Aeschylus. Only seven of his dramas are preserved. He suffered from "shortness of breath," which might have been of cardiac origin. It is said that he died from "shortness of breath" during a public reading of his drama "Antigone."

DISCIPLES OF HIPPOCRATES

Polybus: Disciples of Hippocrates who were under his direct influence adhered at least in part to the teaching of their master. Among these may be mentioned Polybus, the son-in-law of the great Coan.[1]

Polybus opened his book "On Man" by an attack on the physicians who represented the human body as being composed of one substance or being an aggregation of atoms. He showed that those who held the body to be composed of fire, air, water, and earth were not supported by cogent evidence. Polybus turned his attention to the development of a dogmatic humoral pathology; and Thessalus, son of Hippocrates and court physician to Archelaus, King of Macedonia, contended that excessive secretion of bile and phlegm was the primary cause of disease and wrote some books sustaining that thesis. His son, known as Hippocrates III, was an ardent advocate of Plato.

The sons and grandsons of Hippocrates stressed the importance of theoretical conjectures in medical thought and wrote theses containing what now appear as fantastical assumptions regarding disease.

Polybus' work "On the Nature of the Child" and most of the book "On Man," both physiological treatises, are interspersed with anatomical sketches. Polybus is represented as a recluse separated from worldly enjoyments and devoting himself to the study of anatomy and physiology, to the composition of the works of his father-in-law, and to his own studies on medical subjects.

His anatomical sketches were not accurate.[2] He represented the large vessels of the body as consisting of four pairs: the first proceeding from the head and passing by the back of the neck and spinal cord to the hips, lower extremities, and outer ankles; the second consisting of the jugular vessel, and proceeding to the loins, thighs, knee joint, and inner ankles; the third proceeding from the temples by the neck to the scapula and lungs and thence by mutual intercrossing to the spleen, left kidney, liver, right kidney, and finally to the rectum; and the fourth from the front of the neck to the upper extremities, the forepart of the trunk, and organs of generation.[3]

Diocles: The most gifted disciple of the sage of Cos was Diocles of Carystus, the son of Archidamus and a nephew of Hippocrates (350 A.D.). Diocles saw the danger of too much theory and warned his colleagues against philosophical speculations in trying to explain everything. He studied in Athens and traveled extensively to various medical centers[4] to gather medical information.

Diocles was regarded as the greatest physician next to Hippocrates;

like his master, he laid stress on practical experience and actual bedside observation.

Fever was a symptom of morbid conditions, such as wounds, inflammation, and obstruction of the pneuma. He distinguished between pneumonia and pleurisy, and between splenic and hepatic forms of ascites. He regarded the heart as the source of blood and distinguished two main blood vessels: the aorta, extending to the kidneys and bladder, and the vena cava, both giving rise to a system of veins. He recognized more veins than his predecessor. He did not distinguish them, however, from nerves. He pointed out the duct leading from the liver to the gallbladder. He mentioned the *esophagus, cecum, ureters, ovaries,* and *fallopian tubes.*

His physiology appears to have been influenced by the Sicilian school. He looked upon the heart as the seat of the soul, acting as a kind of pneuma which influenced movements and recorded impressions of the senses. The pneuma was renewed by means of respiration and distributed by means of the veins, along with the blood, to the brain and other parts of the body. In this theory, he compromised between the Coan and Sicilian concepts. The blood which was prepared in the liver supplied nourishment throughout the system.

He was inclined towards Cnidism with reference to differential diagnosis of disease and with regard to topical pathology. Digestion, he thought, was a form of putrefaction influenced by the heat in the stomach. The bodily waste was eliminated by the intestines, bladder, skin, sweat, and exhalation. He laid stress on diagnosis and prognosis. He held that no local complaints were curable without taking the constitutional condition into consideration. He ascribed the etiology of disease to impairment of the elementary qualities or disturbance of the pneumatic circulation.

Apoplexy and epilepsy were the results of obstruction of the phlegm. The cause of sterility was attributed to displacement of the uterus. He attributed dystocia (painful or slow delivery) to abnormal presentation, closure of the os uteri, abnormal size of the uterus, defective development, or death of the child. To cure prolapse of the uterus, he advised filling the uterus with air and, after it was in place, applying a pomegranate soaked in vinegar. Diocles based his knowledge of medicine on anatomy and materia medica. He expressed advanced ideas on embryology and toxicology. He wrote books on poisons and pharmacology. His work on herbals contains important instructions concerning the origin, recognition, nutritious value, and medical use of plants; it was freely used by late authors.

Diocles mentions opium as a remedy for toothache; his contemporary Diogoras thought it acted badly on the special senses and was therefore to be avoided in affections of the eye and ear. Two inventions have long survived under the name of Diocles—a bandage for the head and a remedy for toothache containing opium, galbanum, and pepper. Some of his works were still extant in the thirteenth century A.D.

John Actuarius has copied from Diocles the following prescription for a laxative: figs, 30 drachms; soda, 24 drachms; saffron, 3 drachms; rub in honey q.s.; divide in three parts; Sig. One part to be taken once daily.

While Diocles committed errors by following the Sicilian pneumatic-theory and the concept that mental disorders are localized in the heart, such doctrines had no influence on him in his practical medical procedure. In this he followed strictly his master Hippocrates.

According to Pliny, Diocles was second only to Hippocrates in point of reputation. He devoted his time to comparative anatomy, correcting many errors of his predecessors. His greatest critic, Galen, who in one place denied that Diocles was proficient in anatomic pursuits, credited him in another work with being the first to write a manual on the subject of dissection of dead bodies, an art which was confined in those days to a select few and was communicated only to students who were able to keep it secret. Diocles, while following the footsteps of Hippocrates in practical proceedings, blended the practice of medicine with the mythical concept of Pythagoras as taught by the Dogmatics. He subscribed to the science of numerology and to the wonderful properties of number "7" and its various combinations. Diocles issued a number of works; three are ascribed to Hippocrates.

Praxagoras: The successor of Diocles among the Dogmatics was his disciple Praxagoras of Cos (c. 350 B.C.), teacher of Herophilus. He was distinguished for his anatomic knowledge. He is credited with dissecting a human body which, as has been intimated, was rather rare in those days. He believed that the origin of the nerves was in the heart. He demonstrated the absence of cotyledon in the human uterus. He thought the heat of the body was acquired, not inherent. He was one of the few in those days who did not associate the veins with the arteries, but he supposed that the arteries contained air or the vital spirit.

Praxagoras of Cos maintained the existence of eleven different humors. He developed the study of etiology and differential diagnosis and localized the seat of fever in the vena cava and mental disease in the heart. Epilepsy, he thought, was caused by obstruction of the arteries by phlegm.

According to Coelius Aurelianus, Praxagoras recommended massage to the abdomen, in abdominal obstruction after failure of purgatives, enemas, emetics, and rectal injection of air to remove the cause; and finally he advised laparotomy and suturing of the intestine after the removal of the obstruction. It is not known whether he actually performed the operation or only recommended it as the next measure.[5] He was a strenuous advocate of phlebotomy.

Praxagoras laid stress on the pulse (sphygmology) as being of great diagnostic value in disease, a practice which was rather neglected by the other Hippocratics. He reduced human pathology to a regular system. According to Galen, Praxagoras was a lineal descendant of Aesculapius and a contemporary of Diocles.

THE SICILIAN SCHOOL

The Sicilian school appears to have had a great influence on the Dogmatics. The most prominent members of this school were Acron and Pausanias, pupils of Empedocles and, in a later generation, Philisteon of Locroi, a contemporary of Plato. The last was considered the most prominent representative of the Sicilian school of physicians. The Sicilian school laid the foundation upon which the medical structure of Hippocrates was erected.

From the time of its inception, the members of the school devoted themselves to animal dissection and particularly to the study of blood vessels. They were the first to observe that the arteries, after death, were depleted of blood; they concluded that they were filled with air or pneuma. They viewed the pneuma as the most important regulator of organic life. According to their theory, the pneuma was distributed by the veins mixed with the blood and circulated through the body to temper the bodily heat and assist all sense impressions and movements. In conjunction with the warmth of the stomach, the pneuma stimulated the putrefactive processes to aid digestion. The heart was regarded as the central organ of the pneuma.

This doctrine, founded upon a knowledge of anatomy, was momentous to the study of physiology and pathology. The theory that the heart was the seat of the pneuma was in contrast to that of the school of Cos which taught that the soul was located in the heart; they looked upon mental disturbances as a heart affection.

The Cnidians ascribed the cause of disease to the derangement of the pneuma and the four elements, or their qualities. They held that, as long as the pneuma (respiration) was in normal equilibrium, the individual was in good health; but if the pneuma became obstructed by the accumulation of bile or phlegm, disease set in. Other causes for disease were errors of diet, increase or diminution of the qualities, injuries, and heat.

The Sicilians laid particular stress on diet in their therapeutics, a practice introduced by Pythagoras. The leaders of the Sicilian school, Acron and Philisteon, have written works dealing with diet in health and in disease. Galen considered Philisteon as the best reputed author of the Hippocratic writings. The Sicilian cult should be rated with the Cnidian and Coan schools as the most important contributors to medicine, particularly to the teachings of the Dogmatists.

THE DOGMATIC SCHOOL

The founders of the Dogmatic school were largely located in Cos, a city that attained the zenith of prosperity in the Hellenic Age. As a seat of learning, it rose to be a provincial branch of the museum of Alexandria and became a favorite resort of the children of the princes of the Ptolemaic Dynasty.[6]

Menocrates: One of the students of Cos was Menocrates of Syracuse (360 B.C.). He is chiefly mentioned here because he was one of the few quack physicians in the history of Greek medicine and also because of his letter to Philip of Macedonia. He is reported to have been a physician of considerable skill but conceited and vain. He wore a purple robe with a golden crown upon his head and carried a scepter in his hand, impersonating Jupiter. Previous to undertaking any cure, he stipulated that his patient had to follow him, in the event of recovery, wherever he went.

His letter to Philip is characteristic of the man.[7] It read as follows:

"Menocrates Jupiter to Philip, Greetings: Thou reignest in Macedonia and I in medicine; thou givest death to those who are in good health. I restore life to the sick. Thy guards are composed of Macedonians. The gods themselves constitute mine." To this arrogant vanity, Philip laconically replied that he wished the recovery of his reason. This Menocrates should not be confounded with Menocratus of Zeophleta (34 A.D.), physician to Tiberius, who is said to have left 150 works, including a treatise on pharmacology. The latter was among the early users of escharotics. He insisted that, in writing prescriptions, figures be used instead of symbols for weight. He is also famous for his invention of diachylon (lead) plaster and toothpowder, which was celebrated by the rhyming physician Servillius Democrates.

Crytodemus: Another celebrated physician was Crytodemus, who was attached to the court of Alexander the Great. He is said to have saved the life of this monarch by extracting an arrow from his body.

Other Dogmatics: Other Dogmatics were Xenophon; Roxane (Hippocrates IV), a grandson of the Great Master; and Philotimus of Cos (third century B.C.). Philotimus transmitted to the Alexandrian library the Hippocratic book "On the Endemics," together with the library of the Dogmatic school that was located in Cos. For a long time, royal courts preferred the services of physicians coming from the Coan schools.

Influence of Dogmatism: The doctrine and the practical endeavors of Diocles and Praxagoras won many adherents to the doctrine of Dogmatism. They advanced knowledge in the domain of anatomy, materia medica, and dietetics which formed the basis of later scientific development. Some of their followers were Xenophon and Philotimus of Cos, Dieuches and Mnesitheos of Athens, who were lauded by later authors for their valuable work, and Euenor of Argos who distinguished himself in obstetrics and ophthalmology.

Dogmatism long swayed the minds of Greek medical men. It was so easy to attempt to find explanations of observed facts by conjuring up a simple hypothesis that for many years it was the usual procedure. Experience showed that by those means very great advances in medical studies were made. But the trend of philosophical speculations was away from dogmatism toward rationalism.

Status of Physicians: Physicians, during the Greek classical period, were held in high esteem. They freely mixed in the best circles of society and took part in all social activities. They were freed from the temple and from religion. The doctor was known as "Asclepiad" only by name; the term had no more a religious significance. It was like the present designation of "physician"; it indicated that the physician and surgeon were duly trained, having served a full apprenticeship with a qualified physician, attended lectures in a medical school, and been admitted to the medical guild of physicians.

Theopompus, the analyst (350 B.C.), states that the physicians of Cos and Cnidus were descendants from Aesculapius through Podalirius, that they came from Syrnum-Coria, and that they were called "Asclepiadae." This, however, is now generally abandoned and with it the theory that Greek medicine originated in the temples of Aesculapius.

Learned physicians were greatly honored and rewarded by endowment, exemption from taxation, and decrees of honor, and, in some cases, by gold crowns, statues, and in many other ways. Greek inscriptions show that Onasilus, Euenor, Menocrites, and other prominent physicians were honored by publicly subscribed tablets which were displayed in a public building. Empedocles was reluctant to accept a royal crown because he preferred the practice of the art of medicine.

Gomperz, in his work on "Greek Thinkers," says:

The physicians' profession was amply recognized in Hellas at an early date. Its oldest and most famous seats were the lovely island of Cos and the neighboring peninsula of Cnidus, in the southern portion of the west coast of Asia Minor, Croton, in the toe of Italy, and Cyrene, far away in Africa, where grew the umbelliferous plant silphon, so highly valued on account of its medicinal values, that it formed a royal monopoly. Cities and princes competed with one another for the services of eminent physicians. Democedes of Croton, for instance, was retained one year by the city of Athens, and in the next year by the Commonwealth of Aegina, and in the third year by the tyrant of Samos. His annual salary reached a sum of 16,400 drachmae, equivalent to modern francs. After the fall of Polycrates, Democedes was taken a captive from Samos to Susa, where we presently meet him at the royal table, and as confidential adviser to King Darius (521-485 b.c.). Indeed, so admirably had he treated the king and his consort Atossa, that the Egyptian body-physicans who had hitherto enjoyed the royal favor, fell swiftly in disgrace, and were in actual danger of their lives. Again, about the middle of the fifth century, we find the Cypriot-physician Onasilos and his brothers, who had rendered medical services in the field during the siege of Edation by the Persians, enjoying the highest honors and equipped in a princely style with ample crown property.

Most doctors were content to spend their lives in the daily routine of attending to patients. The more intellectual, however, spent much time in experiments and in research work. Their interest in this was continually quickened by the discoveries and lectures of the principal professors; and in subsequent years, when Aristotle began his lectures, the doctors, as well as all students, felt the inspirational stimuli of the "Master of the men who know."

The status of the Greek physician during the Hippocratic and post-Hippocratic period may be surmised from a vase painting in the British Museum, illustrating a Greek clinic about 500 b.c. The doctor, a young, well-dressed man, is sitting before a large bowl, over which a man extends his arm. The doctor bleeds the patient from the median vein at the bend of the right elbow. In front of the doctor we see a seated patient with his left arm bandaged, awaiting his turn for treatment. At the rear of that patient another is entering the clinic, smelling a bunch of flowers as a preventive against infection. At the rear of the doctor is a middle-aged dwarf, suffering from nervousness, and two men, one with a sore leg and another with a heavily bandaged chest. This picture shows that a private physician's office in Greece at that time closely resembled a modern doctor's, and there was a similar resemblance in the doctor's attitude toward his patients.[8]

Neuburger, speaking of the physicians of that period, says, "The medical profession ranked as a trade and was open to any one having the requisite knowledge, though women, indeed, were excluded and slaves might only treat their own class. This comparative freedom enlisted the services of all grades of capacity, from the highest philosopher to the lowest mountebank."

Three classes of physicians were prominent: (1) the general practitioner, who was regularly trained and employed assistants or apprentices; (2) the consultant, or master physician; and (3) the amateur.

Only the properly qualified men who had undergone a course, practical and theoretical, were recognized as authorities. A diploma was essential in the case of official and state physicians. These were chosen from among the best-established practitioners, and nominated and elected to office by the votes of popular assemblies. They usually held office for a year.

Physicians practiced either in their own homes or by going on circuits like the lawyers. The patients were treated either in their own houses or in medical homes or hospitals, which were also furnished with sickrooms for temporary treatment. These clinics and hospitals were provided at their own cost by the more eminent physicians, or were kept up by the community for the use of the official physicians. There are extant inscriptions showing how special hospital and medical taxes were levied. These hospitals were employed chiefly for operative cases and were fully equipped with instruments, appliances, and supplies. The student-assistants watched the surgeons operate and were often encouraged to operate in simple cases. They also accompanied their chief on his professional rounds.[9]

Evaluation of Hippocratic School: Gomperz, referring to the Hippocratic school, states:

The undying glory of the school of Cos (whence the first class of practitioners was trained) does not rest on their method of research but rather on the insight they displayed in perceiving that the premises for the application of the deductive method were not extant, that they had not even come in view and that fantastic conception was taking the place of requisite and valid induction. The pioneer virtues which distinguish the Coan masters from their opponents were a self-abnegation and a timely renunciation of ambitions, fascinating enough and even exalted in themselves, but out of reach at that era and long afterwards. These virtues entitle them to our ungrudging admiration to this day. We recognize their supreme merit in having developed, with tireless powers of observation and extraordinary faculties of clear sight and strong sense, those branches of the arts of healing which are capable of extension without digging at their foundation more deeply. Above all, we may specify their contribution to symptomatology which, by their endless supply of nice distinctions and accurate observations, are a source of pleasure and instruction to modern students of that branch of learning.[10]

References and Notes

1. He must not be confounded with the monarch of Corinth immortalized by Sophocles in the tragic story of Oedipus.
2. The anatomic knowledge of Polybus does not differ essentially from that of Syennesis, the physician of Cyprus, and Diogenes, the philosopher of Apollonia.
3. Parsons, F. G.: Encyclopedia Britannica, Ed. 11, Vol. 1, p. 922.
4. Galen mentions as leaders of the Dogmatic school (or, as he prefers to call it, "The Rational School of Hippocrates") Diocles of Carystus, Praxagoras of Cos, and the great Alexandrian anatomists.
5. Coelius Aurelianus Acut. 3:17.
6. Ross, L.: Reisen nach Cos. Halle, 1852, pp. 11–29. Patterson, W. and Hicks, E.: The Inscriptions of Cos. Oxford, 1891.
7. Hamilton, W.: History of Medicine and Surgery. London, 1831.
8. Selwyn-Brown, A.: The Physician throughout the Ages. Gerhart-Brown, 1928, Vol. 1, p. 81.
9. Neuburger, M.: History of Medicine. London, 1910, pp. 97–98.
10. Gomperz, T.: Geschichte der Denker. Leipzig, 1911.

21

The Athenians

THE Athenians were best known for their general erudition, religious philosophy, and ethics, not especially for their medical erudition. The Greek medical thinkers came from the provinces of Greece, not from its core.

SOCRATES

The greatest of all Greek philosophers, Socrates was not a physician. He was a moral philosopher, an independent thinker, and a champion of justice and freedom. His contribution to medicine was rather from the viewpoint of ethics than from any advancement of medical science. His familiarity with medicine was a part of his general learning, since medicine was a branch of general culture.

Physiology

In Chapter 6 of "The Memorable Thoughts of Socrates," according to the account of Xenophon, Socrates in his argument with the atheist Aristodemus, shows that he is well acquainted with the structure and function of the body:

Does it not appear to you wisely provided that since the eye is of delicate make, it is guarded with the eyelid drawn back when the eye is used, and covering it in sleep? How well does the hair at the extremity of the eyelid keep out dust, and the eyebrow, by its prominency, prevent the sweat from the forehead from running into the eye to its hurt. How wisely is the ear formed to receive all sorts of sounds, and not to be filled with any to the exclusion of others. Are not the foreteeth of all animals fitted to cut off proper portions of food, and their grinders to reduce it to a convenient smallness? The mouth, by which we take in the food we like, is fitly placed just beneath the nose and eyes, the judges of its goodness; and what is offensive and disagreeable to our senses is, for that reason, placed at a proper distance from them. In short, these things being disposed in such order, and with so much care, can you hesitate one moment to determine whether it be an effect of providence or of chance?[1]

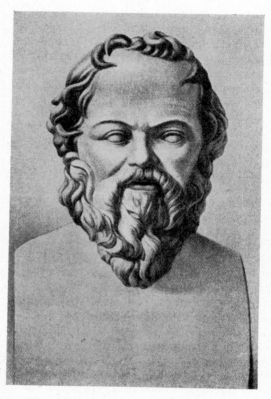

Fig. 121: Socrates (469–399 B.C.). Socrates was born in 469 B.C. near Athens. His father was a sculptor, and he is said to have been trained in the same art. A statue of the Graces at the entrance to the Acropolis was thought to be his work. In 406 B.C., he was a member of the senate of five hundred and refused, at the risk of forfeiting his life, to put an illegal question to vote. He practiced plain living and trained himself to be indifferent to heat and cold, going barefoot and wearing the same clothing the year round.

He repudiated Anaxagoras, who held that prying into the secrets of nature was offensive to the gods.

In Chapter 12 of the same book, Socrates, stressing the necessity of exercise for health and strength, remarks:

To have the body active and healthy can be hurtful to you on no occasion: and since we cannot do anything without the body, it is certain that a good constitution will be of great advantage to us in all our undertakings. Even in study, where there seems to be least need of it, we know many persons who could never make any great progress for want of health. Forgetfulness, melancholy, loss of appetite, and folly, are the diseases that generally proceed from the indisposition of the body; and these diseases sometimes seize the mind with so great violence, that they wipe out even the least remembrance of what we knew before. But in health we have nothing like this to fear, and consequently there is no toil which a judicious man would not willingly undergo to avoid all these misfortunes. And, indeed, it is shameful for a man to grow old before he has tried his own strength, and seen to what degree of dexterity and perfection he can attain, which he can never know if he gives himself over for useless; because dexterity and strength come not of themselves, but by practice and exercise.[2]

Socrates reveals a comprehensive knowledge of the articulation, functions of the nerves, and the phenomena of the special senses:

That my bones are solid and have joints, and that my nerves contract and relax; wherefore that the bones being raised up in their joinings, the nerves, by reason of tension and relaxation, make me to bend my limbs, and that for this reason I now sit here; and so, also, in respect to our conversing, should one assign other similar causes of the phenomena of speech, such as voice, and aerial vibrations, and sounds, and ten thousand other such agencies, all the while neglecting to assign the true reason (of reasons)? While it seemed good to the Athenians to condemn me, it seemed better to me to sit here, and more just to submit to the sentence they had imposed. Since, as I verily believe, had it not been for the last-mentioned reasons, these nerves and bones would long before this have had me away to Megara or among the Boeotians, being set in motion by an opinion of the best, if I had not thought it more just and better to remain than to fly.

Philosophy and Ethics

Socrates, of course, upheld the principle of supremacy of the mind over the body. He regarded the mind as the only worthy object of study. He believed the true self was not the body, but the soul. His philosophy turned men's attention away from the investigation of nature.

The chief reference Socrates made to a physician is in Plato's "Protagoras." He asked a young medical student named Hippocrates this question, "If you had thought of going to Hippocrates of Cos, the Asclepiad, and were about to pay him money and some one were to say to you, 'You are paying your money to your namesake, Hippocrates; what is he that you give him money?'"

"I give money to him because he is a physician-teacher," replied the young Hippocrates.

"And what will he make of you?"

"A physician also."

In his "Phaedrus," Plato has another reference to his master of the medical art. He makes Socrates ask, "Can the nature of the human soul be known intelligently without knowing the nature of the whole body?"

Phaedrus wisely replies, "Hippocrates, the Asclepiad, says that the nature, even of the body, can only be understood as a whole."

While it is true that Socrates makes no mention of a physician when describing the life of "the inhabitants of the state," this, however, does not imply that Socrates was against the physician or the Hippocratic art. It appears that the physicians of Athens in his time did not follow the ethical and practical teaching of the Father of Medicine. "When intemperance and complexity enter into the lives of the citizens," said Socrates, "halls of medicine are always opened and doctors begin to give themselves airs, because not only the rich, but even the slaves, take a keen interest in them."

Socrates' high concept of medical experience might give medical educators of the present time something to ponder about. He was of the opinion that the physician himself ought not to be robust in health and that he should have personal experience with the disease he was to treat in others. In other words, he should have acquired a firsthand knowledge of the pathologic conditions he was to treat.[3]

These remarks have precipitated much criticism from past and present physicians against the Platonic concept of a good physician, but there is obviously more than a grain of truth in these remarks. Frequently the diagnostic technique and the therapeutics would be altered considerably if the physician or surgeon had ever been subjected to these factors himself. In some cases, the diagnostic technique and treatment are literally worse than the condition being treated, more costly than is warranted, and are employed only because they are required by the poverty of the physician's skill. Socrates' remarks were directed at the state and citizens that rendered the presence of physicians necessary, and were not intended as a criticism of the doctor.

Socrates said that he looked upon Aesculapius as a statesman and called his disciples "ingenious sons not because they invented new names for diseases" but because of their skill which he readily recognized and found admirable. "Ought there not be good physicians in a state?" is the question put by Adeimantis and Socrates replied, "Yes, I too, would have . . . good physicians."

The skillful physician, in the opinion of Socrates, would be the one who from his youth had combined, with the knowledge of his art, the greatest possible experience with disease.[4]

In Plato's "Republic," Socrates stated that the treatment of wounds was something that could be entrusted to a comrade in the field if none of the ingenious sons of Aesculapius happened to be present. Where the recovery of health was a question merely of diet, gymnastics, or other regime, it could be well entrusted to "the inferior sort of practitioner and he would be thought to be good enough." But, "when a medicine has to be given, then the doctor should be more of a man." Socrates insisted that the use of such medicine should be restricted to physicians. Private persons had no business tampering with them. Thus, the physician occupied a recognized place in the "Republic" of Plato.

Socrates did not believe that exercise, proper diet, and the *vis medicatrix naturae* alone would suffice to cure or prevent a disease or heal wounds inflicted by accidents or in battle. In the discussion in Plato's *Republic*, about the luxurious state, Socrates speaks of those who "require the help of medicine not when a wound has to be cured or on occasion of an epidemic, but because by ignorance and habits of life such as we have been describing, men fill themselves with waters and winds as if their bodies were a marsh, compelling the ingenious sons of Aesculapius to find more names for diseases, such as flatulence and catarrh." Socrates asks, "Is not this too a disgrace?" When the discussion is turned towards a physician, however, he notes, "and living in this way, we shall have much greater need of a physician than before," signifying that the right kind of a physician would be a bulwark of the ideal Spartan state.

While Socrates praised Anaxagoras for his doctrine of the *nous,* the same gentleman was criticized for not making use of his doctrine in subsequent parts of his philosophy.

Having once heard one reading a book of Anaxagoras, and saying, that *nous* was the disposer and the efficient cause of all things, I was highly delighted with the declaration, and it seemed to me to be admirably said; and I thought, that if *nous* thus arranged all things, everything must be placed in that position in which it was best for it to be; so that no other study remained for man, in regard to both himself and other things, but the investigation of that which was (morally) most excellent and best (or, in other words, moral causes), and that this was the only true science of things . . . But I was greatly disappointed; for as I read on I find the man making no farther use of his boasted *nous*, nor assigning any other cause in the disposal and arrangement of the world than airs, and ethers, and waters, and other similar things many and strange.[5]

Both Socrates and Plato were rigid moralists. Neither would give to the physician the right to use means upon others which he would not use upon himself. The Platonic physician was the type of man who would inoculate himself with a virus or take a new medicine before using such on his patients. Socrates was against quacks and laymen trying to practice the Hippocratic art, "The use of such medicine (to prevent or counteract diseased conditions) should be restricted to physicians; private individuals have no business with them."

Personal History

Socrates was born at Athens during the month of May or June about 469 B.C. Sophroniscus was his father; his mother was a midwife named Phaenareta. After receiving the customary education of that period, he began adult life as a sculptor and exhibited great talent in this art. A group of the "Graces," supposed to be his work, was seen on the road to the Acropolis as late as the second century B.C. It is not known how long he practiced this art, but it appears that he soon gave sculpture up to devote himself to ethics and to promote the welfare and intellectual status of his people.

His domestic life was not a happy one. His wife Xanthippe was proverbially known among the ancients as a shrew. His son Lamprocles was reputedly "dull and fatuous." Xenophon, in his "Memorabilia," states that Socrates' son Lamprocles received from his father a formal rebuke for unseemly behavior towards his mother.

Socrates served five years in the Greek army as a hoplite (in the infantry). His bravery in military campaigns was conspicuous. On two occasions, it is known that he saved the lives of prominent officers. But he had an aversion for political office because this would have entailed the sacrifice of principles. He served a short time as a member of the senate, at which time he made himself unpopular by opposing the idea that the fate of eight generals should be decided by the majority of a single vote of the assembly.

Because of his fearlessness, he was indicted on a trumped-up charge of denying the gods recognized by the state, of introducing new divinities, and of corrupting the youth. Socrates was found guilty by a vote of 280 to 220. He made no attempt to disguise his indifference to the verdict. He proudly maintained that he should have been rewarded for the services rendered to his people as a public benefactor. He refused to take advantage of the advice of a disciple Crito to escape from prison. At the end of thirty days' imprisonment, he was made to drink a cup of hemlock, which ended his glorious life.

Socrates left no writings behind him. What is known of him has been gathered largely from the works of Plato and Xenophon. During his imprisonment, he carried on his customary dialogues. Plato relates in his "Phaedo" how, in his last conversation, he argued that the wise man would regard approaching death with a cheerful confidence, for death was either a dreamless sleep or a new life during which one had the opportunities of testing the wisdom of the heroes and sages of antiquity; in either case there was an advantage for one to die.

PLATO

Plato (427–347 b.c.) was a great admirer of Hippocrates. He held him in high esteem for his ethical and farseeing views of nature. He took his method of deduction as his pattern on many vital subjects pertaining to natural studies, although often not entirely in the sense of the medical savant.[6] His views on physiology were based on Pythagorean ideas and on religious philosophical concepts rather than on the Hippocratic rational grounds.

Plato was acquainted with the writings of Hippocrates and recognized the healing power of nature. He declared that every form of disease was, in a manner, akin to the living being whose complex frame had an appointed time of life and that, in treatment, regimen was always to be preferred to drugs.

Though Plato mentions Hippocrates with respect, his two notices of him are not entirely without what appears like sarcasm. Thus, in the "Protagoras," Hippocrates is introduced as a distinguished doctor who receives pay for his teaching. (This was a favorite accusation against the Sophists.) In another place ("Phaedo"), when the physician's authority is invoked, Socrates is made to reply, "Yes, but must we not compare reason with Hippocrates to see if they agree."

The Platonic concept of a good physician was one who was unsympathetic toward diagnostic procedures made in a haphazard manner and toward operations performed without a careful diagnosis.

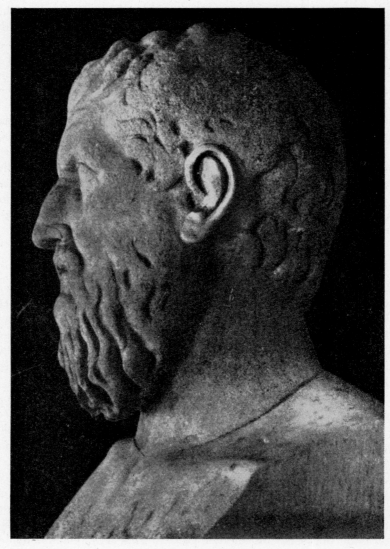

Fig. 122: Plato (427–347 B.C.). Plato was Socrates' most distinguished student, and it is mostly due to him that we know anything about the master's philosophical views. He himself has played a dominant role in all subsequent human thought. (Marble bust in Holkham Hall in England. Photograph by Dr. Frederick Boulson.)

Indeed, many of the painful and dangerous techniques of diagnosis and treatment would be avoided if the Platonic concepts of a good physician were kept in mind. To Plato, if doctors did not cure their patients quickly, they were worse than useless for they only prolonged lives worthless to the state.

In his "Protagoras," Plato satirically tells how the physician examines his patient, "He looks at his face and the tips of his fingers and then he says, 'uncover your chest and back to me that I may have a better view.'" According to Xenophon, diligent practitioners visited their patients twice a day—morning and evening.

Physiology

The physical action of the bodily organs, as well as the moral propensities of man, according to Plato, were governed by a tripartite soul. One part was rational; the other two parts (spirit and desire) were irrational. The rational part of the soul played the most important part in the body and was located in the head; the spiritual part was situated in the chest; and the part connected with desire was located in the abdomen.[7]

Plato sought the ultimate cause of the formation of matter in the idea of God who created out of chaos the four elements: earth, water, air, and fire. All matter owed its characteristics to the combination of these elements. Man was fashioned from these four fundamental elements. The working spirit within him, the soul, was an emanation from the Absolute Intelligence. The link that connected the body to the soul was the appendage, the brain, which was spherical like the heavens and perfectly formed. As the instrument of the soul, according to Plato, the eyes were first formed.

Bodily function was governed by the head. Hence, it was placed at the top of the person and the reason faculties were located in it. The spleen secreted and carried off the impurities which could accumulate and produce disease. The intestines were coiled in order that the food would not pass too quickly through the body and so cause a rapid desire for additional food. Plato's idea of nature was deduced a priori for human needs and predilections.

Plato defined the soul as the force that moved itself and other things without being moved by anything else. The soul, being essentially immortal and divine in its origin, was bound up with the very being of God, and was therefore not dependent for its existence upon any passing association which it might have with matter.[8]

Plato gave to the doctrines of the soul a scientific form. It was the only explanation of the mysterious phenomena of the universe.[9] God, to Plato, was only understood if regarded as being the Soul of the Universe. The Platonic Doctrine of the Soul became the foundation upon which many religious beliefs were built.

It is not difficult to surmise the reason that prompted Plato to drop the theory of a monistic vital entity and to substitute a tripartite soul dominating the bodily activities, for it must have become evident, even to the casual observer, that the food and drink consumed daily had some vital connection with bodily motion and sensation. Undernourished persons were undoubtedly observed to lose bodily power and have their special senses impaired. Plato, therefore, ascribed bodily functions to subordinate spirits coming into existence from the introduction of food into the body. That vegetables and plants possessed spirits responsible for their growth was an old Greek belief. The process of nutrition coming from without to promote bodily function was believed by Plato to be controlled by the soul proper.

Plato's physiopathologic speculations were based upon the teachings of earlier philosophers and upon the Hippocratic principles of medicine. He regarded the world of our senses as embodying the world of ideas and struggling constantly towards a greater perfection. He was always searching for an ultimate force in matter which he believed led to the principle of goodness and beauty, and ultimately to the disclosure of God. Life was combined with fire which was kept burning by the pneuma and was inherent in the streaming blood. The organs of the body were nourished by the theory of the "attraction of likes."

Plato elaborated upon the humoral pathology of Hippocrates. The world, he thought, was composed of four elements: fire, consisting of pyramidal substance; earth, of cubical substance; air, of octagonal substance; and water, of twenty-sided atoms. The marrow consisted of triangles, and the brain was the perfection of marrow. The soul dominated the marrow and the separation of the two caused death. The purpose of the bones and muscles was to protect the marrow against changes of temperature.

Plato taught that the heart was the origin of the blood vessels and, as the seat of the mind, received through them the commands of the superior soul. The lungs, which received through the trachea, a portion of the drink in addition to the air, served to cool off the heart. The liver was smooth as glass and shiny and was composed of sweet and bitter principles derived from the bile. Plato described the liver as being nourished by bile derived from the head, and digestion as due to the action of inspired fire. The liver served the lower desires. The spleen furnished an abode for the impurities of the blood and was in intimate relationship with the liver. The intestine was long and tortuous, in order that the food could remain the longer therein, so that the mind need not be disturbed too often in its contemplation by the frequent renewal of the desire for nutriment, which would be necessary if the intestinal canal were shorter. The tendons served to keep the joints in opposition to facilitate their movements. He ascribed diseases that arose from within the body to outside influences such as improper food and sexual imprudence, in addition to causes which will be mentioned later.

Breathing, he declared, took place by inward pressure of the air, for no vacant space could exist in the body. Sight originated in a union of the light flowing out from the eyes with the rays coming from the object looked at; and hearing was a result of a shock of air which was communicated to the brain, the blood, and even to the soul. Taste was due to a solution of rapid atoms by means of small vessels, which conducted these from the tongue to the heart and soul. The olfactory sense, however, possessed no image as its foundation and was therefore very transitory.[10]

Pathology

The Platonic theory of disease was based upon the speculations of Hippocrates, Empedocles, Anaxagoras, Philolaos, Heracleitos, Pathagoras, and earlier writers. The etiological factors were attributed to excesses in dieting and to disproportionate balancing between eating and exercise, as well as sexual intemperance. The underlying causes of disease were thought to be formed from strange displacements of the pneuma, bile, or phlegm, and in disproportionate mixtures of the four elements. Plato, in later life, was greatly influenced by the opinions of the Sicilian dogmatic medical writer Philisteon, who had a large medical practice in Athens, and his friend Eudoxos of Cnidus, who was practicing medicine in Athens at that time. It was through Eudoxos that Plato acquired some of the medical principles of the Cnidian School.

Plato taught that disease originated in a disturbance of both the quantity and quality of the humoral fluids. The immediate cause of disease was the downflow of mucus and acridity; the most dangerous was corruption of the marrow. Another cause was an unbalance of the yellow and black bile, through which inflammations arose.

Continued fever was occasioned by fire, quotidian fever by air, tertian fever by water, and quartan fever by earth. The mixture of phlegm with bile was the cause of epilepsy. Disturbance of the phlegm itself was the cause of diarrhea. Mental diseases were the result of corporeal evils or of bad education. Aside from bodily exercise and diet, remedies were effected by drugs which combated disease. Plato stated that physicians had to be rulers of the sick, in order to cure them, but they should not be mercenary.[11]

Plato distinguished between the training of those who were to become mere assistants to free doctors and those who were to become free doctors themselves. He referred to two methods of practice: one, mechanical and impersonal; the other, rational and humane. "These assistants, whether they are freeborn or slaves, acquire their art under the direction of masters by observation and experience, but not by the study of nature; yet it is by the study of nature that freeborn doctors have learned the art themselves and instruct their own students." (Laws 720–B.)

Personal History

Plato was born in the year 427 B.C. and lived to the age of eighty. He was the son of Ariston and a descendant of Cordus. His mother's family claimed descent from Solon. He was well-bred and well-to-do. His real name was Aristocles, but he was nicknamed Plato (because of certain peculiarities: the breadth of his shoulders, his style of speech, and the size of his head).

According to Hermodorus, Plato and other Socratics took refuge with Euclides in Megara to escape the prejudice that prevailed against their master in Athens. He appears to have returned to his native city about the year 394. Then he set out to travel, and is said to have visited Cyrene, Magna Graecia, and Sicily. According to Diogenes Laertius, he traveled to Egypt where he conversed with the priests of that country. At Syracuse, he made acquaintance with the tyrant Dionysius, through his friend, Dion, the brother-in-law of the tyrant.

It is related that Dionysius, taking offense at remarks made by Plato, delivered him to a certain Pollis, a Spartan, who sold Plato in the market place of Aegina as a prisoner of war. He was ransomed later by Anniceris of Cyrene. The friends of Plato wanted to repay the ransom money, but his liberator refused and suggested that the money be spent for the purchase of the garden of Academus in Athens. This eventually became historic ground.

Whatever truth there may be in this tale, Plato appears to have returned to Athens about the year 387 and established there his Gymnasium and afterwards the garden near the school, which became known as The Academy. Here he lived most of his life, conducting his discourses and writing his dialogues and his then famous works.

In his early years he studied the natural philosophy of Heracleitus, his theory of the "flux," and the doctrine of Socrates. In his maturity, Plato was not only a philosopher, but also a man of science. His metaphysical theory of ideas carried with it the physical theory of "natural kinds" and provided a basis for zoology and botany. Plato was a prolific writer and possessed a fine style. He is the author of a large number of books, some of which became the basis of numerous religions. Plato died in the year 347. His nephew Speusippus succeeded him as head of the school he founded.

ARISTOTLE

The best known of Plato's disciples, fellow students, and friends was Aristotle (384–322 B.C.). He came from a family of physicians for three generations preceding him, but he himself never practiced medicine. He was in principle a Hippocratic but, like his master Plato, with whom he was connected for a period of twenty years, his medical ideas were colored by philosophical deductions. They were frequently in opposition to those of Hippocrates.

Anatomy and Physiology

After the death of Plato, he became interested in natural history, and his medical concepts accordingly were influenced by his biological investigations. It is doubtful whether Aristotle ever dissected a human body. It is known that he dissected a large number of animals of different species and noted the anatomical variation in them. In consequence of his studies of animals, he is considered the founder of comparative anatomy and physiology. He also investigated the anatomy of fishes and reptiles. He watched the fetal changes during the incubation of bird eggs.

Embryology: He described carefully the development of the embryo chicken and detected on the fourth day after the laying of the egg the presence of the heart like a speck of blood in the egg, beating and moving as though endowed with life. His views on the subject of embryology and genetics held sway up to the early part of the seventeenth century.

Aristotle, while admitting that both parents had a share in embryonic development, rejected the Hippocratic doctrine that both sexes contributed equally to formation of the embryo. He compared the menstrual fluid to a block of marble, the seminal fluid to the sculptor, and the fetus to the statue. He regarded the male semen as the most important contribution to the formation of the embryo, "This fluid endows the child with the faculty of motion, sensation and thought and gives form and the very soul to the future person. The female's

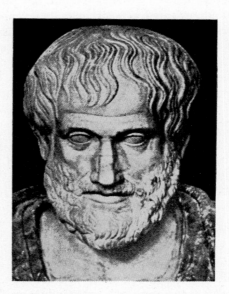

Fig. 123: Aristotle (384–322 B.C.). Aristotle, the foremost disciple of Plato and teacher of Alexander the Great, remained until the end of the Middle Ages the infallible guide in all branches of science.

share in the embryo which arises from the menstrual fluid contributes the material part to the person but adds nothing to the spiritual part."[12] Aristotle opposed the idea that prevailed among Greek philosophers and laymen of that period that a female conceived without the agency of a male.

He believed in spontaneous generation of lower forms of life, a concept previously held by Anaximander (611–547 B.C.), who was of the opinion that eels and other aquatic forms were produced directly from lifeless matter. His pupil Anaximenes (588–524 B.C.), according to Osborn ("From the Greeks to Darwin"), "introduced the idea of primordial terrestrial slime: a mixture of earth and water, from which, under the influence of the sun's heat, plants and lower forms of animal life, are directly produced." Diogenes and Xenophanes, the first to recognize the true nature of fossils, also believed in spontaneous generation. Aristotle fostered this idea so strongly that it has persisted for more than twenty centuries. He taught that many creatures sprang from dung hills and putrid water, that certain bugs arose from moisture, and that some insects took their origin from the dew upon the grass.

For ages after Aristotle, the idea prevailed that shellfish of all kinds were without parental origin, that eels sprang spontaneously from the Nile, that caterpillars were the spontaneous products of the leaves on which they fed, and that winged insects, serpents, rats, and mice were capable of being generated without sexual contact.

The idea that certain living things originate directly from lifeless matter has been widely accepted even to the present time by many unscientific people. The term "spontaneous generation" ("abiogenesis") is most commonly applied to this concept, which does not differentiate as to whether the spontaneous appearance of life from lifeless matter occurred only at the beginning of all life or still occurs today.

As has been intimated, Artistotle derived his knowledge of anatomy and physiology from observations on animals. Aristotle's writings mention over 500 different animals, but his references are of very unequal value. Many of them are mere allusions without any detail; many are mere repetitions of traveler's tales or of legendary lore; but many of them show an accuracy and a minuteness which imply close personal observation. He seems to have dissected some fifty different kinds of animals. He probably never dissected a human body, but did to some extent dissect the human embryo. He obtained his animal material from herdsmen, hunters, bird catchers, apothecaries, and, above all, from the fishermen of the Aegean. His local references are chiefly to two regions—Macedonia and Thrace.

Findings from Animal Dissection: Since his dissection was confined to lower animals, he made errrors in human anatomy and physiology. Aristotle's description of the human body was inferior to his careful biological observations. He confused the functions of the arteries and the veins. He believed that the veins carried the blood from the heart and distributed it throughout the system. He did not explain the return of any blood to the heart. Evidently, he thought that the heart was a self-supplying organ or an inexhaustible fountain. He coined the name "aorta" believing that this vessel contained air. He confounded the nerves with the tendons and ligaments. He thought that the nerves proceeded from the heart, and that the purpose of the diaphragm was to separate the heart from the contaminating influence of the intestine. The brain, he believed, was nothing more than a mass of earth and water, without blood or sensation, the function of which was merely to balance and correct the heat of the heart.

The liver, spleen, and kidneys, according to his opinion, served chiefly to keep the veins in their position. He had peculiar ideas of the functions of the digestive organs. At times his ideas concerning the anatomy of animals were confused. He believed that the bones of a lion had no marrow and that their necks, as well as those of wolves, were devoid of flexibility. He was familiar, however, with the internal viscera and distinguished the jejunum and the cecum. He understood the function of the mesentery. He was first to mention the lymphatic vessels in animals. His description of the aorta and its branches was correct. The word "rectum" in the present sense was coined by Aristotle. He admitted having no knowledge of the internal parts of the human body. He could only judge from their supposed resemblance to animals.

In physiology, he was of the opinion that the heart, being the seat of the soul and the place where passion originated, was the controlling force over all functions. Aristotle believed that the soul was the prime mover of all bodily activities. He recognized, however, the fact that external cosmic influences through the special senses played an important part in human physiology. In his "De Anima," he critically summarized the opinions of earlier Greek philosophers regarding the nature, essence, and attributes of the entity commonly called the "soul." He opposed the opinion of his predecessors who made the soul independent of the body. He distinguished between soul and mind. He identified the soul with the vital principle possessed by both man and animal, declaring that "nothing which has perception is without a soul." He made a distinction between matter and form:

Matter exists, form exists, and the two exist together. Matter represents potentialities, while form gives it attributes and the capacity for actuality —ability to fulfill the end of its existence, so to speak. Body and soul bear to one another the relationship of matter and form; the soul giving functions, or self-realization, to a body which has in it the potentiality of life, that is, to a body possessing organs. For the sake of analogy, if the eye were an animal, eyesight would be its soul, in the absence of which it would no longer be a living eye.

Cosmic Doctrine: The cosmic doctrine of Aristotle was that the world was a living being having a soul. Since everything created was for some particular purpose, the body of man was evolved as the habitat of the soul. Matter was composed of five elements: earth, air, water, fire and ether. Every element should be looked upon as living, since it was pervaded by the soul of the universe. There was an unbroken chain from the simple elements through plant and animal up to man, the different groups merging by insensible shades into one another; plants were inferior to animals, since they did not possess a single principle of life or soul but many subordinate ones, as was shown by the circumstance that when they were cut to pieces each piece was capable of independent growth or life.

Physiological Doctrine: Aristotle tried by logical and scientific method to build up a system of human physiology at a time when the world had little scientific knowledge; many of his physiologic conclusions, therefore, are at present obsolete. Some of his physiologic doctrines were as follows: The intelligence of an animal was in proportion to its bodily heat; thus aquatic animals were of no intelligence. Man, on the other hand, whose warmth was pronounced, possessed a much more excellent soul and therefore a higher intelligence. The soul received the various sensations and issued forth the bodily motion. The soul coordinated all the functions of the body. It was the energy of the active essence. Having neither body nor magnitude, it could not have extension; nor could it be said to move in space. He compared the soul to a motionless sailor in a moving ship. The blood was as essential to the activity of the soul as it was for bodily nutrition. The heart was the source of the blood, the source of innate heat. The heart, not the brain, was the seat of sensation and thought. Thus, he disagreed with Alcameon and Hippocrates, who claimed that the seat of intelligence was located in the brain.

He considered the brain a large gland devoid of blood and, therefore, the coldest organ of the body. By this token, he felt that it could not be severely diseased, an idea which hampered medical progress for many centuries. Its function was to secrete cold humors which prevented an overheating of the body by the fiery heart. The pulsation of the heart and the blood vessels, he thought, was due to a bubbling of the blood, caused by the action of the vital heat. All animal activities were influenced by the heart, which contained the principle of life.

Sensation could be compared to the impression of a seal on wax, the wax receiving form only, but no substance or matter. Imagination arose from the impression made, which endured for a length of time. This was the origin of memory. Man alone possessed recollection. Animals possessed only memory. The latter was unintentional and spontaneous, requiring no voluntary exertion. Aristotle theorized that the soul existed only in so far as it was necessary for the realization of form.

Aristotle's description of the heart and its functions was by no means accurate. "All hearts," he stated, "have three chambers . . . the apex points forward, the largest chamber is on the right and highest up; the smallest on the left; that which is intermediate in size is between the two; the aorta springs from the middle chamber." Aristotle made no mention of the communications between the chambers. However, while reading his "De Anima," one cannot help but get the feeling that Aristotle appreciated the idea of circulation.

Aristotle considered the heart as the source of the vital heat. The air united with the heart in the following manner: "Air is taken into the lungs and from there by the pulmonary vein into the heart, which it serves to cool." The blood was also cooled by the pneuma or spiritus drawn by the lungs. If the vital heat was in the heart, it was clear that this organ was also the origin of emotions, such as pain, pleasure, and desire. He thought that the arteries contained air. He did not explain why the pulses were located in the arteries. He claimed that the nerves originated from the heart and that the liver, spleen, and kidneys had no other function but to supply their veins with blood. He was of the opinion that the arteries conveyed motion to the limbs.

His knowledge of respiration was equally imperfect. He was right that innate heat depended upon the constant supply of air taken by the lungs, just as a burning candle required the presence of air, but he believed that air was necessary to life because it cooled the vital combustive processes and prevented too rapid burning, for the warmer the animal, the greater its need for cooling. He added a fifth element —spirit, or pneuma—to the accepted elements of fire, air, water and earth. He taught that digestion was the result of coction by heat which was also the cause of secretion of mucus, tears, and pus.

Criticizing the views of respiration held by earlier naturalists, he pointed out that "the main reason these writers have not given a good account of the facts is that they had no acquaintance with the internal organs and that they did not accept the doctrine that there is a final cause for whatever Nature does. If they had asked for what purpose respiration exists in animals, and had considered this with reference to the organs (that is the gills and the lungs), they would have discovered the reason more rapidly." Here the insistence on the need for observation of anatomical structures before the framing of views on the functions of organs was sound, although the insistence on an inquiry into final causes was dangerous.

He compared nourishment through the blood vessels with absorption of water by plants, their nourishment seeping in through their roots.

He laid much stress upon environment, variation in the weather, and seasons of the year as causes of disease. He held that phthisis, ophthalmia, plague, and the itch were due to contagion which he attributed to some morbific cause in the air. He upheld the doctrine of Plato's teleology that every organ of the body had an ultimate purpose and predominant reason for its existence. All these views were, for ages, held to be divine truth and caused a long delay in the progress of medicine.[13]

Personal History

Aristotle was the son of Nichomachus, friend and court physician of Amyntas, King of Macedonia, who belonged to the School of Asclepiadae. Aristotle was trained in the medical arts by his father from his early youth. At the age of eighteen (367 B.C.), he came to Athens (and joined the Academy) as a pupil of Plato, who was forty-three years his senior, and with whom he formed a close friendship throughout life.

In 347 B.C., when Plato died and was succeeded by his nephew Speusippus as head of the Academy, Aristotle left Athens at the invitation of his friend and fellow student Hermias, Lord of Assos, whose relative he married, following which he settled in Mitylene.

In the year 343 B.C., Aristotle received an invitation of the Macedonian court to undertake the education of Prince Alexander, then thirteen years of age. He received as a pecuniary grant an amount equivalent to 15,500 pounds sterling a year, which defrayed the expense of his scientific researches. He occupied this position for a period of three years (343–340). After Alexander ascended the throne of Macedonia and was about to start on his Asiatic expeditions, Aristotle left Macedonia and returned to Athens (335). He found Speusippus dead and Xenocrates installed as leader. Aristotle thereupon organized a rival school of his own, The Lyceum, on the ground of the temple Lyceum Apollo. He drifted to natural sciences in which he attained the great honor of being known as the Father of

Biology. There he spent twelve years teaching advanced classes in the morning and making discourses to the general public in the afternoon. From his habit of walking to and fro while he delivered his discourses, the members of his school were called "peripatetics."

There is one significant tradition about Aristotle which suggests circumstances likely to have produced in early life a considerable influence upon his habits and pursuits. His father is said to have been an "Asclepiad,"—that is he belonged to that distinguished caste who claimed to be the descendants of Aesculapius. Now we have it, on the authority of Galen, that "it was the custom in Asclepiad families for the boys to be trained by their father in the practice of dissection, just as regularly as the boys in other families learn to read and write," so we may safely conclude that he received from his father preparation for physiological study.

Aristotle aroused in young Prince Alexander, while he tutored him, an interest in natural history. The latter furnished Aristotle with material for dissection. Thousands of men are said to have been placed in almost every part of the world to collect and transmit to Aristotle whatever they thought unusual in nature. Consequently, Aristotle became the greatest collector and systematizer of knowledge. He left no branch of knowledge unexplored. With the aid of young Alexander, he established the first known museum of natural history. The greatest biologist of modern times, Darwin, thus said of Aristotle, "Linnaeus and Cuvier have been my two gods though in very different ways: but they were new school boys in one field to old Aristotle."

When Alexander died (323 B.C.), the anti-Macedonian party of Athens was prejudiced against all who were favorably disposed to Alexander and they trumped up charges of impiety against Aristotle. Perhaps remembering what happened to Socrates, he left Athens promptly and retired to Chalcis in Euboea where he died the following summer (322). There are some of the opinion that he drank a cup of hemlock that caused his death.

Influence of Aristotle

Some years ago, Dr. Waldstein, an archaeologist, claimed that he had discovered the tomb of Aristotle near Eretria. The greatness of Aristotle was not fully appreciated until the early Middle Ages when the Arab physicians based their structure of medicine and science on the Aristotelian writings, while the church borrowed from him the framework of its theology, and civilized Europe began to see in his writings the epitome of science. Dante hailed him as the master of "those who know."

Aristotle profoundly affected the evolutionary thought of his—and later—times by his dogmatic concept of a guiding intelligence which had as its goal the realization of potentialities leading to perfection. "Nature does nothing without an aim," and "She is always striving after the most beautiful that is possible" are two quotations in point. The guiding principle, the aspiration to the best, was, in later years, seized upon as evidence of special creation: Man was guided by a Creator; man was the best, the highest, the most perfect, for he was in the Creator's image. For almost 2000 years this dogma held undisputed sway.

Writings

He wrote on "Metaphysics," "Ethics," "Politics," "Rhetoric," "The Art of Poetry," and natural sciences, especially natural philosophy, physiology, histology, anatomy, embryology, psychology, the philosophy of the senses, and, above all, natural history.

Aristotle was the high-water mark in ancient Greek biological thought. He was succeeded by Theophrastus who, in turn, was succeeded by Strato.

References and Notes

1. Bysshe, E.: The Memorable Thoughts of Socrates. Cassell Publishing Co., New York, p. 38.
2. Ibid., p. 140.
3. Alleyul, S. F., and Goodman, A.: Plato and the Older Academy. 1876, Vol. 9, pp. 58–69.
4. Jackson, H.: Encyclopedia Britannica, Ed. 11, Vol. 25, pp. 332–338.
5. Rhetoric 2:15.
6. Gordon, B. L.: The Romance of Medicine. F. A. Davis Company, Philadelphia, 1944, p. 82. The writer has occasionally used, in this chapter, sentences and phrases taken from that book.
7. Ibid., p. 83.
8. Burnett, J.: Translation of Plato. Oxford, 1901–1906.
9. Gomperz, T.: Die Philosophie der Griechen. Leipzig, 1869–1871.
10. Elliott, J. S.: Greece and Roman Medicine. William Wood & Co., New York.
11. Allen, T. H.: Science History of the Universe. The Current History Publishing Co., New York, 1909, Vol. 7, pp. 133–134.
12. Cited by Du Bois, A. M.: Ciba Symposia (Nov.) 1939.
13. "The Romance of Medicine," pp. 572–574.

22

The Peripatetics, Epicureans, and Stoics

THE PERIPATETICS

Theophrastus: The successor of Aristotle in The Lyceum of Athens was Tyrtanius of Lesbian-Eresus (330–225 B.C.), named "Theophrastus" by Aristotle. The latter presided over the Peripatetic school for thirty years, during which time two new schools, the Stoic and Epicurean, came into existence. Under his guidance, the school flourished. There were at one period over two thousand students.

Theophrastus had first been a student of Plato; and after his death, he attached himself to the school of the Peripatetics. The friendship between master and student became so great that Aristotle bequeathed to him his library and the originals of his works. He also designated him as his successor at the Lyceum when he removed to Chalcis.

Theophrastus' place in medicine is particularly marked in the field of pharmacy. He collected a large number of plants gathered by the scientific staff that accompanied Alexander the Great in his Asiatic campaign. He described and classified them. His botanical treatises, "Historiae Plantarium"[1] (nine books) and "Causis Plantarium" (six books), afford a striking proof of his attainment as a botanist, of his power of observation, and of his caution in using the testimony of his informants. He described all the plants known at his time, and this work was looked upon as the standard work on botany for almost twenty centuries. It contained the most valuable indications of the therapeutic value of many plants.

In his history of plants, he related that a certain Thrasayas had invented a compound consisting of hemlock mixed with poppy seeds, a small dose of which would cause a painless death within a period of from one or two minutes to a year, depending upon the quantity administered. Theophrastus presented an advanced view for his time, namely that the higher orders of plants were reproduced sexually, a fact which, owing to the opposition of Aristotle, lay dormant until Andria Cesalpini revived it during the Renaissance. Because of Theophrastus' work in botany, he was named the "Father of Botany." The first Latin edition of his work was published at Treviso in 1483, and the first Greek edition at Venice in 1492. His great work "Physical Opinion," of which only a fragment has been preserved, was the fountain from which many generations after him have drawn their knowledge. It extends over the whole range of contemporary knowledge. In natural history, he made no innovation in the work of his master. He shared his opinions on anatomy, physiology, and biology. He was alive to the difficulties that beset many Aristotelian definitions, which leaned towards a materialistic interpretation, in contrast to his colleague, Erdemus, who inclined more to Platonic philosophy.

Regarding the nature of life and the human soul, he showed independence; he considered the souls as well as the bodies of all animals (including human) as made up of like elements, sensation, passion, desire, and reasoning, though in man these elements attained a higher perfection.

Strato: The natural tendency of the school reached its climax in Strato, the most independent and the ablest of the early Peripatetics. Strato of Lampracus followed Theophrastus as head of The Lyceum, over which he presided from 288–270 B.C. He was known as "the physicist." He ascribed the evolution of the world to natural forces and dispensed altogether with the hypothesis of a transcedent deity. He took corporeal forces, heat, and cold as his elements. Strato argued that without empty interspaces, the passage of light or heat or any corporeal property through air, water, or bodies in general, would be inexplicable.

Strato asserted, "In considering the soul one must adhere to the same conditions as when we deal with what is corporeal; if the body needs a substratum so also does the soul." He denied any separation between sense and reason:

Sensation is conditioned by thought, since often when we are thinking of something else we do not feel impressions of sense. The pain one feels in the part affected is merely a delusion, the same as when one thinks he hears sounds at a distance. The carrier of the impression to the central organs (which he placed between the eyebrows) is a current of breath, spirit, or pneuma; if this connection is broken, we never feel the pain.

Strato had a mechanical conception of the universe. Cicero attributed to Strato the saying that one does not require the arts of gods in the construction of the universe. He reduced the formation of the world to the operation of natural forces; he recognized nothing beyond natural necessity. He explained all the functions of the soul as made of motion, denying the separation of reason from the faculties of sense perception. He appealed in this connection to the statement of Aristotle that we are unable to think without a sense image.[2]

With the death of Strato in 270 B.C., the work in the famous school declined.

THE EPICUREANS

Epicurus: Another Athenian naturalist whose philosophy was related to medicine was Epicurus (342–270 B.C.), the founder of the school of Epicureanism which also was known as "Solidism." The gist of his doctrine was originally advanced by Leucippus (fifth century B.C.) and Democritus but was further elaborated upon by Epicurus.

The basis of Epicurus' philosophy was that all that existed in the universe was corporeal, but that certain minute things such as atoms were too minute for our subtle senses to detect. "While we must indeed accept our feelings, we must also believe much which is not directly testified by sensation if only it serves to explain phenomena and does not contravene our sensation."

Atomic Theory: With reference to the composition of matter, he disagreed with the Ionic school that matter was composed of four elements. The fundamental postulate of Epicureanism was that there were infinite multitudes of indestructible, indivisible, and absolutely compact atoms in perpetual motion in infinite space. These atoms, differing in size, configuration, and weight, perpetually moved with equal velocity at a rapid rate. As they moved, they gave rise to new worlds which perpetually tended toward dissolution and toward a fresh series of creations.

The human body, as well as all other substances in the universe, consisted of atoms and interspaces, or pores; these atoms in the state of health were in perpetual motion. They kept circulating in the pores of the body, especially in the alimentary canal where they were most active in order to maintain normal physical function. If these atoms became stagnant because of contraction of the interspaces, disease resulted.

Processes of Sensation: The various processes of sensation, notably vision, he explained on materialistic principles as follows: From the

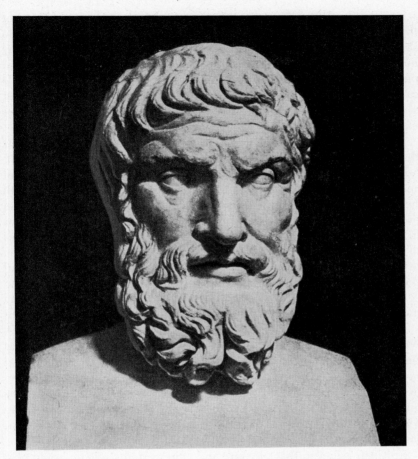

Fig. 124: Epicurus (342–270 B.C.). The famous Greek philosopher Epicurus was born in Samos in the year 342 B.C. He was the son of Neocles, a school teacher. He was known as "The Philosopher of the Garden" because he conducted his school in a garden which he purchased when he returned to Athens. He was a prolific writer. It is related that he left three hundred works on natural philosophy, the atomic concept, the vacuum, love, justice, and many other subjects. Only three letters and a few fragments of his works are extant. What is known of him is through the works of Cicero, Plutarch, and Leucretius. He died in Athens in the year 270 B.C. (The Vatican, Rome.)

surface of all objects there were continually flowing filmy images exactly copying the solid body whence they originated. These images had a direct impact on the visual organs and so produced vision. The purpose of Epicurus was to eliminate the common idea of divine interference. He did not deny the existence of gods, but they were themselves the products of nature, a higher species than humanity but not the rulers of man, nor the makers, nor the upholders of the world. Men should worship them, but they did not have to be inspired either by hope or by fear. "Natural phenomena may be explained in many ways; only let us have no myths of divine action. To assign only a single cause for these phenomena, when the facts familiar to us suggest several, is insane and absurd from a people who dabble in the vanities of astrology."

Physiology and the Soul: Epicurus' idea of human physiology was that all bodily functions were controlled by the soul. The soul itself, however, was corporeal. The soul was a compound of four different species of fine fiery atoms, a kind of warm breath or wind mixed with heat, distributed throughout the frame but more densely massed in the breast.[3] Portions of this subtle substance could leave the body as in sleep, or unconsciousness, yet recover by receiving new quantities of soul substance from the outside. Epicurus' theory abolished the dualism of mind and matter in the human body, which was an essential point in the systems of Plato and Aristotle.

The mobility of the soul was shown in thought, feeling, and bodily motions which it originated. The relation of the two corporeal substances, soul and body, were explained by Epicurus as follows: A person derived sensation or feeling mainly from the soul but also from the body; for the soul would not be sentient without the body; and being so related, it conferred this quality on the body. The body, however, did not share in the other functions of the soul, such as memory and thought. At death the lifeless corpse ceased to function. The soul, too, when separated from the body, could no longer retain sensation and dispersed in the air.

Epicurus believed that pleasure and pain were the sole and only possible motives for our actions, "That pain must be avoided and pleasure pursued is a dictum as plainly evident as that fire is hot, and ice is cold. Every animal as yet uncorrupted by false opinion naturally and instinctively pursues pleasure and seeks to ward off pain." Pleasure could be called the highest good and pain the worse evil. By good was meant simply the end sought for its own sake.[4]

Epicurus held that all mental pleasure was related to bodily pleasure. He contended that mental pleasure extended to past and future objects, while bodily pleasure was confined to the present. Past pleasures stored in the memory continued to be enjoyed.

World Processes: The Epicureans who followed the atomic teaching of Democritus, adopted a purely mechanical view of the world processes. Lucretius was evidently an Epicurean when he regarded the primitive atoms as the seeds out of which individual things developed. In the fifth book of his poems, he traced the progressive genesis of vegetable and animal forms out of Mother Earth. He said that many races may have lived and died out and that those which still existed had been protected by craft, courage, or speed. Thus, he vaguely anticipated the modern idea of survival of the fittest.

Personal Life: Epicurus was born in Samos about the year 342 B.C., seven years after the death of Plato. His father was Neocles, a native of Gorgettos, a small village of Attica. At the age of eighteen, he went to Athens, where the Platonic school flourished under the leadership of Xenocrates. When Antipater banished some 12,000 of the poorer citizens from Samos, Epicurus joined his father at Colophon. It is possible that he listened there to the lectures of Nausiphanes, a Democritan philosopher, and was influenced by the Democritan writings; in time he began to formulate his own doctrine.

In 307 B.C., he returned to Athens, after it had been restored to independence and there he gathered around him a number of disciples. Because of his outspokenness against religion, Diogenes stated that he was disliked by the Athenians. They accused him of licentious conduct. According to Diogenes, the Stoics, who sought to refute the views of Epicurus, appealed to his antecedents and habits rather than facts. Contrary to the picture presented by Diogenes, other trustworthy authorities pointed to the statues which the city of Athens raised in Epicurus' honor and to the number of his friends as indications that the Athenians held him in high esteem.

He lived a simple life, contenting himself with barley bread, one half pint of wine, and water daily. He had warm affection for his countrymen. He united his followers by the charm of his personality. He never entered public life. He died in the year 270 B.C. from a calculus (perhaps in the bladder).

Epicurus may justly be ranked among the promotors of medical progress, particularly for the eagerness with which his tenets were adopted by the school of Empirics in opposition to the Dogmatists who largely followed the views of the Stoics.

THE STOICS

Old Ionian Theory: The Epicurean idea that both body and soul were corporeal and composed of atoms did not satisfy the Stoics, for the Epicureans did not explain the primary constitution of the atom, of elementary solids, nor of their compelling movements. To the Stoics, everything that existed, even the smallest particle, should possess two characteristics: it should be capable of acting and of being acted upon. They went back to the old Ionian theory that matter was composed of the four elements: earth, air, fire, and water. They regrouped these four elements into classes, such as mind and matter, active and passive, soul and body, the first constituent of these pairs being more or less closely associated with "fire." A distinction was made between elemental or creative fire and the destructive fire of the domestic hearth. But, although these various dualisms had a place in the Stoic system, they were all subject to a higher monism, that of the one elemental stuff, the pneuma. Thus their theory tended to reconcile the elemental with the pneumatic theory, the material, and the spiritual. They held that the body was combined with soul in its varying grades by the principle of pervasive mixture. Nowhere was there an absolute line of demarcation between body and soul; and, since all beings had proceeded from the Supreme Intelligence, so they would all be absorbed into the Supreme Spirit.

The Nature of Man: The most important chapter in Stoic physics was the one that dealt with the nature of man. It considered man as a universe on a small scale (microcosm). Each human soul was a fragment of the universal divine force, yet not completely sundered from its parent-stock, the body. The soul was the ruling part of man, and was possessed of reason; it was spread throughout the whole man and was found in all grades, even the lowest. The five senses—sight, hearing, smell, taste, and touch—were all functions of the soul, each working through its appropriate sense-organ. The eye, ear, nose, tongue, and skin thus afforded men knowledge of the outer world. Speech, motion, and procreation were functions of knowledge and action. Breathing and digestion were functions of action alone. Thus human nature consisted of knowledge and action and was guided by reason and will. The highest philosophy was to recognize that reason and will were ultimately one.

Pneumatic Theory: With the decline of the Peripatetic school, Hellenic philosophy received a fresh impetus from Stoicism which attempted to blend opposite tenets into one system by elaborating the idea of "pneuma." The doctrine of pneuma (vital breath, or spirit) was not new in medicine. The Hippocratics ascribed the maintenance of bodily heat to respiration which furnished air within the organism.

When Praxagoras discovered the difference between the veins and arteries in the corpse (the first containing blood and the second being empty), the pneumatic theory was enhanced. It was declared that through the empty vessels pneuma was being conveyed to the different parts of the body, supplying them with vitality. When the vital air reached the brain and heart, it transmitted thought and organic movements.

The peculiar character of air was recognized by the Stoics as something intermediate between corporeal and incorporeal. It will be recalled (Chapter 16) that when Diogenes of Apollonia revived the old Ionian theory that all matter contained life, in opposition to the dualism of Anaxagoras, he declared that air was the one element typical of matter in a gaseous state. The Stoics united the two conceptions into one. The system of the Stoics was held in the highest esteem by the Roman physicians when, in the first century B.C., a small body of physicians under the leadership of Atheneus of Italia endeavored to introduce the doctrine of pneuma in medicine. Their aim was to apply the fundamental idea of Stoic philosophy in order to explain physiology, pathology, and the etiology of disease, thus conciliating the two divergent lines of thought of the Methodists and Empiricists.

The Stoics recognized one single world power, conceived on the one hand as being world reason, and on the other as being identified with the original element of fire, breath of life, or pneuma. "Pneuma is the original matter from which all individual things have emanated, by which all things pervade and rule. The human body was formed from crude elements and pervaded by the warm breath of life which is an emanation from the world-soul." It endowed the body with reason and brought forth speech, imagination, and desire. It was the vital spark of all physiological functions; its chief seat was the thorax.

Stoic psychology held that the soul was corporeal, for otherwise it would have no real existence and would be incapable of holding the body together. The Stoics stood in sharp contrast to the Epicureans who maintained it was the body which confined and sheltered the "light atoms" of the soul and of the body. These corporeal things were identical with reason and mind. The Stoics maintained that mind and body were inseparable.

The Cosmos, according to the Stoics, should be conceived as a single whole, its variety being referred to varying states of condensation of the pneuma, for everything in nature contained pneuma. The soul at first is devoid of content; in the embryo it has not developed beyond the nutritive principle of a plant; at birth the "ruling part" is likened to a blank tablet, although prepared to receive writing. This excluded all possibility of innate ideas or any faculty akin to intuitive reason.

"The source of all our knowledge is experience and discursive thought. Our ideas are copied from the stored-up sensations."

The Stoic system viewed the body as vegetable growth, "for even the lowest parts of the body, the hair and the nails, possess vegetable growth." The embryo, according to the Stoics, was a vegetable; at death man was parted in two, the higher developments of soul finding their way to an ultimate reunion with the Deity, the lower, sinking to vegetable and inorganic life and ultimately disappearing in the four elements. From either point of view individuality after death was lost. In the Roman period, when the hope of a future life was cherished for the maintenance of individual personality, the Stoic teachers dashed this hope with an increasingly firm negation.

According to most ancient thinkers, there was a parallel between the macrocosm and the microcosm: Just as the soul of the world filled and penetrated the universe, the human soul pervaded all the body with the air or pneuma breathed, informing and guiding it, and stamping the man with his essential character of rationality. In the microcosm, the soul was situated in the heart at the center of the body, not in the brain. The universal soul was situated high up in the heavenly sphere.

Founding of Stoic School: The Stoic school of philosophy was founded at the close of the fourth century B.C. by Zeno.[5] The name "Stoic" was derived from stoa, a painted corridor on the north side of the market place at Athens, which the celebrated painter Polygnotus had adorned with frescoes of the Trojan wars. This school was not considered strictly a product of Greek intellect, but rather an offspring of the cultural activities of both the East and West, brought together by the conquests of Alexander the Great. Most Stoics lived outside of Greek territory. Many of them were natives of Alexandria; some lived in Tarsus and Rhodes. Stoicism received its crowning triumph when it was brought to Rome, where it became a powerful creed for two centuries. Stoicism played upon the imagination of cultured men and exerted a wider influence than Platonism. It was a practical philosophy, the main dictum of which was the concept that there was no being save the corporeal. In Stoicism, medicine, philosophy, and science were united; but to the average Greek, medicine was an art entirely separated from science.

Qualifications of Physicians: In ancient Greece, anyone could practice medicine who thought himself qualified to do so and who could find patients. The only exception to this rule was for those who held a state appointment. These men had to be distinguished in their pro-

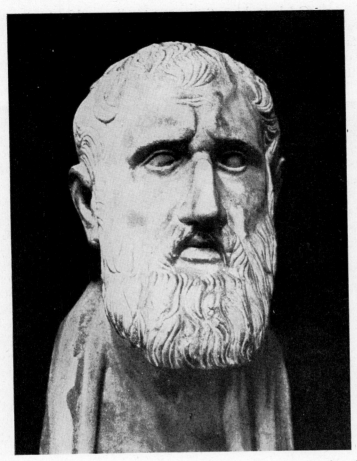

Fig. 125: Zeno, the Stoic (third century B.C.). Zeno, the founder of the Stoic philosophy, was born at Sitinium in Cypress. He was a contemporary of Epicurus. At thirty years of age, he was shipwrecked, losing all his earthly possessions. He accepted the doctrine of the Cynics, which taught contempt for riches. He eventually opened a school of his own where he developed his own ethical philosophy, which included a reverence for moral virtues, simplicity, patience, and fortitude. His philosophy was studied particularly by many Roman nobles. Athens honored his memory with a gold crown and a public burial. His countrymen erected a monumental pillar in his honor. Only a few fragments are left of his numerous writings. (National Museum, Naples.)

fession. In Athens, an applicant for such a position had to give an account of his abilities and course of education before the assembly.

Practically every physician began as an apprentice, often to his own father. Medicine, perhaps more than any other art, has been an inherited

profession. Celebrated practitioners naturally would attract numerous
followers; thus schools arose in Croton, Cyrene, Rhodes, Cos, Cnidus,
and later in Alexandria.

Classes of Physicians: There were three classes of physicians: ordinary
practitioners, teachers of the arts, and amateurs. The last group was

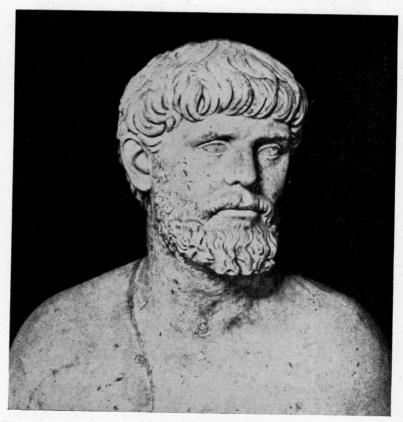

Fig. 126: Apollodorus (c. 140 B.C.). He was a pupil of Penetius, the Stoic.
(The Glyptothek, Munich.)

the most numerous. Having finished his education, it was customary
for the young doctor to travel and settle in any city which seemed to
afford a favorable opening. In an inscription of the year 304 B.C., the
Athenian assembly decreed that Pheidias, son of Apollonius the Rhod-
ian, was to be praised and crowned because, "to show his good will
to the city," he volunteered to act as public medical officer without pay.

Aside from philanthropic motives, he might have had another object in view, namely to build up a practice by treating the poor, gratis.

Offices and Dispensaries: Next to his office, the physician attended to his *iatrion,* or, as we would call it, "surgical dispensary and consulting room." Here the doctor gave his advice, performed operations, and compounded his medicine. Every large city had such an *iatrion;* in some cases, they were supported by special tax as may be seen from an inscription found in Delphi.

Women in Medicine: Since Homeric days Greek women were interested in the practice of medicine. The mother of Socrates was "a midwife brave and burly." A sister to Pyrrho the philosopher was in the same profession. In the Hippolytus, the nurse told Phaedra that, if her disorder was one which could not be revealed to men, there were women who understood those matters. Women probably practiced among their own sex.

ALEXANDER THE GREAT

The decline of Greek culture in the homeland did not prevent its spread in other lands. In the little country of Macedonia, north of Athens and beyond Thessaly, which gave birth to Aesculapius, was born another personality destined to advance general culture and spread medical knowledge all over the world—Alexander the Great. Although his real talent was military, he deserved credit as a promotor of the arts and sciences.

Along the marches of Alexander the Great on his conquests of new territory, he carried to the East that Greek culture which was already spreading westward over the Mediterranean, and in return he brought Babylonia and Egypt into closer touch with Europe. As has been mentioned, his staff collected vast stores of facts in geography and natural history. Thus began three centuries of Hellenism, from the death of Alexander in 323 B.C., to the establishment of the Roman Empire by Augustus in 31 B.C.; during that period, Greek culture, having passed its zenith in its original home, spread to other lands and dominated the known world. The Greek language was spoken "from Marseilles to India, from the Caspian to the Cataracts." The upper classes, from Rome to Asia, accepted Greek philosophy and the Greek outlook on life. Commerce became international, and thought was free as it was not to be again until recent days.

The increased knowledge of the world led to more curiosity about natural things and a more scientific attitude of mind. This great change gained momentum with the founding of Alexandria.

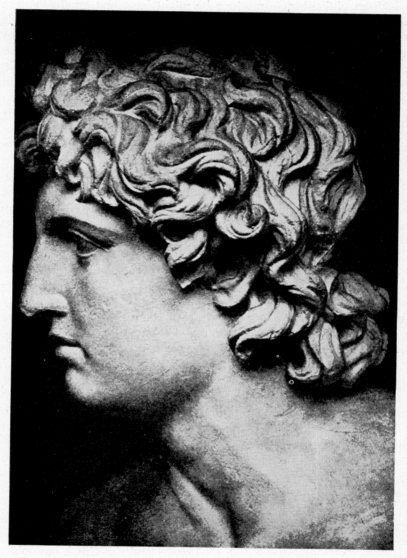

Fig. 127: Alexander (356–323 B.C.). Young Alexander's meteoric career captivated his generation and every succeeding age. His picture remained a motif in art. Lysippus was his fortunate court portraitist, but many others also made likenesses of him. (Here is shown the head of a Hellenistic marble statue, now in the Glyptothek, Munich.)

Alexander the Great, when he selected the present site of Alexandria for the city that bears his name, foresaw the unrivaled advantage of that location, which is situated at the point of union of three continents —Europe, Asia, and Africa. He realized that the city near the Delta of the Nile would become the greatest cultural center of the world. If his dreams were not realized during his short life (for he died at the age of thirty-two, of fever, in Babylonia), they were achieved after his death when the empire he founded was divided among his generals, and Alexandria fell to Ptolemy and his successors.

References and Notes

1. Historiae Plantarium, Lib. 9, C. 17.
2. Tod, M. N.: Encyclopedia Britannica, Ed. 11, Vol. 21, p. 163.
3. Zeller: Philosophy of the Stoics, Epicureans, and Sceptics; English translation by Reichel, O. J.: 1870, Cassel: Epicur, der Philosoph.; Berlin, 1892. Wallace, W.: Epicureanism; London, 1880.
4. The Book of Ecclesiastes expresses a similar sentiment: Ecclesiastes 2: 24.
5. Pearson, A. C.: The Fragments of Zeno and Cleanthis. London, 1891.

23

Alexandrian School

UNDER this title are generally included certain strongly marked tendencies in literature, science, and art which took their origin in the
Egyptian city of Alexandria. The city was founded by Alexander the
Great about the time when Greece was losing some of her intellectual
vigor (c. 300 B.C.). The great natural advantages that Alexandria enjoyed were increased to an enormous extent by the new liberal policies
of the sovereigns of Egypt.

PTOLEMY SOTER

Alexandrian Library: Ptolemy Soter (reigned 323–285 B.C.), to whom,
in the general distribution of Alexander's conquests, the kingdom of
Egypt had fallen, began to draw around him from various parts of
Greece a circle of men eminent in literature and philosophy. To these
he gave every facility for pursuing their learned researches. Through
the inspiration of his friend Demetrius of Phalerum, the Athenian orator, pupil of Theophrastus, and a Peripatetic statesman and philosopher,
Ptolemy laid the foundation of the great Alexandrian library and
prompted the keen search for all written works which resulted in the
formation of a collection such as the world had seldom seen before
the modern era. The library at first contained 50,000 volumes and finally grew to 700,000 manuscripts.

One may imagine what a difficult task it was to bring together such
a tremendous collection; for manuscripts were rare and often few copies
of a given work were in existence, sometimes only one. Indeed this
library alone would have immortalized the founder of the city.

There was only one other large library in existence at that period. It was sponsored by another of Alexander's lieutenants named Eumenes, governor of Pergamos, who gathered 200,000 volumes for his collection.[1]

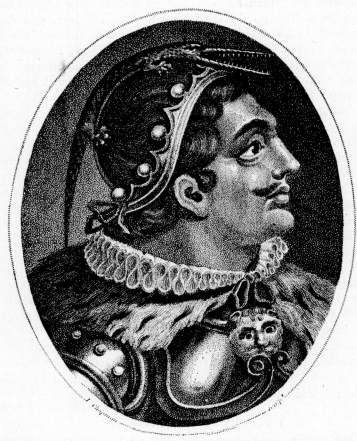

Fig. 128: Ptolemy Soter (376–283 B.C.). Ptolemaeus (the warlike) Soter, known also as the son of Lagus, was the founder of the Ptolemy dynasty of Egypt. He was a great patron of letters, and the library for which Alexandria was famous owed its inception to him. He was the founder of the museum and of the medical school of Alexandria. The head of the medical school, Herophilus, was his court physician. Two years before his death, he abdicated in favor of his youngest son Ptolemy II, Philadelphus, who, like his royal father, was a great patron of letters.

Ptolemy and Eumenes were the only two rulers of Alexander's vast empire who did not devote all their attention to military campaigns. There was much rivalry between the cities of Alexandria and Pergamos; each one tried to excel the other in cultural activities. Alexandria, however, won the greater prestige.

Ptolemy Soter built a museum which attracted a large number of learned men for whom he provided comfortable dormitories in the neighborhood. The good work begun by Ptolemy Soter was carried on vigorously by his descendants and particularly by his two immediate successors, Ptolemy Philadelphus (285–247 B.C.) and Ptolemy Euergetes. Philadelphus' librarian, the celebrated Callimachus, purchased the Aristotelian collection of books and a number of Jewish and Egyptian works. Among these was the Septuagint.

The name "Septuagint" is derived from the story of its translation by seventy, or more exactly seventy-two sages, reported in a letter sent by Aristeas to Philocratis. The story is as follows: Demetrius Phalerum, keeper of the Alexandrian library, proposed to Ptolemy II (Philadelphus) to have a Greek translation of the Jewish law made for the library. The king carefully considered it and, realizing that he had in his domain 100,000 Jewish captives who were anxious to read their law, sent an embassy with rich presents to the high priest Eleazer of Jerusalem, asking him to send six worthy and learned men from each of the twelve tribes to translate the law for him at Alexandria. Eleazer readily sent him the seventy-two men with a precious scroll of the law. They were honorably received at the court of Alexandria, whence they were conducted to the island of Pharos that they might work undisturbed and isolated. When these seventy-two men came to an agreement upon a section of the law, Demetrius wrote down their version. The whole translation was finished in seventy-two days. The Jewish community of Alexandria was allowed to have a copy but accepted it in an unhappy mood; indeed a curse was laid upon the introduction of any change from the original tongue.[2]

PTOLEMY EUERGETES

Ptolemy Euergetes (reigned 247–222 B.C.) enhanced the library greatly by seizing the original editions of the dramatists, the works of Sophocles, Euripides, and Aeschylus, for which he paid 1500 talents or 3000 pounds sterling. These had been deposited in the Athenian archives. He also compelled all travelers who arrived in Alexandria to leave a copy of any work they possessed.

This intellectual movement extended from about 323 B.C. (the foundation of the Ptolemaic Dynasty) to the final subjugation of Egypt by the Romans about 200 A.D. During this period, Alexandrian intellectual activities were of a purely literary and scientific nature.

The First University: It is stated that the rulers themselves took part in the literary forums conducted at the museum (derived from the "Muses") which were called "Feasts of the Museum." The museum founded in the year 332 B.C., was really the first university in the world.

With the growth of the museum and the library of Alexandria, Athens ceased to be the center of learning. It was in Alexandria that Euclid worked upon his geometry and that Eratosthenes measured the size of the earth, coming within a few hundred miles of the correct answer; it was in the city of the Ptolemies that Hippoachus made his astronomical studies; and it was here that Archimedes worked upon his engineering problems.

Alexandria became the ancient Oxford. It was sufficient for one to state that he studied in Alexandria to gain the respect of a community. Ammianus Marcellinus stated: "It is a recommendation for any medical man to say that he was educated at Alexandria." Even as late as the time of Galen, the reputation of Alexandria was great; to have studied there and even to have resided there a short time was tantamount to obtaining the reputation of being a good physician. Nearly all scholars during a period of five centuries received their instruction in the Alexandrian schools.

What had previously been achieved only sporadically and only under the greatest difficulties, owing to the lack of centralization of scientific pursuit, now became available to the sincere student under the domination of wise rulers. All practical and scientific means which were at the disposal of the scholar in the schools of Cnidus and Cos existed in Alexandria along a line of systematic investigation laid down by Aristotle.

Clinical Material: As a medical center, the growth of Alexandria was enhanced by the large supply of clinical material. Sick and debilitated persons from all over the ancient world flocked to Alexandria in search of medical advice, for Alexandria possessed the most eminent physicians of that period.

Here was the first and only place where anatomical investigations could be carried out on human bodies without fear. There were various reasons why Egypt should have been the first place where dissection on human cadavers could be performed. First, in Egypt, embalming was practiced from time immemorial which tended to weaken the old religious fear of the corpse. Secondly, the great interest in the advance of science taken by the liberal rulers tended to outweigh the influence of those averse to dissection.

HEROPHILUS

One of the doctors who contributed to the reputation of Alexandria as a medical center was Herophilus of Chalcedon-Bythinia (c. 335–320 B.C.), a grandson of Aristotle and pupil of Praxagoras and Crysippus, the most renowned philosophers, scientists, and physicians of their period. In medicine, the pupil surpassed his masters. He has been considered by many authorities as second only to Hippocrates. Like Hippocrates, he did not strive for a particular system of medicine but centered his interest entirely on his patient. He was fond of saying,

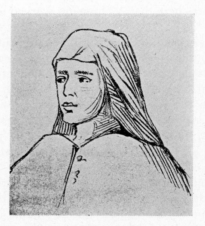

Fig. 129: Herophilus of Chalcedon-Bythinia (c. 335–280 B.C.). Herophilus was a grandson of Aristotle and a pupil of Praxagoras. He was considered a second Hippocrates, but he excelled the Father of Medicine in his knowledge of human anatomy and surgical technique. He is the first medical obstetrician on record. (From an ancient Italian print.)

"Without health, no achievements can be attained in any domain of science." He was an unbiased investigator and followed his own experience in the treatment of the sick. He held aloof from all useless speculative theories, clinging to the principle of Hippocrates to depend on clinical experience by exact methods.

Anatomy: Herophilus was the founder of the school of anatomy in Alexandria that attracted so many students of medicine and he was the first known in history to have performed post-mortem examinations. Unfortunately, only a few fragments of his medical works have survived. What is known of him was derived from his contemporaries who spoke of him as a great anatomist.

He was first to study anatomy of the brain and spinal cord. He was perhaps the first to insist that the brain was the central organ of the nervous system and the site of intelligence, an opinion contrary to that of Aristotle who maintained that the central organ of thought and intelligence was the heart. He was first to distinguish between the cerebrum and the cerebellum. He followed the course of the nerves from the brain to the spinal cord and recognized them as implements of will power and sensation. According to Rufus Ophesus, Herophilus divided the nervous system into two groupings: (1) voluntary nerves ("real nerves") which originated in the substance of the cerebrum and cerebellum (organs of sensation and motion which were spread throughout the system); (2) involuntary nerves that communicated sensation at the command of the will (these could be traced to the encephalon or the spinal marrow which was a continuation of the brain).

He knew that paralysis was caused by defects in the nerves. He went beyond the Hippocratic writings in differentiating between nerves and blood vessels. The calamus scriptorius ("writer's pen," a space at the floor of the fourth ventricle between the restiform bodies) and the torcular Herophili ("the wine-press of Herophilus", the dilated point of the confluence of the superior sagittal, straight, occipital, and two transverse sinuses of the dura mater) are still named after him. He described the meninges and their blood vessels, the choroid plexus, and the ventricles. He believed that the fourth ventricle was the seat of the soul. He observed the lacteals without determining their functions. He knew the vitreus humor, and he described three coats of the eye—the horny, shaggy, and reticular—which served as a protection for the optic organ. He described the optic nerve as having a cavity (optic pores) not observed in any other nerve. He mapped out the abdominal organs, the stomach, the duodenum (which he named), and the rest of the intestinal canal. He was aware that the nerves carried sensation to the nervous centers of the brain, and he knew the difference in function between the motor and sensory nerves. He knew of the lymphatics but not of their origin or function.

He carefully observed the pulse, and he grasped its significance as a gauge for health and disease. He carefully watched the systole and diastole; the pulse rate, strength, regularity, and uniformity of action; and made deductions from these factors. He observed the rhythm produced in the arteries by the beating of the heart, and he compared the different varieties of pulse action to the rhythm of music giving them special names. One of his classifications, the "goat-leap pulse," still survives. Thus, Herophilus may be said to have been the Father of Cardiology, who gave a rational explanation of the pulse.

Pliny, lauding Herophilus for his mastery of the pulse, stated, "To detect its exact harmony in relation to age and disease one needs to be a musician and even a mathematician." Under the name "pulse of the heart," Herophilus described a complaint of rare occurrence in his day, which occasioned sudden death. It was perhaps the anginal syndrome acompanying coronary occlusion.

Herophilus described the liver, salivary glands, pancreas, and the genital tracts of both sexes. He operated upon the liver and spleen and looked upon the spleen as of little consequence in the animal economy. He considered dislocation of the hip joint as incurable when the ligamentum teres femoris was ruptured. He attributed sudden death without any visible cause to weakness, nerve affection, paralysis, and lack of nerve force. He warned against rash extraction of teeth for toothache, since he had seen this procedure followed by death.[3]

Vivisection on Humans: Celsus reported that the Ptolemies gave Herophilus permission to do vivisection upon criminals in order to study during life "the position, color, shape, size, arrangements, hardness, softness, and smoothness of the tissues and to examine the outer surface as well as the prominences and caves of the individual organs." Pliny stated that the Ptolemies themselves took part occasionally in the anatomic dissections.

Celsus, while condemning the practice of vivisection on humans, gave arguments to defend it in certain cases. Instances of human vivisection have been reported in modern times. In the year 1550, the Duke of Tuscany handed over a condemned criminal to the medical faculty of Pisa "to kill after their own fashion and anatomize." Fallopius gave an unfortunate man two large doses of opium, but it may be questioned whether anyone would have interfered even had he followed the supposed example of Herophilus without giving any sedatives. As a matter of fact, tortures equally great or even worse were daily inflicted in the name of law and religion.

Tertullian appears to have had a religious prejudice against Herophilus. He wrote:

Herophilus that physician or butcher who dissected six hundred men in order to find out nature, who killed men in order to learn the structure of their frame, could not by these means come to a perfect knowledge of the internal structure of man since death produces a great change in all parts, so as to render their appearance after death different from what it was before, especially since they did not die a natural death but expired amidst all the agonies of death to which the curiosity of the anatomists had subjected them.

Galen stated that Herophilus was an accomplished man in all branches of physics, excelling particularly in anatomy, which he learned "not from the dissection of beasts alone as physicians usually do, but principally from that of man."[4]

Physiology and Pathology: The knowledge of anatomy of Herophilus, however, had no influence on his conception of physiology and pathology. These subjects remained a field for dogmatic speculation. He himself adhered to the humoral theory for want of a better one.

Writings: Herophilus' investigations were embodied in a work of at least three volumes, one of which was devoted to diseases of the eye. He wrote a commentary on Hippocrates, a book on dietetics, and another on obstetrics in which he pointed out the causes of difficult labor, mentioning malposition, narrowness of the cervix or os, thickness of the fetal membrane, retention of the amniotic fluid, general weakness, and weakness of the uterus, hemorrhage, and death of the fetus. He stated that delivery could occur without rupture of the membranes. Thus, in addition to his great experience as an anatomist and cardiologist, he was also an obstetrician.

It is related that one of his female students of midwifery, named Agnodice, who returned to Athens to practice midwifery, disguised herself as a man to evade the law prohibiting women and slaves from practicing medicine. Due to the envy of male competitors, she was arrested on the charge of corrupting females. At her trial, she surprised her accuser by disclosing her sex. She was, nevertheless, declared guilty on a charge of practicing contrary to the laws of the state but was finally released through the intercession of her female patients.

In his medical works, Herophilus endeavored to link up the teachings of the Coan and Cnidian Schools with the new learning in the Alexandrian schools. He was a strong advocate of clinical studies and deprecated ephemeral speculations. The medical learning of Herophilus was directed toward the evidence of the senses upon reflective thought and upon the superiority of the teaching of experience over conclusions of speculative thought. He attached great weight to symptoms as a basis of diagnosis and prognosis; the pulse beats and the general aspects of the patient's body were his guiding forces in diagnosis. He wrote a special treatise on diagnosis through knowledge of pulses, the rhythmic changes being measured by a clepsydra, or waterclock. With regard to the administration of drugs, he was accused of using them with unnecessary profusion.

Herophilus criticized the old medical classics in the light of the new anatomical and pathological knowledge and the rich experience he had gained in his large practice. His wide studies and philosophical approach enabled him to reconcile the new and old in such a manner as to facilitate greatly the practice of medicine. Fallopius, a fifteenth century anatomist, said, "to contradict Herophilus on questions of anatomy is to contradict the Gospel."

Ancient physicians were in the habit of quoting many of his sayings. One of his famous witticisms was, "The most perfect physician is he who distinguishes between the possible and the impossible."

ERASISTRATUS

The Cnidian school of medicine in Alexandria was represented by Erasistratus of Julis on the island of Chios (310–250 B.C.). He was the son of the physician Cleombrotos and Crotixel.

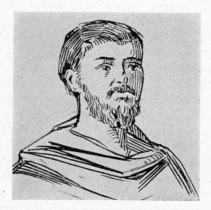

Fig. 130: Erasistratus (310–250 B.C.). Erasistratus was the son of a physician and a pupil of Metrodorus. He was a follower of the school of Cnidus in his pathological studies. In the earlier years, he was court physician to Seleucus Nicator. (From an ancient print.)

Erasistratus received his medical training largely from Metrodorus who was himself a pupil of the philosopher Crysippus (280–206 B.C.), son-in-law of Aristotle. Before Erasistratus became the head of the school of Cnidia in Alexandria, he was court physician to Seleucus Nicator of Antioch. He came to Alexandria evidently because there were no restrictions on dissection under the Ptolemies.

Writings: His writings, even in the time of Galen, were fragmentary. They dealt with anatomy, physiology, hygiene, dietetics, pharmacology, etiology, toxicology, and pathology.

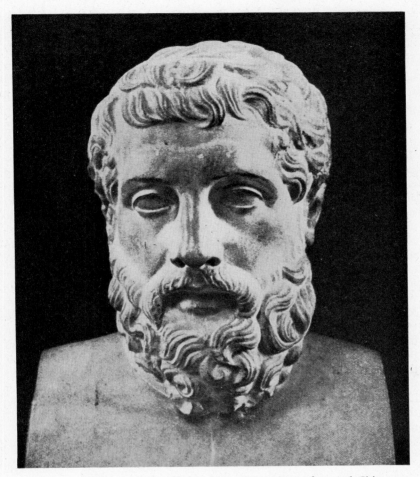

Fig. 131: Metrodorus (c. third century B.C.). Metrodorus of Chios was a pupil of Nessus. Some believe him to have been a disciple of Democritus. He was a sceptic. He accepted the Democritean theory of atoms and voids and the pleurality of the world but held to the theory of his own that the stars were formed from day to day by the moisture in the air acted upon by the heat of the sun. One of his favorite sayings was, "We know nothing; no, not even we know or not." He maintained that everything was to each person only what it appeared to him to be. Metrodorus was the friend of Pyrrhon and the teacher of Anaxarchus. He was probably a contemporary of Epicurus.

Pathology and Anatomy: Under the term "pathology," he referred to many varieties of fever, paralysis, abdominal disease, ascites, and podagra. Like his older colleague Herophilus, he traced the origin of the nervous trunk to the brain and distinguished between motor and sensory nerves; the latter he believed to be hollow. He also differentiated between the structure of the cerebrum and cerebellum and the convolutions of the brains of man as compared with those of beasts. He located the soul in the cerebellum.

From the following passage, it is sufficiently evident that Erasistratus made a careful study of the dissected brain and formed a fairly correct idea of its function and importance:

We examined what the nature of the human brain was; and we found it divided into two parts, as it is in all other animals. Each had a ventricle or cavity of a longitudinal form. These ventricles had a communication with each other, and terminated in a common opening, according to the contiguity of their parts, reaching afterwards to the Cerebellum where there was also a small cavity; but each part was separated from the other, and shut up in its proper membranes; and the Cerebellum in particular was wrapped up by itself, as well as the Brain, which, by its various windings and turnings, resembled the Intestinum jejunum. The Cerebellum was in like manner folded and twisted different ways, so that it was easy to know, by seeing it, that as in the legs of swift-running animals, as the Deer, the Hare, and some others, we observe the tendons and muscles well calculated for that purpose; so in Man, who has a larger share of understanding than other animals, this great variety and multiplicity of foldings in the Brain was undoubtedly designed for some particular end. Besides, we observed all the apophyses, or productions of the nerves which come from the brain; so that, to state all at once, the Brain is visibly the principle of every thing that passes in the body; for the sense of smelling proceeds from the nostrils being pierced, in order to have communication with the nerves; the sense of hearing is also produced by the like communication of the nerves with the ears; the tongue and the eyes receive also the productions of the nerves of the Brain.[5]

He taught that the arteries (which he believed contained air) originated in the heart. He believed that the great vein, the vena cava, was the great reservoir of the blood, while the aorta was the recipient of the spirit. He could not understand why there should be two distinct vessels for the conveyance of the same fluid; and in order to reconcile this apparent superfluity, he maintained that the arteries carried air. He attributed the bleeding that followed cutting of an artery to the fact that, when an artery was cut, not only the vital spirit escaped, but also the blood, having reached the artery by collateral communication with the veins. In the state of health, however, he believed that the arteries contained only air; he was of the opinion that any hindrance in the action of the pneuma which caused the overflow of blood into the arteries resulted in disease. Thus, he gave plethora as the cause of sickness.

He correctly described the heart, its valves, and the chordae tendinae. He discovered the action of the tricuspid valve. He thought that the function of the mitral valve was to prevent the vital spirit from leaving the heart except by way of the aorta. He named the trachea. He connected the hardness of the liver with ascites. He described the liver, the bile duct, spleen, kidneys, and intestines.

He learned the pathology of pleurisy from post-mortem examination and was of the opinion that pleuritic exudates might cause effusion into the heart. In his opinion, the pneuma was the essence of life; the function of the blood was to nourish the body; and every organ was supported by three kinds of vessels—veins, arteries, and nerves. The function of the brain was to transmit blood to the body; of the arteries, to carry the vital spirit from the heart to the organs; and of the nerves, to conduct the animal spirit from the brain to the various parts of the body. Both arteries and veins arose from the heart.

Treatment Methods: Curiously enough, he did not advocate the treating of disease by bloodletting. He preferred treating his patients by starvation and by bandaging their limbs.

He stated that bloodletting presented the following difficulties: (1) The vein was often hard to locate; (2) there was danger of opening an artery by mistake; (3) there was difficulty in ascertaining the precise quantity of blood which should be taken; and (4) there was futility in venesection to relieve inflammation of the arteries occasioned, as he imagined, by a coagulation of the venous blood in their orifices. Noticing that wounds were often followed by inflammation, he assumed that this was also due to a passage of blood into the arteries, and when it involved the larger vessels, it produced fever and disease. Sickness was thus generally due to an overfullness of the veins, or "plethora," which compelled some of the blood to pass into the arteries. He probably acquired his abhorrence of venesection, from his teacher Chrysippus of Cnidus, who had spent months with the Egyptian priests and had learned from them the doctrine that "blood is life" or, as Chrysippus called it, "the food of the soul."

Like many modern physicians, he disliked purgation and substituted emetics and enemas as his routine procedure. He stated that enemas should be mild in quality and sparing in quantity, and he totally rejected the copious and irritating enemas in general use. He recommended abstinence and exercise. He entertained a high opinion of the value of chicory in diseases of the liver and other viscera. In treating

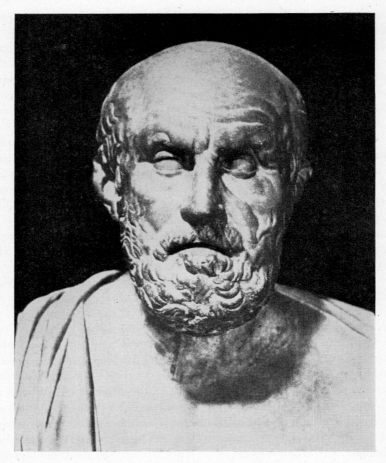

Fig. 132: Chrysippus (280–226 B.C.). Chrysippus was the third Greek leader of the Stoics of Sali in Cilicia. He studied under Zeno in Athens. The dominant note of his philosophy was comprehension rather than originality. He defended Zeno and Cleanthis, his teachers, against attacks of the Academy. Diogenes Laertus said, "If the gods use dialectics, they can use none other than those of Chrysippus." He composed 150 treatises; only a few fragments of these have withstood the ravages of time. (From an old Florentine bust.)

disease, he depended chiefly on diet and regimen, aided occasionally by topical applications. He denounced complex prescriptions and fanciful hypotheses. In hemorrhage of the limbs, he used bandages. In hemoptysis, he gave salted articles with food.

According to Erasistratus' theory of circulation, the blood was prepared in the liver, entered the right side of the heart by way of the vena cava, and thence flowed through the pulmonary artery to the lungs. The valves directed the blood into the veins and the air into the arteries; the left side of the heart received the pneuma from the lungs, whence it was distributed into the blood by the aorta. It is evident that this theory of circulation was confusing. There appeared to be no door-way open for the blood to leave the lung.

His explanation of the circulation of the pneuma was as follows: The pneuma, entering the lungs, penetrated the heart, where it formed the vital spirit; thence it was carried by the arteries to the brain, where it was transformed into the animal spirit, which was transmitted by the nerves to all organs of the body. He correctly regarded the brain as the center of psychic functions. His theory of communication of the blood from the veins to the arteries by small blood vessels was a step nearer to Harvey's discovery, albeit in a reverse direction.

He disagreed with the Hippocratics on the theory of humoral pathology. His studies of anatomy led him to believe that the cause of disease lay in the changes of the solid parts of the body. He followed Heroph-ilus with regard to medicaments. He favored, in most cases, vege-tables, which he called "hands of God."

He directed his attention to the study of symptoms resulting from functional disturbance and endeavored to discover their exciting causes. He considered digestive disturbances to be secondary causes. He looked upon fever as a symptom of inflammation which arose from blood ob-structing the pneuma in the arteries. Among other methods of treatment, were bodily exercise, bathing, fasting, cleansing, massage, diuretics, and diaphoretics. Erasistratus was given credit for being the inventor of the catheter. The writings of Erasistratus dealt with general prin-ciples of physiology, anatomy, etiology, hygiene, food, drugs, special pathology, and therapeutics. He described many varieties of fever, abdominal affections, paralysis, podagra, dropsy, and their treatment. His textbooks on anatomy, especially, contained names given by him to various organs of the body.

In the practice of surgery, he appeared, in some instances at least, to have been a bold and successful operator. He did not hesitate, in cases of hepatic tumor, to make an incision through the skin and muscu-lature into the cavity of the abdomen and apply his remedies directly to the part affected. Yet, notwithstanding this radical method in cases of hepatic disease, he wholly disapproved of tapping in dropsy; he felt that the liver, being in an inflamed and cirrhotic state, would be more pressed upon and injured by the adjoining parts after the water was drawn off and that the operation, in consequence, would be more likely to cause the death of the patient. He likewise objected to the extraction of teeth when much force was required.

Like many of the great teachers before him, he decided, after qualifying to practice medicine, to spend many years in travel and research. He mastered the Hippocratic writings, their commentaries, and the textbooks of his contemporaries, and he visited the famous anatomists and surgeons to learn their technic. Due to his erudition and familiarity with all medical and surgical techniques, he was appointed, for a time, as court physician to the ruler at Antioch. It was while employed in this capacity that he became involved in a romantic love episode.

It is related by the historians, Plutarch, Appian, and Lucian, that he was called to attend to Prince Antiochus, the son of Seleucus Nicator by an early marriage to the Persian Princess Apama. Nicator, it should be remembered, became master of Babylon after the untimely death of Alexander the Great. This prince, who was heir to the Babylonian throne, became madly in love with his young stepmother, the beautiful Stratonice, daughter of Demetrius The Besieger. The young prince knew that it was wrong to be in love with his father's wife, and he tried to suppress his passions. He consequently became melancholy, refused food, became negligent about his person, and would not talk even to his intimate friends. The court physicians were at a loss to ascertain what troubled the young prince. Seleucus, seeing that his son was pining away from day to day, sent for Erasistratus whose reputation extended all through the Near East. The famous Erasistratus watched the young prince several days without any clue as to the cause of his condition. One day, while holding the prince's pulse, he observed that his pulse suddenly began to beat fast; and looking around, he saw Stratonice entering the room. Thus discovering the secret of Antiochus, he revealed it to the king, who immediately arranged a marriage between his son and Stratonice. Galen, who was a bitter critic of Erasistratus, referred to this story sarcastically, "There is no such thing as a lover's pulse."

Medical Reputation: The medical reputation of Erasistratus may be conjectured from the statement of Pliny:

Ptolemy paid to Erasistratus for medical service a fee equivalent to twenty-four hundred pounds. The amount of this fee of course must be exceptional. The average doctor's fee ranged from one to two drachmas (nine to eighteen pence). Sometimes patients remembered the physicians in their will as did the philosopher Lykon, who bid his heir to "satisfy" his medical attendant. "He deserves it more for his zeal than for his ability."

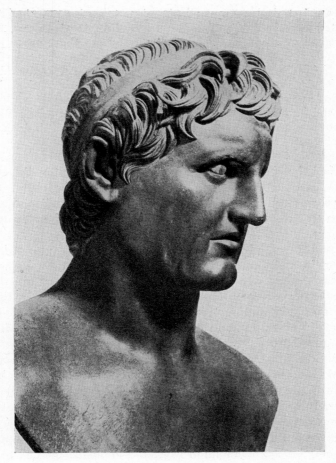

Fig. 133: Seleucus Nicator (c. 350–291 B.C.). Seleucus employed Erasistratus as his court physician. He was the son of Antiochus. As a young man, he accompanied Alexander the Great into Asia (333 B.C.). After Alexander's death, he became master of Babylonia. He was assassinated by Ptolemy Ceranus. (National Museum, Naples.)

Galen, who had an almost superstitious attachment to the memory of Hippocrates, was most intolerant of everyone who appeared to rival his fame. He was particularly bitter against Erasistratus. Galen devoted almost a chapter of his work "The Natural Faculties" to attacking Erasistratus for ignoring Hippocrates in his writings:

For some reason he referred at great length to certain other foolish doctrines and passed over the views of Hippocrates. The opinion of Erasistratus

in his treatise on deglutition was neither rhetoric nor logic . . . he said urine
is secreted from the kidneys but does not say how, in what way . . . but if
Erasistratus kept silent, I wouldn't do so, for I know if one passes over the
Hippocratic view and makes some other pronouncement about the function
of the kidneys (ignoring attraction) one cannot make onself more ridiculous.
It was for this reason that Erasistratus kept silent and the Asclepiadae lied.
They are like slaves who have had plenty to say in the early parts of their
careers and have managed by their excessive rascality to escape many and
frequent accusations, but later, when caught in the act of thieving, cannot
find any excuse.

The fact that Galen did not mention that Erasistratus dissected living criminals condemned to death suggests that the charge against
him, as reported by Celsus and repeated later by Tertullian, should not
be taken seriously. Galen surely would not have spared Erasistratus from
any charge.

The practice of "physic" about this period, according to Celsus, became for the first time divided into three distinct branches—medicine,
surgery, and pharmacy—each of which was pursued as a separate and
independent profession. Hitherto it had been the custom for the same
person to exercise all three functions. Occasionally, when a division of
practice took place, it usually consisted of a separation of medicine from
surgery and pharmacy.

Erasistratus in later years settled at Samos, where he died about 250–
240 B.C. He seems to have committed suicide. He took poison because
of an incurable ulcer. His last words were, "It is well that I should remember of my country." Incidentally, suicide in old age was not an uncommon practice in that part of the world.

His countrymen gave him a grand funeral and erected a monument in
his memory on the mountain of Mycale overlooking the city of Samos
where he was buried.

DISCIPLES OF HEROPHILUS

The schools of Herophilus produced many distinguished men who
carried on the principles of their master. Herophilus was succeeded by
Eudemus, who did much to advance anatomical knowledge. Other
disciples of Herophilus were Bakcheis of Tanagra, a voluminous writer
on medical subjects; Manteas, a skillful surgeon and gynecologist; De-
metreus of Apamea, a renowned obstetrician and writer on clinical
observations; Andreas of Carystos, who wrote a work on materia medica
that was widely read for centuries after; Dioscorides, and Phakas, the

famous court physician of Cleopatra. The doctors of the Alexandrian age pursued medicine from altruistic motives; only quacks and charlatans were mercenary.

The Herophilean school came to an end toward the close of the first century of the present era, but the Erasistratean school maintained a dominant position for a century longer. Strato, Apollophanes of Seleucia, Apollonius of Memphis, Plotomaius, and Martianus were the principal teachers of this school and distinguished themselves by original research and writing. Less is heard of the Erasistratean school than the Herophilean because it strongly opposed the teachings of the Hippocratics and other early masters and thus was continually embroiled in disputes with other medical schools.

GOLDEN AGE OF MEDICINE

The period of Herophilus and Erasistratus was the Golden Age of Medicine, not only of Alexandria but of the entire medical world. Physicians then lived in a period of intellectual as well as social activity. Great progress was made in other branches of science in Alexandria in the latter part of the third century B.C.

Younger Contemporaries of the Period

Among the younger contemporaries of that period may be mentioned Eratosthenes, who was born at Cyrene about 273 B.C. and died at Alexandria about 192 B.C. He was librarian of the museum and the first great physical geographer. He calculated the circumference of the earth by estimating the latitudes. Eratosthenes argued, from the similarity of the tides in the Indian and Atlantic Oceans, that those oceans must be connected, that the inhabited world of Europe-Asia-Africa formed an island, and that it was possible to sail from Spain to India around the south of Africa. He also conjectured that the Atlantic might be divided by land running from the north. This idea was reflected by Poseidonius, who, underestimating the size of the earth, proclaimed that a man sailing west for 70,000 stadia would come to India, a theory which laid the foundation for Columbus' discovery of the New World.

The mathematician, physicist, inventor, and astronomer, Hipparchus, was the founder of algebraic solutions of equations of the first and second degree and worked out many formulas for calculating area and volume. He struck upon an important principle when he pointed out that the line of a reflected ray of light was the shortest possible path.[6] He was chiefly remembered for his mechanical contrivances, including a siphon, a thermoscope, an air pump, and the earliest steam engine, in which the recoil of steam issuing from a jet was used to make an arm carrying the jet revolve about an axis.

The most distinguished scientist of that period was the astronomer Claudius Ptolemy,[7] who must not be confused with the kings of Egypt of the same name. He taught and made observations at Alexandria between the years 127 and 151 A.D. His great work, later called by its contracted Arabic name of "Almagest," was an encyclopedia of astronomy, which was based on and supplemented the work of Hipparchus. This remained a standard treatise until the days of Copernicus and Kepler.

A book on optics was also attributed to Ptolemy. It contained a study of refraction, including atmospheric refraction, which was described by Sarton[8] as "the most remarkable experimental research of antiquity." The author found that when light passed from one medium to another, the angles of incidence and refraction were proportional, a relation which was approximately true for small angles.[9]

References and Notes

1. A smaller library was established in Serapion. During the attack of Julius Caesar on Alexandria, the Alexandrian library was accidentally destroyed by fire. The Serapion library was enriched by Cleopatra, who presented the library with 200,000 volumes she received from Mark Antony which he had removed from Pergamos.
2. This letter was edited by H. St. Thackery in Swete, H. B.: Introduction to the Old Testament in Greek; 1906. Josephus: Antiquities; 12:12. The Talmud repeats the story, adding that Ptolemy built a basilica for the seventy-two sages and provided seventy-two golden chairs for them.
3. This statement is not supported by Galen who is the most noted authority on Alexandrian medicine. Tertullian supported the statement of Celsus; but since he lived 500 years after (137 A.D.), his testimony does not merit any credence.
4. De Dissect., Ch. 5.
5. Cited by Hamilton, W.: History of Medicine, Surgery, and Anatomy. Vol. 1, 1831.
6. Sarton, G.: History of Science. Vol. 1, p. 208, 1927. Isis, No. 16, 1924.
7. Bunberry, E. H., and Brazley, C. R.: Encyclopedia Britannica, Ed. 11, Vol. 22, pp. 618-626.
8. "History of Science," Vol. 1, p. 274, 1927. "Isis," No. 16, p. 79, 1924.
9. Dampier, Sir W. C.: A History of Science. New York, 1943, pp. 52-54.

24

Empiricism

EMPIRICISM in the primary sense signified the method or habit of judging things from observation or trial. In the modern sense, Empiricism denotes a system of reasoning based upon hasty and inadequate observation, neglecting scientific principles and precision, in other words conclusions based upon mere experience or a practice without knowledge of the theory of the subject discussed. It applies particularly to one of the ancient medical cults of Alexandria which maintained that practice or experience alone without theory was the foundation of the science of medicine, that is was idle to speculate on remote causes or on anatomy and pathology of disease.

This school was inaugurated by Philinius of Cos and Serapion of Alexandria to counteract the methods of the Dogmatists, who treated diseases according to fixed theoretical rules. The Empirics claimed to be the followers of Hippocrates. They originally paid some attention to the symptoms of disorders. They considered the idiosyncrasies of their patients as affected by climates and localities. They employed the therapeutic measures which had been found effectual in analogous cases.

PHILINIUS

The originator of this school, Philinius of Cos (c. 250 B.C.), had been a student of the Herophilean school but later rebelled against the teaching of his master, who stressed the importance of anatomy in the diagnosis and treatment of disease. Philinius came out with the statement, "The anatomical knowledge I derived from Herophilus has been useless to me in treating the sick." He advised his followers to direct their aims to careful personal observation of the sick and to the accumulated

609

experience of others in their practice; to discard all physiological, anatomical, and pathological hypotheses; but to depend entirely upon clinical observations and tried remedies.

By their revolutionary methods, the Empirics reduced the science of medicine to a system of therapeutics. They taught that the physician's first duty was to find ways of removing the symptoms by drugs used in similar cases.

SERAPION

The younger contemporary of Philinius, Serapion of Alexandria (c. 220 B.C.), also a student of Herophilus, was even more militant. He denounced all physicians, from Hippocrates down, for their hair-splitting speculations. He despised anatomy and asked, "What is the use of knowing the shape and position of the brain and liver?" He rejected entirely the dogmatic physiology and pathology. His favorite motto was, "It is not the cause but the cure of sickness that concerns the physician, not how we digest but what is digestible." He reduced the art and science of medicine to a system of therapeutics and he said the physician's duty was to search for specific remedies, not for a correct diagnosis.

Serapion laid down three cardinal principles upon which medical practice should be based: (1) personal experience gained by design or accident (autopsy); (2) experience of others or the knowledge that has come down by tradition (history); and (3) analogy. If the first two principles did not suffice to institute proper treatment, then the third principle could be utilized by deductions made from similar cases.

GLAUCIUS

A later Empiric, Glaucius of Taras (170 B.C.), incorporated the doctrine of Serapion into a philosophical system and designated it "the tripod." He maintained that the method taught by Serapion should be attained by inductive methods and be employed for therapeutic purposes. Later, a fourth leg was added to the tripod, namely the physician could base his internal diagnosis on external signs; for instance, if the physician found a scar on the patient's head, he was justified in attributing the cephalalgia to the injury of the head.

PYRRHON

Another prominent Empiric was the sceptic Pyrrhon of Elis (c. 360–270 B.C.). Pyrrhon was a follower of Democritus and Epicurus in his philosophy and concepts of physics. He gathered many of his ideas while following Alexander the Great on his military expeditions. One of his teachings was, "If it is impossible for one to gain true knowledge, the wise man should withdraw into himself, avoiding distress and emotion which belongs to the contests of vain imaginings." Personally, he passed a life of solitude. He was the most thorough agnostic in the history of thought. His ethico-philosophical teaching was a mixture of that of the Epicureans and the Stoics. Little is known of his medical learning except that he was against Dogmatism and was inclined toward Empiricism while treating the sick

HERACLIDES

The Empirical school reached its zenith in the person of Heraclides of Taras (c. first century B.C.). Galen called him "most excellent physician" giving him the praise for never preferring the interest of his party to the truth. His nephew Soranus considered him the only worthy Empiric known. Only a few fragments of his work survive, but it is known that he wrote a commentary on Hippocrates and an apology for his Empirical ideas. He was particularly assiduous in inquiring into the remote causes of disease. His description and treatment of phrenitis, cholera, tetanus, and other dangerous diseases appear, from what is recorded in the work of Coelius Aurelianus, to have been "judicious." He made copious contributions to the materia medica of his day. He wrote on dietetics, surgical diseases, the diagnostic value of the pulse, the preparation of drugs, and poisons and cosmetics. His records were much quoted by his colleagues and used even by opponents of the Empiric school. His methods of treatment, in contrast to other Empirics, were founded on tests. He paid attention to the preparation of remedies and the indications for their uses. Among his favorite remedies were cinnamon, pepper, balm of Gilead, and opium.

Heraclides was not fond of controversy. His mild manners and gentle character led the Empirics to accuse him of relapsing into Dogmatism. He did not seek notoriety by abusing his colleagues or by introducing new, startling remedies. On the contrary, he endeavored to weed out the already overgrown garden of Empiric nostrums.

His work "On the Preparation and Proving of Drugs" represents what was the best in Empiricism. It contains nothing but what he himself had examined and tested. He left prescriptions containing opium for cases of sleeplessnes, spasm, colic, cough, and cholera, using a large dose of the drug in hydrophobia.

Heraclides described phrenitis, tetanus, croup, and ileus. Brain fever he divided into three forms—inflammatory, gastric, and cerebral. He treated the last condition by placing the patient in a darkened room, by applying cold compresses to the head, by bloodletting, and by the use of enemas. In acute fevers, he stated fluids were not to be withheld from the patient.

He was scarcely less distinguished as a surgeon than as a physician. He invented instruments for the reduction of dislocation of the hip joint. Perhaps he utilized some of the inventions of his contemporary Archimedes in his methods of reduction of dislocations and treatment of fractures. He also invented a mechanical method of separating the lids from the eyeball to prevent adhesion after an injury. His method was employed for many centuries after. He devised an operation for ankyloblepharon and polypus of the ear.

His reputation as a physician and surgeon was so high as to obtain from Coelius Aurelianus the title of "The Prince of Empirics." His work on materia medica[1] was a great contribution to medical science.

After the death of Heraclides, a decline took place in the pharmaceutical branch of medicine. Henceforth, the researches of medical men were directed chiefly toward the discovery of remedies calculated to counteract the deleterious effect of poisons.

DEMOCRITES

In contrast to Heraclides, who carefully tested the preparations which he ordered for his patients and prescribed only those which in his opinion had merits, Democrites, who flourished at about the same period, introduced in his practice a variety of most complex prescriptions. Among others may be mentioned mithridatum ("Democratic confection"), a formula exhibiting a strange mixture of not less than forty-four ingredients. The formula for this heterogeneous conglomeration may be found at the Royal College of Physicians, in the pharmacopeia of the year 1746.

The theriaca andromachi of the same pharmacopeia was still larger, occupying nearly three-quarters of a page and exhibiting a list of not less than sixty-one, distinct, component parts. Somewhat similar to this complex composition was the celebrated anodyne, invented about the same time by Herennius Philo, a native of Tarsus (the metropolis of Sicily), which was named after him, "Philonium." The chief ingredients consisted of opium and euphorbium, mixed with various aromatics and formed into a confection. In the pharmacopeia mentioned, a preparation under the name of "Philonium" is pre-eminent, the formula of which is as follows:

Philonium Londinense
  R Piperis alba
    Zingiberis
    Seminum carui, singularum, P.: uncias duas
    Opii colati, P.: drachmas sex
    Syrupi e meconic, ad mellis spissitudinem cocti; triplum omnium
      pondus
    Opium vino solutum syrupo, calefacto curiose
      immisce: tum adde caetera in pulverem redacta[2]

NICANDER

Among the Empirics of the same period (c. 135 B.C.), the name of Nicander (second century B.C.) of Colophon who flourished in the time of Attalus, King of Pergamos, deserves to be mentioned. He enjoyed a high reputation as physician but a still higher one for his general attainments as a poet and a grammarian. Two of his books have survived the ravages of time.

EMPIRIC VIEWS AND METHODS

Celsus, in his discussion of the Empirics, stated:

They admit that evident causes are necessary, but deprecate inquiry into them because Nature is incomprehensible. This is so because the philosophers and physicians who have spent so much labor in trying to search out causes cannot agree amongst themselves. If reasoning could make physicians, the philosophers should be most successful practitioners as they have such abundance of logical words. If the causes of diseases were the same in all places, the same remedies ought to be used everywhere. Relief from sickness is to be sought from things certain and tried, that is from experience which guides us in all other arts. Disquisitions can have no connection with medicine, because physicians whose opinions have been directly opposed to one another have equally restored their patients to health; they did not derive their methods of cure from studying the causes about which they disputed, but from the experience they had of the remedies which they employed upon their patients. Medicine was not first discovered in consequence of reasoning, but the theory was sought after the discovery of medicine. Does reason, they ask, prescribe the same as experience, or something different? If the same, it is unnecessary; if different, it must be mischievous.[3]

The Empirics followed some of the Hippocratic teachings but never acknowledged it. They paid attention to clinical observations, but they made no attempt to arrive at general laws from isolated facts. They were guided almost exclusively by experience in therapy. They directed their energies to practical aims. They abandoned all speculative and controversial concepts and maintained that philosophical, dogmatic, and theoretical discussions could be of no help to the patient. Anatomy, which Hippocrates, Herophilus, and Erasistratus considered indispensable to the practice of medicine, was regarded by the Empirics as useless. They maintained that the organs of the dead body behaved differently than those of the living body. Of course, vivisection was out of the question. The Empirics looked upon such practices with horror. The only way one could gain some knowledge of anatomy and physiology was by observing surgical operations, and surgery at this period was not a developed art. Little abdominal surgery was done. Surgery was largely confined to occasional operations for scrotal hernia, the removal of vesical calculi, and the couching operation for cataract. Galen, in his commentary on Hippocrates, inveighed against the Empirics who claimed that Hippocrates belonged to them "while in truth, he (Hippocrates) avails himself on all occasions of logic and of anatomy to which he was much devoted."[4]

Some of their maxims as quoted by Celsus were:

Disease is not cured by talk but by drugs.
Husbandmen and navigators are not trained by disputation but by practice.
The important question is not what causes but what dispels disease.
    Not the hidden cause of disease will benefit the sick but the information derived from the existing morbid condition immediately at hand.

If the antagonism of the Empirics towards the study of elementary medical subjects had not been so extreme, Alexandrian medicine might not have suffered such a decline, for there were some merits in their doctrine. In the beginning, the Empirics made important contributions to medical progress. They treated fractures and dislocations in a much improved manner. Their method of reducing scrotal hernia was commendable. Their technic of dressing wounds was praiseworthy, and their art of bandaging was progressive. A certain Amyntas was credited with introducing a special device for fracture of the bridge of the nose, and Ammonius invented a "lithorite" to crush large vesical calculi which could not be removed by ordinary extraction. The most commendable achievements of the Empirics were made in the domain of pharmacology. A number of their contributions to this subject were employed down to the last period of antiquity. They added a number of new drugs to the pharmacopeia. They particularly increased the knowledge of poisons and their antidotes.

Valuable contributions to materia medica were made by Crotonas, the court physician of King Mithridates to whom he dedicated his writing. The king himself made contributions to the study of poisons and antidotes. In passing, it should be mentioned that at this period there was a tendency of wicked rulers and others to use poison to get rid of their enemies as well as to protect themselves against revolutionary elements. Mithridates' experiments with poisons and their antidotes culminated in "Mithridatum," which was employed for centuries. This poison consisted of a mixture of the blood of Pontine ducks with toxic substances; by gradually increasing the doses, toleration of the poison ensued and a large dose could be taken with safety. Incidentally, when Mithridates was poisoned by an enemy with his mixture, it did not affect him. He did not, however, die a natural death. When the report reached him that an enemy was about to take his life, he asked a Gallic soldier to stab him with a spear.

Mithridates cultivated in his garden other deadly drugs, such as eupalous and scordium. According to Plutarch, the last king of Pergamos grew many poisonous plants in his yard, such as henbane, hellebore, hemlock, aconite, and dorycinium. A number of prescriptions handed down by medical authors were ascribed to Cleopatra. Two of them relating to cosmetics have been lost. One remedy for diseases of women has survived.

OTHER NOTED EMPIRICS

Other Empirics of note were Apollonius Biblas ("the book worm," c. 180–160 B.C.), Zeuxis (commentator of Hippocrates, c. 250 B.C.) and Zophyros, who classified drugs according to their therapeutic action and who discovered ambrosia, the supposed antidote for all kinds of poison; and Herodotus of Tarsus, a city which next to Alexandria was distinguished for its schools of learning.

Among the Empirics of a later date was Theodas, or Thudas, of Laodicea, a Jewish osteologist, a student of Alexandria, and last of the Empirics. The doctrine of Theodas and his method of observation will be dealt with in the chapter on Talmudic Medicine.

INFLUENCE OF EMPIRICISM

History is indebted to Celsus, not only for a description of the teaching of the Empiric cult, but also for the exposure of its policies. Albutt is of the opinion that the Empirics as well as the Methodists were in some way a continuation of the Cnidian and Coan schools, the latter considering the whole patient and his environment and the former, the locality of the disease and the local treatment. The Cnidians and the Empirics merely listed symptoms without coordinating them and were, in consequence, only haphazard therapeutists.[5]

Alexandrian Empiricism might have served a good purpose if the followers of Philinius had been able to shake off the human weakness of going to extremes. As it was, they were compelled to indulge in subtle reasoning in order to agree upon the treatment of cases where experience was of no aid. Rejecting the study of anatomy and physiology rendered the localization of many diseases impossible. Differences of opinion resulted in disputation and acrimony. The spirit of scientific investigation which distinguished the early medical schools of Herophilus and Erasistratus gave way to hairsplitting and subtle scholasticism.

In time their cardinal principle, depending exclusively on observation, was pushed so far as to engender the wildest fantasies. Hence confidence in their treatment of disease waned, and the medical schools of Alexandria lost their supremacy and finally broke up.

The remnant of medical prestige that was left in Alexandria was swept away about the middle of the first century B.C., during the reign of Ptolemy Physkon, who expelled all scholars from Alexandria. Many of the medical celebrities moved to Pergamos and Laodicea, and some came to Rome. A half century later, Alexandria regained some of its medical prestige, but it was a mere shadow of its former self.

The literary centers that were founded in Rhodes, Syria, and in many cities of Asia Minor, although retaining certain Alexandrian characteristics, differed considerably from the older Alexandrian schools. What was left of Empiricism was only the name, and even this has lost its former significance. It has now become a term signifying a doctrine opposed to science and rational practices.

ROME—NEW EDUCATIONAL CENTER

After the defeat of Cleopatra in Egypt, particularly after Egypt fell to Rome and under Augustus (30 A.D.), Rome developed into a world educational center. Many works on the Greek and Alexandrian arts and sciences were carried over to the Roman capital. The speculative philosophy of the neo-Platonists, the doctrine of the agnostics, and the teaching of the Stoics and Epicureans attracted students from the Mediterranean shores and Asia Minor to the new world capital. These students eagerly embraced the occasion of coming to this new center of culture and opportunity.

The end of Egyptian independence signalized the end of Alexandrian medicine. Rome became the center of world culture and the heir of Greece in medicine, and philosophy, and the arts.

The absorption by the Romans of the Ptolemean kingdom, whose capital Alexandria had long been the scientific world center, produced, however, no creative scientists. Rome was a distributor and disseminator of Greek medicine rather than a producer of scientific geniuses. The Romans were practical men. They did not take to philosophy; they were not given to academic arguments about the essential nature of things which was the basis of Greek scientific literature. Slow to appreciate the scientific attitude, they accomplished few scientific results. Hellenism began slowly to influence Roman thought after the Punic War, around 214 B.C., and during the period between 200 and 189 B.C., when Rome broke the power of Alexander's successors and established her protectorate throughout the eastern Mediterranean. The influence of Greek ideas began to grow with the triumph after the battle of Pyda, 168 B.C. Numerous educated Greek hostages came to Rome. The library of the Macedonian kings was brought with them. They formed a nucleus for the infiltration of Greek wisdom into Roman society.

Although the Romans' relation to science improved as time went on, and educated men learned the Greek language and were affected by Hellenic philosophy, the general scientific principles of the Greek physicians as expressed in the writings of the Hippocratic, Aristotelian, and Alexandrian schools were seldom understood even by educated Romans. The prevalent attitude towards nature among the Latin-speaking upper classes, whether Italian or provincial, was expressed by the Stoic creed. That system, based on a rigid conception of the interrelation of the different parts of the world, provided little stimulus for the acquisition of new knowledge or for anything in the way of research. Thus, in place of knowledge accumulating progressively on a basis of a broad theory, there was either a type of exact but intellectually aimless observation or a rejection of all knowledge not of practical importance.[6]

There have been various attempts to explain why the Romans did not continue the scientific work of the Greeks. It is a strange phenomenon, for the value of the experimental method was still being demonstrated by the achievements of the Alexandrians. That school continued its activities in a restricted way under Roman rule and was the ultimate source of the only important Latin medical work that has come down to us, the "De Re Medica" of Celsus. The explanation may be attribu-

ted to the fact that the Romans were given to immediately useful studies
and not to speculation.

References and Notes

1. Withington, E. T.: History of Medicine. London, 1904.
2. "History of Medicine," p. 128.
3. De Med., Praefat.
4. Elliott, J. S.: Outlines of Greek and Roman Medicine, New York, 1934.
5. Albutt, T. C.: Brit. M. J., 1449–1505–1598, 1901. Greek Medicine in Rome;
    London, 1921.
6. Singer, C.: The Legacy of Rome. Oxford University Press, 1940, p. 266.

25

Roman Medicine

THE native Roman medical system was of an animistic nature, devoid of scientific elements. The Romans inherited folk medicine from the Etruscans and other aborigines of prehistoric Italy. The healing profession was in the hands of priests, magicians, elders of the family *(pater familias)*, old women, eccentric persons, and particularly those marked with physical deformities, such as hunchbacks, epileptics, and cross-eyed persons.

MEDICAL DIVINITIES

Roman medicine remained in a primitive state for 800 years after Greek medicine began to emerge from the sea of superstition and natural therapeutics took the place of spiritual healing. There were, in ancient Rome, innumerable healing divinities; they governed all kinds of ailments, each of whom bore the name of the disease over which it ruled.

The sexual processes of women from courtship to lactation were governed by no less than eighteen different divinities.

The power of Mars was exercised over pestilence. In one of the works of Cato the censor (234–149 B.C.), there was an incantation which read, "Let no war and pestilence come on thy people, fierce Mars." The goddess Salus, identified with the Greek deity Hygeia whose function was the preservation of health, was worshipped with rites borrowed from the Egyptians in the temples of Isis and Osiris. Carna was the protectress of the intestine to whom "Carnalia" prayers were offered. Ovid mentioned her as a practitioner of the magic art, who practiced exorcism upon young children attacked by the bloodthirsty Striges. Carna

619

touched the doorsteps of the children's house three times with an arbu-
tus twig, following which she sprinkled the threshold with water while
holding the entrails of a two-month-old pig.

The deity of malarial fever, a disease which raged in the plain of the
Tiber, was known as "Febris." Three temples in Rome were dedicated
to the goddess Febris. She was addressed as *Febris diva, Febris sancta,*
and *Febris magna.* There was an ancient sanctuary erected to her on

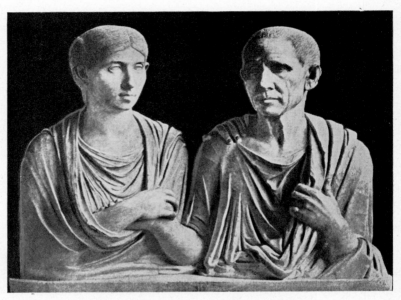

Fig. 134: So-called "Cato and Portia." (Double bust, Vatican, Rome.)

the Palatine Hill where she was worshipped. In later times, this
goddess governed two forms of the disease, *Febris Tertiana* and
Febris Quartana. An inscription to her on a votive tablet has been
preserved.

The Romans worshipped Mephitis, the goddess of putrefaction. Foul
odors were invoked in her name. A temple was erected at a place where
asphyxiating fumes emerged from the earth. They paid homage to An-
geronia, the deity of plague. They honored Mania, the goddess of insanity. They performed religious services to Uterina, the goddess who
made difficulties for women during labor; and they honored Lucina,
Diana, Opifera, and Nemi, the goddesses that played an important
part in the general life of women. Lucina was the goddess of birth.

Carmenta governed abnormal birth. The god Farcinus and the goddess Rumina controlled the sexual processes of women up to the time of conception. The god Mutunus ruled over sterility, and women made sacrifices to her as did young bridegrooms if they were impotent. Ossifragi took care of the development of the child. The young mother could address her appeal to no less than fourteen gods from Juna Lucina down to Prosa and Pertvorta. Minerva, Memor, and Medica, the goddesses of wisdom and particularly of medical science, were revered.

The Romans also canonized the goddess Ossipaga, who presided over the growth of the bones, and the goddess Carna, in whose care were the viscera and to whom offerings of bean broth and bacon were made, for these substances were considered to be among the most nutritious articles of human diet.

Such was the heterogeneous collection of medical divinities whom the lively imaginations or superstitious fears of the Romans called into fictitious existence and to whose unsubstantial guardianship they were content to confide their health. The entire pantheon of disease and physiological functions was presided over by *Dea Salus* whose temple was on one of the summits of *Quirinalis;* she was the deity who took the public health under her supervision.

Generally speaking, the ancient Romans were more prone to learn the superstitions of other people than to acquire for themselves useful knowledge.

According to Pliny, "The Roman people for more than 600 years were not indeed without medicine but without physicians." They relied mostly on religious rites; the average Roman citizen had a household god, for a variety of diseases, to whom he paid homage in case of sickness. Aside from the household gods, temples were erected in Rome as early as 467 B.C., in honor of the healing god Apollo, and as early as 460 B.C., in honor of Aesculapius. A temple was built in 450 B.C. in honor of the goddess Salus, when a pestilence struck Rome.

The Etruscans had a considerable knowledge of primitive medicine; and to these people, as well as to the Sabines, the ancient Romans were indebted for their knowledge. A few simples of questionable value constituted their entire materia medica to about 187 B.C. Numa Pompilius, who was king of Rome (c. 715 B.C.), is reported to have studied physical science. This monarch, in his "Lex Regia," ordered the performance of Cesarian section on women who died during labor. The law of the twelve tablets of Numa forbade the burning or burial of bodies within the city walls and also referred to dental operations. Livy related that Numa Pompilius was struck by lightning and killed as the result of his experiments.

In 399 B.C., the first *lectisternium* (a festival of Greek origin) was held in Rome to combat pestilence. It was a gathering for the purpose of sacrifice and prayer; the images of the gods were laid upon a couch, and a meal was spread on a table before them. These festivals were celebrated as occasion demanded. Driving nails into the temple of Jupiter to ward off "the pestilence that walketh in the darkness" and "destruction that wasteth at noonday" was practiced as late as 360 B.C. The low degree of surgical knowledge (according to Livy) was evident from the fact that, after a battle in 309 B.C., more soldiers died of wounds than were killed in action. An epidemic in the year 291 B.C., which baffled their medical skill and threatened destruction of the population, compelled the Roman citizens to seek other succor than their own defective knowledge supplied.

Versions as to the story of the presence of Aesculapius in Rome were given by the historian Livy (59 B.C to 17 A.D.) and the poet Ovid (43 B.C. to 17 A.D.). According to Livy, the Roman people had no special patron-god of medicine before the year 292 B.C., at which time a pestilence occurred throughout the empire causing consternation. The Sibylline Books were consulted as to what should be done. The books indicated to send an embassy to Greece to procure the aid of Aesculapius, the god of healing.

Ovid's version of the plague and his graphic descriptions of the symptoms of those suffering from the plague were interesting and will be reproduced here in full:

The Island surrounded by the channel of the Tiber introduced the son of Coronis into the sacred rites of the city of Romulus. A dire contagion had once infected the Latian air, and the pale bodies were deformed by a consumption that dried up the blood. When wearied with so many deaths, they found that mortal endeavors availed nothing, and that the skill of physicians had no effect, they sought the aid of heaven, and they repaired to Delphi which occupies the center spot of the world, the oracle of Phoebus, and entreated that he would aid their distressed circumstances by a response productive of health, and put an end to the woes of a City so great . . .

Ambassadors were then sent to Epidaurus to demand the god; the people refused to part with him but he appeared to one of the Romans in sleep and consented to go, saying:

Lay aside thy fears; I will come, and I will leave these my statues. Only observe now this serpent, which with its folds entwines around this staff, and accurately mark it with thine eyes, that thou mayest be able to know it again. Into this shall I be changed; but I shall be greater, and I shall appear to be of a size as great as that into which heavenly bodies ought to be transformed.[1]

On his arrival at Rome, the epidemic ceased, and the temple was built in his honor. For a long time, it was customary for the sick to sleep on the portico of the Aesculapian temples, hoping that the god of healing might inspire them in a dream as to how to cure their illness. Sick slaves were left there unattended by their masters to die. As the number of unfortunate people increased Emperor Claudius put a stop to the crude practice.

EARLY ROMAN PHYSICIANS

There existed in ancient Rome many medical cults, chief of which was that of Epidaurus; incubation sleep was administered, and sacred snakes and dogs were exhibited to the sick. The Church of St. Bartholomew now stands on the ruins of the Temple of Aesculapius. Aside from religious rites, which consisted of prayers, magic, and prescriptions from the Sibylline Books, crude surgery was practiced.

Notwithstanding Pliny's statement that for a period of 600 years the Romans had no physician,[2] Rome was not altogether without medical practitioners. The *Lex Aemela,* as early as 433 B.C., ordained punishment for doctors who neglected a sick slave. Plutarch, in the Life of Cato, wrote of a Roman ambassador who was sent to the king of Bithynia in Asia Minor to have his skull trepanned. Roman medicine of later days was borrowed from Greece. After the destruction of Corinth in 146 B.C., a large number of Greek prisoners of war, many of whom were physicians, came to Rome. These captives, needless to say, had no particular love for their captor. The Roman word for doctor, or physician, was *medicus.* The term was used liberally, applying even to drug peddlers.

Medicine, in the earlier periods of Roman history and possibly as late as the time of the emperors, was of Greek origin. It appears to have been practiced chiefly, if not exclusively, by slaves and freedmen, upon whom the title of *medicus* was indiscriminately conferred, in the same manner as the Iatraliptae of the Greeks were not infrequently dignified with the appellation of *physis*. In fact, all medicine from Hippocrates to Harvey was Greek medicine whether it was found in Alexandria, Rome, Baghdad, Salerno, or Paris. Everything in medicine, worthy of its name, was Greek in origin. The importance of the services of the *medicus*, both to individuals and to the state, gradually raised them to their due rank and estimation in society and obtained for them, in a multitude of instances, the honors of citizenship and the grant of various privileges and immunities.

Pliny complained, "People believe in anyone who gives himself out for a doctor, even if the falsehood directly entails the greatest danger. There is, unfortunately, no law which punishes the medicus if through his fault someone dies. It is permitted to him by our danger to learn for the future, at our death to make experiments, to set at naught the life of a human being."[3]

It may be inferred from Pliny that the *medici* he referred to were largely foreigners, "The dignity of the Romans," wrote Pliny, "does not permit him to make a profession of medicine, and the few Romans who begin to study it are venal renegades to the Greeks." Pliny was against these foreign healers. "The Roman people," he stated, "in extending its empire, has lost sight of its ancient manners and, in that we have conquered, we are the conquered; for now we obey the natives of foreign lands, who, by the agency of a single art, have even outgeneraled our generals."

Oculists: Many of these healers occupied themselves with diseases of the eye *(medici ocularii)*. Most were in reality eye-ointment vendors. Rome of that period could boast of only one celebrated oculist, Demosthenes Philalethes, who flourished at the time of Nero. He wrote a textbook on diseases of the eye which was in use down to the fourteenth century.

The discovery of about 230 ancient seals in the northern and western provinces of Italy showed that the Roman oculists employed salves widely. The seals, found attached to jars of ointment, bore the names of the ointment, of the oculist who discovered it, and of the manufacturer, and stated the purpose for which it was to be used, together with the directions for use. The ointment consisted mainly of zinc and calamine. Some depilatories and tweezers for pulling out hair, possibly for trichiasis, were also found.

One inscription on a seal read, "The incense salve of T. Attius Divixtus against attacks of ophthalmia" *(T. Atti. Divixti. Dia. Libanu).* The signa directed, "To be ground up with an egg" *(Ad. Imp. Ex. Ovo).*

On at least one seal, there was an inscription indicating that some oculists specialized in surgery. The inscription read, "Medicus clinicus chirurgicus ocularis."

Martial poked fun at the eye doctors in the following words, "Now you are a gladiator who once were an ophthalmist; you did as a doctor

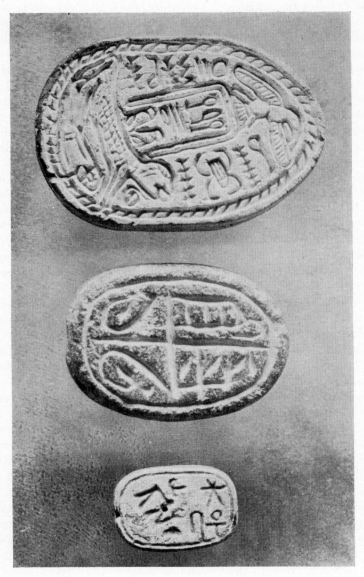

Fig. 135: Roman medical seals. These seals were discovered some years ago in the northwestern provinces of Italy. They were found attached to ointment jars. Some bear the names of the ointments and oculists who discovered them, and some bear the manufacturers' names and the purposes for which they were prescribed. The salves mainly consisted of zinc and calamine. One inscription reads, *"Medicus clinicus chirurgicus ocularius."*

what you do as a gladiator. . . . The blear-eyed Hylas would have paid you sixpence, O Quintus; one eye is gone, he will still pay threepence; make haste and take it, brief is your chance; when he is blind, he will pay you nothing."[4]

Archagathus: According to Cassius Hemma, quoted by Pliny, the first Greek physician to practice in Rome was Archagathus (219 B.C.), He was an immigrant from Peloponnesus and was the son of Lysamius. He was honorably received in Rome for his notable skill in the treatment of wounds and ulcers. The senate of Rome bestowed upon him the right of citizenship and secured for him a *taberna* in a busy district of the city.[5]

This *vulunerarius* (wound surgeon), disregarding his surgical limitations, soon undertook to do serious operations. It was not long before his unskilled surgery aroused the ire of the people, and in derision he was named *carnifex* (butcher); in consequence thereof, he and all other foreign physicians were expelled from the country.

Cato: Generally speaking, Roman healers at that period did not belong to a distinct class. The profession was open to all who wanted to practice it. With many, medicine was a sideline.

As a typical example may be mentioned Marcius Percius Cato (234–149 B.C.), surnamed the "censor." Cato was born in the small town of Tusculum. He came from an ancient plebian family noted for their military service. He was raised as an agriculturist, to which profession he devoted himself when not in military service. Owing to the influence of a Roman statesman, he was introduced to a prominent Roman official, through whose influence he received his first political appointment as a supervisor of public buildings and market places. A short time after (in 198 B.C.), he was promoted to magistrate; and three years later (in 195 B.C.), he was appointed consul. In that position he represented the government in various places. He was a strict administrator of public affairs, opposing all social reform and strictly enforcing public morality as he saw it. While in Spain, he quelled revolutionary tendencies and crushed all opposition with great cruelty, for which he was rewarded with military honors. After he established his reputation as a soldier and a statesman abroad, he served the state at home.

In Rome, he particularly took upon himself to oppose Hellenic culture, which he thought threatened to destroy the rugged simplicity of conventional Roman life. It was while discharging his office of censor, that he opposed all foreign culture. He imposed heavy taxes upon dress and personal adornment, especially of women and young slaves purchased as favorites. He was against any new ideas and vehemently urged the dismissal of the Greek philosopher Diogenes, who came as ambassador from Athens, because Cato thought that Diogenes' views were dangerous.

He particularly abhorred Greek physicians. He accused them of poisoning and killing the sick.[6] To his son Marcus, he wrote, "The Greeks are a hard and a perverse race; believe me, when I tell you that each time this nation brings us new knowledge it will not merely corrupt Rome but will be much worse. They have sworn to kill all the barbarians by means of drugs. They call all the Romans barbarians. Remember, I forbid physicians for you." According to Plutarch, Cato stated "Hippocrates refused treatment to the king of Persia, saying, 'I will never make use of my art in favor of barbarians who are enemies of Greece.'" Cato believed that all Greek physicians were bound by this rule and animated by this motive. Cato not only used his position as censor against physicians but tried to impose his own medical ideas, which consisted of magic and folklore, upon the community.

During the last period of the republic, slaves, barbers, and phlebotomists assumed the role of physician and practiced the profession without restriction. Slaves were taught the art of healing, and the fees they collected belonged to their owners. A medical slave, who had been taught to dress a wound, concoct a remedy, or mix a poison in order to get an enemy out of the way, fetched a better price than a eunuch.

In his book "De Re Rustica," he recommended many remedies. Cato assures us that the ancient Romans were healthy without medicos. He advised that a sick ox be given three grains of salt, three laurel leaves, three rue leaves, and various other threes three times a day for three consecutive days, both patient and physician fasting and the drug being given with both standing erect.

His panacea for all human diseases was his favorite vegetable, cabbage. He prescribed it internally and externally as a poultice, raw, or cooked. He declared that it would even cure cancer. He injected its juice into sinuses and fistulas by means of a syringe composed of a bladder tied to a reed. He stated that if a slave was ill and failed to respond to the cabbage cure, he should be gotten rid of at once, for it was a bad procedure to feed a man who could not work. One of his prescriptions was, "Keep the urine of one who is wont to eat cabbage; warm it; immerse the patient into it; you will soon cure him by this treatment; it has been tried." Another of his teachings was, "If you wash small children with urine, they will never become weak . . . and if there is any bruise, it will break it up and heal it if you apply mashed cabbage, and if an ulcer or cancer arise in the breast apply mashed cabbage; it will heal it."

Cato prided himself that his knowledge of medicine was far superior to that of the Greek physicians. He considered ducks, geese, and hares a light and suitable diet for the sick.

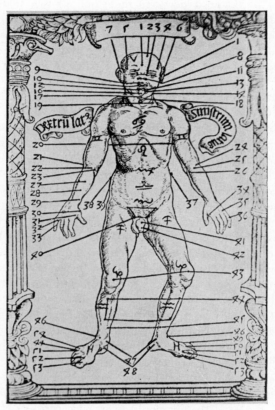

Fig. 136: A fifteenth century drawing, showing suitable locations for vene-section according to the zodiac. (Courtesy of Funk and Wagnalls Co.)

His conception of medicine was evident from his treatment of fractures and dislocations, "Split a divining rod up the middle, trim off the fragments of wood, bind it to the injured part, and do not fail to chant, 'huat, hanat, huat, ista, pista, sista, domiaba, damnaushra, et luxato'." Even though the split divining rod might conceivably be interpreted as a splint, the babbling of meaningless utterances in effecting the cure showed Cato in his proper light.

Cato's antagonism to the Greek physician of his time, however, was not altogether undeserved. While there were among them some competent doctors, many of them came to Rome to enrich themselves in disregard of all ethical principles. This, however, did not apply to the Greek physician only. Native healers do not appear to have been any better.

The corruption of medical practice was due to the fact that the Roman physician had no training. He acquired his medical knowledge as an apprentice of a Roman healer; and if the master physician were poorly trained, it followed that the student would not excel his teacher professionally or ethically.

Greek science hardly penetrated below the upper classes. Thus in medical works of the fourth and fifth centuries of the Christian Era, we still encounter numerous survivals of the older material. There are many references in St. Augustine's "De civitate dei" which show that ancient beliefs were widely current even among the well-to-do of his day. After the fall of the Empire, unscientific beliefs lingered among the barbaric peoples that entered into its heritage. Even the prescriptions and practices of Pliny, of Marcellus Empiricus, and of Sextus Placitus Papyriensis could be traced to the folk customs and folk beliefs of ancient Rome and still persist in the sayings and doings of continental peasantry.[7]

After Cato's death, a decree was published ordering the banishment of all Greeks (161 B.C.). The senate particularly forbade residence to philosophers on the pretense that the Greek philosophers were undermining popular religion and infecting Roman youth with the poison of skepticism. As medicine was to a large extent a branch of philosophy, physicians were excluded from the country. This was not the first time that "wise men" of foreign lands were excluded from Rome. In 319 B.C., Cornelius Hispollus ordered the Chaldean astrologers from Rome to leave Italy within ten days. A similar edict was again issued in 33 B.C. by Marcus Agrippa.

Asclepiades: The first Greek physician to make an impression upon the Roman people was Asclepiades (born 124 B.C.) of Prussa-Bithynia in Asia Minor. He studied medicine and rhetoric in Athens and in Alexandria. He traveled to many lands. In Rome, he began his career by teaching rhetoric, a field in which he exhibited natural ability. He was a friend of Cicero, Crassus, and Mark Antony, by whose advice he turned to the art of medicine.

According to Neuburger, Asclepiades was first to express his antagonism towards the teaching of the Hippocratics. He condemned all those who thought that anatomy and physiology were the foundation of medicine. He was against the humoral theory and opposed the concept of *Vis Medicatrix Naturae* of Hippocrates. He asserted that the physician should actively interfere with nature, "Not only is nature useless, it may even be harmful; natural healing power is a delusion.

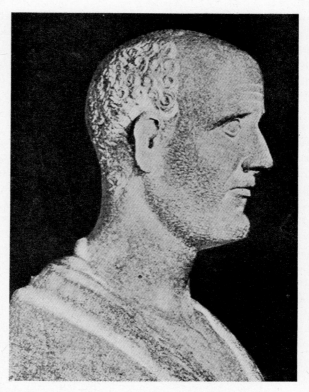

Fig. 137: Asclepiades (born 124 B.C.). Asclepiades of Bithynia was the first physician who contributed to the establishment of Greek medicine in Rome. This bust is presumably a copy of an older statue of Asclepiades which was dug up in Rome near Porta Capena and which bears the inscription "Asclepiades." (Capitoline Museum, Rome.)

It is the physician's duty to cure safely, quickly, and pleasantly." Pliny was perhaps justified in regarding him a charlatan whose only ambition was to build up a reputation for himself abroad.

Asclepiades based his medical system on a modification of the atomic or corpuscular theory of Democritus, according to which disease resulted from an irregular or disharmonious motion of the atoms of the body. His remedies aimed at the restoration of harmony. He had no faith in drugs. He advocated change of diet, frequent baths, massage, and exercise. He favored the liberal use of wine, undiluted or slightly diluted (these kinds of prescriptions suited his more Epicurean patients). Furthermore, he used emetics occasionally and bloodletting[8] rarely. He always insisted upon kindness to his patients.

Asclepiades divided diseases into acute and chronic. He paid much attention to chronic diseases, which were numerous in the large and prosperous community of Rome. These conditions had been somewhat neglected by the Hippocratics. He gave a correct description of malaria and recommended scarification in the region of the ankles in cases of dropsy. He advised that, when tapping, the opening be made as small as possible. He practiced bronchiotomy. He once observed a spontaneous dislocation of the hip joint. He observed psychic complications in pneumonia and pleurisy. He was the first to treat mentally diseased patients with gentleness. He ordered them to be moved into the sun and provided with music and songs instead of having them incarcerated in dark cells.

Among the interesting fragments which survive of the writing of Asclepiades is the following:

That the joints of patients suffering from chronic disease may be dislocated without external violence is testified by Hippocrates in his "De Articularis." I have met with two such cases; one in a Persian who, without blow or fall, began to have pain in the hip and often he had lain in bed for three months; the head of his thigh bone was drawn and dislocated outward, I suppose through the excess of the pain. The other case was that of a young tragic poet whose thigh bone was also dislocated outward by the influence of the muscles drawing aside the bone and forcing it from the place. (Here he appears to have agreed with Hippocrates.)[9]

Fevers and inflammatory disorders he accounted for upon the hypothesis of obstruction; while he ascribed syncope, languor, dropsy, and similar complaints to a preternatural relaxation of the pores. He imagined dropsy to proceed from an infinite number of small holes in the flesh that converted all the food received into water; the precise manner in which this miraculous hydrogenation, or transmutation, to water took place, he prudently left unexplained. He ascribed hunger and more particularly that enormous appetite which the ancients termed "bulimia" to opening of the larger pores and thirst to the dilatation of the smaller pores of the stomach and abdomen. His description of diseases and their division into acute and chronic classes evinced accuracy of discrimination and acuteness of perception.

He proposed, by means of various kinds of exercise, to relax the pores in those complaints which he referred to obstruction. Thus he facilitated the free transmission of the interrupted atoms or molecules. He laid down this extraordinary paradox as an established maxim: One fever was to be cured by another and it was necessary to subject a patient to the endurance of thirst. This last regulation he enforced rigorously. However great their craving, he would not permit his patients to touch so much as a single drop of water during the first two days of illness. With a view to opening the pores, he had frequent recourse to frictions, especially in dropsy and in inflammatory affections of the brain, if for no other reason than for the purpose of inducing sleep.

In fevers, after their violence was somewhat abated and even in cases of phrenitis, he not only permitted but enjoined the use of wine, carried even to the extent of intoxication, believing that such a practice would promote sleep. He deemed sleep essential to persons laboring under cerebral inflammation. He also employed wine in cases of lethargy, with the diametrically opposite view of rousing and stimulating the patient. To these various proceedings, according to Celsus, he added a most severe system of abstinence in all ailments during the first days of the attack. On the fourth day, he permitted the moderate use of food.

He was no friend to emetics or cathartics and usually substituted enemas for the latter. He was not averse to bleeding. He placed his chief reliance upon diet, regimen, and frictions. Among his favorite medications, was cold water used internally as well as externally. One might surmise that his principle of "quick-sure-and-pleasant" for which he was popular among the Romans was due chiefly to the free use of wine which he prescribed where others withheld it. His popularity among the Roman nobility was due to his Epicurean philosophy. He was honored and beloved by Crassus and Mucsius; Atticus and Cicero were his great admirers; and the Persian emperor Mithridates invited him to his court.

The popularity of Asclepiades among the Romans may be inferred from the following tale by Lucius Apuleius: On one occasion he broke up a funeral procession to the astonishment of a large gathering of friends when he called out, "I am Asclepiades and I say take down the corpse from the pyre." He extinguished the fire which was intended for the cremation of the supposed dead body and stopped the funeral banquet. He had recognized that the alleged corpse was not dead; and in the presence of the entire party, he removed the supposed dead to his home, where he administered restoratives and soon revived him.[10]

Pliny was not impressed with Asclepiades, "There is, however, one thing and one thing only," he states, "at which we have any ground for indignation—the fact, that a single individual, and he belonging to the most frivolous nation in the world, a man born in utter indigence, should all on a sudden and that, too, for the sole purpose of increasing his income, give a new code of medical laws to mankind."[11] Pliny related that Asclepiades wagered that he would never die of disease. He won the wager, for he lived to an old age and died from an accident.

Galen, who was a bitter foe of all who differed from Hippocrates, attacked Asclepiades and his theories, "Asclepiades did not know that urine enters the bladder through the ureters; he never saw a stone passed by one of these sufferers or observed that this is preceded by a sharp pain in the region of the kidneys, as the stone traverses the ureter, or that when the stone passes the pain stops." Galen sarcastically remarked that Asclepiades was so ignorant that he thought the fluid which was drunk passed into the bladder by being resolved into vapors and that, when these had been condensed, it thus regained its previous form and turned from vapor into water. "He simply looks upon the bladder as a piece of wood."[12]

Galen further criticized Asclepiades as follows:

He holds that nothing is naturally in sympathy with anything else, all substances being divided and broken up into inharmonious elements and absurd molecules. He was ignorant of nature's faculties . . . thus he invented some wretched nonsense to explain blood production and *anadoset*. From the point of view of treatment, he was not able to cure kidney ailments, nor jaundice, nor disease of the black bile . . . must we not, therefore suppose that he was either mad or entirely unacquainted with the practice of medicine?[13]

Asclepiades may be ranked as the first foreign physician who contributed to the establishment of Greek medicine in Rome. Asclepiades' actual merits are difficult to estimate for his writings have been lost. Although there were widely divergent views as to his medical prowess, the general judgment about his professional skill was favorable. Celsus admitted that he learned much from him. Apuleius called him a "second Hippocrates." Even Pliny, who indignantly remarked that a poor man sprung from the most vulgar of nations should not give laws of health to mankind, did not withhold his admiration from him entirely. Galen's opposition was because he had attacked the Father of Medicine and was the precursor of the Methodists.

The literary work of Asclepiades is estimated to have been about twenty volumes; only fragments of them are found in later literature. Many of them have been collected by G. Gompert; they deal with such subjects as the pulse, respiration, fever, heart disease, dropsy, ulcer, regimen, climate, drugs, and preparations of remedies.

Asclepiades was almost forgotten by the approach of the fourth century A.D., partly owing to his antagonism against Hippocrates but chiefly because of the dislike of Pliny, who regarded him as a self-seeking charlatan, and because of prejudice against him on the part of Galen, who resented his opposition to the Father of Medicine. Asclepiades died at an old age through a fall from a stairway. He did not wish to be his own physician. In the year 1700, a bust was dug up in Rome near the Porta Capena, bearing the inscription "Asclepiades," which was taken to be that of the Bithynian.

Antonius Musa: After Asclepiades, the most celebrated physician in Rome was Antonius Musa (c. 50 B.C.), through whose influence Julius Caesar bestowed citizenship on Greek physicians. After Caesar's death, following his military campaigns in Egypt and Spain, his successor Augustus, who was successfully cured by Antonius Musa from a severe inflammation of the liver, showed his appreciation to the medical profession by exempting all physicians from taxation. As a personal token of appreciation, he ordered the erection of a statue of Musa near that of Aesculapius and presented him with a signet ring of knighthood. These factors, however, did not change the medical standards of Rome because no examination was necessary to practice medicine.

Antonius Musa's fame was largely due to his social connection with Roman royalty. He claimed the discovery of a remedy which enabled him to maintain the good health of Caesar and Maecenas. His secret remedy was probably sulfur baths, for Horace tells of having obeyed Musa, the physician of Caesar, who had recommended sulfur baths to him.

Musa is said to have introduced lettuce, chicory, and endives into the pharmacopeia. He prescribed the excrement of dogs for angina. He regarded herbs, particularly lettuce, as a sovereign remedy for all diseases, and he claimed the ability to pulverize a stone in the bladder. Galen mentioned a number of remedies recommended by Musa, which were still in use in his day.

Scribonius Largus: The first Latin medical author after Celsus was Scribonius Largus (c. 47 A.D.), who dedicated his prescription formulas to the Emperor Claudius. He was physician to Empress Messalina, and he accompanied the Emperor on his expedition to Britain (43 A.D.).

He followed the school of Empiricism; and his method of classifying disease was by the position of the organs in the body, which is a very ancient method that may be traced to Egyptian medical papyri (c. 1700 B.C.).

Scribonius described the use of vibration, which he obtained by the friction of two objects, in the treatment of headache and similar diseases of a nervous nature—a sort of electric physiotherapy. He also described a method of obtaining opium. He is the earliest writer known to mention the Hippocratic Oath.

He traveled extensively, utilizing his journeys in extending his knowledge of medicaments and aiding his collection of prescriptions. His work, containing 271 prescriptions arranged according to the parts of the body, from the head to the foot, had in addition to rational remedies, many magical, secret, and housewives' remedies. Some of these he collected during his travels by paying big sums of money to famous physicians, dilettantes, and quacks at health resorts. His success as physician was largely owing to the fact that he followed the methods of Herophilus of using drugs, contrary to the practice of Asclepiades and the Orthodox method of his contemporaries, of healing disease by diet. His formulary portrays him as lacking the scientific spirit possessed by his precursor Theophrastus.

Neuburger, after pointing out the shortcomings of Scribonius, remarks, "nevertheless there is, particularly in the introduction of his little work, a strain of consciousness which evokes sympathy and which is in keeping with his eloquent lament over the moral and intellectual decline of his contemporaries."[14]

Pedanius Dioscorides: The scientific spirit, which was not apparent in Scribonius, was much in evidence in Pedanius Dioscorides (c. 40— 90 A.D.). What Hippocrates was to medicine in general, Dioscorides was to materia medica. He freed it from the superstition collected throughout the ages and from the rhizotomists, or root-cutters, who in his own time gathered roots and herbs and sold them as remedies in conjunction with magic rituals. Dioscorides animated the subject of materia medica with true scientific spirit and encouraged careful investigation of all vegetable, animal, and mineral substances that were to be used to combat diseases.

In his work "De Universa Medicina," published in five volumes, he described the properties and physiological actions of over 600 plants and plant products. Only about 150 of these were known to the Greek physicians in the time of Hippocrates. Dioscorides was free from the Dogmatism and Empiricism of his predecessors. He held himself as

far aloof from superstition as was possible in those days. He was the
first to make a comprehensive and scientific study of plants. Hence
he was known as "the Father of Materia Medica." He was methodical;
he created an exact terminology; he gave an accurate description of
remedies derived from the vegetable, animal, and mineral kingdoms;
and he described reliable means for their preservation, testing, medi-

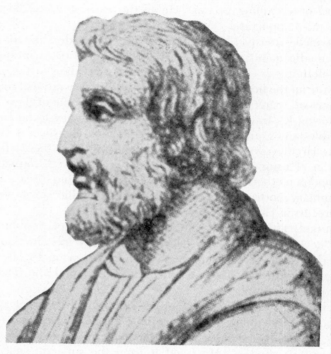

Fig. 138: Dioscorides (40–90 A.D.). Dioscorides is considered the father
of materia medica. His description of ancient plants enables one to identify
them. He is said to have collected 958 different remedies. His position as
surgeon in the army of Nero enabled him to study the plants of many countries.

cal use, dosage, and action. He classed the remedies according to the
diseases which they were supposed to cure, such as for example, diuretic
diaphoretics, digestives, and laxatives, and noted the places where each
plant came from, what it looked like, and for what purpose it was to
be used. His work contained a list of poisons and antidotes. Most of
the plants mentioned can still be recognized from his descriptions.

Of particular interest are the facts that he was familiar with the medicinal plants of Arabia and that his work contained the first reference to the chemical preparation of metallic agents.

Dioscorides was the first to describe scientifically opium preparations. He pointed out the fact that they allayed pain, induced sleep, were useful in coughs, and in overdoses brought on lethargy and death. He told how various preparations were made from the opium poppy. Dioscorides was first to mention aconite and ammoniacum and to discuss the therapeutics of aloes. He coined the name "hydrorgyrum" (meaning fluid silver) for mercury. He described the method for preparing elatorium and gave the technic of making vinegar of squills. He referred to the astringent properties of iron and to the use of aspidium for tapeworm. He showed how to detect adulteration of drugs and recommended drugs for sterility as well as birth control. Galen's objection to the materia medica of Dioscorides was that he ascribed too many virtues to one drug.

About 100 of his remedies are still found in the modern pharmacopeia. His "work" became known as the "herbal" and has been consulted by physicians and laymen for a period of 1500 years. A translation of this work is still employed by certain Muslim scholars. He exercised as much authority in materia medica as Galen did in the practice of medicine. For almost fifteen centuries, he was followed blindly.

Pedanius Dioscorides was born in Anazarba near Tarsus in Cicilia. At an early age, he settled in Rome, where he became surgeon in the army of Nero. He accompanied the army on various military expeditions, utilizing his journeys to gain botanical and pharmacological knowledge.

His materia medica remained as he left it for almost 1000 years without any progress. The Arab physicians somewhat enlarged the number of drugs but followed his system. Galen often quoted him. In the third volume of Paulus Agina (Sydenham Society edition), are recorded about 90 minerals, 600 plants, and 168 animal substances used therapeutically by Dioscorides.

Crateus: The work of Dioscorides was revived a century later by Crateus, the physician of Mithradates VI, King of Pontus. Crateus' pioneering work consisted mainly of drawing pictures of plants so that the plants, which were to be used as remedies, could be recognized instead of getting lost in a maze of magic spells.

LATER ROMAN MEDICAL EDUCATION

Notwithstanding the large medical field that the Western Empire provided and the wide acceptance of Greek medicine by the upper classes, it is remarkable that the Latin-speaking peoples produced no eminent physician.

During the Republic, medical education had been entirely a matter of private teaching. The relation of pupil and master, exhibited by the Hippocratic oath, was evidently that which prevailed under the early Empire. The initiate declared:

> I will reckon him who taught me this Art as dear to me as those who pro-created me. I will look upon his offspring as my own brethren and will teach them this art, if they would learn it, without fee or stipulation. By precept, lecture, and every other mode of instruction, I will impart a knowledge of this Art to my own sons, and to those of my teacher, and to disciples bound by a stipulation and an oath, according to the Law of Medicine, but to none other.

The very form of the oath suggests the arrangements which were gradually made for medical instruction at Rome. The first important teacher was the Greek Asclepiades of Bithynia. He founded a regular school at Rome which continued after him.

At first, the school was the mere personal following of the physician, who took his pupils and apprentices with him on his visits. At a later stage, such groups combined to form societies, or colleges, where questions of the art were debated. Towards the end of the reign of Augustus or the beginning of that of Tiberius, these societies constructed for themselves a meeting place on the Esquiline, the so-called "Schola medicorum." It had a president with the title of *archiatrus* and a secretary known as the *tabularius,* or *scriba.* Finally, the emperors built halls, or *auditoria,* for the teaching of medicine. The professors at first received only the pupils' fees. It was not until the time of Vespasian (emperor 70–79 A.D.) that medical teachers were given a salary at public expense.[15] The system was extended by Hadrian (117–138) and Alexander Severus (222–235).[16]

The office of the Order of Archiatri perhaps dates from the days of Xenophon of Cos, one of the later members of the family of Asclepiades. Xenophon was praised by the people of Cos as a public benefactor. He had done creditable work in the army for which he had gained the spear and gold crown for distinguished conduct in the field, in spite of the fact that he broke the oath of his guild in participating in the murder of his master. In the early empire, physicians were often tempted to help get rid of a cruel, unscrupulous dictator, for many physicians were still in the position of slaves in the hands of an Agrippa. Herodian relates that the first act of Caraculla was to order the execution of the court physicians, because they had refused at his request to hasten the death of his father Severus. Tacitus and some modern critics question the story of the guilt of Xenophon, accused of poisoning the Emperor Claudius. The story is mentioned by Archdeacon Farrar, who holds up Xenophon as a "hideous" example of pagan depravity contrasted with Christian virtue; "cynical" and "atheistic" are among the milder epithets.

The following was the formula for investiture of a "count" of the *archiatri* under Theodoric:

> We invest you henceforth with the countship of the archiatri, that among the masters of health *(salutis magistros)* you alone may be preeminent and that all who have disputes in medical matters may yield to your judgment. Become the arbiter of a noble art, and decide its conflicts which are commonly only settled by the event; by so putting an end to harmful quarrels you will, in a way, benefit the sick. It is no mean office to rule over the wise and prudent and to be reverenced by those who are themselves reverenced by others. May your visits bring health to the sick, strength to the weak, and sure hope to the despairing.

Then in his master's name he continues:

> Dwell in our palace, enter with confidence into our chamber, privileges which others obtain only at a great cost, for they enjoy them merely as servants. You may chasten us with fasting, you may impose rules which counteract our tastes, you may prescribe for us things we abhor, in a word you may exercise over us an authority which we could not righteously exercise over others.[17]

The position and name of *archiatrus* was of Greek origin, and was mentioned by Herodotus. The title was applied to physicians of the eastern kings, such as that of Mithradates of Pontus. In Rome, it received a more prominent significance.

Xenophon was known as *archiatrus,* or chief physician, to "the August divinities," a term perhaps meant to include Agrippa and Nero. He was succeeded in that office by Andromachus, inventor of a famous theriac, or antidote.

There were also communal physicians who received the title *archiatri popularis* or *comes archiatrorum,* who were permitted to practice privately, but their chief duty was to attend to the poor and to instruct pupils in the art. Antonius restricted the number of these physicians from five to seven and ten to each municipality, depending upon the size of the city; they were chosen by the municipality.

The first duty of the *archiatrus* was to take care of the monarch himself. At the court of Constantinople, the *Archiatri Palatini* formed a distinct body whose chief had the title of "count," and the members of the guild ranked among the *perfectissimi*.

In the year 378 A.D., an *archiatrus* was appointed by each of the fourteen districts of the city of Rome by the decree of Emperor Valentinian. The German *Arzt* is derived from *archiatrus*.

There were also special physicians for the colleges and gymnasiums at Rome and for the vestal virgins who continued until the fifth century. The greatest care was taken in the election, which was preceded by some kind of an examination. These government physicians had no control of the physicians in general. The practice in Rome as in Greece was open to anyone. Naturally, those who had aspired for the position of *archiatri* were careful in their course of study. Gradually, qualified teachers increased, and medical schools opened in various localities, some of which as at Beneventum and Avranches lasted till the beginning of the Middle Ages. Finally, they had to be legally recognized; this carried with it many privileges which tended to raise the social status of the profession.

There were also head midwives in each district who treated the poor free. It appears from the appointment of Valeria Verecunda as chief midwife of her district that the midwives were already registered. Pliny spoke of them as *nobilitas obstericum*. In the Justinian code, they were frequently alluded to as *medicae*. They often attended to medical matters. Scribonius Largus told of a matron who cured epilepsy in Rome with a "specific" consisting chiefly of animal blood. These *medicae* were unscrupulous in their practice. They were ready to assist in criminal abortions and all kinds of wicked practices.[18]

In the age of Augustus, culture in Rome reached its highest level. This monarch, who established a constitutional form of government (27 B.C.), also introduced ordinances which improved the sanitary and hygienic conditions of the land. These ordinances were enforced by the *archiatri*.

Because of their importance to the welfare of the citizens, Augustus recognized the State physicians as a privileged class. He regulated the number of physicians employed in the army. Each military regiment had a staff of twenty-four surgeons. The North Sea naval squadron also had an ophthalmologist. These military medical practitioners were under the direct command of military officers and had no "surgeon general." In contrast to the civil physicians, who received fair remuneration for their services, military physicians were poorly paid.

It is not clear to what extent malpractice was controlled by the Romans of that period. Judging from the steps taken to punish criminal abortion, it may be assumed that the practice of medicine was well-regulated.

LEGALIZATION OF MEDICAL PRACTICE

Not until the reign of Lucius Septimius Severus (reigned 193–211 A.D.) was medical practice definitely legalized. He introduced a system of licensure and made the medical practitioner responsible to the State for his actions. Criminal practices, such as the administration of abortifacients, were punished by fines and revocation of license.

SOCIALIZED MEDICINE

The Romans were probably the first to experiment with socialized medicine. There were State, circuit, and municipal physicians, as well as school physicians. The poor received free medical treatment.

Neither time nor tide affects human nature. The fact that wealthy persons not infrequently feigned poverty in order to receive free medical attention will strike a familiar note with present-day practitioners. Galen, who had a large private practice in Rome, complained of the annoying experiences he had with certain rich patients. They frequently deceived him in order to test his ability as a diagnostician. This medical genius, however, readily detected a liar by feeling his pulse.[19]

SURGEONS

In the time of Galen, medicine was separated from surgery. Galen, who formally attended to both branches of medicine wrote: "Since I lived in Rome, I had to make many concessions to the custom of the capitol and leave most of these things to the so-called 'surgeons'." Rome had many skilled surgeons among the numerous specialists. An idea of the surgical work may be derived from the instruments which have been recovered in Pompeii and Herculaneum. Included among the 200 instruments that were discovered in Pompeii and the 40 in Herculaneum are 90 pairs of bronze forceps (most of them for removing superfluous hair), 45 probes of various shapes and sizes, 13 iron bis-

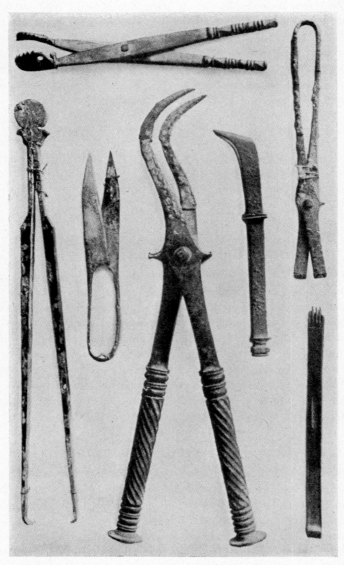

Fig. 139: Surgical instruments from Pompeii. (From Dr. K. Sudhoff's collection.)

touries, the same number of cupping instruments, a lancet with a silver blade and a bronze handle, an "s"-shaped catheter, and a uterine and an anal speculum.

At Rheüms, eighteen surgical instruments were discovered, including forceps, spatulas, scalpels, and syringes, all in bronze. With these, was the seal of an ophthalmic surgeon.[20]

HOSPITALS

The great contribution of Rome to medicine was the hospital system. It was a scheme that naturally arose out of the Roman genius for organization and was connected with the Roman military system. Among the Greeks, the *iatreia* (surgeries) were well known; they were, however, the private property of the medical man.

Columella (first century A.D.) spoke of *valetudinaria* (infirmaries) for sick persons. Seneca told us that *valetudinaria* were in use even by free Romans. The excavations at Pompeii show that a physician's house might even have been built somewhat on the lines of a modern "nursing home." There are passages in Galen which seem to imply that it was in the provinces that private institutions first developed into subventioned public hospitals.

This development of public hospitals early affected military life. At first, sick soldiers had been sent home for treatment. As the Roman frontiers spread ever wider, this became impossible, and military hospitals were founded at important strategic points. The sites of several such military hospitals have been excavated. The earliest that has come to light is of the first century, at Carnuntum, about twenty miles from Vienna. The best explored is at Novaesium, on the lower Rhine near Düsseldorf.[21]

References and Notes

1. Ovid: Metaphysics. Vol. 2, 15:64-67, English translation by Riley, H. T.
2. Pliny the elder gives a dark picture of the physicians of his time. They had the opportunity to administer poisons, to make wills, and manage intrigues. Historia Natura, Lib. 29:8.
3. Elliott, J. S.: Outlines of Greek & Roman Medicine. New York. 1934, p. 6.
4. Gordon, B. L.: The Romance of Medicine. F. A. Davis, Co., Philadelphia, 1944, pp. 534-536.
5. Strange as it may seem, no Greek writer appears to know anything about Archagathus. It is likely that he was a lower class surgeon who, having failed at home, thought that he might make his fortune among the "barbarians."
6. Pliny: Historia Natura, Lib. 29:1.
7. Singer, C.: The Legacy of Rome. Oxford University Press, 1940, p. 281.

8. Puschmann: History of Medical Education. Translated and edited by Hare, E. H., London, 1891.

9. Oribasius: Lib. 47.

10. Lucius Apuleius: Florida, Book IV, Chapter 19. Cited by Castiglione, A.: A History of Medicine. Alfred Knopf, New York, 1941, p. 199.

11. Cited by Robinson, V.: The Story of Medicine. New York, 1936, p. 93.

12. Galen: On the Nature of Faculties. 1:3. English translation by Brook, A. J.: William Putnam Sons, New York, 1916.

13. Ibid.

14. Neuburger, M.: History of Medicine. London, 1910, p. 221.

15. Alexander Serverus had seven court physicians, only one of whom was paid. The others received only three rations a day.

16. "The Legacy of Rome," pp. 281-282.

17. Withington, E. T.: Medical History from the Earliest Times. The Scientific Press, Ltd., London, 1894, pp. 111-112.

18. Ibid.

19. "The Romance of Medicine," pp. 537-538.

20. Milne, T.: Surgical Instruments in Greek and Roman Times. Oxford, 1907.

21. "The Legacy of Rome," pp. 293-294.

26

The Methodic School

THEMISON

THE most gifted student of Asclepiades was Themison of Laodicea (123–43 B.C.). Themison elaborated the theory of Solidism taught by Asclepiades into a new system which he named "Methodism"—a school that insisted on more rigid doctrine than Asclepiades but was less extreme than either the Dogmatic school of Cos or the Emperic school of Alexandria. Themison discarded the study of remote causes of diseases which concerned the Dogmatists. He distinguished different disorders by their symptoms as did the Empirics. He placed no stock in the humoral theory and the critical days of Hippocrates. He accepted the division of diseases into acute and chronic classes as listed by Asclepiades. He abandoned the principle of differential diagnosis of individual diseases.

Themison declared that if physicians observed the symptoms that various diseases had in common they would learn that in all or nearly all cases there was an increase or diminution of the secretion or excretion. He added this concept to the theory of Asclepiades.

By and large, he accepted the arbitrary principles of Asclepiades, according to which diseases were caused by constriction, fluxion (relaxation of the pores), or by mixed forms, irrespective of age and climate. He explained the mechanism of human physiology and pathology on the theory that the body was composed of minute particles or atoms and interspaces, or pores. These particles in the state of health were in perpetual motion. They kept circulating within the pores of the body, especially in the intestines, where they were most active and thus maintained the normal physiologic functions.

Disease was occasioned either by clogging of the pores and stagnation of the little solids, caused by contraction of the tissue *(status strictus)*, or by relaxation of the pores which caused the solids to move too freely *(status laxus)*. The therapeutics of this system consisted of relaxing and astringent remedies; for example, if the atoms became motionless and the pores of the tissues constricted because of a cold, then measures, such as bloodletting, leeches, cupping, scarification (opposite the affected side), poultices, warm baths, reduction of diet, and occasionally restriction of sexual intercourse, were employed. Occasionally, laxatives and diuretics were employed. On the other hand, when the body was in a relaxed condition, remedies, such as cold air, cold baths, wine, diets, vinegar, or alum, were employed. If contraction occurred in one part of the body and relaxation in another part (that is *status mixtus)*, antagonistic remedies were applied to the different parts of the body at the same time.

All that was necessary was a general knowledge of the ailment and the circumstances common to most complaints.

Themison was of the belief that first the patient should be weakened by abstinence from certain foods and afterwards stimulated in order to repair the damage done.

It is evident that Themison's system did away with many difficult theories and a large number of drugs which had been used traditionally. His therapeutics consisted of laxatives, astringents, and regimen. Such a system greatly simplified the study and practice of medicine. Because of this, Methodism was quickly accepted by a large number of the profession. In a certain sense, this system was an improvement over Dogmatism, which, after all, placed blind reliance on the wisdom of Hippocrates. It surpassed Empiricism with its complete dependence on one's own experience.

Methodism taught that diseases were to be judged from their symptoms only and not from their causes and that it was unnecessary to consider the individual peculiarities of a case, when once the case was classed under a certain group of diseases. Like the Empirics, they objected to the study of anatomy. They held that most ailments were general and the locality of the disease-manifestation was unimportant; for constriction and relaxation were the same and, no matter where they occurred, required the same treatment. Remote causes were not necessary, since all illnesses were produced either by constriction or relaxation. Thus, like the Empirics, they reduced medicine to a very simple system of treatment. Themison, so to speak, reversed the aphorisms of Hippocrates that "life is short and the art long"; the art became short and simple under his guidance.

Themison himself, who was trained in the old schools, realized that the fundamental principles of Methodism, although very simple, had to be modified frequently because of the deficiencies which the doctrine presented. His theory did not provide for the treatment of surgical diseases, for the removal of foreign bodies, for the reduction of fractures and dislocations, and for the removal of tumors and abscesses. It failed to take prophylaxis into consideration. It did not even take care of all internal diseases, such as, for example, empyema and ascites. The intelligent Methodist had to modify the system of Themison when called upon to treat some diseases.

His system in general consisted first in weakening the patient by abstinence from certain important foods and afterwards pushing stimulants in order to repair the injuries done. According to Juvenal, Themison was not held in high esteem by the more thinking classes, as may be seen from the following satire:

> How many sick in one short autumn fell,
> Let Themison, their ruthless slayer, tell.[1]

Themison however, enjoyed a considerable reputation among the populace.[2] Themison, before he was influenced by the doctrine of Asclepiades, was the first to describe the symptoms of rheumatism. He was a pioneer in the use of leeches and is reported to have written a book on elephantiasis. It is related that he was eager to write a treatise on hydrophobia because he had such an attack in his early childhood; but whenever he started to write, the disease impressed his mind with so much fear that the mere thought manifested in him symptoms of hydrophobia.

The Methodist sought to escape the traps of Dogmatism and Empiricism and fell into a worse trap. He did not agree with Empiricism and the blind administration of drugs, yet his own explanation of pathology was worse. The Methodist disagreed with the Dogmatic system because it investigated the primary causation and localization of disease and established the etiology and symptomatology of disease. The learned Methodist physician also had to depend upon symptoms to diagnose disease and was obliged to base his treatment on the cause of disease in spite of himself. The average student who received his medical training from a Methodist physician was frequently at a loss, when searching for a diagnosis, because he lacked a knowledge of anatomy, physiology, and particularly pathologic anatomy.

Apropos the theory of Methodism, Celsus merely said that the members of this school asserted that the knowledge of causes bore the least relation to the methods of cure and that it was sufficient to observe some general symptoms of distemper. He stated that they classified disease as: (1) bound; (2) loose; and (3) a mixture of these.[3]

Themison divided surgery into four distinct classes (communities): (1) foreign bodies (coming from without); (2) fractures and dislocations; (3) tumors and abscesses; and (4) arrest of development. The treatment, respectively of each, was: (1) to be withdrawn; (2) to be replaced; (3) to be removed or incised; and (4) to be made good.

Lacking the requirements of elementary subjects, such as anatomy, physiology, and remote etiology, the elimination of individual symptomotology, pathologic anatomy, and a large part of materia medica, the study of medicine was so abridged that it tempted untutored persons to take up medical arts. Cobblers, tanners, butchers, bakers, dyers, blacksmiths, farmers, and weavers dropped their trades to become "doctors." It was this factor that deteriorated Methodism to its lowest level.

THESSALUS

One of these Methodists was Thessalus, the son of a weaver of Tralles, Lydia. Thessalus dropped his loom and hurried to Rome to become a doctor. What Thessalus lacked in medical knowledge, he made up with ego and demagogy. Said Pliny:

No mountebank ever attracted more crowded audiences or gaping admirers than this impudent pretender, who proposed to make his pupils proficient in the whole science of medicine in the space of six months' time. By this means, he attracted to himself a multitude of pupils from the lowest ranks of society, who accompanied him on his visits to his patients for the space of time specified. At the expiration of this time, he conferred upon them the privilege of practicing on their own accounts.

Both Pliny and Galen referred to Thessalus as insolent and vain— a man who swept away all precepts of his predecessors and denounced with a burning passion the physicians of every age.

Thessalus announced publicly that medicine surpassed all other arts and that he himself surpassed all other physicians. He proclaimed himself a medical reformer and disregarded all medical authority, even that of the Methodists. To quote Pliny again, "He flouted ancient and contemporary authorities and asserted that no physician before and after him accomplished anything worthwhile." He derided the aphorisms of Hippocrates; he ridiculed the Alexandrian sages, particularly Erasistratus; he rebelled against his own school; he even opposed the teaching of his master Themison, forming dogmas of his own.

The primary contribution of Thessalus to Methodism was a method which he presented as a new idea to the effect that the state of the whole body and especially the parts affected could be changed.

He succeeded in elevating himself to the highest circle of society by dedicating his writings to Nero. His writings dealt, among other things, with diet, chronic diseases, and surgery and he wrote a violent polemic against Erasistratus, the sage of Alexandria. He opposed the humoral pathology of Hippocrates; he denied the action of drugs upon the liver and kidneys; and he rejected all agencies which were supposed to dispel the bile and phlegm, claiming that their irritation gave rise to such secretions.

That he succeeded in convincing his townsmen that he was the founder of a new and true system of medicine may be seen from the memorial on his tombstone, which was erected by the side of the Appian Way and which refers to him as "the conqueror of physicians."

Thessalus left only one certain monument to his credit. He is said to have been the first to give bedside instructions to his students. The purpose of such a performance, however, might have been the unholy one of making an impression upon his students and patients, both groups of which readily acclaimed him as the most celebrated physician in the world. The retinue of students, no doubt, while impressive, was disturbing to nervous patients. Martial satirizing these healers, had this to say about them:

> Faint was I only, Symmachus, 'til thou
> Backed by an hundred students, throng'dst my bed;
> An hundred icy fingers chilled my brow:
> I had no fever; now I'm nearly dead.[4]

Thessalus modified the reduction cure of his predecessors. He presented various degrees of fasting, ingestion of hot drinks, pepper, mustard, squills (thinning), wine, massage, baths, sinapism, and irritating plasters. This was followed by restorative remedies, stimulating foods, and other appropriate measures. The method of treatment was carried out commonly in periods of three days each, occasionally in longer periods of eleven days. In these methods, one may see that he followed in a measure the "critical days" of Hippocrates, although he publicly denounced the Father's authority.

GALEN'S OPINION OF METHODISM

Galen relates that a certain Pausanias, a celebrated Sophist, had complained of loss of sensation in the fourth and fifth finger of his left

hand. The Methodist physician who attended to him considered the
condition caused by "constriction," and he applied poultices locally
but without effect. He (Galen), who was summering at that place,
at once recognized that it was not a constriction. On inquiry, he found
the Sophist had been thrown from his chariot some hours before and
had struck his back on a stone. He therefore applied counterirritants
to the region of the origin of the brachial plexus, and the patient recovered to the confusion of the Methodist and to his own triumph.
Galen repeated the story three times in his writings.

The city of Rome, at the beginning of the Augustan Age, was inhabited by over a million people. It was not a desirable place for
medical practice; for the large lower classes were degraded and thrift-
less, and the small upper classes were debauched, tyrannical, and cruel.

Drug vendors sold poison for a high price for the purpose of doing
away with enemies. Drugs to destroy hair on the body were much in
vogue and were usually composed of a mixture of arsenic and unslaked
lime; depilatories were used to pull out the roots. This was first practiced by women but in later years also by effeminate men. The tweezers
discovered at Pompeii were suitable for pulling out hair, and the depilatories may have been applied after the use of tweezers.

The imperial city swarmed with doctors who received their diplomas
after six months of training under Thessalus or who had no training
at all; they were divided into specialists with high-sounding names.
Galen stated that in his time large cities, such as Rome and Alexandria,
swarmed with specialists who traveled about from place to place.

SPECIALISTS AND QUACKS

Medicine itself was separated into various branches, as indicated by
the complaint of Galen, who said, "Since I lived in Rome, I had to make
many concessions to the customs of the capitol and leave most of the
things that are so-called 'surgical'."

Cicero makes Crassus observe that all arts are degraded by subdivision, "Do you suppose that in the days of the Coans and Hippocrates, there were special physicians—some for wounds and others
again for the eyes?"

The Latin epigramist Marcus Valerius Martialis (b. 38 A.D.) described the performance of some of the specialists, "Casselius removes
or cures bad teeth. Hyginus cauterizes ingrowing eyelashes which
irritate the eye. Fannius removes enlarged uvulae without cutting. Eros
eradicates brandmarks from the skin of slaves. Hermes is reckoned the

best surgeon for fractures."[5] Several epigrams by Martial indicate how medicine was abused in his time:

> Diaulus, who was once a surgeon,
> Now assists an undertaker.
> Here at length he finds the office
> To which alone his skill is suited.[6]

The following quotation is interesting for the light it throws upon the clinical teachings and state of medical practice of the period:

> Last night Andragoras was well and hearty,
> The merriest guest at all our dinner party,
> And dead this morning! What was his attack?
> He dreamt he saw Hermocrates the quack. (vi. 53)[7]

EYE DISEASES

Eye diseases formed a prominent specialty in Rome in the time of Nero. They were divided into two classes: *medicae oculari* and *chirurgi oculari*. Eye diseases were largely in the hands of an ignorant class of oculists. The so-called "eye doctors" of Rome used ointments exclusively.

Demosthenes of Marseilles may be mentioned as an example of the one celebrated ophthalmologist.

Galen, referring to diseases of the eye, said that it was useless to write of the eye scientifically, for the oculists would not understand. They treated a corneal abscess by shaking the patient's head until the abscess burst. It cannot be argued that the *medicus* specialized in various branches because it was easier to be proficient in one branch than to pay attention to the entire field of medicine; for the therapeutics of all branches, with the exception of the eyes, were practically the same and consisted of dietetics, hydrotherapy, massage, gymnastics, wine, milk, honey, and certain herbals.

Galen, attacking the greed of his Roman colleagues, bitterly declared that the only difference between a robber and a physician was that the former's misdeeds were done in the mountains and the latter's in Rome.

REMEDIES

Scribonius Largus, who was the author of a formulary, mentioned a matron who cured epilepsy in Rome by a secret remedy consisting chiefly of animal blood. He also noted an African *medica* who had a wonderful remedy for colic, compounded of burned horn, snails, and wine, the secret of which he bought at a great expense. He recommended many fantastic popular remedies.

Even as great a man as Archigenes advocated the use of amulets in certain cases. According to the satirist Martial, the doctors were ever ready to assist in poisoning, abortions, and other wicked practices. There were a few physicians who were honorable and who did not sell their inventions for profit; as an example Heracleides of Tarentium may be mentioned. He dedicated his treatise on treating nosebleed to Antioch, and his method was copied by Galen. Theodore Prisciaon published a gynecological work for public use. But the weight of medical mysticism, which was seemingly uprooted forever by Hippocrates, shot up once more in Rome and began to choke the healthy growth of enlightenment.

STATUS OF PHYSICIANS

In the days of Julius Caesar, Greek physicians were granted citizenship. Augustus, who felt that his life had twice been saved by physicians, issued liberal laws pertaining to medical practice. Tiberius and Nero, who well-nigh destroyed the aristocracy of Rome, were very friendly to the slaves and freedmen. The social position of the physician was greatly enhanced under their reigns, as may be seen by reading Quintilian, who recommended as a rational topic a subject which would probably have disgusted an earlier generation of Roman aristocracy. The question was, "Which is the most useful member of the state, orator (that is lawyer and politician), physician, or philosopher?" In the postulated case, a man left three sons, a philosopher, an orator, and a physician, but he divided his property into four parts and left the extra share to the one of his sons most useful to the state. The fact that a physician was held in a category comparable to the orator and philosopher shows the advance made in later Roman times.

Another cause which contributed to the rise of medicine in the social scale was the establishment of the office of *archiatrate*.

Rome was the happy hunting ground of quacks who gave themselves high-sounding names. There were drug peddlers who hawked their medicine in the city and country.

Most of the best practitioners in the time of Augustus were either freedmen or slaves. The master of a great household selected a slave for his ability and had him trained to be the medical advisor of his family. The skill shown by him sometimes gained for him his freedom.

These physicians were sometimes called upon to mutilate slaves.[8] The price of a slave physician was fixed at sixty solidi.[9] The freedmen physicians had booths in which they prescribed and compounded medicine, and they were aided by other freedmen and slaves who were either assistants or pupils. But even in the golden days of Rome under the Caesars, and particularly under Augustus Caesar, when the Methodists were at their height and were admitted into the best circles of society, they had not attained the same dignity as the Greek physicians.

Celsus, who held the balance between Empiricism and Dogmatism, said there was no rightful place for Methodism. He called the Methodists "cow doctors" and "savages," declaring that the old physician knew all about the "communities" (the four classifications of disease) but was not content with them. When Celsus was asked how the Dogmatists, Empirics, and Methodists differed from the Eclectics, he answered, "Why these sects employ the same remedies and pursue very much the same course of treatment. They only differ in their reasoning of disease."

DECLINE OF METHODISM

At a later period, Methodism declined; most Methodist practitioners had recourse to personal systems of practice or became immersed in sterile Empiricism. The more enlightened exponents of the system, regardless of the schools with which they were affiliated, turned to the accumulated mass of valuable practical experience. Many of them became interested in surgery. Others advanced the study of obstetrics. The later Methodists, while still adhering to party affiliation, departed considerably from the teaching of the sect.

While it was true that the Methodists suffered a great decline after Themison and Thessalus, it should not be construed that Methodism ceased as a system of medical practice. It did not disappear even after the spread of the doctrines of the Pneumatic and Eclectic cults. It had the support of no less an authority than Soranus of Ephesus, whose works and memory were revered far into the Middle Ages.

SORANUS

Soranus flourished during the reigns of Trajan and Hadrian (98–138 A.D.). He was a celebrated surgeon, gynecologist, obstetrician, and pediatrician. According to Suidas, Soranus practiced in Alexandria at first and subsequently came to Rome. He is credited with two medical works which are extant—one on fractures, "Physice et Medici

Minores" (published in 1841), and the other on "Diseases of Women" (published by Rose in 1882)—and a biography of Hippocrates.[10] The most important of his works is on acute and chronic diseases. Unfortunately, only a few Greek fragments of this monumental work are extant. A complete Latin translation was made by Coelius Aurelianus, himself a Methodist and the author of a book bearing the same title.

In his biography of Hippocrates, Soranus states that Hippocrates was among the few citizens of Athens who were honored with a crown of

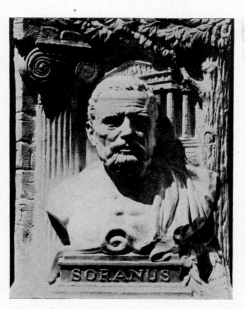

Fig. 140: Soranus of Ephesus (98–138 A.D.). Soranus practiced medicine in Alexandria and subsequently came to Rome. He was the leading exponent of the Methodist school. His most important work was "On Acute and Chronic Diseases." He also was the author of the "Life of Hippocrates."

gold and a place for him in the prytaneum, the greatest honor that could be conferred on anyone by the Greeks. Soranus passed in silence over the story told by Galen that Hippocrates cured the plague of Athens, which had been introduced from Ethiopia, by means of fire, in which was thrown sweet-smelling herbs and flowers, along with perfumes, which purified the air. Soranus merely observed in general terms that Hippocrates predicted the pestilence and took the necessary steps to prevent the cities of Greece from infection.

His work, "The Life of Hippocrates," which probably formed one of a collection of biographies of physicians, is referred to by Suidas. It is said to have been the only authoritative biography of the great physician.

Diseases of Women and Children

Soranus was perhaps the first physician of antiquity to deal scientifically with diseases of women and children. His writings contained, not only what had already been known at that period about these subjects, but far more. His work had a far-reaching influence many centuries later. His work on obstetrics which was intended for midwives who were the sole obstetrical practitioners at this period, was also accepted as a textbook by physicians. It was written in simple Greek. Perhaps owing to his early training in Alexandria, his writing was free from superstition and prejudice. He disregarded all legends and fantastic notions that prevailed about women during pregnancy and the puerperal state. He discarded all rough manipulations of women to facilitate labor, such as running, shaking the body, and climbing stairs, all of which were advocated by the Cnidian school. His description of the uterus, its ligaments, and the displacements to which the organ was susceptible, revealed that he had a profound knowledge of the female generative organs. He denied the then popular belief that the uterus kept migrating about the abdomen. He was aware that the os uteri opened during coitus and menstruation and describes the clitoris scientifically. He was, however, unaware of the existence of the hymen.[11]

With reference to embryology, Soranus taught that the embryo was nourished through the umbilical cord. He denied the possibility of predicting the sex of the child by means of observing the intrauterine position of the fetus. As a measure of preventing conception, he recommended closure of the os uteri with a particular preparation. He warned that inducement of abortion should only be undertaken during the third month of pregnancy, and then only on strong women, and that puncture of the membranes to induce labor was a very dangerous procedure. His account of obstetrics revealed that the art was well developed in his time.

He attributed difficult labor (dystocia) to the following causes: advanced age, poor health, abnormalities of the generative organs, obstruction of the vagina by a tumor, contracted pelvis, dead fetus, and abnormal position of the child. Separation of the placenta was facilitated by the introduction of the hand into the uterus. Vaginal examination was carried out by means of a speculum. The oiling of the fingers prior to vaginal examination was indicated.

The only normal position was head presentation. The most common abnormal position was foot presentation. Labor pains were stimulated by pressure on the abdomen or traction on the child. The perineum was protected by holding a linen cloth in front of it.

Difficult labor, particularly in deformed or fat women, was often accounted for by a transverse, "knee-elbow" position. The bladder and rectum were evacuated to facilitate labor. Version was performed in abnormal presentations. If, for some reason, normal delivery was impossible, in order to save the mother's life embryotomy should be performed. The instruments used included a short ring and a blunt hook.

The umbilical cord was divided with a knife, and the cautery was not permitted. After delivery, the child's eyes were irrigated with clean water and its body anointed with warm oil. The meconium was removed by inserting the little finger in the anus. After a thorough inspection of the newborn, its entire body was swathed with a wool binder and the baby was placed in a basket (on wheels). The baby was put to the breast on the third day. During the intervening time, it was given cooked honey.

If a wetnurse was employed, she had to undergo an examination. Her nipples were carefully examined and her milk tested. This test was accomplished by mixing the milk slowly with water. If curdling ensued, the milk was declared unsuitable for nursing. It was stipulated that the wetnurse should be between twenty and forty years of age; and while nursing, she was required to abstain from wine. Her diet and bowel movements had to be regulated, and moderate exercise was urged. If for some reason, the child could not be suckled from the breast, it was nursed with equal parts of honey and goat's milk.[12]

Soranus discussed the significance of crying in infants. He stipulated that the baby should be nursed until one and one-half to two years of age, after which it was weaned. He described treatment for teething, diarrhea, skin eruptions, and fever in children. In his book on the etiology of disease, he opposed the popular belief of demoniacal causation. He warned midwives against superstitions regarding the interpretation of dreams, divination, and other mysteries.

The midwife, in whose care the lying-in woman was placed, had to be trained, not only in the practice of midwifery, but also in materia medica and dietetics. It was necessary that she should know how to perform version when necessary. Particular attention was paid to her character. She had to be free from all corrupt and criminal practices, temperate and not avaricious. Delivery was accomplished on a "labor stool" which consisted of an armchair with a straight back. The mid-

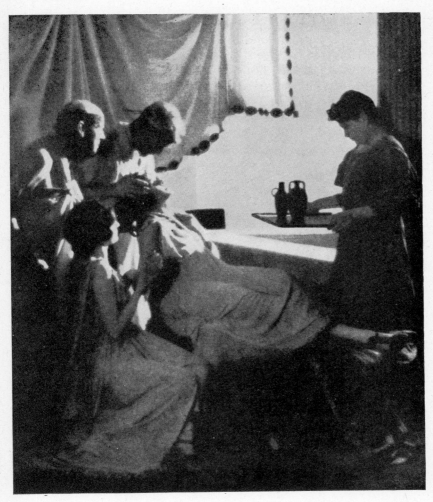

Fig. 143: Paul of Aegina (625–690 A.D.). Paul of Aegina was an able surgeon and one of the foremost writers of the late Greek period. His "Epitome" gives a description of eye surgery in antiquity and furnishes many interesting details on the use of sutures. Woolen threads were employed for suturing the eyelid, the ends being fastened to the forehead under tension with plasters. He suggests that "a medium be observed as to the consistence of the thread, for that which is too soft is itself first broken." (Courtesy of Davis and Geck, Inc.; as depicted by an artist.)

pain is mitigated and dispersed by the trembling and palpitation of the heart."[14] He also mentioned the use of music therapeutically in epilepsy and credited this form of therapy to Hippocrates.

ECLECTICS

There were in ancient times, as at present, physicians of independent minds who did not adhere to any system and who tried to select the best of all systems. These men, not being able to establish general rules, tried to decide practical questions according to their fancy or their reason. They assumed the name of "Eclectics," or "Episynthetics." They adopted no exclusive system but selected from each that which seemed to them best. They did not constitute a sect, for they had no dogmas or immutable theories. They were not committed to any person or doctrine and could judge a subject impartially.

References and Notes

1. Juvenal, *Decimus Junis* (c. 60-140 A.D.): Translation by Housman, E., 1905.
2. Hamilton, W. B.: History of Medicine, Surgery and Anatomy. Henry Colburn and Richard Bentley, London, 1931, Vol. 2.
3. De Medicina, Libra 1.
4. Selected Epigrams of Martial. Translated by Post, E.: Ginn & Co., Chicago, 1908, Chapter 5.
5. Ibid. Martial 10:56.
6. Withington, E. T.: Medical History From the Earliest Times. London, 1894.
7. Ibid.
8. Paulus: Aegintus. Vol. 2, p. 371.
9. Christ, W.: Geschichte der griechischen Litteratur. 1898.
10. Dechambre, H. J.: Encyclopedie des Sciences Medicales. Third Series.
11. Ilbeg, J.: Die Ueberlieferung der Gynokologie des Soranos von Ephesos. Leipzig, 1910.
12. Ibid.
13. "Geschichte der griechischen Litteratur."
14. De Morbis Acutis et Chronicis, Lib. 5.

27

The Encyclopedists

It has been pointed out already that early Roman medicine was largely a heritage of earlier times and was practiced by the elders of the family or the community, by old wives, and by eccentric or deformed persons. The amateurish Roman interest in medicine arose to some extent from the desire to be independent of strangers, particularly from Greek physicians.

The knowledge of medicine of that period was a part of the liberal education of poets, philosophers, and statesmen. Greek was the classical language of the literati. Prominent Roman writers who were not particularly attached to the medical profession were interested in medicine as a part of general literature.

TITUS LUCRETIUS CARUS

Among the first of these writers, was the poet and philosopher Titus Lucretius Carus. Lucretius was perhaps also the first native Roman philosopher who wrote in his native Latin language. His atomic doctrine on natural phenomena was perhaps influenced by Asclepiades, who was his older contemporary or his predecessor by a few years. Lucretius was a great admirer of Epicurus (4th century B.C.) whose philosophy of life was popular among the cultured Romans of that period. Like Epicurus, he attributed the origin of the world to the interaction of atoms without the intervention of any creative intelligence.

In his first two books, he attempted to show that the world was not governed by a capricious agency but had come into existence, continued in existence, and would ultimately pass away in accordance with the primary condition of the elemental atoms, which, along with empty spaces, were the only eternal substances.

661

He attributed even mental phenomena to atomic origin:

There is no existence, save atoms and voids. . . . Nothing is ever begotten
of nothing by divine will. . . . Everything springs from *semina certa* (deter-
minate units). The genesis of all things is typified by generation of organic
beings, and the species of plants and animals give us models for all
processes and natural laws.

The conception of generation had its converse, "things cannot ever
be turned to naught." Such an attitude expressed the law of indestruc-
tibility of matter on which modern physical and chemical knowledge
is based.

The atomic theory led Lucretius to the opinion that diseases were also
brought about by atomic influence. Describing the plague of Athens
(430 B.C.), he asked, "What is its cause?" and he answered, "just as there
are seeds *(semina)* of things helpful to our life so, for sure, others fly
about, that cause disease and death."

It may be of interest to point out that, seventeen centuries later,
Girolamo Fracastoro (1483–1553 A.D.), pondering over the nature of
epidemics, developed the theory of Lucretius that such "diseases were
due to *seminaria* (seed stores). These semina, or seeds, reproduce their
like in infected victims whose bodies they enter by fomites or foci of
infection."

Some writers have seen in Lucretius the beginning of the theory of
evolution. He exhibited a *scala naturae* (a ladder of life) somewhat
similar to the evolution theory which may also be discerned in the
writings of Aristotle. He stated, "the earth produces out of herself first
plants, then animals of ever higher and higher types . . . even as down
and hair and bristle are first formed on the limb and breast, so the newborn earth raised up herbage and shrubs first, and thereafter produced
the races of mortal things."

In these remarks, may be seen the principle of the origin of species
in a rude form. It had to wait eighteen centuries for a Darwin to put
it into a scientific form.

In his third book, he applied the atomic principle to explain the nature of the human mind and the vital principle of man, giving his view
that the soul perished with the body. In his fourth book, he discussed
the Epicurean doctrine as to how objects were perceived, namely that
images were cast off from all bodies which acted on the senses by the
direction of the mind. In the fifth book, he explained the origin of life
and the gradual advance of man to a civilized being. In all his works,
he presented a group of speculative ideas, applying them to the inter-

pretation of human life and nature. He also presented his views of anatomy, physiology, and hygiene. He discussed the effect of diet and climate on health. His encyclopedic mind embraced all sciences known at his period and led him to proffer logical explanations for such phenomena as thunder, lightning, natural springs of water, volcanoes, suffocating vapors, and pestilence.

According to the account of Jerome, Lucretius was born in the year 95 B.C.; and while still of tender age, he became mentally unbalanced in consequence of the administration of a love philter. He wrote his works during his lucid intervals, and he died by his own hand in his forty-fourth year. The statement of Jerome has been questioned by Cicero and other writers. They pointed out that work characterized by such strength, consistency, and continuity of thought was not likely to have been composed in the interval of madness.[1]

Lucretius' most important work was "De Rerum Natura."

MARCUS TERENTIUS VARRO

Even more characteristic of the interest of Roman authors in medicine was Marcus Terentius Varro (116–27 B.C.), whose researches extended into all realms of learning. Varro held that a knowledge of medicine was necessary for a complete education. He discussed medicine in both of his works; his "Disciplinarum" (encyclopedia) and his "De Re Rustica." His works were the prototype of numerous medical works on the liberal arts. "De Re Rustica" was written in the eightieth year of his life. According to Caelius, Varro, when he was seventy years old, estimated that he had written 499 books on various subjects.

Because of his great learning and fluency of pen, he received the title "encyclopedist." In "De Re Rustica," he ascribed to bad hygiene and poor sanitation the outbreak of an epidemic in the city of Corcyra. He related how, upon one occasion when a severe epidemic broke out, he helped to abate the epidemic by ventilating the sick room and rebuilding the houses on a sanitary principle.

The most remarkable of his medical observations was with regard to malaria. He imputed it to invisible organisms prevailing in marshy districts:

In building houses you must avoid the neighborhood of marshy places, because when the marshes begin to dry, they engender a multitude of invisible insects which are introduced into the mouth and nostrils with the inhaled air and occasion serious diseases. . . . Precaution must also be taken in the neighborhood of swamps, because small creatures invisible to the eye fill the atmosphere in marshy localities and, with the air inspired through the nose and mouth, penetrate into the human body, thereby causing dangerous diseases.

Varro was not surpassed in the scope of his writings by any ancient authors, including the later Greek philosophers. He was born at Reate in the Sabine country. He received his early education from Laelius Stilo, the famous critic, philosopher, and philologist. He later went to Athens where he became a pupil of Antiochus of Ascalon, a Platonist.

In politics, he was a follower of Pompey. His literary taste was admired by Caesar, who employed him to select books of Greek and Latin literature for his library which he intended to erect. His work was enlivened by humor; his style was lucid. His works were collected, soon after the invention of print, and published and circulated widely. The first edition of his "Res Rustica" appeared in Venice in 1472.

AURELIUS CORNELIUS CELSUS

By far the most native Roman medical writer was Aurelius Cornelius Celsus (25 B.C.–50 A.D.), who lived around the time of Themison, or shortly thereafter. Celsus preferred to be known as a follower of Asclepiades; but unlike his master, he was a great admirer of Hippocrates and was among the foremost to introduce his teaching among the Romans; hence he became known as the "Latin Hippocrates."

He believed in his humoral theory and many more of his doctrines but was thoroughly independent in his medical thoughts; he was not bound to any system. While he was influenced by Asclepiades, he opposed Methodism. He adopted many concepts of the Alexandrian school but rejected Empiricism. He revered the teaching of Hippocrates, but he was against Dogmatism.

His literary interest was encyclopedic in character. His work, bearing the title "Artes," embraced rhetoric, history, philosophy, the arts of war, agriculture, government, law, and medicine. Medicine was the only part of his work that survived. In the introduction of "De Re Medica," Celsus gave a historical review of medicine up to the time of Asclepiades and Themison. He pointed out that therapeutics were divided in Alexandria into three branches: (1) curing by diet (dietetics), (2) by drugs (pharmacology), and (3) by hand (surgery). He passed an unbiased opinion on the three systems of medicine.

His criticism of Methodism was most interesting. His work "De Re Medica" has taken its place with the "Corpus Hippocraticum" and with the work of Galen as a monument of ancient medicine. From his work, many other writers have drawn their material up to comparatively recent times.

His "De Re Medica" was divided into eight books. The first two dealt with diet and with general principles of therapeutics and pathology; the third and fourth books discussed internal medicine; the fifth and

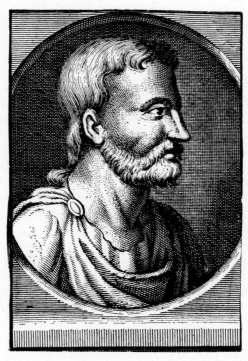

Fig. 144: Aurelius Cornelius Celsus (25 B.C.-50 A.D.). Celsus was the most prominent Roman medical author to write in the Latin language. Little is known of his private life beyond the fact that he lived in the Augustan Age when learning in Rome was at the highest level and that he was born of a patrician family known as the *Cornelii*. Celsus was a man of profound culture, but his main interest was medicine and natural sciences. His "Artibus" (25 and 35 A.D.) was the most complete work on the arts and sciences known in his age. The sixth book of "Artibus," "De Remedica," dealt with medicine and was the first book on general medicine to be printed.

sixth, external diseases; the seventh and eighth books, surgery, were perhaps the most valuable.

Celsus dealt briefly with anatomy and physiology; but although his anatomical description was brief, it was clear and well presented; only the parts necessary to understand disease were mentioned.

He described the sutures of the skull, the foramens, the maxillary and mandibular bones, and the teeth. He gave a good description of the perforated plate of the ethmoid bone. He mentioned the semicircular canals of the ears. He gave the correct number of the vertebrae and the ribs. He described the situation of the scapula, humerus, radius, and ulna, the bones of the pelvis, the extremities, and even the carpal bones. He understood well the structure of the joints, pointing out that the cartilage was part of their formation. He did not describe the muscles individually. He knew the topography of the liver, spleen, kidneys, and stomach, and he distinguished the arteries from the veins.

In describing their relationship, he stated, "The vein is in close proximity with the artery, and the nerve passes between the two." The term *venae* in his work signifies vessels in general. He distinguished air-conducting *arteriae* and blood-conducting *venae*. The term *nervi* in his work, at times, signified nerves and, at other times, muscles or tendons. He noted that arteries could spurt blood when cut.[2]

Although the writings of Celsus showed that he cultivated anatomic knowledge, it did not appear that the science of anatomy was very much studied by the Romans. There is good evidence that after the decline of the school of Alexandria, anatomy was neglected and languished in obscurity.

The arguments of Celsus, against taking the pulse as a criterion in disease, were interesting. The pulse, he said, was an uncertain indication of the state of health of a person because its frequency varied much with sex, age, and constitution of the patient, while temporary derangements of the organs of digestion gave it an appearance of weakness. At the time when the general health of the system was impaired, as at the beginning of a fever, the pulse could be weak, making it appear of extreme debility; but in fact, a violent exacerbation was just but beginning and the patient could gain sufficient strength to carry him through the paroxysm and conduct him to uneventful recovery. Again, the pulse was often full, quick, and strong from exercise, exposure to the sun, or other temporary exciting causes, such as passion of the mind. It was also affected by the arrival of the physician and the patient's anxiety to learn his opinion. For these reasons, the patient's pulse should not be examined on the doctor's first arrival. The physician should sit down with the patient first, establish a cheerful mood, and allay his agitation. Then he could engage in lively conversation and, with guarded inquiries, delve into the state of the patient's health. Following this he could examine the pulse.

Speaking of serpent poison, he recommended extracting it from the wound by sucking, provided the person who performed the operation had no wound or ulcer in his mouth. He believed that the venom of a serpent was not injurious when swallowed and was lethal only when absorbed into the wound. He recommended immersion in water as a cure for hydrophobia, "The only remedy is to throw him into a fish pond and if he is unable to swim, keep him for some time immersed, so as to make him swallow a portion of the water and then raise him out of it alternately, immersing and emerging, but if able to swim, he should be kept in the water . . . by which means the thirst and the dread of the water will be effectively subdued."

In epilepsy, he recommended cupping around the occiput or scarifying in two places—over the occiput and over the first vertebra of the neck. This was done to produce a "copious brain." Dropsy, he stated, was more easily cured in the case of slaves than free persons because those who were most easily compelled to submit to the abstinence and privation necessary for cure were more speedily relieved than those whose exemption from restraint prevented cure.[3] In dropsy, he restricted the quantity of drink to that amount which was indispensable for the maintenance of life, preferring such a treatment to the use of drugs with diuretic properties.[4] Celsus felt that it was better to keep the bowels open by diet than by purgative medicine.[5] He pointed out the propriety of attending to the excretion of the urine and of being certain that the quantity voided was equal to or exceeded the amount of liquid consumed. If the balance was in favor of urinary output, cure of the disease could be hoped for.[6] In sciatica, following the advice of Hippocrates, Celsus recommended that three or four eschars should be made on the hip and kept discharging.

In the seventh book of "De Re Medica," Celsus spoke of breaking up a stone in the bladder in order to facilitate its removal. The method was originally ascribed to Ammonius, who coined the name "lithotomist." Celsus advised bleeding more sparingly than did Hippocrates, lest he should exhaust the patient too much at one time. He employed cupping and scarifying cautiously. He recommended abstinence during the early stages of disease. In the later stages, he ordered liquid diets, cautiously regulated so that the patient should not overload his stomach.

Celsus, in the preface of "De Re Medica," demonstrated that he was not altogether free from some of the popular beliefs of his day, especially with regard to the causation of disease. He referred the etiology of some diseases to the anger of the gods. He considered epilepsy to be a mysterious disease, advocating the blood of a slain gladiator, followed by periods of fasting; and like most healers, he recommended hygiene and hoped for good luck, "If these do not suffice, the head is to be shaved, then anointed with oil, adding vinegar, nitre and salt, effused over it." There was no evidence that he looked upon epilepsy as a sacred disease in quite the same way that it was viewed by all ancients, beginning with the Egyptian papyri. He did not prescribe incantations or other magical cures for epilepsy.

While he was against human vivisection, he favored dissection. In his time, dissection of the human body was permitted in Rome. At the end of the introduction, he stated:

It is both cruel and superfluous to dissect the bodies of the living, but to dissect those of the dead is necessary for learners, for they ought to know the position and order, which the dead show better than the living and wounded, but even the other things, which can only be observed in the living, practice itself will show in the cures of the wounded, a little more slowly, but somewhat more tenderly.

His knowledge of physiology was that taught in the Alexandrian schools.

In his introduction to Book II, he stated, "I shall not hesitate to rely on the authority of the ancients and especially of Hippocrates." He followed Hippocrates with reference to the etiology, symptomatology, and prognosis. Symptoms indicating impending disease were sweat, salivation, fatigue, or sudden increase or loss of weight. Celsus divided disease into two classes: general and local. He rejected the division by some of his predecessors into acute and chronic forms.

Celsus' description of malarial fever cannot be surpassed. He described the symptoms of each of the three forms, quotidian, tertian, and quartan, in detail. His view that fever was an effort on the part of nature to eliminate morbid material from the body was far in advance of his time. His studies of urinary diseases were comprehensive; he held that slow micturition and hematuria, with pain in the pubic region, were symptoms that indicated disease of the bladder. When the urine was viscid, containing a heavy sediment, arthritis was foreshadowed. Blood spitting, when not accompanied by fever, headache, and pain in the chest, indicated that the lesion was either in the nose or esophagus. If the blood was foamy, it signified that the lungs were affected. When the sputum was whitish and thick, the prognosis was favorable. On the other hand, if it was purulent and accompanied by fever, thirst, and loss of appetite, the prognosis was unfavorable.

Diseases of the liver were marked by vomiting and hiccup. The treatment consisted of laxatives and, if the disease was due to an abscess, incision and drainage had to be made promptly. Celsus coined the term *cardiacus* for morbid conditions of the heart and *insania* for insanity. He graphically described the prodromes of insanity and consumption. For the latter, he recommended change of climate (that is a sea voyage or a long visit to Egypt), warm baths, massage, and a diet largely consisting of milk. He prescribed turpentine and honey as a medical measure.

The symptoms of nephritis were pain in the region of the kidney, pale and watery urine, polyuria, and blood or gravel in the urine. Headache was a symptom which appeared in many diseases. He suggested mustard plasters and massage for its relief. He described diseases of the stomach in great detail. He recognized forty different kinds of skin disease. Some dermatological conditions still bear his nomenclature, such as alopecia areata and lichen agrius. He classified remedies according to their physiologic action, such as laxatives, purgatives, diuretics, diaphoretics, and emmenagogues.

Celsus was the first Roman writer to give a comprehensive account of surgical procedure. He gave a description of an ideal surgeon:

A surgeon ought to be young, or at any rate, not very old; his hand should be firm and steady and never shake; he should be able to use his left hand with as much dexterity as his right; his eyesight should be acute and clear, his mind intrepid and so far subject to pity as to make him desirous of the recovery of his patient, but not so far as to suffer himself to be moved by cries; he should never hurry the operation more than the case requires; not cut less than is necessary, but do everything just as if the other's screams made no impression upon him.

Celsus devoted the last two books in his "De Re Medica" to surgery. He concerned himself with the treatment of wounds, injuries, fractures, dislocations, osseous caries and necrosis, fistulas, ulcers, tumors, hernias, amputation, and trepanation. He gave methods for stopping hemorrhages and discussed ligatures. Celsus recommended that an injured vessel should be tied in two places and divided between the two ties.

Celsus was rather free in the use of the lancet. He suggested many major operations, such as, for example, lithotomy, and the operation for crushing a stone in the bladder. He described plastic operations for the repair of the nose, lips, and ears. He stated that a dislocation should be reduced before inflammation set in. If union of a fracture failed, he suggested extension and the rubbing together of both ends of the broken bone to stimulate union. If these measures also failed to promote union, he recommended an incision down to the ends of the bones and open reduction. "The fracture will heal soon." He was against amputations. "The last-said remedy is lawful only in cases of gangrene." Celsus, as did Hippocrates, thought that the circular incision should not be made in living tissue, lest a fatal syncope should ensue.

He recommended reduction of hernia by taxis and operation. A part of the operation was cauterization of the canal. He warned against giving purgatives in case of strangulated intestines. He advised an operation for extirpation of goiter, removal of tonsils, and wiring of teeth. He gave an account of a reflector which perhaps was a dental mirror. He recommended resection of ribs for the cure of sinuses in the chest walls. He employed the couching operation for cataract. His description of inflammation was taken from Hippocrates: the cardinal signs of inflammation were redness, swelling, heat, and pain (rubor, et tumor, cum calore et dolore). Among the instruments mentioned in "De Re Medica," were scalpel, cup, sound, hook, forceps, speculum, trepan, amputation saw, spatula, and various special bandages, including one for hernia.

In the introduction to his work, there was a description of the evolution of medicine up to his own time. He enumerated more than seventy Greek and Graeco-Roman physicians whose works have since perished. He gave an account of the Alexandrian schools, the part played by Hippocrates, and the contribution of the Asclepiadae to the doctrine of the Methodists. Celsus venerated the great men of the past. Eighty physicians were mentioned in his book belonging to different periods and different schools, some of whom we know only through his book. The "De Re Medica" was used as a textbook for students up to comparatively recent times, both as a source of information and as an excellent piece of literature.

His work has remained free from all corruption and interpolation of text from which his predecessors' works have suffered. He had an open mind and availed himself of the labors of his illustrious predecessors. He did not hesitate to criticize Hippocrates' critical days in disease, which he regarded as a relic of the doctrine of numbers, introduced from the east by Pythagoras.

Very little is known of Celsus' private life beyond the fact that he lived in the Augustan Age when learning in Rome was at the highest level, and also that he was a patrician of a class that considered the practice of medicine beneath its dignity. He himself most likely never practiced the healing art. This may have been the reason why he did not have any pupils and why he was not cited by his contemporaries or by many later writers.

Pliny referred to him as a literary man and not as a practicing physician, but he was magnetically attracted towards the healing art. His work was a collection from prominent Greek authors. It was probably intended as a handbook of general knowledge, requisite for landowners who employed a large number of slaves and had use for reference works on medicine as well as agriculture.

For that matter, Celsus himself might have held a position as overseer of such an estate and used his "De Re Medica" for the bedridden slaves in the infirmary. His diction was elegant, and his thought was concise. His ethical tone was high, and the line of treatment marked considerable progress. Although his work was virtually unknown in the Middle Ages, his was the first classical book on medicine to be printed. It appeared in Florence in the year 1478.

GAIUS PLINIUS SECUNDUS

In contrast to the critical mind of Celsus, free from all sorts of bias and interpolation, was Gaius Plinius Secundus (23–79 A.D.), generally known as "Pliny" (the elder). Like many other Romans of the period of the early empire, he studied the philosophy of the Stoics. He was devoted to nature and to moral and ethical teachings. Pliny's views of religion showed that he was also influenced by the Epicureans. "Only the weakness of humanity," he declared, "has embodied the being of God in many human forms and endowed Him with many human faults and vices . . . the existence of a divine providence is uncertain,[7] but the belief in its existence and in the punishment of wrong doing, is salutary."[8].

Pliny was inconsistent in his writing. Although he stated that it was wrong to inquire into the future and to do violence to nature by resorting to magic,[9] he did not deny the significance of prodigies and portents. He questioned the belief in a god but accepted everything he was told without question or criticism. During his long travels, he took copious notes of what he saw and heard but was naïve to the point of accepting everything he was told without criticism or investigation.

Pliny was not a physician. In fact he was against physicians and particularly those of Greece, whom he accused of all sorts of ethical violations and moral weakness. "Medicine, in spite of all lucrativeness," said Pliny, "is the art of these Greeks that the serious Roman thus far has refused to cultivate; our fellow citizens have not been willing to touch it and even if they do so, they desert it at once to the Greeks."

Pliny complained that victorious Rome was culturally enslaved by the Greeks. This appears to have been the general sentiment among the cultured Greek, for Horace expresses the same sentiment, "Captive Greece had taken captive her rude conqueror."

Pliny adhered to the opinion that every plant had some medicinal value, and if the therapeutic value of each plant were determined, there would be a cure for every disease. Pliny believed that everything in creation had a useful purpose and was created for the benefit of man-

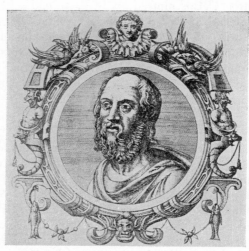

Fig. 145: Gaius Plinius Secundus (23-79 A.D.). Pliny was born at Verona of a wealthy family. He was educated in Rome under the best tutors. At the age of twenty-three, he entered the army. Returning to Rome in 52 A.D., he practiced at the bar for a short period but found the practice of law so unattractive that he devoted himself to writing and reading. He amassed material enough to fill 160 volumes of manuscript, which he bequeathed to his nephew of the same name. His "Historia Naturalis," in thirty-seven books, is the only one of his works that has come down to us. Pliny extended the meaning of natural history also to include the history of medicine and fine arts. (From an ancient print.)

kind. This doctrine was an outgrowth of *teleology*, an early Greek con‑ cept which contended that everything had a purpose. Pliny recorded, in his "Historia Naturalis," remedies for fractures, dislocations, hemor‑ rhages, ulcers, abscesses, tumors, stomach disorders, malfunction of the liver, kidney diseases, phthisis, dropsy, asthma, tonsillitis, erysipelas, rheumatism, gout, malaria, jaundice, lethargy, melancholia, poisoning, toothache, and tapeworm.

The remedies for these morbid conditions were, like the rest of his information, a mixture of folklore, magic, and religion, collected from various people and different countries. His remedies consisted not only of herbs but also of disgusting substances, such as saliva, dung, semen, milk of various animals, and a host of magic and religious cures.

Pliny had a great influence on the popular mind of his time, although he appears to have had little actual knowledge about medicine. He claimed to be a practical man, following only experience. He was against theories; but from some of his writings, it is manifest that he did not know the meaning of the words "practical" and "experience." He was rather gullible and uncritical. An example of Pliny's cry for experience in medicine may be seen from his report about the herb *dittany*, which he claimed had the power of extracting arrows from the body. He based his assumption on the alleged report that stags, when struck by an arrow, were cured when fed on this plant. Pliny took this information from a spurious text of Theophrastus and transmitted it as a fact (he omitted to mention the author). Pliny cited other strange stories, such as that the Icetides assured him that quartan fever could be cured by sexual intercourse, provided the woman was just beginning to menstruate, and that hydrophobia could be cured by placing a cloth saturated with menstrual fluid under the drinking cup of the patient. He reported men whose feet were so large that they held them over their heads like parasols to shade themselves from the sun; and persons who had but one eye in the middle of the forehead.

His statements with reference to menstruating women were amusing for their absurdity:

On the approach of a woman in this state, must will become sour, seeds which are touched by her become sterile, grafts wither away, garden plants are parched up, and fruit will fall from the tree beneath which she sits. Her very look even dims the brightness of mirrors, blunts the edge of steel, and removes the polish from ivory; dogs licking the discharge are seized with madness, and their bite is venomous and fatal. . . . If the menstrual discharge coincides with the eclipse of the moon and sun, the evils resulting from it are irremediable and no less so when it happens when the moon is in conjunction with the sun, the congress with a woman at such a period being noxious and attended with fatal effects to a man.

It is, however, unfair to judge the merits of his natural history by his failure to verify his statements. Few men in his days or for centuries thereafter searched for proof.

As a writer, this erudite and much traveled man exhibited great industry and an interest in natural phenomena that was quite uncontrolled by any real scientific standards. Learned and curious, Pliny was entirely devoid of a critical faculty. In his "Historia Naturalis," he collected an

enormous amount of material, entirely unsifted, and this work his
nephew rightly spoke of as an "opus diffusum, eruditum, nec minus
varium quam ipsa natura." By Gibbon, it was described as "that immense register where Pliny has deposited the discoveries, the arts, and
the errors of mankind." It was drawn from about 2000 works—most
of them now lost—by 146 Roman and 326 Greek authors.

Pliny's "Historia Naturalis" consisted of thirty-four volumes, with
a table of contents, a preface, and a list of authors quoted. His principal
authority was Varro.

The main thought that went through Pliny's book was that nature
served man. Natural objects were hardly described as such but only
in relation to man. All things had their uses:

Nature and the earth fill us with admiration. . . . It is mere folly to
inquire into the nature of God . . . ridiculous to suppose that the great head
of all things regards human affairs.[10]

While other animals have an instinctive knowledge of their own powers
. . . only man is helpless without instruction. He alone desires honors and
possessions . . . he alone provides for his grave and even for his future after
death. . . . All other animals live at peace with their kind . . . but verily with
man, most of his misfortunes are man's doings.

Pliny described a botanical garden kept by a Roman for the purpose
of ascertaining the medical and allied properties of herbs. In his descriptions of living creatures, Pliny went back to Aristotle and Theophrastus; but he had no system, and he was scientifically far inferior
to his sources. He held the view that all plants had their own special
medical powers. He thought that nature existed for man. His philosophy, which accorded in general with the Stoic scheme, was largely
drowned and lost in his love of detail and was often submerged in
rhetoric.[11]

The medical collection of Pliny, which was to be a substitute for the
works of the "wretched Greeks," consisted of a vast series of remedies,
built supposedly on the firm ground of experience and not on theory.
Actually it was not founded on experience. However, it was perhaps
the prototype of practices that echoed for centuries after him down to
the Middle Ages.

According to his nephew, Pliny the younger:

He began to work long before daybreak. . . . He read nothing without
making extracts; he even used to say that there was no book so bad as not
to contain something of value. It was only the time when he was actually in
his bath that he was exempted from study. When traveling, as though freed

from every other care, he devoted himself to study alone. . . . In short, he deemed all time wasted that is not employed in study.

In his preface, Pliny claimed to have read 2000 books. His works indicated, however, that he had not been a good judge in the selection of books, nor was he able to distinguish well between fact and fancy. The subject matter in his book showed he had neither the temperament for investigation nor the time for independent thought. His natural history, which was intended to serve as an encyclopedia of all physical knowledge, consisted of fact mingled with legend, indiscriminately put together, without any effort on the part of the author to distinguish the one from the other. His work was more of the superstition of Cato than the science of Varro, who was his principal authority.

Medicine, however, is indebted to Pliny for furnishing information as to the scope of medicine in his time, particularly with reference to the various systems of medicine; and because of the historical data on prominent physicians which he presented, he merits the respect of the medical profession. In "Historia Naturalis," he gave a detailed account of the old system of medicine, explaining it as best he could, and he listed scores of physicians whose names would have been lost if it were not for his faithful records. Even the magical remedies he collected are of historical value.

Finally, it must not be forgotten that it was his scientific curiosity that led to his premature end at the age of fifty-six while watching the eruption of Vesuvius. While in the Bay of Naples, commanding the Roman Fleet, he observed the volcano of Vesuvius beginning to erupt; wishing to get a closer view, he sailed for the shore on a small boat. Sulfur fumes which choked him could not stop this spirited man. The slaves who accompanied him brought him water but fled in the face of the fumes and molten lava which flowed down the mountains, but this did not deter Pliny from his eagerness to observe the volcano in action at close range. Pliny kept on climbing the mountain and disappeared from view, never to be seen alive again. Two days later, when the volcano had quieted down, his companions came back to search for him and found his body at the foot of Vesuvius. There were no injuries on his body. Thus came to a close the life of an indefatigable writer, who, in search of knowledge, brought destruction upon himself.[12]

THE PLAGUE OF ROME

The account of the plague of Rome by the poet Ovid showed how the Romans of the Augustan Age were familiar with medical phenomena.

Ovid (Publius Ovidius Naso, 43 B.C.–17 A.D.), gave a vivid description of a pestilence that ravaged during his time in Rome:

While the calamity seemed natural and the baneful cause of so great destruction was unknown it was opposed by the resources of medicine. But the havoc exceeded all help, which now lay baffled. At first the heaven encompassed the earth with a thick darkness, and enclosed within its clouds a drowsy heat. And while the moon was four times filling her orb by joining her horns, and, four times decreasing, was diminishing her full orb, the hot south winds were blowing with their deadly blasts. . . . It is known for a fact that the infection came even into fountains and lakes, and that many thousands of serpents were wandering over the uncultivated fields, and were tainting the rivers with their venom. The violence of this sudden distemper was first discovered by the destruction of dogs, and birds, and sheep, and oxen, and among the wild beasts. The unfortunate ploughman wonders that strong oxen fall down at their work, and lie stretched in the middle of the furrow. And while the wool-bearing flocks utter weak bleatings, both their wool falls off spontaneously, and their bodies pine away. The horse, once of high mettle, and of great fame on the course, degenerates for the purposes of victory; and, forgetting his ancient honors, he groans at the manger, doomed to perish by an inglorious distemper. The boar remembers not to be angry, nor the hind to trust to her speed, nor the bears to rush upon the powerful herds. . . . A faintness seizes all animals; . . . in the woods, in the fields, and in the roads, loathsome carcasses lie strewed. The air is corrupted with the smell of them. I am relating strange events. The dogs, and the ravenous birds, and the hoary wolves, touch them not; falling away, they rot, and, by their exhalations, produce baneful effects, and spread the contagion far and wide. With more dreadful destruction the pestilence reaches the wretched husbandmen, and riots within the walls of the extensive city. At first, the bowels are scorched, and a redness, and the breath drawn with difficulty, is a sign of the latent flame. The tongue, grown rough, swells; and the parched mouth gapes, with its throbbing veins; the noxious air, too, is inhaled by the breathing. The infected cannot endure a bed, or any coverings; but they lay their hardened breasts upon the earth, and their bodies are not made cool by the ground, but the ground is made hot by their bodies. There is no physician at hand; the cruel malady breaks out upon even those who administer remedies; and their own arts become an injury to their owners. The nearer at hand any one is, and the more faithfully he attends on the sick, the sooner does he come in for his share of the fatality. And when the hope of recovery is departed, and they see the end of their malady only in death, they indulge in humors, and there is no concern as to what is to their advantage; for, indeed, nothing is to their advantage. All sense, too, of shame being banished, they lie promiscuously close to the fountains and rivers, and deep wells; and their thirst is not extinguished by drinking, before their life is. Many, overpowered with the disease, are unable to arise thence, and die amid the very water; and yet another even drinks that water. So great, too, is the irksomeness for the wretched creatures of their hated beds, that they leap out, or, if their strength forbids their standing, they roll their bodies upon the ground, and every man flies from his own dwelling; each one's house seems fatal to him: and since the cause of the calamity is unknown, the place that is known is blamed. You might see persons, half dead, wandering about the roads, as long as they were able to stand; others, weeping and lying about on the ground, and rolling their wearied eyes with the dying movement. They stretch, too, their limbs towards the stars of the overhanging heavens, breathing forth their lives here and there, where death has overtaken them.[13]

OTHER ENCYCLOPEDISTS

Among other widely learned men who were deeply interested in medicine was the blind philosopher Sirnaeus Seneca (3 B.C.–65 A.D.), the author of "De Immatura Morte," who ascribed the cause of disease to luxury and debauchery. He asserted that excessive bathing, sweating, and drug-taking were some of the causes, and that fresh air and moderation induced longevity. He condemned the behavior of the charlatan of his day and praised the faithful and vigilant physician for his beneficent service, which could not be evaluated in monetary terms.

Another encyclopedist was Lucius Junius Calumella (first century B.C.), a scholar of note and a writer on agricultural subjects. He gave as his theory of the etiology of disease the inhalation into the system of certain invisible beings.[14]

Another who favored the study of medicine was Gellius (130 A.D.), who declared that a minimum knowledge of medicine was indispensable even to the laity. Plutarch held that every man should know his own pulse and recognize things harmful or beneficial to him. Athenaeus, the originator of the Pneumatic sect, insisted that medicine should be made a subject of general instruction, since a knowledge of it was requisite to every calling. Every man should be his own physician.

Vitruvius, in his work "De Architectura," dwelt upon the importance of hygiene, pointing out the necessity of selecting a mountainous place for erecting a house:

It should not be exposed to wind, mist, heat, or great cold, (and should be) away from marshes, the poisonous exhalations of which exert a morbid influence on man. . . . Those who work with lead, such as for example, those who deal with aqueducts, have the disadvantage of being subject to lead poisoning. The daylight in a person's room is to be regulated according to use. Signs as to whether a particular locality is salubrious or not may be detected by examining the liver of a recently slaughtered animal; if this organ is found to be greenish-yellow in color, the locality is not fit to live in.

References and Notes

1. Mason, J.: Atomic Theory of Lucretius. 1884. Sellar, W. Y.: Encyclopedia
    Britannica, Ed. 11, Vol. 17, pp. 108-109.
2. Celsus: De Re Medica. Book 2, Chapter 10, Section 15.
3. Ibid., Chapter 21, p. 161.
4. Ibid., Chapter 1, p. 162.
5. Ibid.
6. Ibid., p. 163.
7. Historia Naturalis, 29:1.
8. De Universa Medicina. Gunther, R. T.: English Translation, Oxford Univer-
    sity Press, 1934.
9. Historia Naturalis, 2:114.
10. Cited by Singer, C.: The Legacy of Rome. Oxford University Press, 1940, p.
    276.
11. Ibid., p. 277.
12. Sandys, J. E.: Encyclopedia Britannica, Ed. 11, Vol. 21.
13. Ovid: The Metamorphoses. Vol. 7, pp. 510-537.
14. Cited by Preuss, J.: Biblische-talmudische Medizin. S. Karger, Berlin, 1911,
    p. 159.

28

The Pneumatics and Eclectics

ATHENAEUS

THE doctrine of the Pneumatic school was based on the idea that the pneuma, or vital spirit, was the source of health and disease. This theory was revived in Rome by a small body of scientifically minded physicians who sought to find a more comprehensive theory of health and disease than had hitherto been advanced. The founder of this medical cult, Athenaeus of Cilicia, who practiced in Rome during the middle of the first century A.D., was a Stoic and based the foundation of his theory on Stoicism. The Pneumatics became the strongest opponents of the Methodists.

Athenaeus believed that all physiological processes were influenced by the pneuma, or "vital air," and that perfect health depended upon the normal condition of the pneuma. The *tonus* that maintained such a normal condition was recognizable in the pulse. Disease, on the other hand, was the result of an imperfect condition of the pneuma, which was caused, in turn, by a faulty condition of the elementary qualities. The nature and gravity of the illness depended upon the degree of disturbance of the pneuma: Since the pulse mirrored changes in the pneuma very closely, according to the Pneumatics a knowledge of the pulse was essential in diagnosis; and as the pneuma was affected by diet, a knowledge of the therapeutic actions of food was also essential.

Pneumatic Theory

The theory of pneuma embraced the four elements and their qualities: The union of heat and moisture maintained health; heat and dryness caused acute disease; cold and moisture caused chronic disease;

and cold and dryness caused mental depression. The Pneumatics believed that the source of the pneuma was the heart whence it was carried by the arteries to every part of the body. It was on this basis that the pulse was such an excellent diagnostic indication. Dilatation of the arteries drove the pneuma onward, and contraction drove it in the opposite direction. The fluctuation of the pulse was ascribed to the exhalation of the spirit from the heart and arteries.

It should be mentioned that the Pneumatics did not ascribe all diseases to a change in the pneuma. Some they attributed to humoral and elemental changes. For example, fever was thought to be the result of corruption of the cardinal humors. Quotidian fever was considered to be dependent upon cold and moisture and was influenced by cold and moist humors, such as an excess of phlegm. Tertian fever depended upon warmth and dryness and was influenced by a change in the yellow bile. Quartan fever was caused by alteration of the black bile, which was produced by cold and dryness. They viewed humoral pathology as a second cause. The season of the year, age, and location were held responsible for febrile attacks. Quotidian fever occurred in the winter when the air was cold, in cold climates, or in old age. Tertian fever attacked the young in the summer time; hot and dry climates were particularly conducive to it. Quartan fever occurred in the autumn.

The Pneumatics divided the etiology of disease into extrinsic causes, such as overeating, and intrinsic causes, such as stone in the bladder. Plethora was considered an extrinsic cause because it was attributed to overindulgence in food. Search was made, not only for apparent causes, but also for hidden causes. Diagnosis, as has been intimated, depended largely upon the pulse, which they studied carefully. They recognized ten varieties of pulses.

Their therapeutics was based on the principle of *contraria contraribus curantur*. Contraries were deemed necessary to counteract dyscrasia of the elements and humoral and pneumatic changes. Cold was combated by warm drinks or applications. Moist lesions were treated by dry remedies and vice versa.

Eclecticism

Although the Pneumatics also took notice of the humoral theory, their method of treatment differed from that of the Dogmatists. They relieved morbid conditions far less by drugs than by physical or dietetic methods, such as bodily exercise, baths, and mineral springs. With regard to therapeutics, the Pneumatics were not bound by any single system. Their method was Eclecticism, although they held themselves to tradition with regard to the etiology, pathology, and symptomatology. They paid careful attention to the quality of foodstuffs, water, air, sun, and the patient's topographical environment.

Athenaeus' Theories

Athenaeus gave directions to men and women, young and old, on how to live a normal life. He laid stress upon the simultaneous development of body and mind. He taught that early education should be mixed with exercise and play. He recommended that, after twelve years of age, when more scientific instructions were given, the greatest attention should be paid to bodily exercise, partly to suppress the growing sexual urge.

The education of women he urged to be mainly domestic, such as cleaning, baking, and attending to all the housework, since such work, he stated improved appetite and produced a healthy complexion. He endeavored to reform the prevailing abuses of the medical profession. He was of the opinion that the knowledge of medicine should constitute an essential part of the education of youth, and that every man should be a physician. The Pneumatics made scientific progress, despite their theory, and recognized many diseases not hitherto known. They were self-opinionated, according to Galen, "The Pneumatics would rather betray their country than abjure their opinions."

According to Orabasius, Athenaeus was a prolific writer. He mentioned one work consisting of thirty volumes and quoted from volume twenty-nine of this work. His works covered the entire range of medicine. Unfortunately, only extracts, dealing with dietetics, physiology, embryology, pathology, and hygiene, remain. His reputation as a physician arose largely from his inquiries regarding diet.[1]

ARCHIGENES

Another Pneumatic was Archigenes, son of Philippus, a prominent pharmacologist. He lived in Rome during the reign of Emperor Trajan. Archigenes was considered one of the ablest medical authors of ancient Rome. He was born in Apameia and went to practice medicine in Rome. He wrote extensively on the pulse; he distinguished as many as eight or ten different varieties of pulse with various subvarieties. He referred to the pulse's rapidity, fullness, slowness, tenseness, rhythmicity, and regularity. Galen wrote a commentary on his book on pulses. He suggested that different kinds of pain could indicate the regions affected. Archigenes classified fever according to the location of the corruption of the pneuma in the fluids or solid parts and according to

other causes. Fevers were described as intermittent or continued. He
often based his description on speculative theories and not on practical
experience and observation. He was first to draw the distinction between primary and secondary symptoms in disease. He introduced
opium for treatment of dysentery. He accurately described the symptoms and progress of abscess of the liver. He wrote the best contemporary account of leprosy and had a knowledge of diphtheria. He
attempted to locate the pathology of disease according to the variety
of pain.

He was a surgeon of note, and special mention should be made of
his limb amputations, an operation which was dreaded by the early
Greeks, partly because of the formidable hemorrhage, and partly because they looked with horror on any form of mutilation. Hippocrates
only mentioned amputation in case of gangrene; but in the hands of
Archigenes, the operation assumed a quite modern aspect. The indications for the operation included severe injury and deformity.

He operated for cancer of the breast and for morbid conditions of
the uterus. He employed ligatures to check hemorrhage when pressure
(tourniquet) above the point of the operation was impractical. Archigenes indicated the sites for amputation. He employed actual cautery
to arrest hemorrhage. He used a vaginal speculum for examination of
the female organs.

According to Heliodorus, he operated upon injured skulls and practiced trephining. He treated surgically cases of empyema, hypospadius,
and exostosis. He performed resection of ribs and was familiar with
flap-cutting. He described the roller and split bandages. He was
one of the few who escaped unscathed the stinging pen of Juvenal.
Galen seems to have drawn material from his writings and was inspired
by him. The only criticism Galen had was the following:

It should have been the special duty of Archigenes, who appeared on
the scene next in order after the most illustrious physicians, to infuse more
light into medical teaching. Unfortunately, he did the opposite; for we who
have grown old in the exercise of the art and should therefore find it easy
to comprehend what is written about medicine, are at times unable to understand what he says. Such being the true state of affairs I propose to undertake what Archigenes failed to accomplish.

Archigenes found time, amidst his busy professional life among
prominent Romans, for considerable literary activity. He wrote, in
popular form, the fundamentals of the Pneumatic theory and harmonized them with the best of Empiric and Methodic medicine.

HELIODORUS

Heliodorus (second century A.D.), the celebrated surgeon, who
flourished during the reign of Trajan, belonged to the Pneumatic school.
All the surviving fragments of Heliodorus' writings deal with surgery.
He was especially famous for his knowledge of the treatment of wounds
and injuries of the head, and for his operation of hemorrhoids. He was

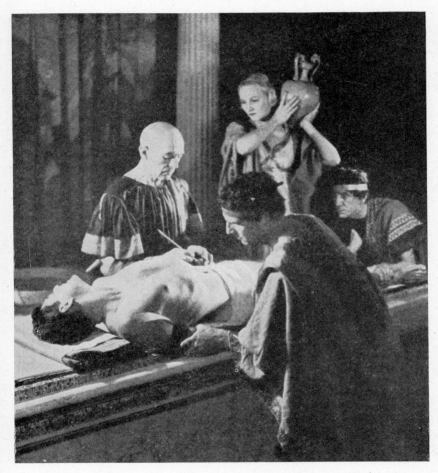

Fig. 146: Heliodorus (second century A.D.). Heliodorus practiced in Rome
during the reign of Trajan (98-117 A.D.), and he was the first to describe ligation
and torsion of blood vessels. He ligated varices of the scrotum before operation
and was one of the first to treat urethral stricture by internal urethrotomy. He
also described various head injuries, the operative treatment of hernia, and flap
amputation, employing ligation of the larger vessels. (Courtesy of Davis and
Geck, Inc.; as depicted by an artist.)

the first perhaps to treat urethral stricture by internal urethrotomy. But he is particularly to be recommended for his description of the ligature to check hemorrhage. The Hippocratic writers knew nothing of ligatures and treated hemorrhage by cold, pressure, styptics, and sometimes by actual cautery. Ligatures were introduced by the Alexandrian surgeons.

Heliodorus gave a first account, not only of the terminal ligatures, but also of the supposedly modern invention of torsion. Speaking of the hernial operation, he said to ligate the large vessels, but as for smaller ones to catch them with hooks and twist them. With reference to amputation, Heliodorus stated:

Amputation above the elbow and knee is dangerous owing to the size of the vessels. Some operators in their foolish haste cut through all the soft parts with one stroke, but it seems to be better to first divide the flesh on the side, away from the vessels and then to saw the bone so as to be ready at once to check the bleeding when the large vessels are cut, and before operating, I want to ligate as tight as possible above the point of the amputation.

Heliodorus, describing the technique of removing a supernumerary digit, stated that a circular incision was made around the digit near the base; from this, two vertical incisions were made opposite one another; thus laid bare, the digit was removed by cutting forceps, and the flaps were then brought together and sutured.

PHARMACOLOGY

The father of Archigenes, Philippus, was a pharmacologist. It is not known whether he was a physician. Pharmacology and toxicology were not separate branches of medicine at this period. Both were part of the duties of the medical profession. The physician frequently prepared his own remedies from the herbs he had planted in his own garden, but pharmacology aroused the keenest interest of *dilettanti*. A prominent pharmacologist of that period was the rhizotomist Cratevas, who lived at the court of Mithradates VI and was the author of two important works: an illustrated herbal, and a treatise upon pharmacology in general.

ORIGIN OF THE ECLECTICS

The Eclectics originated in the attempt made by Claudius Agathinus of Lacedaemonia, a pupil of Athenaeus, to reconcile the doctrine of his preceptor with the concepts of the Empirics and the Methodics. He elaborated upon the work of his master with reference to the pulse.

He differed from his master in the administration of warm baths, preferring cold ones instead. He recommended these for children of all ages. He experimented upon dogs to determine the action of hellebore. Eclectism was also a counterpart of Stoicism; it sought illumination from philosophy. Eclectism declared itself free to accept what was best in the systems of Empiricism and Methodism.

The merit of raising the Eclectics into a sect, however, largely belonged to Aretaeus (50–130 A.D.), who, starting with the doctrine of the Pneumatic school, reduced the theory of its founder to a more scientific form and reinforced it with a number of valuable observations.

ARETAEUS

One of the most consistent followers of Hippocrates among the Graeco-Roman school of physicians was Aretaeus. Owing to the extreme modesty in his writings, which excluded everything of a personal character, very little is known of his life history. Even the period in which he flourished is a matter of conjecture.

The Ionic dialect in which he wrote indicated, according to philologists, that he lived during the second century A.D. The fact, however, that he subscribed in such a large measure to the Pneumatic theory was taken to indicate that he probably lived in the middle of the first century A.D., during the reigns of Nero and Domitian (about 54 to 81 A.D.). The place of his birth was indicated by his surname "the Cappadocian." It is believed that he received his education in Tarsus, which was the nearest city of academic repute at that period. That he lived for a time in Egypt was indicated from the numerous references to Egyptian medicine and habits. His references to Egyptian diseases and therapeutics conveyed the idea that he studied in Alexandria which still retained its prominence as a medical center.

Only a small part of his writings remain intact, the chief of which is his "De Causis et Signis Morborum."[2] What is left of the rest of his work is of a fragmentary nature, derived from quotations in books of other authors. In all his medical works, he manifested individuality, both in content and style. The fact that his work is in accord with some of the fragments of Archigenes of Apameia indicates that he drew from some of the same sources as his predecessor. The honesty and modesty of his writings are apparent to all who have studied his works. It is also apparent that he improved upon the concepts of his predecessors both in content and refined method of expression. His designation by his contemporaries as the "incomparable Aretaeus" shows that he was above reproach.

He took as his model the sage of Cos, as his work indicates. Hippocrates is the only name mentioned in his book. Like "The Father of
Medicine," he was thoroughly emancipated from superstition and free
from arbitrary speculation. Like Archigenes, he belonged to the school
of Eclectics. In fact, his work contains what he thought the best of all
systems. He supported his medical arguments by scientific reasoning
and keen observation and did not sacrifice medical experience for
speculative theory.

Aretaeus considered a knowledge of anatomy of the internal structures of great importance to judicious appreciation of treatment. He
began every chapter with the structure of the organ he was about to
discuss, treating it more fully than any other ancient writer. Aretaeus,
like the Pneumatics, regarded the heart as the principal organ in which
the soul and nature of man resided. In physiology, he believed
with Aristotle that respiration was the process by which the pneuma
reached the lungs and thence the heart, the seat of life. The blood he
thought was prepared in the liver, the bile in the gallbladder; in the
large intestine, a secondary digestion took place; in the spleen thick,
coagulated blood was to be found; the seat of the soul was the heart.
He knew that the content of the arteries was light-colored, that of
the veins dark. The heart, being situated in the center of the lungs,
excited the desire for fresh air and thus influenced respiration. He
regarded the nerves (some of which he believed to branch off from
the spine) as the source of sensation and motion. The lungs, being
composed of a loose kind of tissue with "rough cartilaginous arteries,"
were not provided with muscular tissue and only furnished with fine
slender nerves not susceptible to pain. "Hemorrhage from the lungs,"
he thought, "is particularly dangerous, although patients do not des-
pair even when near their end. The insensibility of the lungs to pain
appears to me to be the cause of this, for pain is more dreadful than
precarious, whereas in the absence of it, even serious illness is un-
accompanied by fear of death and is more dangerous than dreadful."

Typical of his keen observation was his vivid description of phthisi-
cal persons with "curved nails, shrunken fingers, slender sharpened nostrils, hollow glassy eyes, cadaverous look, prominent bones, the scapulas
standing off like the wings of a bird, thin veneer-like frame, the limbs
like pinions, prominent throat, and shallow chest." He adds that "moist
and cold climates are the haunts of this disease."

While Aretaeus based his medical studies on the structure of the
body, anatomy was rather his weak point. He held with Erasistratus
that the liver was the blood-producing organ "which is the root of the

veins" and, on this account, was little else than a factory and store-house of blood. With reference to bodily physiology, he considered the stomach to preside over the sensations of pleasure and uneasiness; and from its proximity to the heart, he thought it a common source of all the faculties contributing greatly to the strength and composure or defection of the mind and soul.[3] Of stomach disorders, he said: "Such disorders are common to those who toil in teaching, whose yearning is after divine instruction, who despise delicate and varied diet, whose nourishment is fasting and whose drink is water." As a "purge of melancholy," he prescribed "a little wine and some other more liberal sustenance." The bile, he wrote, was distributed from the gallbladder to the intestines; and if the intestines became too engorged with it, the bile was thrown back into the veins and by them diffused over the system.

In his essay on "brain fever," he described the powers acquired by the soul before dissolution in the following words:

Every sense is pure, the intellect acute, gnostic powers prophetic; for they prognosticate to themselves, in the first place, their own departure from life; then they foretell what will afterwards take place to those present who fancy sometimes that they are delirious; but these persons wonder at the result of what has been said. Others also talk to certain of the dead, perchance they alone perceiving them to be present, by virtue of their acute and pure sense, or perchance from their soul seeing beforehand, and announcing the men with whom they are about to associate. . . . For formerly they were immersed in humors, as if in mud and darkness; but when the disease has drained these off and taken away the mist from their eyes, they perceive those things which are in the air, and, through the soul being unencumbered, become true prophets. [4]

He looked upon the nerves as the organs of sensation and the source of the action and motion of the limbs. "Tetanus is a disease of the nervous system as is gout and phrenitis." He was aware that the nervous function of sensation was distinct from that of motive power; that either might cease and the other continue. He made a curious statement in regard to paralysis, namely that if the membrane of the "spinal marrow is injured below the head, the parts on the right side will be paralyzed if the nerve towards the right side be hurt, and conversely, if the left side; but that if the heart itself be so affected, the inverse law of consequence holds concerning the parts related, since each nerve passes over to the other side from that of its origin, decussating each other in the form of the letter X."

He believed with the Pneumatics that the pneuma, which was situated in the heart, controlled the physiology of man and influenced all the functions of the body, such as digestion, circulation, and respiration. He gave a splendid description of psychic depression and excitement. He was the first to reveal familiarity with the tubules of the kidneys and the ramifications of the portal vein and the bile ducts. He considered syncope to be a cardiac affection, "for those who fall on the ground and faint, possess a small and weak pulse and palpitation of the heart may be observed." Under the name of "Syriac, or Egyptian ulcer," he was first to describe pharyngeal diphtheria. His descriptions of pleurisy with empyema, asthma, tetanus, apoplexy, hysteria, epilepsy, and paraplegia, have been praised by many writers. He gave a systematic description of diabetes. Other diseases mentioned by him were dropsy, jaundice, various diseases of the stomach and intestines, diseases of the liver, leprosy, and spermatorrhea.

He stated that ancients attributed epilepsy to lunar influence as a punishment upon wicked people for their crimes, whence it was called "sacred disease."[5] Aretaeus was against the popular belief that epilepsy was a sacred disease. He regarded it as resulting from natural causes, having its seat in the brain, whence a cold phlegm or pituita was secreted and passed down the blood vessels; there it encountered the pneuma, causing coagulative obstruction, thus producing a convulsion. Even the Hindu Hippocrates Susruta, 700 B.C., suggested a fanciful treatment for epilepsy. He used the bile of a lizard, of an elephant, of a special deer, and of a bear cooked in oil. Epileptic seizures were regarded in Greece as manifestations of the activities of the gods. The therapy was largely a matter of purification and sacrifice to appease these supernatural powers.

Aretaeus' work was divided into two parts: (1) the causes and signs of acute and chronic diseases, and (2) the curative treatment of acute and chronic diseases.

The doctrine of the pneuma, or ethereal principle, existing in the microcosm, by which the mind performed all the functions of the body, held a more prominent position in the works of Aretaeus than in those of any of the other authorities.[6]

His work exhibited strong traits here and there of the Pneumatic school. Regarding the blood, he stated it was the warming principle of all the parts. He classified diabetes as a sort of dropsy exhibiting the watery principle. He declared that the effect of white hellebore was that of fire, "so that whatever fire does by burning, hellebore effects still more by penetrating inwardly." The last remark shows that Aretaeus did not hesitate on occasion to give vent to his imagination, which also figured in some of his pathological descriptions. Allowing for such overstrained touches here and there, he generally avoided extravagant ideas and rested chiefly on accurate observation and common sense. He hardly ever quoted an authority, and although much of what he stated was taught before, he dealt with his subject matter as the common property of science proved by his own experience. The freedom with which he followed or rejected earlier opinions has occasioned him to be classed by some among the Eclectics.

His therapeutics were simple and rational, guided mainly by experience. Like Hippocrates, he paid attention to regulation of mode of life, fresh air, exercise, and proper diet. He used only a few drugs, mostly those that were mild in action. When strong measures were called for, he prescribed drugs cautiously. He was first to introduce cantharides as a counterirritant. He ordered opium to quiet pain. He employed emetics and purgatives, and insufflation powder in affection of the larynx. He was in favor of bloodletting, cupping, vesicants, cautery, inunction and stimulating salves.

His boldness of treatment on occasion was exemplified in his selection of the veins to be opened in certain cases; those of the arm, ankle, tongue and nose were all listed. He was the first to mention the use of leeches, which Themison is said to have introduced.

In respect to surgery, his resources appear to have been in advance of Celsus. He was familiar with the operation for stone in the bladder, the use of the catheter (where its insertion was not contraindicated by inflammation), and incision into the neck of the bladder (where catheterization was contraindicated).

Aretaeus condemned the operation of tracheotomy first proposed by Asclepiades. He held that "the heat of the inflammation becomes greater from the wound and contributes to suffocation and the patient coughs; and even if one escapes the danger, the lips of the wounds do not unite, for both are cartilaginous and unable to grow together." His surgical writings appear to have been lost. There is every reason to think that he brought to bear upon external medicine the same good sense which he applied to internal affections.

His work "De Causis et Signis Morborum" passed through editions in various languages. The English edition of Adams was published by the Sydenham Society.

MARINUS

The most prominent anatomist of that period, also of the Eclectic school, was Marinus, who flourished during the reign of Nero (37–

68 A.D.). Marinus was mentioned by contemporary authors as remarkable for his anatomical inquiries. Galen spoke highly of him as the reviver of a branch of knowledge which before him had suffered undeserved neglect. Galen also stated that Marinus gave an accurate description of the muscles, that he particularly studied the glands, and that he discovered the glands of the mesentery. He fixed the number of cranial nerves at seven, and he observed the *palatine* nerves, which he classified as the fourth pair. He described the fifth nerve as the auditory and facial, which he regarded as one pair, and the *hypoglossal* as the sixth pair. Marinus discussed many physiological problems, some of which were whether fluid penetrated into the lungs, whether blood was contained in the arteries, and whether the brain exhibited pulsatory movements.

Of the twenty volumes he is reported to have written, only the table of contents has survived. What is known about his anatomy is an extract drawn up by Galen. Galen mentioned also a list of his pupils, among whom were Quintus, the famous teacher of Lycos of Macedonia; Numisianos of Corinth; Satyros of Pergamos; and Pelops of Smyrna. Among other famous physicians of this period, Galen recorded the name of Alianos the younger, Heracleianos, and Julianos.

RUFUS

One other prominent writer of comparative anatomy was Rufus of Ephesus, a Greek physician who flourished in Rome during the reign of Trajan, 98–117 A.D. He and Marinus recorded the status of the subject of anatomy in Alexandria before Galen. According to his own statement, his knowledge of anatomy was derived from dissecting monkeys. He complained that, in his day, anatomy was confined to animal dissection and, at best, some human surface anatomy on slaves; whereas in earlier times, human bodies had been dissected for teaching purposes. He traced a number of nerves from their origin in the brain to their distribution in the body. He ascribed to the nervous system sensation, motion, and coordination. He distinguished between nerves of sensation and those of voluntary motion. He exhibited the decussation of the optic nerve at the infundibulum and described the capsule of the crystalline lens under the name of "lenticular membrane." His book on anatomy was intended for beginners. His "Study of the Pulse" appears to have been based on the work of Herophilus. He discussed the places where the pulse was to be taken, the beating of the pulse, and its variations in disease and at various ages. He distinguished many kinds of pulses according to rate, strength, volume, and contraction of the arteries. He regarded the heart as the seat of

life and the organ of the pulse. He pointed out the difference in structure and capacity between the right and left ventricles. The left ventricle he considered thinner and smaller. He believed the spleen had
no function. He explained that the term "carotid" (from a Greek word
associated with the idea of "deep sleep") was applied by ancients to
the arteries of the neck, because they believed that when these vessels
were strong, one was inclined to sleep and lose the use of the voice.[7]

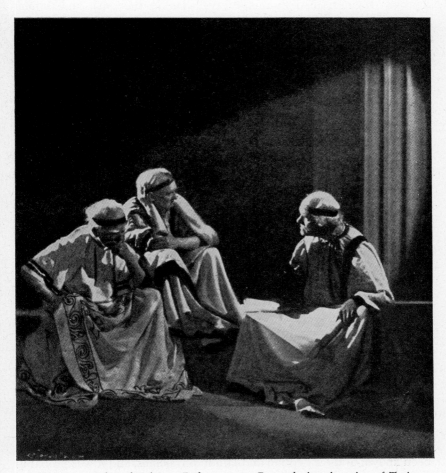

Fig. 147: Rufus of Ephesus. Rufus came to Rome during the reign of Trajan
(98-117 A.D.). His works mentioned that traumatic aneurysm might result from
wounds of the arteries, and he discussed various methods of hemostasis, including
digital pressure, pressure by bandage, astringents, torsion, cold applications, and
complete severance of incised or eroded vessels. Bleeding of the larger vessels
was controlled with ligatures. Caustics were resorted to only in putrid or gangrenous wounds. (Courtesy of Davis and Geck, Inc.; as depicted by an artist.)

He warned against using enemas and diuretics. Rufus forbade the use of a catheter in bladder inflammations. He ordered mild and soothing treatments, such as baths, poultices, and pressure over the bladder. He described vesicle calculi, vesicle hemorrhage, paralysis of the bladder, and prostatic abscesses, and recommended therapy for all of these.

Rufus was among the oldest authors to discuss bubonic plague and leprosy. He described traumatic erysipelas, epithelioma, and tumors of the tendons; and he outlined measures of checking hemorrhages by pressure, torsion, cold applications, astringents, ligatures, and severance of the incised vessels. He gave a description of dysmenorrhea and discussed hygiene during pregnancy. He discovered many medical compounds. One was a purgative colocynth.

He understood that pressure on the neck nerves (not on the carotoid arteries!) could cause loss of voice, and he was of the opinion that the nerves proceeded from the brain. He stated that there were two kinds of nerves—motor and sensory. The heart he considered the seat of life. He demonstrated the investing membrane of the crystalline lens of the eye. Galen, who, as has been indicated, was not in the habit of throwing bouquets to other writers, especially on anatomy, spoke of Rufus as a skillful physician who devoted much time to anatomy. Rufus wrote a treatise on gout, consisting of thirty-seven chapters. Only fragments are left of this momentous work. None of his works mentioned by Suidas is extant.

SURGEONS OF LATE ANTIQUITY

Antyllus

Among the surgeons of late antiquity, none surpassed Antyllus in skill; he flourished during the reign of Trajan (second century A.D.). What Aretaeus achieved in medicine, Antyllus accomplished in surgery. His historical sketch of the treatment of cataract is most interesting. He said when the lens of the eye was opaque, it could be removed from the axis of vision in at least four different ways:

1. It could be simply depressed or "couched" (reclinatio lentis). The operation, though now abandoned, is of great antiquity, having been known to the Egyptian and Hindu physicians, and it was probably the main one in use up to the present era.

2. It could be extracted completely, a method first mentioned by Galen, apparently as a recent invention, for he said, "some have taken in hand to remove cataract by paracentesis."

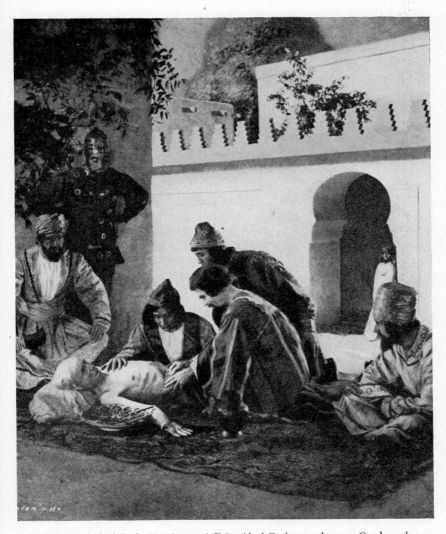

Fig. 148: Abul Casim (936-1013 A.D.). Abul Casim was born at Cordova during the Arabian investment of Spain. He brought advances to surgery, which
were employed for over five centuries. In his thirty-volume "Altasrif," a chapter
is devoted to methods of suturing and differentiating between small and large
wounds. The former were approximated with a series of figure-of-eight stitches.
For intestinal wounds, small threads of intestinal tissue were used. (Courtesy of
Davis and Geck, Inc.; as depicted by an artist.)

3. The lens could be broken up and left to be absorbed. Celsus noticed the division of cataract, though only as a preliminary to couching.

4. The lens could be broken at once and removed by suction. This operation was long practiced in Persia, and according to Abul Casim was invented there in his time (eleventh century). Rhazes, who was himself a Persian, attributed the earliest mention both of extraction and suction to Antyllus, remarking that Antyllus said, "Some also have made an opening under the pupil (iridectomy) and have extracted the cataract. This can be done when the cataract is small but if large it cannot be extracted for the humors come out with it and some have used a glass instrument, *concilum vitreum*, and by sucking it have sucked out the cataract and the humor with it."[8]

Unfortunately his work "De Medicamenti" has not survived the ravages of time. We are indebted to Oribasius and later writers, such as Rhazes and others, who preserved some fragments of his work, for the knowledge that he was perhaps the greatest surgeon of antiquity.

Antyllus was particularly famous for his operation on aneurysm, which is still known as the "Antyllus operation." His technique was to ligate the artery above and below the pulsating sac, following which he opened the aneurysm and emptied its contents. He described two kinds of aneurysms: those that resulted from a local distention of the artery and were cylindrical in form and those that came from a lesion of the vessels and were round. He advocated the operation of bronchotomy when suffocation was threatened. He performed skillful herniorrhaphies.

Leonidas

Aëtius listed Leonidas of Alexandria as another surgeon of note. His method of operating for fistula did not differ materially from the present system. He removed cancer of the breast by amputation and cautery. His views on hydrocele, glandular swelling, orchitis, hernia, and ulcer showed sound judgment. He investigated the subjects of fracture of the skull and of bone surgery. He also was familiar with the fact that the guinea worm *(Dracunculus medinensis)* was endemic in India and Ethiopia.

FAMOUS ECLECTICS

The designation "Eclectic" has been applied to the greatest physicians, such as Hippocrates, Galen, Heracleides, and others. The medical Eclectics, however, formed a school which had many divisions. Some

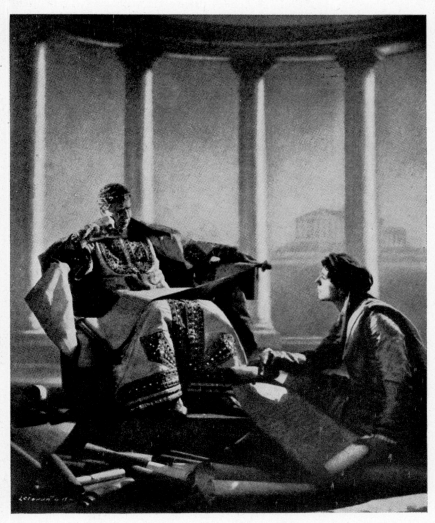

Fig. 149: Aëtius of Amida (c. 500 A.D.). Aëtius was royal physician to Justinian I and lord high chamberlain at the court of Byzantium. His works, though essentially compilations of ancient teachings, are of interest historically. He described the method for treatment of aneurysm at the elbow, known later as that of Anel (1710). This consisted of double ligation of the brachial artery three or four fingerbreadths below the axilla, followed by opening the sac, which was allowed to heal by suppuration. (Courtesy of Davis and Geck, Inc.; as depicted by an artist.)

like Archigenes, founded a system of their own, but some who claimed the title of "Eclectic" were a hindrance to medical progress. They advanced their own theories for selfish motives. Most of them showed an unfortunate tendency either to dilettantism or compilation.

The greatest compiler of medical history was Oribasius of Pergamos, physician and friend of Emperor Julian, at whose suggestion he compiled seventy medical books. Only about one third have survived. These works are of great value, because he mentioned the authors and quoted them with exactness. To Oribasius we owe our knowledge of Antyllus and Archigenes. He died about 400 A.D.

References and Notes

1. Neuburger, M.: History of Medicine. London, 1910, pp. 226-227.
2. See Greek with English translation by Adams, F.: Sydenham Soc., London, 1850.
3. De Causis et Signis Morborum Acutorum, Chapter 1.
4. Locher: Aretaeus aus Kappadocien. Leipzig, 1847.
5. De Dinturnis Morbis. Chapter 4. Cited by Biblical, Theological and Ecclesiastical Cyclopedia, Harper Bros., New York, 1894, Vol. 6, p. 32.
6. Adams: Preface to Aretaeus, pp. 10-11.
7. Hamilton, W.: History of Medicine, Surgery, and Anatomy. Vol. 1, London, 1831.
8. Rhazes: Continence 2:3. Cited by Withington, E. T.: P. 94, Chapter 2:3.

29

Galen

As THE second century of the Christian Era rolled on its way, a distinguished physician, medical writer, and teacher made his presence felt on the medical scene. This man, whose teachings remained authoritative for fifteen centuries, was Claudius Galenus, commonly known as "Galen." His works are noteworthy as a medical encyclopedia, wherein are recorded his own studies, the medical knowledge of his time, and a review of the works of his predecessors. The history of his life is better known than that of any other Graeco-Roman physician, partly because modesty did not keep him from telling all he knew of himself and of his accomplishments, and partly because his contemporaries, with whom he was at loggerheads, also wrote about him.

PERSONAL HISTORY

Galen was born in the year 131 A.D. at the city of Pergamos, in Mysia, a city celebrated for its temple dedicated to Aesculapius, for its school of medicine, and for its ancient library. His father Nicon, from whom he received his early education, he described as remarkable, both for excellence of natural disposition and for mental cultures; his shrewish mother, on the other hand, appears to have been a second Xanthippe.

When Galen reached the age of fifteen, he was taught the sciences, logic, and the philosophies of the Peripatetics, Stoics, Platonists, and Epicureans. He was acquainted with the idealism of Plato, the realism of Aristotle, the skepticism of the Epicureans, and the materialism of the Stoics. The following incident led Galen to the study of medicine: When Galen was still fifteen years old, his father, who desired him to be a philosopher, dreamt that he saw Apollo who urged him to influence his son to study medicine. Consequently, in 147 A.D., when he was about

697

sixteen years of age, to please his father he left Pergamos for Smyrna in order to place himself under the instruction of the anatomists and physicians, Pelops and Satyros, as well as under the Peripatetic philosopher Albinus, all of whom he soon outstripped by his universal attainments.

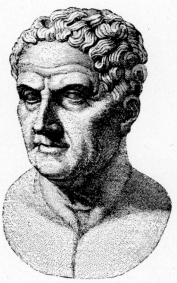

Fig. 150: Claudius Galen (130-201 A.D.). Claudius Galen, a celebrated Greek physician, was born at Pergamos, Mysia. He studied medicine in Alexandria and in other places and was physician to the school of gladiators in his native city for six years. He then went to Rome, where he gained a great reputation, attended the emperor Marcus Aurelius and his two sons, and later, the emperor Severus. Of his works, eighty-three genuine treatises still exist. He gathered all the medical knowledge of his time. His medical work continued to be the authority for centuries. He probably died in Sicily.

When Galen was twenty years old, his father died. By that time, Galen had already acquired all the medical knowledge which his native country had to offer. Since it was customary in those times for physicians to travel in order to gain knowledge from the leading physicians in various countries, Galen set out on his ten-year medical expedition. He went to Corinth (to study under Numisianos and to Cilicia, Phoenicia, Palestine, Crete, Cyprus, and Alexandria. In those days, Alexandria still retained some of the ancient fame it had acquired during the days of Herophilus and Erasistratus.

When Galen arrived in Alexandria, human dissection was no longer permitted; only human osteology could be acquired from the skeletons

left from olden times. The student had to content himself with learning the internal organs of the body with information derived from the
dissection of hogs and apes. Galen, being thus deprived of human dissection, assumed that human organs were identical with those of lower
animals, an error which unfortunately hindered the progress of human
anatomy for centuries.

On his return to his own country (157 A.D.), he was charged by its
ruler with the treatment of the wounded gladiators in the great circus.
This provided him with the opportunity for displaying his anatomical
knowledge and surgical skill. After remaining at home for three years,
he went to Rome (161 A.D.), where his brilliant talents in elocution,
his great medical skill, his accurate logic, his profound erudition, and
his versatility soon secured for him the highest place in the community.
There he was introduced to Eudemus, a celebrated Peripatetic philosopher, who was his countryman. He cured the philosopher of a serious
malady which had defied the best efforts of the local physicians. Ere
long, his learning and unparalleled success as a practical physician
earned for him the titles of *Paradoxologus*, the wonder-speaker, and
Paradoxopoeus, the wonder-worker. He attracted considerable notice
as teacher, medical writer, and practitioner.

A strong spirit of rivalry prevailed at this time among the Dogmatists, Empirics, Methodists, and other medical sects, each of which was
supported by numerous and zealous partisans. The schisms among
the Dogmatists had greatly weakened their strength; some of the
Dogmatists followed Hippocrates; other, Erasistratus; and still others,
Asclepiades. This enabled the Methodists to gain the ascendancy, and
they held first place in the public estimation. The Empirics, with
their idle pretensions, their vanity, and their irrational practices, had
fallen into the contempt they more or less deserved.

Galen's attempt to purge the healing art of the many errors which
had deteriorated the teachings of Hippocrates, his efforts to free medicine from the multitude of absurdities and superstitions which dis-
graced it, his great popularity, his professional success, and especially
his vanity, his self-acclaim, and his disdain for his colleagues, gained
him the enmity of nearly all physicians of the Roman capital and made
his life in Rome unbearable. In his work on "Prenotions," he accused
his colleagues of base jealousy and stupid ignorance, calling them
"thieves" and "poisoners." He closed by saying that, after having un-
masked them, he would leave them to their evil designs by abandon-
ing the great city to seek a home in a smaller place, where the surroundings would be more congenial. His departure was perhaps also

precipitated by the fear of being poisoned by his enemies. His critics
accused him of running away from the pestilence which raged in
Rome at that time. It is unlikely, however, that Galen would have
deserted his patients at such a time.

He returned to his home town Pergamos, where he remained only a
short while. He was soon called to Aquileia in Venetia by the Emperors
Lucius Verus and Marcus Aurelius, whose confidence he enjoyed while
in Rome. Upon the death of Verus (of apoplexy), Marcus Aurelius,

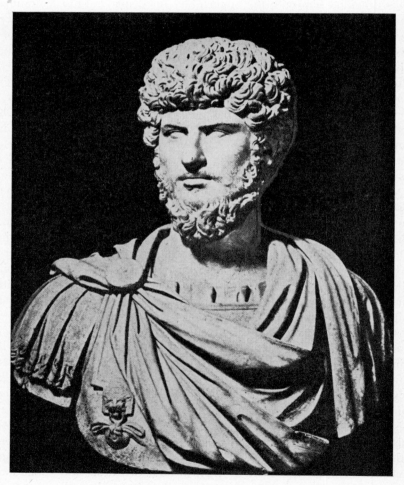

Fig. 151: Lucius Verus (died 169 A.D.). Lucius Verus was the adopted son of
his uncle Antonius Pius, as was Marcus Aurelius. These two men were corulers
of the Roman Empire from 161 to 169 A.D.; at the latter date Verus died.

who was away from his capital in order to prosecute the war on the
Danube, ordered Galen to return to Rome to be the guardian of his
son Commodus, during his absence. He ascribed the circumstances
that brought him back to Rome to divine guidance, "this was the will
of Aesculapius."

About that time (170 A.D.), Galen prepared for Marcus Aurelius his
famous theriac, to be taken daily in small quantities. This preparation
was also used by Septimus Severus, whose court physician Galen was
for a period of thirty years.

After the return of Marcus Aurelius from his campaign against the
Germans (175 A.D.), he was ailing and took, in addition to his usual
morning pill of theriac, a dose of bitter aloes, the *hiera picra* of Galen.
In spite of this, his disorder so increased that, on the following evening, a message was sent to Galen requesting him to sleep at the palace.
Hardly had he arrived, when he was summoned to the emperor's bed-
room, where he found three army surgeons feeling his pulse and diagnosing the case as an early stage of fever. The following text of Galen is
interesting, because it affords an example of Galen's idea of a clinical
history:

I was summoned also to spend the night in the palace, a messenger coming to fetch me, by order of the emperor, just as the lamps were being lighted.
Three physicians had seen him in the morning and at the eighth hour, and
two had felt his pulse, whilst to all did it appear the beginning of an attack.
I, however, remained silent; then the emperor, perceiving me, asked why
I had not, like the others, felt his pulse. I replied: Two have already done
this, and from their experience upon the journey with thee are better able to
judge of its present condition." As I said this he called on me to feel him,
and as the pulse, taking into consideration the age and constitution of the
patient, seemed to me inconsistent with an attack of fever, I declared that
none was to be feared, but that the stomach was overloaded with nourishment
which had been coated with phlegm. This diagnosis called forth his praise
and he thrice repeated: "Yes, that is it, it is exactly as thou sayest; I feel that
cold food is disagreeing with me." He then asked me what was to be done.
I answered him frankly that if another than he had been the patient I should,
following my custom, have given him wine with pepper. "With sovereigns
like thyself, however, physicians are in the habit of employing the least
drastic remedies, therefore it must suffice to apply wool saturated with warm
spikenard upon the abdomen." The emperor replied that warm ointment on
purple wool was his usual remedy for pain in the stomach, and called
Peitholaos to apply it and let me go. This being done and his feet warmed
by rubbing with heated hands, he demanded Sabine wine, threw pepper
into it and drank, after which he said to Peitholaos that now at least he had

a physician and a courageous one, repeating that I was the first of physicians and the only philosopher; he had tried many, not only the covetous but those greedy of fame and honor and those filled with envy and malice. As I have just stated, this is the most remarkable diagnosis I have made.[1]

On Galen's second sojourn to Rome, he remained for a number of years and greatly extended his reputation as a physician. He no doubt found the practice of his profession lucrative; he is said to have received, for curing the wife of Consul Boethius, a sum equivalent to $1750. At that period, he wrote some of his more important treatises, such as "The Diagnosis of the Diseases of the Eye," "The Anatomy of the Uterus for Midwives," and three books on "The Movements of the Lungs."

When he returned to his native town after years of practicing in Rome, he stopped at the Island of Lemnos, where he learned the method of preparing a certain concoction called *terra lemonia*. It is not certain whether he ever returned to Rome. There is some doubt as to the time and place of his death. According to Suidas, he died in 200 A.D., during the reign of Septimus Severus, at the age of seventy. However, Abu-l-Faraj states that he died in Sicily in his eightieth year.

WRITINGS

Galen was a voluminous writer, not only on medicine, but also on philosophy, logic, ethics, and grammar. Eighty-three of his works are still extant and are acknowledged to be genuine. Nineteen treatises ascribed to him are questionable; forty-five books that bear his name are undoubtedly spurious. He left also nineteen fragments and fifteen commentaries on different works of Hippocrates.

Cabanis observed that "Galen was a genius sufficiently comprehensive to embrace all the sciences and cultivate the whole of them with equal success, who, rapidly distancing every competitor, soon divided the admiration of the world with Hippocrates and became the oracle of physic."

He wrote fifteen books on anatomy, of which at least six are now extant in Arabic translations; two copies of each are preserved in the Bodleian Library at Oxford. Most important of these works are "On Anatomical Administrations" and "On the Use of the Parts of the Human Body." "On Anatomical Administrations" covers dissection and consists of fifteen books, six of which have been lost. "On the Use of the Parts of the Human Body" consists of seventeen books, all of which have been preserved. He also left eleven other works on anatomy, handed down in a more or less imperfect state; four others have been lost.

Galen gathered up all the medical knowledge of his time and arranged it on such a firm basis that it continued to be authoritative for fifteen centuries following. In general principles, he may be considered a follower of Hippocrates. His method was to reduce all knowledge to general principles by observation of facts. Although he regarded those who took the title of an individual school (such as Hippocratics, Paraxagoreans, or Herophilists) as slaves, his predilection for Hippocratic writings was well marked, and he always spoke of Hippocrates with profound respect, professing to act upon his principles and to expound his doctrine. Thus, he revived the Hippocratic system of medicine that had been tarnished and debased by the worthless dross with which the Dogmatists had too successfully alloyed the precious ore.

Galen never forgot his own individuality and importance. In one of his books, he wrote:

No one before me has given the true method of treating disease. Hippocrates, I confess, has here before shown the path but as he was first to enter it, he was not able to go as far as he wished . . . he has not made all necessary distinctions and is often obscure as is usually the case with ancients when they attempt to be concise. He says very little of complicated disease; in a word he has begun what another was to complete; he has opened the path but left for a successor to enlarge and make it plain.

But while Galen "infinitely surpassed both Hippocrates and Aretaeus in point of erudition, as a pathological observer he fell considerably below the level of either, not so much from any deficiency in his powers, as from his yielding to the delusions of specious although worthless theories."[2]

Galen attached little weight to other medical celebrities. He regarded himself as the logical successor to Hippocrates, but he did not often follow his footsteps. As Bostock aptly remarks:

While he was the admirer of Hippocrates, always speaking of him with great reverence, professing to act upon his principles and expounding his doctrine, in reality there are few writers whose work both as to substance and manner are more different from each other than those of Hippocrates and Galen, the simplicity of the former being strongly contrasted with the abstruseness and refinement of the later.[3]

Indeed, Galen himself, does not wholly escape the charge of contributing his share to the adulteration of the genuine text, as Cabanis expressly declares:

What is gained in his hands must be allowed to have more appearance of dress and ornament than of real solid acquisition. The observations which had been collected, and the rules which had been laid down, by Hippocrates, in assuming a more splendid and systematic form, lost much of their original purity; Nature, whom the Coan Physician had always followed with so much accuracy and caution, became obscured, and as it were overwhelmed, beneath the foreign pomp of various sciences and dogmas; and the art of medicine, overloaded as it already was with subtle and superfluous rules, became entangled in new and needless difficulties.

GALENIC ANATOMY

Dissection: Galen's description of dissection shows him to have been a master of this art. He advised the use of a probe in dissecting out the portal vein as the surrounding tissue was cut away, so that finally

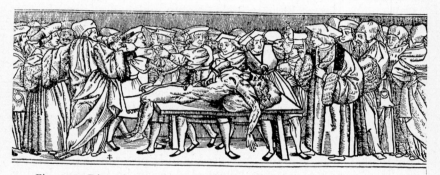

Fig. 152: Dissecting scene from the title page of Galen's "De Anatomicis Administrationibus." A crowded room contains about twenty-five figures in academic dress. On a table in the foreground, lies a body, the abdomen of which has been opened. A discussion is in progress. A young enthusiast is excitedly demonstrating, with one hand in the abdomen and the other raised in gesture. An older lecturer stands at the head of the dissecting bench. He is making a point. Another youth hands some of the viscera to a yet older academic. There are no books in the scene. (Translated into Latin by Johannes Guenther of Andernach and printed at Paris in 1531 by Simon de Colines.)

the minutest branches were exposed. He described the use of a blow pipe and other instruments employed in dissection. He envied those that had the opportunity to dissect human bodies, as may be deduced from his statement, "The doctors who attended Marcus Aurelius in the German wars dissected the dead bodies of the barbarians," leaving the impression that he himself did not have this unusual anatomical experience. He believed, however, that the anatomy of man could be learned from studies on animals. He did not appreciate the fact that the internal organs of beasts differed anatomically from those of human organs, just as their external aspects varied. For long past a millennium, physicians, following the teachings of Galen, held that the human sternum, or breast bone, was divided into sections like that of an ape, that the human womb had two long horns like that of a dog, and that the hip bone was spread out like that of an ox. Galen chanced to observe only two human bodies; one was a corpse washed out of its grave by the Nile and the other was that of an executed criminal left for the birds to devour. Both of these bodies only afforded him an opportunity to observe the skeletal system, since the soft tissues had decayed.

Skeletal Examinations: In his monograph on the skeleton, Galen recommended to the student that the bones be seen and handled, not merely studied from books. He advised students to go to Alexandria, where they could see human skeletons, and not to trust merely to the descriptions in books. He gave the following account of the manner in which he availed himself of his meager opportunities to study human anatomy:

I have examined human bones, when decayed tombs or monuments have fallen in my way. A sepulchre, slightly built on the brink of a stream, having suffered from the violence of the torrent which had overflowed it, the body carried away by the force of the current, stopped at last in a kind of harbor, bounded by pretty high banks. I had an opportunity of seeing this body, the flesh of which was already rotten, although the bones still adhered to each other; so that it resembled a skeleton prepared for the use of the student. At another time I saw the body of a robber lying on a mountain, remote from any public road. He had been killed by a traveller whom he attacked, and the inhabitants of the vicinity, conceiving so wicked a man a proper prey for the vultures, refused him the rights of burial; and, two days after, his bones were stripped of their flesh, and dry, like those prepared for students.

Interest in Anatomy: Galen strove hard to awaken an interest among contemporaries in the structure of the human body but was not able to overcome their indifference. In the 400 years that elapsed between Herophilus, Erasistratus, the founders of the Alexandrian schools of medicine, and Galen, the zeal for dissection had cooled off. The schools of the Methodists and Empirics did not consider a knowledge of anatomy necessary to practitioners of medicine.

Galen's Anatomic Concepts: Galen's anatomy was based partly on the Alexandrian anatomy and partly on that of his immediate predecessors, Marinus and Rufus Ephesus, but especially on his own dissections. He missed no opportunity of pointing out the importance of anatomy to medicine and declared that, although he seldom operated himself, he often saved his colleagues by timely warnings of surgical disaster. He told the story of a certain surgeon who unintentionally divided the median and ulnar nerves and the brachial vessels because of his ignorance of their position. The operator was so terrified that he only ligated the vessels, and the partially paralyzed patient avenged himself by following the surgeon on the street, calling after him, "You cut my nerves!"

He collected and collated all the knowledge of anatomy of his time and added numerous observations of his own for coming generations. He carefully described all the organs of the body; and although sometimes inaccurate for the reasons mentioned, his descriptions generally were a great advance over those of Hippocrates, Aristotle, and the Alexandrian anatomists.

The main difficulty with Galen's anatomic concepts was that he often made the structure of the human body fit his erroneous theories of physiology and the religious philosophy of his day. He believed in the concept of teleology, which assumed that the structure of every part of the functioning body was preconceived and followed a certain intelligent, purposeful plan. "In my view," stated Galen, "there is nothing in the body useless or inactive, but all parts are arranged to perform their offices together and have been endowed by the creator with specific powers."[4]

This school of teleology was by no means unanimously accepted, even by the Church. St. Augustine, for example, questioned the intelligence of placing the organs of reproduction between the organs of defecation and urination. As to modern scientists, Helmholtz, perhaps the greatest investigator in the field of physiologic optics, thought that the construction of the visual organs fell far short of perfection.

Galen's anatomic studies, however, were the best among ancient anatomists down to Vesalius in the sixteenth century. Even the latter hesitated to contradict him. When Vesalius demonstrated that the Galenic description of the hip bone was wrong, he apologized for deviating from Galen's teaching by stating that man had changed shape by wearing tight trousers.

Galen's osteology could hardly be surpassed. He counted over 200 bones in the human body. He divided the spinal column into cervical, dorsal, and lumbar regions and gave correct descriptions of the number of vertebrae and the articulations of each. He named the bones, the sutures of the cranium, and other structures.

From Galen's own words, it may be observed that he regarded comparative anatomy merely as an introduction to human dissection, without which the latter could not, in his opinion, be studied with sufficient advantage.

"It is easier," he observed, "for an experienced anatomist to detect at a glance what is familiar to his observation, and what is not, than for a novice to discover by close application what is most obvious."

Anatomic Terms: He introduced many new terms in osteology, one of which was *symphysis* for the point of junction of the fibrocartilage between bones. He named and described the styloid, squamous, mastoid, sphenoid, and ethmoid bones, and he described the malar, maxillary, and nasal bones, and nasal cartilages. Very little has been added to his descriptions in modern textbooks.

The muscles were less complete in the Galenic description, but they were nevertheless carefully reported. He was the first to introduce the names *platysma myoides* and *popliteus* and to describe these muscles. He correctly set forth the maxillary group of muscles, the six muscles of the eyeball, the two muscles of the eyelid, the muscles of the spine, head, neck, and extremities, the frontalis muscle, and the muscles of the body proper. Many of his descriptions and names have been adopted as standard and included in modern textbooks. He described the heart as having the appearance of a muscle; he erred, however, in the description of the structure of the heart, for he believed that there were pores in the interauricular and interventricular walls. Because of preconceived physiological concepts, he believed that the uterus had two cavities and that the glands were simply receptacles for excrementitious humors from excretory vessels. In his description of the intestine, he took the liberty to effect a compromise between the intestinal structures of the *carnivora* and *herbivora*, thus showing that he knew the difference between the two.

Circulatory System: His morphology of the circulatory system was that of his predecessors; the arteries he believed took their origin from the heart and the veins from the liver; the latter he considered a hemopoietic organ. The blood, he taught, flowed from the liver to the veins and entered the left ventricle. From there, it was distributed by the arteries to all parts of the body.

He rejected the idea that the arteries contained air. Galen gave a description of two meninges. He had no knowledge of the arachnoid membrane of the brain. He recognized seven cranial nerves. He knew that section of the optic nerve (through which the pneuma passed from the head to the eye) caused blindness, while severing the nerves of the intraocular muscles interfered with the mobility of the visual organs. He was of the opinion that the spinal cord was a sort of a lesser brain which served the lower part of the body. He identified spinal pathways.

The function of the nervous system, he believed, was to carry the pneuma or the vital spirit to all parts of the body. He taught that the nerves of sensation sprang from the brain; those of motion, from the spinal cord. He knew that the brain was the central organ of the nervous system.

In the anatomy of the blood vessels and lymphatics (angiology), he surpassed his predecessors and contemporaries. He described the aorta and the jugular veins. He recognized that the arteries had three coats. In his main work on anatomy and physiology "De Usu Partium," he stated, "The arteries and veins anastomose with each other throughout the whole body and exchange with each other blood and spirit, by certain invisible and exceedingly minute passages." Thus, he revealed a premonition of the capillaries.

GALENIC PHYSIOLOGY

Galen greatly assisted the advance of physiology by recognizing that every part of the body existed for the purpose of performing a definite function. His philosophy was greatly influenced by the teachings of Aristotle and Plato, who taught that "Nature makes nothing in vain." Galen's praise of the structure of man sounds more like "a religious hymn in honor of the Creator, who has given proof of His Omnipotence in creating everything perfectly conformable to its destination," than the view of a naturalist.

Galen followed the Ionian idea that matter was composed of the four elements—air, fire, earth, and water; he also favored the atomic doctrine that a body was composed of atoms and interspaces; and like his predecessors, he believed that the life-giving principle was invested in the soul, *pneuma*, or *spiritus*.

Pneuma, frequently occurring in Galen's writing, was used in two senses: (1) It referred to the inspired air which was drawn to the left side of the heart and thence carried all over the body by the arteries; here it was analogous to the modern concept of oxygen in respiration; (2) it also was used to refer to the vital principles carried by the veins and presided over by the subconscious vegetable life "nature," or *spiritus naturalis,* which was practically equivalent to nature itself.

Galen seems to have accepted most of the current theories as to the etiology of disease. He agreed with the doctrine of the four humors— the blood, the phlegm, the yellow bile, and the black bile. He accepted the existence of three kinds of spirits—the natural, the vital, and the animal. These served, in his opinion, as instruments to as many sorts of faculties, residing in the respective parts where these faculties were formed. The first of these was the "natural," the seat of which he supposed to be in the liver, where it presided over generation, growth, and nutrition. The next, the "vital," dwelt in the heart, whence it dispensed warmth and life to every part of the body, through the medium of the arteries. The third and noblest, the "animal," in conjunction with the governing or reasoning faculty, was lodged in the brain, where it presided over all the faculties and communicated the power of motion and sensation to every part of the body, through the medium of the nerves.

The blood was perfected in the heart, where it was supplied with the *calidum innatum* (innate heat) and then passed through the body. The pulse arose from an active dilating force, "pulse force," communicated to the arteries from the heart.

The heart was the seat of passion and courage. The brain was the seat of the rational soul and an organ for the secretion of mucus and for cooling the heart. The lungs also served to cool off the heart. The liver was the place for the preparation of the blood and the seat of love. The "animal spirits" were the cause of the soul's activity. They originated from the blood, but in the brain became the "animal spirits." From the origin of the "animal spirits," the dependence of mental impressions (and disturbances) upon the bodily condition was also explained. Galen divided mental disturbances into mania, melancholia, imbecility, and dementia. The origin of all these, he traced, like Hippocrates, to the first great cause.[5]

Respiration: Galen proved that quiet respiration was performed mainly by the diaphragm, but forced breathing by the intercostals as well, and that by inspiration the air entered mechanically into the expanded chest cavity. He was led to misinterpret experiments, to maintain that the pleural cavities were normally filled with air, whereby expansion and contraction were facilitated. According to Galen, respiration was shared by the heart and the entire arterial system, as well as by the lungs, the arteries receiving air through the skin in diastole and excreting "soot" through the same in systole. Accordingly, pulse and respiration served an identical purpose. He concluded that arterial pulsation was the result of power transmitted from the heart.

Nervous System: He believed that the brain was insensitive, that it possessed a movement synchronous with respiration, which served to drive the pneuma out of the ventricles into the nerves. The meninges were a support and covering and united the blood vessels. The spinal cord conducted sensation and movements. It was a sort of smaller

brain, controlling the parts below the head and sending out nerves
in streams.

If the cord was cut between the third and fourth cervical vertebrae,
respiration stopped; if between the cervical and dorsal, the animal only

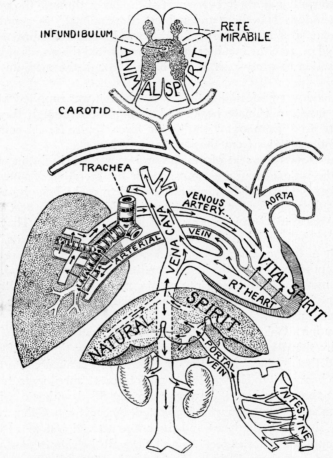

Fig. 153: Diagram illustrating Galen's physiological scheme of circulation.

breathed through the diaphragm and upper trunk muscles. Pressure
upon the brain induced stupor; injury to the fourth ventricle or upper
portion of the spinal cord was fatal. The seat of the soul was the
cerebrum. Pneuma played the chief part in the physiology of the senses.

Galen's chief physiological work was his investigations of the nervous
system, in which he made extensive use of vivisection. He distinguished

sensory, motor, and mixed nerve trunks. He traced the connection between the vagus and the sympathetic and showed the importance of
the recurrent nerves in the production of voice. Above all, he declared
that the nerves had no power in themselves, but merely conducted impulses to and from the brain and spinal cord. This knowledge gained
an advantage for Galen over the hated Methodics.

Pneuma: His idea of pneuma, however, differed from previous conceptions in that it could be interpreted as being composed of a material
element instead of a metaphysical substance, as understood by his predecessors. According to Galen, the pneuma was not a fixed entity blown
into the body at the time of birth or conception but something that
had to be constantly renewed through the inspired air of the world-
soul. He used the word "spirit," not only in a figurative sense, but also
in the generally accepted sense.

Galen's explanation of the physiology of digestion and nutrition was
very complicated:

The food enters the stomach; after it has undergone "coction", it proceeds
to the liver where it is changed into blood. From the liver it is carried to the
heart, whence a sufficient quantity of blood necessary for nutrition is expelled
through the pulmonary artery into the lungs; a smaller portion passes through
the (imaginary) pores of the heart septum into the left ventricle, where it is
mixed with the pneuma that entered the heart through the pulmonary veins
during diastole. No blood returns from the lungs to the heart; all of it is
used up for the nutrition of these organs. From the left side of the heart, the
blood mixed with the pneuma proceeds through the aorta to be transferred
finally into the veins by pore-like anastomoses at the termination of the
blood vessels. The nutrition of the body is thus supplied by the veins. The
remainder of the blood returns to the right side of the heart by a kind of ebb
tide in the venous circulation.

He knew that the systole forced the blood out of the heart cavity
and that the diastole drew blood into it. He compared the mode of
nutrition to the irrigation of a garden by a canal.

The function of respiration was to cool off the heat produced by the
heart and to introduce the pneuma, which passed from the lungs through
the pulmonary vessels. It is evident that Galen went beyond Aristotle
in the concept that the function of the pneuma was to maintain physiological body temperature.

The pneuma, "spirit," or life-giving principle, which in the body
formed the soul, was constantly taken from the renewed world-soul by
the act of respiration. It became the animal spirit when it came in contact with the brain and nerves; it became the vital spirit when it reached

the heart and arteries; and the natural spirit when it reached the liver and renal veins. These three physiological faculties kept in operation all the functions of the body.

Physiological Forces: Galen designated the forces upon which nutrition, assimilation, secretion, and muscular action depended as (1) attractive, (2) repulsive, (3) retentive, and (4) secretive. He described sixty "hard" motor nerves arising from the spine and seven "soft" sensory nerves originating from the brain. He also recognized the sympathetic nerves to which he ascribed the sensibility of the intestines. This complicated physiologic system was regulated and governed by a prmal force, the soul. Galen may be said to have been the first (down to the time of Servetus) to give a comprehensive theory of the circulation of the blood and to put the physiology of the nervous system on a scientific basis.

The Eye: Galen accepted the Alexandrian teachings. The crystalline lens was considered by him most essential to vision. He thought this to be proved by the fact that, in cases of hypochyma (cataract), in which a pathologic humor was formed between the cornea and the lens, vision was impaired. He characterized the lens as divine—*divinum oculi.* By other Greek physicians, it was known as *anima oculi,* the spirit, or soul, of the eye. Galen conceived the thought that the dark retina lined the posterior surface of the lens, thus forming a mirror from which objects were reflected, and on which impressions were registered and transmitted by the visual spirit via the hypothetically hollow optic nerves to the brain. Returning, the visual spirit followed the same route, coming from the brain to the lens and thence to the pneuma (the air which he believed to be in the anterior chamber) and to the cornea, where the process ended, and in some mysterious way vision took place. The mysterious third ventricle, the abode of the soul, was believed to be that part of the brain which translated this impression into vision. Reflection was the keynote of Galen's explanation of the visual phenomenon.

Because of the supposedly great importance of the lens to vision, Galen elaborated his theory that nature had located the crystalline lens safely between the soft and the watery humors, so that it was protected against injury from without by strong tunics and doubly fortified in front by the cartilaginous lids.[6] All the structures of the eye were provided only to safeguard this precious crystal.

The name "crystalline" was first mentioned by Celsus (25 B.C.–50 A.D.). "Under this," said Celsus, "is a drop of humor from which proceeds the faculty of vision, called by the Greeks 'chrystalloides'."

According to him the lens was separated from the cornea by a space which he called *locus vacuus*. This empty space, he thought, was the location of cataract, known as *suffusio*, and was believed by the ancient ophthalmologists to be caused by a diseased humor descending from the brain. The entire ancient world thought of the lens as a candle within a magic lantern, the rays of which were supposed to proceed outwardly to illuminate the dark path of the person.[7] Even as keen-

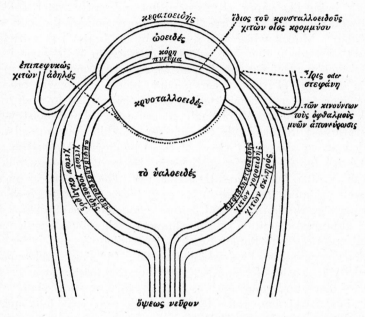

Fig. 154: The eye as described by Galen. (Reconstruction by Magnus.)

minded a person as Euclid,[8] the first to explain the visual act scientifically by mathematical diagrams and to point out that light emanated from the eye in the shape of a cone, "the visual cone," could not detach himself from such erroneous ideas.[9]

The Senses: The pneuma likewise occasioned smell by forcing its way into the anterior ventricles of the brain, which were the seat of this sense. Hearing originated in the penetration of the pneuma, in the form of waves, into the course of the nerve of hearing. He compared the propogation of sound to a wave.[10]

Temperaments: In direct opposition to what had been said concerning mental activity and its cause and seat, he explained the temperaments by the mixture of the elements and therefore divided them into

(1) the dry and warm (choleric), (2) dry and cold (melancholic), (3) moist and warm (sanguine), and (4) moist and cold (phlegmatic). The sensations again were dependent upon the animal spirit.

GALENIC PATHOLOGY

The Galenic view of pathology was founded upon the four elements, to which were attached the primary qualities. Fire represented hot and dry; air, being like vapor, represented hot and moist; water, cold and moist; and earth, cold and dry. To these, corresponded the four cardinal humors. Mucus, which was secreted by the brain, had in itself the element of water; yellow bile, which had its origin in the liver, had in itself the element of fire; black bile, which was formed in the spleen, had in itself the element of earth; while blood, which was prepared in the liver (an error committed by all ancients) had in itself a uniformly mixed element. Accordingly, mucus was cold and moist; yellow bile, warm and dry; black bile, cold and dry; and blood, warm and moist.

Galen accepted various views of the Dogmatists, Methodists, and Pneumatics, but he also was an Eclectic. He gave a foremost place to the four cardinal humors and their qualities. The doctrine of pneuma occupied an important place in his pathology. Galen attached more importance to the impurity and plethoric anomalies of the blood than to the abnormal condition of other humors, "whereby a way is paved to the transition from humoral to haemopathology."

Galen described four kinds of inflammation: (1) simple inflammation caused by an excess of blood; (2) inflammation arising as a result of excess of blood and pneuma; (3) erysipelas inflammation when yellow bile gained admission; and (4) cirrhosis or cancerous inflammation when phlegm was present.[11]

Causation of Disease: The causes of disease were divided into three classes: (1) remote causes (primitive or exciting); (2) antecedent, or predisposing; and (3) synectic (proximate, or conjunct). The first were external causes and included mechanical injuries and abnormalities, such as were associated with air, food, drink, rest, exercise, sleep and waking, excretions and retentions, and affections of the mind. The other two causes were internal. The second was due to a morbid condition of the body, which was antecedent to disease, and the third coincided with the disease. When the cause was present, the disease was also present and vice versa.[12]

To adopt a modern nomenclature, the exciting cause of disease (for example, in gout) could be due to overexertion or an excess of some kind. The predisposing cause was a morbid state of the humor which could be inherited. The proximate cause was the actual deposit of morbidity in the joint.

Diseases could be acute or chronic. Chronic diseases arose mainly from disorders of the phlegm and black bile. Acute diseases originated from anomalies of the yellow bile and blood. He rejected the Hippocratic division of disease into stages of crudity, coction, and crisis. He accepted coction of humors, crisis, and lysis, but not as stages of disease. He also accepted the doctrine of critical days, which he developed into a complete system; the most important day was the seventh. The concept of critical days was adhered to by physicians up to recent years.

Galen defined medicine as "a science which teaches what is sound and what is not so; and what is of an indifferent nature, or holds a middle place between what is sound and what is the reverse." In another of his books, which treated of the establishment of medicine, he defined it as an art which taught the preservation of health and the cure of disease.[13]

Symptoms of Disease: From the consideration of the causes of disease, he proceeded to the symptoms of disease, which he defined to be signs of "preternatural affection caused by or following a disease as a shadow does a body." He recognized three kinds of symptoms, the first and most numerous of which resulted from an injury, or interruption, of the action of the parts; the second, from a change of quality, unattended by any disturbance of function; and the last, from defects of excretion and retention.

The signs of disease he arranged under the heads of "diagnostic" and "prognostic," the former being employed to point out the distinctions between the several kinds of disease; the latter, collected from the species, violence, and peculiar character of each, enabled some opinion to be formed as to its probable duration, effects, and termination. The diagnostic symptoms he divided into pathognomic, or unvarying, symptoms, which, being peculiar to certain complaints, and uniformly present in their attacks, served as infallible marks of distinction; and adjuncts, or those which were common to many complaints, and served only to distinguish such as belonged to the same family, or genus.

Galen did not greatly advance in semeiology. He laid, however, much stress on the pulse. He wrote many elaborate treatises on this subject. His sphygmology stressed the motion, rapidity, force, tension, frequency, rhythm, regularity, and volume of the pulse. Of course, he employed the sense of inspection to its limits, observing all possible changes in the patient's body.

He also mentioned direct auscultation with reference to the hissing noise heard in case of penetrating wounds in the chest. Inspection of urine was also a routine practice. Of course, it was not with the intention of making a chemical examination. Attention was paid to the secretions and excretions with reference to color and sediment.

Doctrine of Indication: Galen promulgated the doctrine of "indication," which term comprised "whatever enables us to draw conclusions from as to treatment apart from experience"—a concept which the Empirics rejected entirely; to them, experience was the only rule of treatment. The Methodists reduced the method of treatment to one rule only, namely the restoration of the normal state of the pores by the use of contraries.

The first and the greatest indication was to remove the cause of disease or to prevent its action. A second indication arose from the symptoms, any of which could form a ground for treatment; if against nature, by "contraries;" if according to nature, by "similars."

Other sources of indications were the temperament of the patient, the season of the year, extreme circumstances generally, and the patient's dreams. He held that some drugs, such as emetics, purgatives, poisons, and their antidotes, acted through their whole substance and were in a sense specifics. Most drugs, according to Galen, acted through one of their elementary qualities, heat, cold, moisture, or dryness, which they possessed in a potential form; thus pepper and opium were potentially hot and cold respectively; each quality was divisible into four degrees. This theory has been worked by medieval physicians *ad absurdum*.

Prognosis: Galen's prognosis was based upon a scientific foundation. He utilized his knowledge of anatomy and physiology, and used his logical mind to foretell the outcome of a disease. With more piety than modesty, he said, "With the help of the deity, I have never been wrong." To his skill of prognosis, he owed much of his success as a practitioner. That his prognosis was generally accurate may be ascribed also to the careful clinical histories he kept.

Diseases: Galen observed a large number of diseases. Of those affecting the gastrointestinal system, catarrh, colic, dysentery, cholera, and intestinal parasites could be mentioned. He ascribed dysentery to intestinal ulceration, which was produced when the inner surface of the intestine was eroded by morbid juices. Cancerous ulceration was present when the stool had an ichorous appearance. Cholera was recognized by acute onset, thready pulse, cramps, and, in the later stages, unconsciousness. Intestinal worms were generated by putrefying material in the intestines in the presence of bodily heat. Jaundice was due to obstruction of the bile duct. Owing to the anatomic structure and the physiologic activity of the liver, it was subject to obstruction. Indigestible and raw foods were often the exciting cause.

Dropsy resulted from affection of the liver, spleen, kidneys, lungs, and intestines, as well as from retention of menstrual blood. Ascites produced shortness of breath and cough, by upward pressure of the fluid and by the collection of fluid under the diaphragm, as well as by secondary pressure on the lungs. The pulse in ascites was small, frequent, hard, and tense. Galen called attention to the so-called *morbus cardiacus,* often mentioned in ancient medical works. He objected to the name "colic" which signified an affection of the colon, since this pain could occur in any part of the abdomen.

He distinguished pneumonia from pleurisy and described the differential diagnosis. The former, he stated, was marked by dyspnea and bloody sputum, and he advised the physician to pay attention to the appearance of the sputum in the different stages of the disease. The nature of the sputum disclosed the humor causing the inflammation. Green, black, or foul-smelling excreta were favorable signs. The pulse and respiration were to be watched. The pulse could be full, abundant, frequent, at times hardly perceptible, and irregular. An intercurrent pulse was a sign of danger. The breathing in pneumonia was superficial and rapid; the more the air passages were obstructed, the greater the dyspnea.

On the other hand, in pleurisy, the pain was of a stitching character. The pulse was quick, frequent, of medium size, and the arteries were tense and hard. To differentiate it from liver disorders, attention should be paid to the stools, which in the latter were characteristic.

The treatments for pneumonia and pleurisy were almost identical. Poultices, blood letting, and purgation were the chief methods of treatment. Diarrhea was a bad omen and was an indication for the use of opium and diuretics. A light diet and wine were indicated when the excreta were scant. Galen did not treat the complication of pleurisy by empyema as fully as Hippocrates did.[14]

Galen held that nature had to be preserved by that which had relation to nature. Galen listed three sorts of principles in men: spirits, humors, and solids. He thought that between perfect health and disease there were three kinds of temperaments, or imperfect mixtures, compatible with the exercise of the functions of life. He agreed with

Hippocrates that diseases were cured by their contraries *(contraria contraribus curantur)*. He also agreed with the sage of Cos in the doctrines of coction, crisis, and critical days.

Galen distinguished an inflammatory and ulcerative form of phthisis and an insidious variety. As causes of phthisis, he mentioned laceration of the lung tissue and continued coughing and blood spitting. He differentiated stomach hemorrhages from those of the lungs by the fact that blood vomited from the stomach was dark in color and was expectorated without coughing, while blood coming from the lungs was bright and frothy and was expectorated with coughing.

As treatment for phthisis, he mentioned bandaging of the limbs, inunction, diets (preferably barley water), fruit, rest, and drugs to promote sleep as well as to reduce secretion. Here again, he laid stress upon the pulse which he described as small, weak, soft, quick, and "hectic."[15]

Salt sputum, diarrhea, and loss of hair were bad omens. In such cases, nourishing food (such as milk), relief from constipation, such remedies as balsamics, and such astringents as myrrh, turpentine, and Armenian bolus, were indicated. The best curative measure, however, was change of air through a sea voyage or a trip to Egypt. He urged residence in dry and elevated localities.

It is interesting here to note that Galen realized the infectious nature of consumption when he said, "Consumptives emit foul emanations and fetid odor into the room they inhabit. It is a matter of experience that those who sleep in the same bed with consumptives fall into consumption and that those who live long with them, eat and drink with them, or wear their clothes and linen attract the disease."[16]

Inflammation of the kidneys was an illness which could last throughout life. Deficiency of secretion of urine was caused by obstruction of the urinary passages, dense urine, coagulated blood, inflammation, paralysis of the bladder, or irritative urine. In overretention, Galen advised the use of the catheter. Renal calculi came from the same origin as gout.

The treatment of stone in the bladder and gout demanded the use of asses' milk, urine with honey as a diuretic, and such drugs as myrrh, parsley, caraway, ammoniacum, and the powder found in sponges. Renal colic could be differentiated from intestinal colic by the use of purgatives. In intestinal colic, the pain would disappear; in renal it would not. Galen believed that diabetes was due to a loosening of the kidneys, hence the frequent micturition.

The treatment of gastric disturbance consisted of emetics, covering the head and stomach regions with hot cloths, twenty-four hours of fasting, and under certain conditions cold compresses to the epigastrium.

Headache was caused by humoral derangement, strong odors, drinking unwholesome water, or the penetration of air into the veins. Migraine was due to abdominal affections, such as gas and morbid humors, entering the veins and penetrating the head. The seat of the pain was in the ventricles of the brain. Vertigo was mostly cerebral in origin. Apoplexy was influenced by plethora and accumulation of phlegm in the ventricles and in the substance of the brain. Respiratory paralysis led to death.

Epilepsy was caused by obstruction of the cavities of the brain with phlegm or black bile. It was known as "the disease of Hercules." The treatment consisted of venesection in the regions of the feet, dietetic measures, and the administration of treacle.

Lethargy was localized in the meninges and caused by sluggish phlegm. Galen held this to be a dangerous condition.

Melancholia occurred in two forms. In one, the whole mass of blood was affected; in the other, only that of the brain. Where the whole mass of blood was affected, blood letting was an important part of the cure. Amenorrhea, abstinence from sexual intercourse, grief, and worry were predisposing factors.

Mania owed its origin to watery bilious humors and was distinguished from phrenitis by the lack of fever. Galen ascribed skin diseases to a gouty diathesis.

MATERIA MEDICA AND THERAPEUTICS

Galen delineated the duties of the physician and his behavior in the sick room. Visits should be made regularly but not too often. The physician should not be burdensome through loud speech. He should accommodate himself to the level of the patient's education, inclination, and habits.

In materia medica and therapeutics, Galen was not as proficient as Dioscorides. Galen was in the habit of prescribing many drugs in one prescription. He paid high prices for various nostrums; and strange as it may seem, he placed great faith in amulets. He classified medicines according to their qualities, their inherent dryness or moistness, coldness or heat, and not according to their therapeutic effects. Cistus (rock-rose) he prescribed, for its astringent and gently cooling powers, in all kinds of fluxions. He insisted that in all cases the cause of the disease was to be treated and not the symptoms. Strong remedies were not to be used on weak patients.

Surgery: Aside from minor surgery, such as attendance to abscesses, treatment of wounds, and phlebotomy, Galen conformed to the general custom of the physicians in Rome. He seldom used the lancet. He had but a superficial knowledge of medical and surgical gynecology. He mentioned a variety of surgical instruments, but these were intended for general information, not for use. He gave careful directions for the treatment of wounds and ulcers. Hemorrhage was stopped by cold applications, astringents, sutures, ligatures, and cautery.

His teachings on fractures and dislocations showed many advances over those of Hippocrates. He mentioned a case of resection of the sternum with exposure of the heart. He described resection of the rib in empyema. He set forth a plastic operation in cases of defects of the nose, ears, and lips. His description of the treatment of lymphatic gland abnormalities and fistulas cannot be surpassed. Obstetrics were not fully treated in Galen's works. It is interesting to note that he was of the opinion that presentations other than those of the vertex were rare.

Diseases of the Eye: He had very little to say on diseases of the eye. He mentioned cataract, which he ascribed partly to the cloudiness of lens and partly to the ocular humor, but he did not state by which method the cataract was removed—whether by couching or extraction after incision.

Hygiene: Galen wrote on hygiene but not in such a way as to add materially to that subject. He advocated fresh air, exercise, gymnastics, and hunting. He recommended bathing, especially for the aged, for whom, according to his theory, hot baths counteracted their "cold and dry" natural condition. For the same reason, he advised wine for the aged. Old persons, he stated, required three meals a day. In his work "De Sanitate Tuenda," he stated, "The games which afford relaxation to mind and body are the best."

Drugs: He was the first writer to have turned his attention to the art of obtaining the aroma of plants and flowers by distillation; he left behind him a description of the process. He revealed the curious fact that starlings were fattened upon hemlock, which was poisonous to man. He was aware that animal poisons were harmless to man until mingled with the blood of the person inoculated. He observed that "nothing has the same power upon the human body outwardly as inwardly. Thus, neither the venom of the viper, nor of the asp, nor the frothy spittle of the mad dog, is alike mischievous when it falls upon the skin or enters the stomach, as when outwardly communicated by a wound." In confirmation of this, he adduced the fact that Cleopatra killed herself by introducing the poison of an asp into a wound made in her arm with her own teeth. He mentioned the powerful influence which habit exterted over the system in rendering it insensible to the effects of many of the most virulent poisons, as exemplified in the case of a woman who gradually accustomed herself to the use of hemlock of which she was able to take considerable quantities without the slightest injury. In his book on the art of preserving health, speaking of the influence of music, he stated that "Aesculapius was in the habit of curing those, in whom violent emotions of the mind had induced a hot temperament of the body, by melody and songs."

Diabetes: Diagnosed cases of diabetes appear to have been a rarity among the ancients, since we find little notice taken of it by any of the writers who preceded Galen. Galen himself acknowledged that he met with but two cases of it.

GALENIC CRITICISM OF OTHER METHODS

Galen criticized severely many of the medical and surgical specialists of his own time who acted on the assumption that the whole was merely the sum total of its parts and that, if a patient was ailing and the affected parts were treated individually, the health of the whole organism was affected. His medical system was intended to strike a balance between the excessive learning of the Dogmatists and the loose practicality of the Empirics.

Galen severely criticized the Methodists who looked on disease as something fixed and finite, an independent entity, to be considered entirely apart from its original setting. It is to Galen's merit that he crystallized and brought to focus all the best works of the Greek medical schools which preceded his own time in a form which was essentially Galenic and which, as such, was transmitted to succeeding ages. He laid the foundation upon which subsequent medicine was constructed.

SPREAD OF GALENIC MEDICINE

In the fourth century A.D., the Byzantine physicians of Emperor Julian made the huge mass of Galenic writings available to the ordinary practitioner. Galenic medicine spread throughout Syria and thence was carried by the Nestorians into Persia, where it became implanted, eventually spreading to the Mohammedan world. In the ninth century, Galen was translated into Arabic and was used as a textbook for seven centuries throughout the east by Hebrew and Arabic scholars.

Arabian sovereigns, such as Harun al-Rashid and Abdul Rahman III, were great patrons of Greek learning, especially medicine. They at least partially followed the doctrines of Aristotle and Galen. With the exception of pharmacology, the Arabs made no independent contributions to medicine. They were essentially systematizers and commentators.

Averroes, in the twelfth century, introduced Aristotle to the Mohammedan world. Avicenna (Ibn Sina 980–1037 A.D.), who was the most famous Muslem authority on medicine for a period of 400 years and who in certain respects, overshadowed Galen himself, was a close follower of Galenic medicine. In the eleventh century, Latin translations of the Arabic texts began to make their way into Europe. This undermined the authority of the school of Salerno, a native western school, where hitherto the teachings of Aristotle and Galen had assumed a position of supreme authority. The scholastic philosophy became blended with the schools of Naples and Montpelier, and this intermixture became the final word on the science of medicine. In 1453, Constantinople fell into the hands of the Turks. The Byzantine scholars, when they fled from the Byzantine countries, took along the original versions of the Greek works to Europe, which reawakened a great interest in the study of Galen and Aristotle. Prominent among the humanists' movement was the English physician Thomas Linacre (c. 1460–1524), who, after returning from Italy where he gained an extraordinary zeal for the new learning, devoted the rest of his life to the promotion of humanistic scholarship and especially to making Galen accessible to Latin readers.

Galen's fame kept up to the days of Paracelsus (sixteenth century), who broke away completely from Greek classical medicine. "Let us do away with all authority whatsoever and get back to nature," he cried out at his first lecture as professor of medicine at Basle. He symbolically burned the works of Galen and Avicenna in the presence of his students.

The final collapse of Galenic authority in medicine was brought about by the Renaissance anatomists, particularly those of the Italian school, who finally toppled Galenism to the ground. Among these were Vesalius (1514–1565), Michael Servetus (1509–1553), and Andrea Cescalpino.

SCOPE OF GALENIC MEDICINE

There was scarcely a subject in medicine, and few outside, which was not covered by Galen's versatile genius. His books on all branches of knowledge number over 600. As a philosopher, he was in the tradition of Plato and Aristotle. His writings on this subject were studied diligently and were quoted for ages. In philosophy, as in medicine, he was an Eclectic and did not adhere to any particular school. He selected what seemed to him the best of all schools. Galen's full importance to medicine was not recognized until after his death.

The best and most modern edition of Galen's work is that of Kuhn, published in twenty volumes between 1821 and 1833. There are several German and French translations of the most important treatises. A list of his works is given in Smith's "Dictionary of Greek History and Roman Mythology."

APPRAISAL OF GALEN

There has been a tendency among historians to emphasize a difference in the personality of Hippocrates and Galen—the two greatest physicians in the history of ancient medicine. The following appraisal by Withington, is not complimentary to Galen:

Hippocrates separated medicine from philosophy; Galen reunited them. Hippocrates relied on observation, and little on theory; Galen, if he did not reverse it, at least thought theory was of equal value. Hippocrates believed that medicine was the greatest art; Galen strove to convert it to a philosophy, accepting the Dogmatic motto: "The physician who is also a philosopher, is godlike." Hippocrates related what he observed briefly and simply in order that others might do likewise. Galen introduced his observation either to show how much cleverer he was than his colleagues or at best to exemplify or support some particular theory of his own. Hippocrates or one of his pupils said science and belief were two things; the one begat knowledge, the other ignorance; Galen occasionally held them to be compatible. There can be no question as to who was the greatest of the two men, but had Galen's work been lost there can be little doubt that the Dark Age would have been much darker and prolonged than it was, for the medieval practitioner could not appreciate the higher art.

Galen was the last of the Greeks to carry the banner of medical science and philosophy in the twilight of antiquity. With his death, the dark shadows of stagnation swept over Europe. The transference of the world capital from Rome to Constantinople marked a decline in scientific investigation in the period that followed the fall of Rome. Students contented themselves with blindly following the writings of the Greek and Roman masters. Their greatest ambition was to be able to comment on the texts of the classical teachers. Medicine ceased to be a living issue, and classical antiquity came to an end.

ORIBASIUS

After Galen, the last prominent physician of antiquity, and a great compiler of medical knowledge, was Oribasius of Pergamos, physician and friend of Emperor Julian (360–363). It was at the Emperor's suggestion that he composed a medical collection of seventy books; only about a third of these works have survived.

References and Notes

1. Prenotione ad Posthuman, Chapter 11. Cited by Neuburger, M.: History of Medicine, pp. 248-249.
2. Hamilton, W.: History of Medicine, Surgery, and Anatomy. London, 1831.
3. The Natural Faculties. English translation by Brook, A. J.: Wm. Putnam Sons, New York. Cited by Neuburger, M.: History of Medicine, p. 248.
4. Neuburger, M.: History of Medicine. Oxford University Press, London, 1910.
5. Ibid.
6. Shastid, T. H., in Wood, C. A.: American Encyclopedia and Dictionary of Ophthalmology. Cleveland Press, Chicago, Vol. 11, 1917, p. 8595.
7. Draper, J. W.: The Intellectual Development of Europe. Harper and Bros., New York, Vol. 2, 1876, p. 279.
8. Seligmann: Geschichte der Medizin und Krankheiten. Jahresb. ü. d. Leistung. d. ges. Med., 1:388, 1877.
9. Gordon, B. L.: The Problem of the Crystalline Lens. Arch. Ophth., 14: 774-788, Nov., 1935.
10. Falk: Galenus' Lehre Vom Nerven Systeme. Leipzig, 1871.
11. Draper, J. W.: Cultural Development of Europe. Harper and Bros., New York, Vol. 1, p. 180.
12. Withington, E. T.: History of Medicine. London, 1904.
13. Cited in "History of Medicine, Surgery, and Anatomy."
14. "History of Medicine," pp. 250-251.
15. Ibid.
16. Gasquet: The Practical Medicine of Galen in His Time. Medico Chirurgical Press, 1867.

30

Talmudic Medicine

INTRODUCTION

THE medical literature that has come down to us from the third to the end of the fifth century A.D., with a few notable exceptions, is marked by stagnation and decay. Independent observation, rational thinking, and practical skill were rare. Pathology, that branch of medicine which treats of the essential nature of disease and especially of the structural and functional changes caused by disease, was *terra incognita*. The vast majority of people around the Mediterranean and its hinterlands looked upon disease as a calamity brought about by supernatural rather than by natural forces; and in the event of sickness, advice was solicited from healers supposed to possess divine knowledge. The art of medicine was usurped by priests, and their temples served as hospitals. To the Hebrews, and later to the Christians, the Bible was the source of all wisdom, even though the Bible was not intended to be a medical work.

Christianity took under its wings those that were diseased spiritually and physically. Jesus is referred to as the physician of body and soul. The gospels contain many medical similes, and the care of the sick is enjoined as one of the most sacred duties of Christianity. Later, when Rome succumbed to the onslought of the Northern Barbarians, medicine was compelled by the stress of the time to find asylum in monastic cells. The nature of treatment is shown in St. James, "If anyone is sick among you let him call for the elders of the church: and let them pray over him, anointing him with oil in the name of the Lord and the prayers of faith shall save the sick and the Lord shall raise him up. Pray for one another and ye shall be healed."[1]

725

Alexandria, which was the medical center of the world for over 500 years, had lost its prestige during the reign of a Ptolemy, who expelled the learned masters and their students from the academies; and while Alexandria regained some of its prestige one half century later, it never received enough vigor to assert itself medically. Medicine was mainly dominated by the Empirics, whose views on medicine were narrow and whose knowledge was scanty as compared with the medical leaders of a century back.

Medical Literature: The remnant of Jews in Palestine who were not uprooted by the Roman conquerors rebelled against Roman culture and devoted their intellectual energy to the study of their law. They established academies in Tiberias, Sepphoris, and Caesarea; and those who dwelt in Mesopotamia established academies at Nehardea, Nisibis, Machoza, Pumpeditha, and Sura where all known sciences were discussed (if not directly, at least to illustrate certain points of law) under the leadership of various savants, the most famous of which were Rab and Samuel. The result of the discussions at the academies of Palestine and Babylonia was later incorporated in two large encyclopedic works known as the Palestinian and the Babylonian *Talmudim.*

Pliny refers to a certain physician named Zachalias (perhaps Zachalias, an Alexandrian Jewish physician) who dedicated a book on medicine to Mithridates the Great.[2] Wunderbar refers to Theodus, or Theudas, of Laodicea (70 A.D.), a student of Alexandria and famous in the school of the Empirics, as being a Jew.[3] In his work on medicine, now lost, Theodus of Laodicea classified medical practice into (1) diagnosis, (2) therapeutics, and (3) convalescence. His views on the methods of observation and the value of experience were a valuable contribution to ancient medical literature. He held that observation of an effective remedy in one case was all that was needed to achieve good results in a similar case. Theodus, however, availed himself of the therapeutic experience of others. He was not a worshipper of tradition as the other Empirics were. It is evident that such a personality would arouse the antagonism of the Dogmatics who relied entirely upon tradition.

The Mishna[4] mentions a book on therapeutics called "Sefer Refuoth,"[5] and the Talmud[6] speaks of a work in pharmacology named "Megillath Sammin,"[7] neither of which has survived the ravages of time.

Hebrew literature reveals that the Jews had great faith in medical arts and practices. To quote the author of Ecclesiasticus (second and third centuries B.C.), "If you are taken ill, offer prayers to God and place yourself under the care of a physician."[8] Talmudic teachers urged their pupils not to wait until they were sick to consult a physician, "Be attentive to the instruction of your physician while you are well."[9] "No one should think that the Lord will do miracles for him and cure him Himself."[10] Self cure was discouraged, "One that is chained cannot free himself. . . . It is prohibited to live in a town where there is no physician."[11]

Duties of Physicians: The duties of the patient to his physician and the obligation of the physician to the patient were regulated. "An out-of-town physician has a blind eye[12] (that is lacks personal feeling)." Dispensing free medical services was not approved, "A physician who takes nothing is worth nothing."[13] The physicians' fees, while not regulated by the state, appeared at least in one case to have been liberal, for it is recorded that Tobit paid his physician five silver talents (about ten dollars) for one eye treatment (leukoma).[14] This is the average fee for an eye specialist at the present time.

There were, among the Hebrews, district and communal physicians who were employed to give expert testimony as to the character and extent of physical disability sustained in cases of injury,[15] or in the event the court decreed corporal punishment to an offender, they were to appraise the physical endurance of the person to be punished.[16] District physicians were selected by the elders of the community upon the recommendation of the board of physicians.[17]

The authority to practice medicine was received from the judges of the community after the applicant had served a period of apprenticeship under a reputable medical practitioner. The Talmud names two kinds of physicians: *rophe omman*[18] (skilled physician) and *rophe mumche* (expert physician). The Talmud differentiates between a licensed physician duly authorized by the judge of the community and the physician that practices without authority. It is reasonable to assume that the candidate to whom the judge granted authority to practice had to pass some kind of medical test. The right to practice the healing art was occasionally also transmitted from father to son.[19]

The authority to practice medicine was not granted in the Talmudic academies, although medical subjects were frequently discussed and many of the masters were celebrated physicians.[20] The studies in the academies were usually theoretical in character, and medical subjects were only indirectly alluded to for the purpose of illustrating certain points of law.

Indeed, lay-physicians were often consulted by the academies in order to clarify certain points of law. A famous physician known as Theodorus (Theodus) Harophe[21] was consulted by the academy of Jabneh as to whether or not an animal could live without a uterus. Rabbi Ishmael, the head of the academy, thought that the animal could not live any length of time without that organ and that its flesh, therefore, could not be used for food. Theodorus gave as his opinion that the absence of the womb did not endanger life and that the meat, therefore, could be eaten. He added that all cattle leaving Egypt had their generative organs removed so that the fine species of cattle of Egypt could not be cultivated elsewhere.[22]

Hospitals: It is not clear whether hospitals were provided for the ailing by the ancient Hebrews. The sick were certainly not admitted to the synagogues as was the custom among the Egyptians and Greeks, who believed that disease came from the gods and that there was no better place to reach the gods than in the temples. Perhaps the Jews at the beginning of the present era followed the Babylonian custom of taking care of the indigent sick in the open air.[23] Because of the mild climate of Palestine, open air hospitals were feasible, at least during certain periods of the year.

It is related that one day Rabbi Ishmael and his colleague Rabbi Akiba were administering to the sick in the streets of Jerusalem when a passing peasant, observing their action, asked them, "Aren't you interfering with the ways of the Lord? The Lord punished them with sickness for their sins and you are trying to heal them." "Aren't you doing the same thing?" the sages replied. "God created the earth to provide mankind with food and you don't wait for him to plough, fertilize, and sow, but you do it yourself."[24] Bringing the sick outside to benefit from contact with holy men is reflected in the New Testament, ". . . they brought forth the sick into the streets, and laid them on beds and couches, that at least the shadow of Peter passing by, might overshadow some of them."[25] In later years, it became a custom among Jews to utilize the anteroom of the synagogue for hospital purposes.

Medical Instruction: The method of medical instruction was largely practical. The student accompanied his preceptor as he made the rounds of his patients. In the aforementioned case of Theodorus, it is stated that he took along his students with him. This appears to have been the usual procedure also among the Greeks and Romans.[26] Besides clinical instruction, the Hebrew student also received theoretical teaching. The Midrash mentions at least one case of a student who remarked to his preceptor, "You have long taught me the principles of medicine."[27]

Research: The fanatical adherence to, and high respect for, tradition was a great hindrance to the progress of medicine among all peoples;

tradition and authority were almost worshipped. Independent inquiry and personal observation were generally frowned upon when the results ran counter to ancient authority. Investigation was almost wholly restricted to the study of the writings of Aristotle, Hippocrates, Ptolemy, and Galen. To question their authority was impiety. The highest ambition of a scholar was to be able to explain and to comment on the teachings of the great masters, whose doctrines they followed blindly.

There were, however, among the Talmudists, those like Rab (third century Babylonian teacher), who, while respecting tradition and experience, did not neglect personal investigation and research. It is related that Rab lived eighteen months among shepherds in order to observe diseases of the eye among cattle.[28]

ANATOMY

While the study of human anatomy was still in its infancy, personal observation on human cadavers was not completely excluded from the Talmudic student. The students of Rabbi Ishmael, in spite of the fact that the presence of dead bodies necessitated isolation for seven days, dissected a human body in order to verify certain anatomical teachings.

Osteology

It is related that the students of R. Ishmael (100 A.D.), who doubted the generally accepted tradition that the number of bones in the human body was 248, obtained the executed body of a young harlot, subjected the body to a boiling process in order to get rid of the soft tissues, and found the number of bones to be 252.[29] Of course, neither of the numbers mentioned corresponds to the teaching of modern osteology, but the differences may be ascribed to the youthful age of the subject used for dissection.

The larger number of bones enumerated by the Mishna in no way reflects the anatomic knowledge of the Talmudic anatomists. No two anatomists agreed on this point. Hippocrates, for example, counted only 91 bones in the body; and counting the nails among the bones, he raised the number to 111.[30] Galen counted more than 200 bones, but he did not commit himself as to the exact number. Curiously enough, the celebrated Muslim physicians, Avicenna (1037) and Abulkasim (1106), who usually followed the teachings of Galen, listed 248 bones in the skeleton—the figures given by the Talmud. Modern anatomists, depending on their classification, also differ; the figures run between 200 and 226.

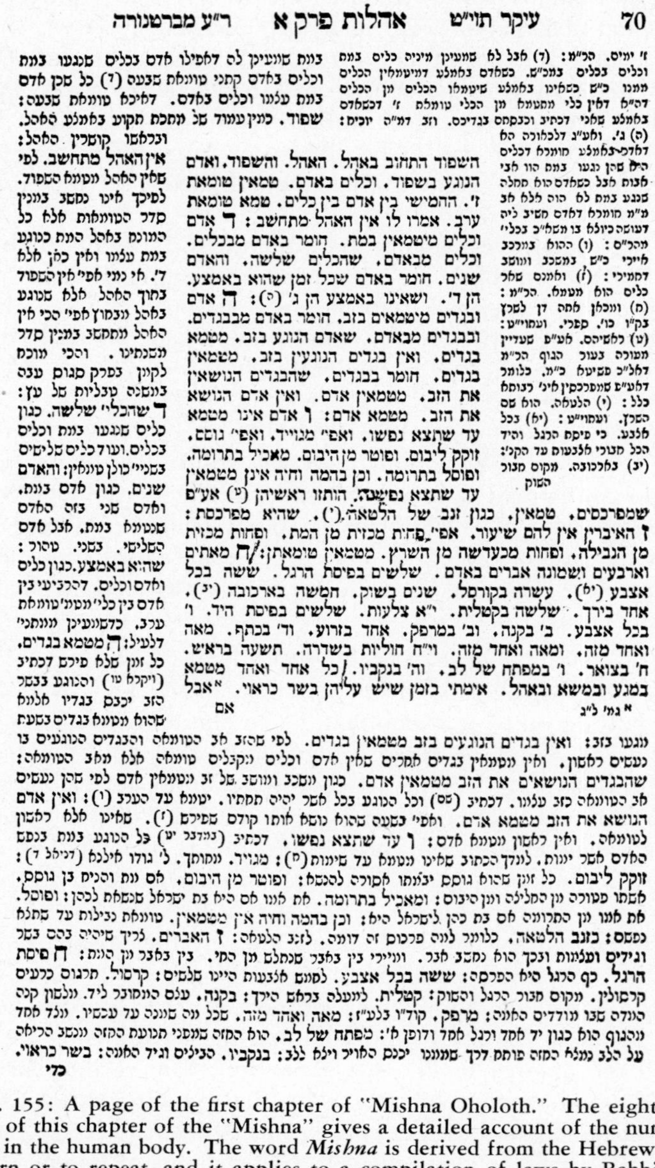

השפוד התחוב באהל. האהל. והשפוד. ואדם
הנוגע בשפוד וכלים באדם. טמאין טומאת
ז. החמישי בין אדם בין כלים. שמא טומאת
ערב. אמרו לו אין האהל מתחשב: ד אדם
וכלים מיטמאין במת. חומר באדם מבכלים.
וכלים מבאדם. שהכלים שלשה. והאדם
שנים. חומר באדם שהכל זמן שהוא באמצע.
הן ד'. ושאינו באמצע הן ג' (ס): ה אדם
ובגדים מיטמאים בזב. חומר באדם מבבגדים.
ובבגדים מבאדם. שאדם הנוגע בזב. מטמא
בגדים, ואין בגדים הנוגעין בזב. מטמאין
בגדים. חומר בבגדים. שהבגדים הנושאין
את הזב. מטמאין אדם, ואין אדם הנושא
את הזב. מטמא אדם: ו אדם אינו מטמא
עד שתצא נפשו. ואפי' מגוייד. ואפי' גוסס.
זוקק ליבום. ופוטר מן היבום. מאכיל בתרומה.
ופוסל בתרומה. וכן בהמה וחיה בהמה מטמאין
עד שתצא נפשם. הותזו ראשיהן (ט') אע"פ

שמפרכסים. טמאין. כגון זנב של הלטאה (י'). ז שהוא מפרכס:
ז האיברין אין להם שיעור. אפי'. פחות מכזית מן המת. ופחות מכזית
מן הנבילה. ופחות מכעדשה מן השרץ. מטמאין טומאתן (ח) מאתים
וארבעים ושמונה אברים באדם. שלשים בפיסת הרגל. שישה בכל
אצבע (יא). עשרה בקורסל. שנים בשוק. חמשה בארכובה (יג'). ו'
אחד בירך. שלשה בקטלית. י"א צלעות. שלשים בפיסת היד. ו'
בכל אצבע. ב' בקנה. וב' במרפק. אחד בזרוע. וד' בכתף. מאה
ואחד מזה. ומאה ואחד מזה. וי"ח חוליות בשדרה. תשעה בראש.
ח' בצואר. ו' במפתח של לב. וה' בנקביו. /כל אחד ואחד מטמא
במגע ובמשא ובאהל. אימתי בזמן שיש עליהן בשר כראוי. *אבל

Fig. 155: A page of the first chapter of "Mishna Oholoth." The eighth paragraph of this chapter of the "Mishna" gives a detailed account of the number of
bones in the human body. The word *Mishna* is derived from the Hebrew *Shana*,
to learn or to repeat, and it applies to a compilation of laws by Rabbi Judah
(c. 200 A.D.), a contemporary of Galen. The "Mishna" is divided into six parts;
the last part is known as *Taharoth*, which deals with cleanliness; *Oholoth* is a
subdivision of this section.

The difference is best seen when certain parts of the skeleton are viewed separately, such as for example the spinal column. Hippocrates knew of 22 but Galen counted 24 bones.[31] The Arabic physicians also enumerated 24 vertebral bones.[32] The school of Salerno, which as a rule followed the anatomy of Galen in this respect, gave the number of vertebrae as 18 as in the Talmud. Modern anatomists count 33 vertebral bones. The differences in these figures may be due to the fact that the older anatomists did not count the vertebral bones of the neck and the lower spine in their figures. R. Hiyah compared the bones to the pillars of a house;[33] if it were not for the bones, men would creep like worms on the ground.

Talmudic osteology divided the body into two parts,[34] namely (1) the trunk, including the four extremities; and (2) the neck and head. The trunk, again, was divided, (a) sagittally, into the two sides, right and left; and (b) coronally, into the back and the front. Hence, arose the following scheme:

I. TRUNK AND EXTREMITIES

A. The Two Sides.
  1. Lower Limbs.
    a. Phalanges 15
    b. Metatarsals 5
    c. Tarsals 8   40 (foot, tarsals)
    d. Malleoli 2
    e. Unidentified 10
    f. Leg (tibia, fibula) 2   (leg)
    g. Patella 1
    h. Inner and outer tuberosities 4   6 (knee)
    i. Femur 1
    k. Ilium 1
    l. Ischium 1   3 (pelvis)
    m. Pubes 1
  2. Middle.
    Ribs 11   (ribs)
  3. Upper Limb.
    a. Scapula 1
    b. Clavicle 1
    c. Acromion process 1   4 (shoulder)
    d. Coracoid process 1
    e. Humerus 1   (humerus)
    f. Olecranon process 1
    g. Capitellum of humerus 1   2 (elbow)
    h. Radius and ulna 2   (forearm)

I. TRUNK AND EXTREMITIES (*Continued*)

i.	Styloid processes	2	
j.	Carpals	8	
k.	Metacarpals	5	30 (hand)
l.	Phalanges	15	
	Total......101 x 2 = 202		

B. Back, or spinal column (exc. cervical vertebrae).

1.	Dorsal vertebrae....................	12	
2.	Lumbar vertebrae...................	5	18 (vertebrae)
3.	Sacrum, coccyx.....................	1	

C. Front, or breast.

1.	Sternum and		
2.	Costal cartilages	6	
	Total of Trunk and Extremities	226	6 (key of heart)

II. HEAD AND NECK

A. Head.

  1. Cranium.

a.	Frontal bones	2	
b.	Parietal bones	2	9 (head)
c.	Occipital bone	1	
d.	Temporal bones	2	
e.	Malar bones	2	

  2. Openings.

a.	Mouth (maxillaries)	2	
b.	Ear (pinna)	2	5 (openings)
c.	Nose (cartilage)	1	

B. Neck.

1.	Vertebrae	7	
2.	Windpipe	1	8 (neck)
	Total of Head and Neck...........	22	
	Grand Total of Skeleton...........	248	

In addition to the 248 bones there were 365 *giddin* (membranes), the meaning of which is not clear but which perhaps includes tendons, nerves, and blood vessels that were not generally distinguished at that period, although Hippocrates, Erasistratus, Herophilus, and particularly Galen knew the difference between them. The Talmud has little to say about the muscles of the body. Muscles were generally included in the *ebarim* (limbs).[35]

The Brain

The Talmud, however, shows profound knowledge of the internal organs of the body.[36] The brain was referred to as *moach* and the

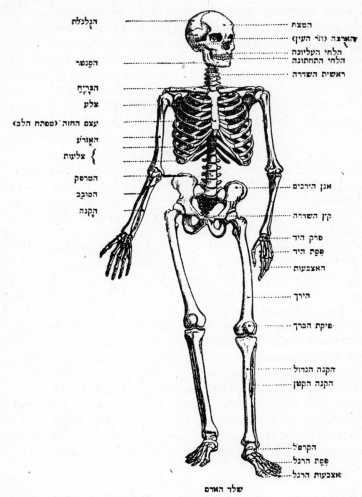

הגֻלגלֹת ⋯⋯⋯ המצח
⋯⋯ הָאַרֻבה (חֹר העין)
⋯⋯ הלחי העליונה
⋯⋯ הלחי התחתונה
הקַנטֹר ⋯⋯ ראשית השדרה
הבְּרְיַח ⋯⋯
צלע ⋯⋯
יעצם החזה (טפחת הלב) ⋯⋯
האֻזרֹע ⋯⋯
{ צלעות ⋯⋯
המרסק ⋯⋯ אגן הירכים
הסובב ⋯⋯
הקֻנה ⋯⋯ קֵץ השדרה
⋯⋯ פרק היד
⋯⋯ פפת היד
⋯⋯ האצבעות
⋯⋯ הירך
⋯⋯ פיקת הברך
⋯⋯ הקנה הגדול
⋯⋯ הקנה הקטן
⋯⋯ הקרסֹל
⋯⋯ פפת הרגל
⋯⋯ אצבעות הרגל

שלד האדם

Fig. 156: Hebrew nomenclature of the bones of the human skeleton.

spinal cord as *chut*. The brain was separated from the spinal cord by two beanlike projections, *pullin*,[37] known as the "occipital condyles." Within the *pullin* was the brain and without was the cord.[38]

The brain was covered by two membranes, the dura and the pia mater. The arachnoid was not recognized. There were three cavities in the skull, occupied by three kinds of brainy matter: cerebral, cerebellar, and pons. Thirty-two nerve branches originated from the brain and spinal cord which were distributed throughout the entire body.[39]

Above the forehead (in the median line) was the fontanel which was soft and pulsating in infants.[40] The brain and spinal cord were interdependent.[41] R. Judah considered the brain as the center of intelligence, as is seen from his sarcastic remark, "It appears to me that he has no marrow in his skull."[42] In an argument between R. Eliezer and R. Joshua, the first emphatically declared that the intellect was located in the head,[43] notwithstanding the fact that the Bible ascribed, to the heart and kidneys, the qualities of thought, emotion, and sensation.

The Heart

The heart was described as consisting of two chambers, *beth halal katan* and *beth halal gadol* (small and large cavities).[44] It was located toward the left.[45]

Amemar cites R. Nachman to the effect that there were three vessels in the chest cavity: One was connected to the heart, *koneh ha-leb* (the aorta); one was connected with the lungs, *vena kaba* (superior *vena cava*); and one was connected with the liver, *vena kaba*[46] (inferior *vena cava*). According to Rab, the smallest perforation in the aorta, *koneh ha-leb,* was fatal. Mar Samuel thought that only a big hole was fatal.[47] Katzenelenson was of the opinion that Samuel held the Aristotelian view that the aorta contained air. A small leak, therefore, was not fatal. On the other hand, Rab knew that the aorta contained blood, and therefore the smallest opening could prove deadly. Both large vessels of the neck were known in the Talmud as *vridin.*

The heart was never at rest like the other organs. It kept continuously contracting and dilating. The "Zohar" knew of the auricles and ventricles, and also the mechanism of the pulse.[48] The heart, because of its great import to life, received careful attention. "The life of all organs depends upon the heart."[49]

The Lungs

The lungs were composed of two "rows" *(arugot)* right and left, attached to the spinal column. There were three lobes *(unnos)* on the right and two on the left side.[50]

Ancient authorities disagreed with reference to the number of lobes of the lungs. Hippocrates mentioned three on each side, while Galen counted only two on each side. This indicates that Galen experimented only on animals that possessed two lobes on either side and that he never saw a human lung with the accessory lobe on the right side. Physicians of the Middle Ages had a difficult time reconciling the opinions of Hippocrates and Galen, both of whom were followed religiously.

They finally justified the Hippocratic statement with reference to the lobes by rationalizing that in the time of the "Father of Medicine," man was stronger and had accessory organs.

The large bronchi *(bet ha-simponot)* entered the inner side of each lobe. Alongside the bronchi, the large blood vessels *(mizrakin)* also entered. The pleura was composed of two layers, an outer rough one and an inner, rose-colored one.[51]

Plato's view that the lung absorbed all kinds of fluid was noted by the Talmudists.[52] Erasistratus was, according to Celsus, the first authority to demonstrate that no fluids entered the lungs.

The air drawn in by the lungs was the source of life.[53] It penetrated the body, as the air of the universe penetrated the atmosphere.[54] The very soul depended upon the air. If there were no air in the body, the soul would be helpless; and if there were were no soul to govern inspiration and expiration, life would be impossible. Life could not exist without air, as a candle could not burn without it. One who put a lighted candle in an attic or small room where another was asleep was committing murder.[55] R. Akiba declared that a sleeping chamber should be at least 4 x 4 cubits (6 x 6 feet) in size.[56] R. Yohanan said, "Save on food and spend on your dwelling place."[57]

The respiratory apparatus consisted of the larynx *(goren)*, which was opposite the nape of the neck *(oreph)*,[58] the trachea *(gargereth koneh)*, and the thyroid cartilage *(koba)*. The trachea had six rings *(hulyoth)*, held together by muscular fibers.[59] Only the large ring had cartilaginous tissue all around it.[60] The trachea was situated in the right and the esophagus in the left of the neck.

The human voice originated in the lobes of the lungs[61] and passed out through the larynx. The human voice had seven different modalities.[62] Castrated males had a clear voice, and women who were born with infantile genitals *(aylonith)* had a heavy and rough voice. The normal female's voice was of a higher pitch than the normal male's.[63]

The Liver

The liver was the source of the blood supply. It was the heaviest of the visceral organs, hence its name *kabed*, meaning "heavy." It was situated near the fifth rib, the region known as *chamesh* ("five").[64] It should be recalled that Abner aimed to stab his foe Asael in the region which was at the center of the liver.[65] The Talmud mentioned *yathereth ha-kabed*, a finger-like projection, or *ezba ha-kabed*,[66] arising from the right side of the liver in animals. The liver was related to the pancreas which was considered an accessory organ of the liver.

The liver possessed seven vessels which distributed blood throughout the body.[67] It was attached to the diaphragm (tarpesha) by a fold of periteneum.[68] It was united also with the gallbladder (marah) by means of a narrow tube (simpona).[69] The liver and heart were considered the basic organs of the body. According to R. Judah, the liver came first because it supplied the heart with blood. Its red appearance was due to its large blood supply.[70]

Because the liver was considered by ancients the source of the blood supply and the "soul of life is in the blood," spiritual powers were attributed to it. Stress was laid upon real or imaginary abnormalities of the liver for the purpose of foretelling future events. Any deviations from the normal, observed in the color, structure, or aspect of the liver, were interpreted as prognostic signs of national or personal import. Those that occupied themselves with the foretelling of events from the appearance of the liver became known as "hepatoscopists." The prophet Ezekiel, referred to the liver as a means of telling future events among Babylonians, "For the king of Babylon standeth at the parting of the way, at the head of the two ways, to use divination; he shaketh the arrows to and fro, he inquireth of the teraphim, he looketh at the liver."[71]

The liver was utilized by ancients for medical purposes. The liver and bile of animals, reptiles, and fish were used for many diseases. In the case of Tobit, the burnt liver of a fish was mixed with the bile and was used to treat a leukomatous condition of the cornea. Diluted reptile bile was used by ancient Egyptians and Babylonians as a remedy for internal and external diseases.

The liver is now known to contain antianemic factors and elements vital to body metabolism, and various liver extracts are prescribed in convalescence. To the man of antiquity, the liver had a greater significance, restoring not only health but the soul itself.

In folk medicine, the liver was considered the organ of anger. A drop of bile (marah) discharged in the liver was thought to quell anger.[72] The Talmud explains that bile was called marah ("bitter") because it sickened the body. Many diseases were ascribed to the bile (machla zu marah). There were two kinds of bile, yellow or white bile and black bile. This suggests that the Talmud ascribed disease to the kind of humors.

Digestive Organs

The digestive organs included the lips (sefatayim), the teeth (shinnayim), the tongue (lashon), and the palate (chek).

The importance of the mouth *(peh)* to the processes of digestion was emphasized by R. Tachlifa of Caesarea, "Come and see the many miracles God does to man and which man does not know. If food had to pass directly into the alimentary canal, it would cause much pain and discomfort, but God created a well in the mouth (salivary gland) that softens the food and makes it go down easily."[73] Another saying was, 'The body contains many fountains, whose waters differ. The water of the eyes is salty, that of the ears greasy, that of the nose fetid and that of the mouth sweet."[74] The saliva *(rir)*, coming from the mouth, was supposed to be tasteless. Thus Job asked, "Is there a taste in the *rir* of healthy persons?"[75]

The saliva, aside from having a mechanical action, also aided digestion. If it were not for this function, food might be rejected (vomited) by the stomach.[76] The tongue and palate were the two organs of taste *(taam)*. The tongue was composed of many layers which made it sensitive. Under it, there was a gland that secreted fluid.[77] Three kinds of teeth were mentioned: molar, canine, and bicuspid. The alimentary canal of man was composed chiefly of the pharynx, esophagus, stomach, intestines, ileum, colon, rectum, and anus. The walls of the esophagus *(veshet)* were made up of two coats.[78] R. Yohanan warned that one should not talk while eating because there was danger that the food would enter the windpipe instead of the pharynx.[79] The lining of the stomach had hair-like projections *(milath)*,[80] said Mar Samuel; there were no such projections below the pylorus.

The gastrointestinal tract throughout its length was covered externally with the peritoneum, except the posterior part of the lower surface of the rectum. The peritoneum formed the greater omentum which was attached to the curvature, or bow, of the stomach.[81]

The stomach, or *kebah*, besides serving the function of grinding the food, also promoted sleep.[82] Among the aged, where the first function became weak, the function of inducing sleep was taken up by the nose so that, when one organ was awake, the other organ induced sleep. When both organs were awake or both were asleep, then death was sure to follow;[83] this was an old Aristotelian idea.

"The end of the digestive period is made manifest by the return of a desire for food."[84] According to Resh Lakish, "Thirst is a sign that digestion has taken place."[85] "The stomach performs a purely mechanical function, that of churning food. . . . The digestion proper *(ikkul)* is carried on in the intestines. . . . Eating when the bowels are full is like building a fire in a furnace from which the ashes have not been removed."[86] "Normal defecation hastens digestion."[87]

A later writer stated: "When one eats or drinks (tasty food) the small gastric orifices open their mouths, cause stimulation of the stomach and promote digestion and absorption of the food."[88] "The gastric juice has the property of curdling milk."[89] "The stomach, because of its fermentation properties, is widely used in the production of cheese. . . . Birds digest their food rapidly; dogs slowly,[90] in about three days."[91] Because in oriental countries dogs received little nourishment, providence allowed their food to remain in the alimentary canal for three days.[92]

The spleen was known at *techol*. Its function was to stimulate laughter.[93] Plato and Arateus, long before, ascribed laughter to the spleen. Seremonis Samonicus (240 A.D.) stated that persons with large spleens had a foolish laugh. Extirpation of the spleen stopped it, and the person developed a serious countenance.

The Special Senses

Of the five special senses, sight and hearing were considered special creations of God. "The seeing eye and the hearing ear, the Lord hath made even both of them."[94]

The Eye: The Talmudic knowledge of the anatomy and physiology of the eye may be briefly described as follows:

The eye (*galgal-ha 'ayin*) is a globular organ situated in the cavity of the orbit (*chur-ha 'ayin*), which is also globular;[95] the eyes are imbedded in a mass of fat within the bony cavity of the skull, secured and protected from injury in front by the lids (*afappayin*), *lashes (risim), and brows (gebinim).* The eyelids are also known as *shemurot* (watchers) because of their function, in common with the lashes, in guarding the eyes against foreign bodies, wind, and the glare of the sun.[96]

Eyebrows were considered an especially important protection for the visual organs. It was customary for ancient people to attempt to promote the growth of long eyebrows in order to prevent the sweat from the forehead from flowing into the eyes.

The word for "eye" *(ayin)* was derived, according to Talmudic authorities, from the homonym *ayin,* "a well" or "a spring."[97] Ancients looked on the eye as the well of the human body[98] because in that organ was situated the fountain of tears.[99] "As a spring," remarked a Talmudic writer, "brings forth water, so the eye keeps up refilling itself, and, as a well becomes useless the moment its sources dry up, so the eye, if the fluids are failing, loses the pleasures of sight."[100]

The "Book of Lamentations" compared the eye to a well, the reflection of vision being brought about by the watery humors.[101]

The mechanism of vision was perplexing to all ancients. The old theory that vision was brought about through reflection by the watery humors of the eye[102] was disputed by Alcameon and Democritus. A far more advanced theory was that of Aristotle, "The perceived objects stimulate a motion in the higher centers of the brain. In consequence thereof the sense organs are acted upon. What we see in the object is color. We see it through the medium of light which sets the color in motion. Without light we see no color, hence no object either."

Perhaps inspired by Aristotle, the Zohar stated, "In the interior of the eye are found many small nerves and blood vessels. The center pillar produces sight. One branch goes up to the top of the head and another branch terminates at the heart."[103]

The eyeball was composed of seven tunics[104] as follows: ocular conjunctival, scleral, corneal, choroidal, retinal, and iritic, and the lenticular capsule.[105]

The sclera *(haloben-shebeayin)* was described as a white membrane, the structure of which was formed of fatty tissue.[106]

The pupil in the Talmud was known as *galgal reina,* the wheel of vision,[107] and also as *uchma.*[108] The center of the pupil was known as *parchuf shebecomet.*[109] In the sacred writings, the pupil was the most essential part of vision because of the common observation that, when the pupil was injured or diseased, vision was impaired.

In the Old Testament, the pupil was termed *ishon* (at times *babat-ayin,* or *bat-ayin*), the diminutive of the Hebrew *ish* (little man) because of the little image seen in the pupil.[110] The iris *(kesheth)* was described as being situated at the inner junction of the black and white coats. The Bible has no word descriptive of the iris. In neo-Persian, it is named *madar-i-ain,* "Mother of the Eye." The neo-Hebraic form *kesheth* signifies a rainbow because of its various colors.

An interesting observation was that the eyes were larger in fat persons and smaller in thin persons.[111]

The presence of salt in the tears was considered injurious to the eye. Thus, R. Simeon ben Yacai, when he emerged from the cave where he had spent twelve years almost buried in the sand, had his eyes irritated by the salty tears and he cried from the pain.[112]

The image in the pupil was taken by ancients as the very soul of the person. The term *bath horin,* or *bath melech,* in the Talmud perhaps refers to some such concept, as in the following passage, "When one strikes the other upon the eye and the *bath horin* (free or noble daughter) escapes and blinds him, he (that makes the assault) is responsible for the damage done to the eyes."[113]

Old age was considered an important cause of impaired vision as well as of other pathologic changes in the eye. R. Simeon ben Chalafta said that in old age, "the eye that sees very far cannot see from near"[114] (a reference to presbyopia).

R. Simeon ben Yochi said, "When the eyes drip, the eyelashes disappear."[115] The steady overflowing of tears in the conjunctival sac irritated not only the mucous membrane of the conjunctiva but also the margins of the lids.

Excessive use of the eyes was an important cause of eye disease. R. Joshua ben Levi stated, "Why is the Torah called *Tushiyah?* Because is weakens the body and the eyes."[116]

Mar Samuel advised daily baths for "an unclean head produces blindness." Among unclean people of warm climates, perspiration, dirt, and vermin from the head entered the eyes and caused conjunctivitis, keratitis, and all forms of ophthalmia.

Vision was ascribed to divine power. This theologic explanation of vision seemed to have been in vogue well up to the eighteenth century. Leading ophthalmologists like Briggs, who discovered the optic disc (1776), and Porterfield, who showed that the blindspot was the place of entry of the optic nerve (1759), explained binocular vision as a reflex act of the soul. Porterfield gave the attitude of the ophthalmologists of his day in the following passage, "The connection between our ideas and motions excited on the retina, optic nerve, and sensatorum is unknown to us and seems to depend entirely on the will of God."[117]

THE EAR

"The ear and the eye are God's gift to man; the other organs are contributed to man by his parents."[118] The anatomical studies of the ear in the Talmud are confined to the external parts. The interior anatomy of the ear was not known. The ear, known as *ozen* (Aramic *udna),* was composed of two parts, the upper, or cartilaginous part *(tenuch haozen,*[119] *gaboth shel ozen,*[120] or occasionally *bedal ozen),* and the lower, or soft part, the lobe *(alia,* or *milath).*[121] The School of Ishmael gave a moral reason for the structure of the ear, "The whole ear is hard and the *alia* is soft so that if one hears a profane word, he shall bend the *alia* over the opening of the ear and lock it."[122]

R. Judah expressed an Aristotelian idea when he stated that perforation in the cartilaginous part of the ear did not heal. R. Meir, on the other hand, thought that it did heal.[123] The idea that a wound in cartilaginous tissue did not heal was discarded by R. Jose ben Nehurai, who told of a sheep that was cured of an opening in the trachea, "Since the cartilage of the ear is of the same structure as that of the trachea, a perforation in the cartilaginous tissue must be curable." The ears figured in the priestly code.[124] Injuries to the upper part of the ear, an opening in the external ear as big as a pea, and gangrene of the ear all disqualified a priest from performing his duties.

Among congenital ear deformities, was mentioned a double ear.[125] An interesting Talmudic observation was that the movement of the external ears among animals was essential to their welfare. It enabled them to receive sounds from inimical beasts at a distance.[126]

There were three kinds of deafness: (1) a deaf-mute; this type of deafness was congenital; since children learned to speak by hearing words, a child deprived of the sense of hearing remained mute; (2) a deaf person able to speak (usually acquired deafness); and (3) a partially deaf person or one who was deaf in only one ear.[127] R. Judah reported the case of the children of R. Yohanan ben Gada who were all born deaf.[128] The Talmudists knew that congenital deaf-mutism could be transmitted from parent to offspring. This is an observation far in advance of the time. In recent years, Graham Bell found, among 22,062 deaf-mutes, that 54½ per cent had other deaf-mutes in their family. Consanguinous marriages are frequently the cause of propogating this defect.

Under the term *cheresh,* the Talmud included deaf-mutes.[129] Rabbah appears to have suspected that deafness was due to pressure on the ear within the head, owing to external injuries.[130] This, of course, applied to acquired deafness.

Cheresh applied to one who could speak but could not hear.[131] *Illem* was one who could hear but could not speak.[132] The deaf-mute, according to the Talmud, lacked normal mentality *(lav bar deah).*[133] He might be able to work but had no intelligent judgment and therefore was not punishable in the eyes of the law. Other Talmudic observations were, "One cannot hear two sounds at the same time."[134] "The ear is an involuntary organ; it hears even when one does not desire to listen."[135]

Deafness could be acquired by a direct or an indirect blow on the head or by an unusually loud noise.[136] The last was an important observation. During the first World War, many cases of deafness were reported as a result of shell shock. Aviators, returned from a combat zone during the second World War, presented a similar condition. The Talmud declared: "If one shouts in the ears of a slave and deafens him he must set him free." Other causes of deafness were sickness, insufficient secretion, and old age. The mystic R. Johanan ben Dehibai attributed deafness, as all other impairment of senses, to sexual sins.

Treatment of the ear consisted of instillations of oil or oil-soaked soft material.[137] Abaye, quoting his mother stated, "The use of the fluid of the kidneys (perhaps urine) is the best remedy for earache."[138] A physician was quoted by Rabba as saying that all fluids were harmful to the ear except water of the kidneys of a goat. An entire page was devoted to the treatment of ear pathology, but most of the therapy was connected with magic.

Incidentally, the ears were used to identify a person's trade. The builder had the sign of a ruler on his ear as a trade mark; the weaver, his wool flakes;[139] the dyer, his sign; the money changer, a coin *(dinar)*;[140] and the writer, his pen *(calamus)*. Earrings served originally as amulets for protection against evil spirits and unlucky stars.[141] Earrings used now for ornamentation thus have a venerable history.

THE NOSE

The nose, aside from being endowed with the sense of smell, was the window through which breath passed in and out of the lungs. The Hebrew term *aph* also signified "wrath," or "anger;" the nose was assumed also to be the organ of anger. The connection between anger and the nose could be due to the fact that the nose turned red, and the *ala* of the nose moved when a person was angered. A curious observation was made by the Talmudists to the effect that animals, when angered, passed a vaporous air through their nostrils. *Ktzar appayim,* or "short of nose," was applied to quick-tempered persons;[142] *erech appayim,* or "length of nose," was applied to those who were slow of temper. The nostrils were known as *nechirayim.*[143] The nose was always considered the principal feature of the face by which one was recognized. Abba said, "One who does not want to be recognized should cover his nose.[144] The inhabitants of Sepphoris, Palestine, during the days of Ursicinus, endeavored to disguise themselves by putting certain plasters on their noses, but they were betrayed and captured.[145] A haughty person was known as *gabath aph,*[146] or *baal ha-chotem.*[147] Among the deformities that disqualified a priest from his prescribed duties were a flat nose, a very short nose, a nose with closed nostrils, and a long nose that hung over the lips. Preuss is of the opinion that all these deformities were the result of leprosy.

Among the diseases of the nose were polyps *(polypus).* R. Muna quoted R. Judah as saying that the touch of the hand (unclean) to the nose could be the cause of polyps; and therefore, such a hand deserved to be cut off. According to the Mishna, marital relations between husband and wife could be severed if any one of the parties had polyps before they married and this fact was not disclosed.[148] The Gamara confined this law only to leprosy but not to polyps. In case of leprosy, it was immaterial whether it was contracted before or after marriage. The meaning of *polypus* was not clear in the Talmud. Mar Samuel thought it was a condition of the nose where a fetid odor (*ozaena*) was emitted.[149] Another pathology of the nose familiar to the Talmudists was epistaxis, or periodic bleeding, of the nose. The treatment for this has always been, and still is among certain peoples, magical.

Ancients attached magical significance to sneezing. They believed these sudden nasal paroxysms marked the passage of an evil spirit from the body. In certain parts of Africa, sneezing is still thought to signify the passing of an ancestral ghost from part of the body. Homer made Penelope overjoyed that her son Telemachus sneezed when she made a wish.[150] Strange to say, this belief is still in vogue. When one tells a story and one of the audience sneezes, the proper remark is, "It testifies to the truth." Xenophon looked upon sneezing as a favorable sign.

Aristotle stated that sneezing was regarded by the Greeks as of divine origin, and those that saw one sneezing remarked, "God preserve you." The Romans greeted the sneezer with *deus te adjuvante*. According to Petronius Arbiter, the word *salve* was used.[151] In the Talmud, sneezing was known by the word *ittush* and was considered a favorable sign of convalescence, a belief shared by no less an authority than Celsus. The Talmud considered sneezing among the seven good omens for the recovery of health. The other six signs were perspiration, watery stools, frequent micturition, seminal emission, sound sleep, and dreaming.[152] R. Zeira said, "If one sneezes during prayer, it is an omen that his prayers will be listened to." Another observation was, "*Ittush* is an involuntary action, is accompanied by pleasant sensation and presages good fortune."[153] The Talmud gave voice to a tradition that in early times man was never sick and his death came suddenly; when on the way to some place or on the street, he would suddenly sneeze and his soul would pass out of his nostrils. Because sneezing was connected with death, it became customary to say *hayim tobim umarphei* (a good and healthful life). The school of Gamliel prohibited such greetings and considered them heathen superstitions. Hippocrates thought sneezing dangerous among persons who suffer from lung disease. Dioscorides reported that, during the time of Valerius Flaccus.

cases of sneezing frequently turned into epileptic fits. Carol Sigon
stated that the customary wishful blessings in sneezing dated from
the year 590, when there was a severe outbreak of bubonic plague in
Rome; the sick died sneezing, and those that witnessed these deaths
prayed for their recovery.

PATHOLOGY

Before taking up the subject of Talmudic pathology, it is important
to bear in mind that the Talmudic teachers did not approach the subject out of scientific curiosity. Their interest in animal pathology was
rather prompted by religio-dietary motives. Their aim was to ascertain
which animals and parts of animals were *kosher* (permitted as food)
and which were *terepha* (forbidden as food). They laid down a rigid
rule that any abnormal condition found in the animal that would have
resulted in its death rendered the flesh of the animal *terepha*.[154] In this
respect, the Talmudists were perhaps the first to advance the theory
that diseases were produced by pathologic changes in the tissues and
structures of the body itself. It must be remembered that the ancient
Egyptians and Babylonians thought that morbid bodily conditions were
due to external and largely supernatural causes, such as for example
evil spirits entering the body and destroying the blood.

The Ionian School ascribed diseases to the changes in the four elements. Hippocrates and the school of Cos attributed the pathology of
disease to changes in the humors. Democritus and his school believed
that diseases were influenced by stagnation of the atoms in the pores of
the body. Indeed, few if any physicians before the nineteenth century
surmised that disease was the result of changes in the organs and tissues
themselves. It may also be noted here that the Hebrews were perhaps
the first to inspect animals intended for dietary use.

The Talmud divided animal pathology into two classes: (1) diseases caused by heavenly or invisible causes, *machla bidei shamayim;*
(2) ailments caused by human or natural agencies, *machla bidei
adam.*

As an example of the first could be mentioned an invisible disease,
such as perforated peptic ulcer with ensuing peritonitis and death.
Such an ailment rendered animal flesh unfit to eat. As an illustration
of the second type, produced by human agencies, could be cited laceration of the throat and severance of the trachea, such as was usually
caused by a knife. The latter was not necessarily fatal in man since
the damage could often be reparable with sutures or the application
of an immovable brace around the neck. In animals, however, where

surgery was not applicable, such an injury was usually fatal because, by moving its head, the links of the trachea could get out of position and block the entrance of air into the trachea, resulting in suffocation. The flesh of such an animal was *terepha*. However, when the trachea was only partly cut, or cut vertically, the injury could heal in a natural way, and therefore its flesh was declared *kosher*.

The word *terefah* applied to meat from animals that had received a fatal injury, those that had suffered incurable diseases, or those marked by some physical abnormality. In other words, it referred to meat from animals that were so diseased or injured that prospects for recovery were slight. In order to determine which flesh of certain slaughtered animals was not taboo, all organs had to be inspected and changes in the tissues carefully noted. The observations and the discussions that followed these investigations afford an interesting insight into an extraordinarily developed knowledge of pathology. The minuteness of the examination was illustrated by the fact that animals unsuitable for food included those where examination revealed perforation of the meninges, pericardium, heart, lungs, pleura, diaphragm, esophagus, stomach, intestines, or gallbladder.

Other abnormalities in the animal's tissue which made its flesh unsuitable for food were fracture of the spine, severance of the spinal cord, fracture of the majority of the ribs, severance of the larynx or the pharynx, and fistula communicating with both bronchi. Black discoloration of the lungs was looked upon as a fatal condition indicating disintegration. Red (hyperemia), blue, and light green discolorations of the lungs were viewed as not necessarily fatal, and the flesh of such an animal was therefore considered edible.[152] Gaseous degeneration of the lung made the animal's flesh unfit for food.

Extirpation of the spleen and absence of the uterus were not considered fatal.[156] Abscess or atrophy of the kidneys was thought to be incurable. A dry and bloodless liver that crumbled under the fingers was considered *terepha*. Partial extirpation of the liver, where enough liver had been left around the biliary duct, was thought not to be fatal. The scope of this work does not permit more numerous illustrations concerning Talmudic pathology. The subject here can only be considered in a general way.

The system of Talmudic pathology was based on a passage of Leviticus 22:8, which reads, "That which dieth of itself or is torn by a beast, he shall not eat to defile himself therewith." The Talmud extended this law to include the flesh of animals affected with any disease which would have later caused the death of the animal.[157] In order to determine the condition of internal organs, each slaughtered animal was subjected to an autopsy.

The Talmudists viewed the condition of the lungs of the slaughtered animal as an index of the animal's health. In any doubtful lung pathology, the respiratory organs were inflated. When air did not enter certain parts of the lungs, it was requisite to ascertain whether the obstruction was caused by hardening of the lung tissue or by the deposit of mucus in the bronchi. If the obstruction was due to mucus, the flesh of the animal was permitted to be used for food because the mucus might have been expelled by a cough. On the other hand, if the bronchial impediment was due to induration of the lung tissue, the animal was considered *terepha*.

The present procedure to determine the patency of the fallopian tubes was employed by the Talmudists to test for perforation of the lungs. Air was blown into the trachea; when it escaped with a hissing sound, the pulmonary system was considered perforated. In collapse of the lungs, the following procedure was suggested: The lungs were to be immersed in water; if the water did not bubble upon inflation of the lungs, it was a sign that the lungs were not perforated. The flesh therefore was *kosher*.

R. Simeon said an animal "is only *terepha* if the opening penetrates the pleura and the lung back to the bronchi." He did not give any explanation for his statement; but to the medical student, it was self-evident that such an injury usually came from without by the piercing blow of a pointed instrument in the region of the lung, or from within by the rupture of a lung abscess or by the opening of a tuberculous cavity into the pleura. In either case, the air entering the lung did not remain there but passed out into the pleura and filled up the chest (pneumothorax). Such a condition was frequently followed by inflammatory changes and effusion of serous or fibrinous fluid (hydrothorax), which filled up the pleural sac, frequently resulting in pyoneumothorax, leading to death because the lung did not expand; and the more effort the animal made to get in air, the more the chest cavity expanded. This open door for the escape of the air from the lungs was fatal, and therefore the flesh of the animal was *terepha*. R. Nachman stated that, when the perforated lung was found close to the walls of the chest (Rashi, "adhering to the ribs"), the flesh was *kosher* because in this case the opening was closed, and the air remained intact in the lungs. If a part of the lungs was found missing, the animal was *terepha*.[158]

The flesh of animals with pleural adhesions, if they could be easily separated with the tips of the fingers, could be eaten; but if the adhesions were firmly developed into bands of connective tissue, the animal was not considered to be in a healthy condition. Dry pleurisy was not considered dangerous. The Talmud refers to a cavernous lung, filled with mucus or phlegm (typical of that observed in tuberculosis, which can be diagnosed at present by percussion and auscultation).

"Perforation of the outer and inner meningeal membranes renders an animal unfit for food" because such an injury was followed by inflammation and secretion of serofibrinous effusion, which, when becoming profuse, penetrated into the brain, the path of least resistance (for the skull above and the scalp were of firmer texture), causing pressure on the vital centers of the brain. This usually resulted in death. If the outer membrane only was found perforated, the animal was declared to be *kosher.*

If, therefore, an animal had been struck on its head, the meningeal membranes had to be examined, for even a small opening could prove fatal. Fracture of the skull without injury to the meninges was not considered fatal because it did not necessarily lead to pathology of the brain, and therefore the flesh of an animal suffering from such a fracture could be eaten.

"A penetrating wound in the heart cavity makes an animal unsuitable for food." Such an opening was generally inflicted by a knife, a spear, or an arrow, and resulted in instant death. The animal died before there was time for slaughter. "If, however, the heart is not penetrated all through its thickness, it is fit for food" because the heart could keep up functioning and the animal could recover. There were also internal causes for heart perforation, such as the last stages of myocarditis when the heart muscle could become so thin that a strong exertion could effect an opening into the heart and instant death would follow.

"Fracture of the spine with severance of the cord is fatal."[159] This presumably applied when the division of the cord was in the region of the neck. The animal died immediately because through this region the respiratory organ was supplied with nerve force; breathing stopped suddenly and the animal died from suffocation. The severance of the cord in the dorsal or lumbar regions was followed by paralysis of the extremities; the animal could live until the nerve supplying the kidneys gave way, when the animal died from uremia. Where only the vertebral bones were damaged, the animal's life was not in any danger, and therefore its flesh was *kosher.*

The case of Rabina, as related in the Talmud, shows that the Talmudists recognized the modern teaching that symptoms of diseases

were merely external manifestations of internal changes in the tissues.
A sheep that dragged its hind leg was brought before Rabina to determine the cause of the animal's abnormality. A previous diagnosis of
ischialgia *(shigrona)*, or gout, in the hip, had been made by another
teacher. Rabina disagreed with this diagnosis and expressed his opinion that the abnormality was due to paralysis caused by the severance
of the spinal cord. An autopsy confirmed his diagnosis.[160]

Extirpation of the uterus was taught by the school of R. Tarphon to
be fatal. This was disputed by some sages of the school of Jabneh.
When Theodus, a famous physician, was later consulted, he gave as his
opinion that an animal could live without a womb. He supported his
opinion by disclosing the fact (as we have already observed) that all
cows leaving Alexandria for foreign countries had their wombs extirpated in order not to give an opportunity to foreign countries to raise
such fine specimens of cattle.[161]

The Talmudic teachers, in their investigation of pathologic conditions
among animals, frequently resorted to experimental methods; and while
they venerated tradition, if it was found that experimental findings were
contrary to tradition, they rejected tradition. Thus, dislocation of the
hip joint in fowls was considered *terepha*, for it was thought that such
a deformity endangered life in a fowl. When it was discovered by R.
Simeon ben Halaphta that such a deformity could be cured by putting
the joint into a splint, the law was reversed.[162] Thus, when R. Haninah
asked R. Judah about the law concerning a dislocated hip in a fowl,
he gave his decision that it was *kosher*. R. Haninah utilized a hen having such a deformity as a specimen for instruction to his students. R.
Simeon ben Halaphta was known for his experiments. He was called
askin bedaborim ("the theory prober"). He once took a hen that had
lost its feathers (which, according to tradition, was *terepha*) to a warm
place, covered her with some garment, and sure enough a new crop
of feathers appeared on the fowl in a few weeks. Thus, he proved that
such a condition in fowls did not necessarily endanger its life, and
therefore it could be used for food.[163]

The above examples, cited at random, show that centuries ago the
study of pathology engaged the serious attention of Hebrew students.
While these searching investigations in pathology were made on animals and perhaps for religious reasons rather than out of scientific
curiosity, the fact remains that a definite approach to the subject of
pathology was made, and scientific methods of investigation were employed. Granting that animal pathology differs in many respects from
human pathology, the difference is primarily one of degree, and the

bridge that connects the human animal with other mammals is not difficult to cross.

HYGIENE AND PROPHYLAXIS

Next to pathology, no other subject received as much attention in the Talmud as hygiene and prophylaxis. It has been shown in a previous chapter that the Hebrews, far back in the twelfth century B.C., had enacted laws for the prevention and suppression of the spread of contagious disease and that, when the diagnosis was certain, they were enjoined to isolate and disinfect the person stricken. These rules, which had already occupied a prominent place in the Old Testament, were further elaborated on in Talmudic literature.

While many of the principles of social hygiene promulgated in the Talmud were beclouded by ethical, religious, and occasionally super-stitious conceptions, most of the ordinances were in harmony with modern science. Extraordinary subtlety of thought was manifested in dif-ferentiating the degrees of impurity and designating the measures neces-sary for purification. To take proper care of the body was a religious duty imposed upon the individual. The rigidity of the Rabbinic law did not apply only to the sick. "Thou shalt live with the law but not die with the law," was a familiar dictum. Baths,[164] massage, and inunctions were recommended to preserve good health. Rules regarding regula-tion of diet were laid down: not only what to eat and what not to eat, but also how and when to eat. A good breakfast and the liberal use of fresh vegetables daily were recommended as affording ideal nourish-ment.[165] The use of water with meals was thought to be essential to digestion, "He who eats without drinking, eats blood."[166] After a meal, a short walk was prescribed. "One must not partake of food which is offered with the (bare) hands." Rabbi Simeon ben Gamliel disapproved of the practice of kissing on the mouth. It was required to clean a cup before and after drinking and to spill out what was left after drinking so that others would not unknowingly use it.

The size of the sleeping chamber was regulated, and it had to be at least 6 x 8 cubits (9 x 12 feet). The height of the room was required to be not less than one half of its length.[167] Windows were not per-mitted to open into dark alleys.[168]

Discussing Talmudic prophylaxis, one must bear in mind that the Jews, like all ancient peoples, understood illness and death caused by violence but could not conceive of them as normal incidents of life. They believed them to be accidents produced by the intervention of extraneous, natural, or metaphysical forces, such as worms, demons, ghosts, and the like. They visualized disease-demons in the air as the cause of disease and left it to the modern observer and the microscope to capture these little demons, culture and visualize them, and build upon them the structure of modern bacteriology.

In considering the etiology of disease, one finds a striking resemblance between the ancient animistic idea of demons and the modern doctrine of biologic pathology. Both concepts agree that the cause of illness is introduced from without. Both concur that the exciting cause is invisible to the naked eye. Both state that the disease-producing factor has a predilection for certain tissues or organs of the body. The difference is only in the concept of the nature of the pathogenic forces, and this may be accounted for by the invisibility of the minute extraneous forces to the ancient healer, who possessed no microscope.

In the light of modern bacteriology and hygiene, the Talmudic conception of pathogenic demons is of much interest. Their mode of attack, their predilection for certain organs, their prevalence in certain localities and during certain seasons of the year, the symptoms they produced, and the measures taken for the prevention and cure of their attacks, might not be out of place in a modern book on hygiene.

Mazzikin (demons) were said to be transmitted from person to person, from animal to animal, and from animal to person. He who occupied himself with the practice of casting out evil spirits was, therefore, careful to keep his mouth closed while carrying out the exorcism lest the demon pass from the mouth of the patient into his own, a precaution taken by the modern physician when examining the mouth of a patient suspected of contagion.

Next to direct contagion, transmission through the air was considered important. According to Talmudic teachers (who usually voiced the prevailing beliefs of the Egyptians, Greeks, and Babylonians), the air was literally filled with spirits, as was evident from the following citations: "They (*mazzikin*, or "demons") hover around the houses and fields. . . . Particularly are they numerous in the lower regions of the air."[169] "They (the demons) exceed us in number."[170] "Each one of us is surrounded by them, a thousand on his left, ten thousand on his right."[171] "A whole legion of them are on the watch."[172] "In public places (synagogues) the air is filled with them. . . . In time of epidemic one must be careful to isolate himself in his house and avoid the street."[173] Vacant houses amid ruins were believed to be favorite rendezvous for evil spirits.[174]

Midsummer (from Tammuz 17 to Ab 9—about July 15 to August 15) was considered perilous to life and health because intense heat was most favorable for the gathering of evil spirits. The Talmud warned persons to avoid the streets during the hot season of the year (particularly from 10 o'clock in the morning to 3 o'clock in the afternoon) because the terrible demon *keteb meriri* roamed in the atmosphere during that period.[175]

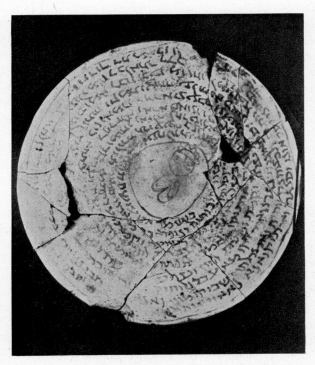

Fig. 157: Aramaic Hebrew incantation discovered in Mesopotamia. This bowl is from the Frau Professor Hilprecht collection of Babylonian antiquities in Jena. Translated by Gordon, C. H.: Archiv. Orientalni, 9: 1937; Orientalia, 10: 1941. (Courtesy of Professor Julius Lewy, Curator of this collection.)

Demons were thought to be particularly malevolent during the night; and for this reason,[176] in eastern countries, it is still believed that exposure to night air produces disease.

Water also was considered a medium for demons. "One that drinks water from creeks and pools, particularly at night," said Mar Samuel (the Talmudic Hippocrates), "takes a chance with his life because *shabriri* (the demon causing blindness) dwells in those waters."[177] Drinking water from uncovered vessels, particularly when exposed to night air, was considered hazardous. "The one who draws water from wells located in dark places draws demons into his system. To walk on places where (polluted) water is spilled is dangerous." The avoidance of spilled water was reminiscent of the modern precaution against contact with saliva or mucous discharges. It was strictly forbidden to drink water handled by one whose hands were not washed in the morning.[178]

Oil was considered a powerful medium for disease. According to the Talmud, there was a specific demon named *Hama* dwelling in oil. One, therefore, was warned not to walk in oily places.

It was necessary to avoid unsanitary places, since most malignant demons were thought to inhabit such locations as drain pipes, pits, and privies.[179] Demons were believed to be abundant in decomposed animal and vegetable material.

Persons weakened by disease were considered particularly susceptible to demonic attacks because it was believed that Satan always struck when resistance was low.[180]

ETIOLOGY

The relationship between Talmudic medicine and the medicine of Greece and Rome may best be shown from the various theories on the etiology of disease. All schools of thought may be detected in Talmudic literature. The theory of the Ionian school that the human body consisted of four elements was expressed by a later rabbi, Rehumai, who stated, "In the body there are four elements, fire, air, earth, and water."[181] A later teacher suggested, albeit vaguely, the humoral theory in his simile, "The body of man is like a kingdom . . ."[182] R. Yochanan interpreted the word *adam* somewhat in accord with the humoral theory: The "A" stood for the Hebrew *adama* (earth); the "D," for *dam* (blood); and the "M," for *mara* (gall).[183] Another rabbi, Eliezer, held that 99 per cent of diseases (internal) were due to *mara*.[184] Reziel stated that "everything in the world" was created from the four elements which were parallel in the human body to the four humors (blood, phlegm, red bile, and black bile) and represented hot, cold, dry, and moist qualities.[185]

Another attempt to explain the vital phenomena of life and its deviation in disease was made by Mar Samuel who stated *hakol baruach* ("all diseases depend upon the pneuma"), a theory which prevailed from the time of Hippocrates down to the sixteenth or seventeenth centuries A.D. The Hebrew *ruach* signified wind and spirit, like the Latin *spiritus* and the Greek *pneuma*.

Heat and Cold: Excessive heat or cold was given as the cause of disease by some Talmudic doctors. "All diseases are caused by heavenly agencies except cold and heat,"[186] conveying the idea that if proper precautions are taken, such conditions could be prevented. The Hebrew terms *zinim upachim* (cold and heat) apply, according to some authorities, to malaria as a specific disease. Disease was also attributed to plethora[187] and extravasation of blood into the tissues. This etiology of disease was first advanced by Erasistratus, who opposed the humoral theory of Hippocrates.

Worms: Since the earliest times, worms have been mentioned as the cause of disease. Cuneiform inscriptions on tablets of remote antiquity unearthed in Mesopotamia depicted worms gnawing at the vitals of humans. Isaiah, speaking of disease and physical destruction, said, "The maggot is spread under thee and the worm covers thee."[188] Job alluded to the worm as the cause of his trouble.[189]

The Talmud, which often echoed the beliefs and practices of the Near East, stated, "A host of worms infest the human body, both living and dead. . . . There are worms infesting the liver[190] *(arkata)*." There is a worm found in the trachea of sheep causing them to cough,"[191] "and there is one in the abdominal cavity named *kirza*."[192] Interesting was the Talmudic description of a worm *murna,* found occasionally between the prepuce and the glans penis, the treatment for which was circumcision, "even Gentiles submit to this operation."[193] The Talmud prohibited the eating of certain vegetables (perhaps lettuce and watercress) possibly because of the human parasites often deposited on them. Amebic dysentery is still an endemic disease in the East.

The term "worm" *(rimah* in Hebrew) was applied by ancients, and for that matter even by moderns, not only to actual worms and elongated crawling creatures, such as the beetle, caterpillar, and the leech, but also to insects, parasites, maggots, and all sorts of larvae.

How worms came to be associated with disease is not difficult to understand. In the East, the presence of worms in the alimentary canals of humans and animals has always been of frequent occurrence. The tapeworm (one of the Cestoda), roundworms (Ascaris lumbricoides, found chiefly in children and occupying the upper portions of the intestines), and threadworm (Oxyuris vermicularis, a common parasite infecting the rectum, the larvae of which entered the body by drinking water or eating vegetables, such as lettuce and watercress) were commonly observed passing through the rectum. It was natural, therefore, to believe that these crawling "demons" were the cause of all disease,

particularly when the "demon" was cast out of the body by vermifuges, and symptoms, such as diarrhea, fever, apparent anemia, ir-
ritability, restlessness, and even convulsions, disappeared.

Worm seeds occupied a most important position in the ancient pharmacopoeia. Some of the vermifuges in the modern pharmacopoeia
have a venerable history and may be traced back to ancient Babylonia.

Overeating: Overeating was given as a cause of disease. The Talmudic teachers, judging from the strict regulation of diet, attributed
many pathologic conditions to gastrointestinal disturbances.[194] They
laid stress on the quality and the quantity of food and on the regularity
and frequency of eating, as is seen[195] from the following quotations:
"Most sickness results from overeating. . . . Do not overload the
stomach."[196] "More sickness results from too much than too little
food."[197] "The end of the digestive period is made manifest by the
return of the appetite."[198] "Eating when the bowels are full is like
making a fire in the stove from which the ashes have not been removed."[199] "One must not eat too much at a time."[200]

One should take time at his meal, eat slowly, and not swallow large
pieces.[201] The food should be chewed well to be mixed with the saliva.
The saliva, aside from its function of moistening the food, added also to
its palatability,[202] and water should form an essential part of the
meal.[203] Too many delicacies were not good for digestion.[204] The
substantial part of each meal should consist mainly of bread.[205] Meats
should be used as little as possible,[206] and it was best to eat them towards evening (because they took longer to digest).[207] Children
should not be fed on meat or wine.[208] Delicate persons could get
along with less food.

Of the three meals, breakfast was considered the most important
(because sufficient time was given to assimilate all previously eaten
food during the night's rest).[209] R. Akiba advised his son Joshua not
to neglect the morning meal.[210] Another statement was, "The morning
meal brings health to the entire body."[211] The main meal, however,
was advised for noontime. A lapse of four hours should be allowed
between meals.[212] The last meal of the day (for scholars at least)
was at six in the evening[213] (evidently because of their inactive life
they needed more time to assimilate the food). Sudden changes in the
kind of diet could lead to sickness.

Sexual Excesses: Sexual excesses were considered by the Talmudists
to be dangerous to one's health. The one who indulged in sexual excesses, said a Talmudic doctor, grew prematurely old.[214] R. Elijah
was of the opinion that intemperate sexual intercourse produced "pod-

agra,"[215] a disease marked by violent pain in the extremities. Rabbi said that sexual imprudence affected the heart. One should not indulge in intercourse soon after returning from a prolonged journey, after a meal, after venesection, and after strenuous exercise. Excessive coitus had a bad effect on a fetus.[216]

Maimonides collected all the fragmentary instructions in the Talmud with reference to sexual abuses and set them down in his famous work "Mishna Torah." "The one that indulges intemperately in sexual intercourse becomes aged before his time, loses his strength, the hair of his head, his eyelashes and eyebrows fall out, his teeth get loose, and he is attacked with violent pains. . . . One, therefore, has to be watchful not to have any intercourse until he feels strong enough." The worst form of sexual abuses has always been that of masturbation. The Talmudic sages interpreted the death penalty of Onan as a punishment for destroying a potential human being. Thus said R. Eliezer ben Jacob, "One that practices onanism (withdrawal) is like one who commits murder."

Intoxicants: Excessive drinking of wine was mentioned as a cause of disease. The one that gave himself up to intoxicating drinks would not reach his seventieth year.[217] Abba Saul said, "I am an undertaker and have often had occasion to observe bones of habitual drunkards; they appear as burned."[218] Intemperance weakened the heart. "One having sexual connection while under the influence of liquor is in danger of heart failure." Another saying was to the effect that children of drunkards acted drunk.[219] The last quotation recalls the remark of Diogenes when he met a stupid youth, "Young man; your father was very drunk when your mother conceived you." Quatrefages observed that children begotten by an intoxicated man often presented signs of obstreperousness and absence of intellect.

Sunstroke: Rabbi Ishmael thought that 99 per cent died through sunstroke.[220] This, of course, applied to those who lived in tropical or subtropical climates.

References and Notes

Owing to the various Talmudic systems, it was deemed advisable to abbreviate the names of the systems. Quotations from the Babylonian Talmud will have no other designation than the book quoted; "J" before the name of the work refers to the *Jerusalem Talmud*; "T" indicates *Tosephtha*; "Mid." is the abbreviation of *Midrash* (Exegesis on the Old Testament).

1. St. James 5:14-16.
2. Historia Naturalis 37:10.
3. Wunderbar: Biblisch-talmudische Medizin 1:25.

4. *Mishna* is derived from the Hebrew *shana* (to learn; to repeat) and applies to a compilation of laws by the Patriarch R. Judah, a contemporary of Galen, who lived about 200 A.D.
5. Talmud; Pesachim 56.
6. The name *Talmud* is derived from the word *limud;* it denotes learning and refers to about thirty-five volumes of legal documents and discussions based upon the *Mishna.*
7. Talmud; Yoma 38-a.
8. Sirach 38.
9. Ibid.
10. Talmud; Shabbath 32-a.
11. Ibid.; Sanhedrin 17-b.
12. Ibid.; Baba Kama 85-a.
13. Ibid.
14. Tobit 2:10.
15. Talmud; Sanhedrin 78-a.
16. Ibid.; Makkoth 22-b.
17. Mid. (Exegesis on the Bible); Exodus; Rabba 46-3.
18. Talmud; Sanhedrin 91-a.
19. J. Talmud; Shekalim 13. Cited by Preuss: p. 17.
20. Among the celebrated physicians of the rabbinical academies may be mentioned Mar Samuel (200 A.D.), Hanina (third century), Tabiyah (third century), Jernte (200 A.D.), Manjomi, Binjamin, Ama, Bar Nathan Hiyah, and Abayye.
21. Kethuboth 4; Sanhedrin 93-a. See also Oholoth 4:2.
22. Talmud; Bekhoroth 4:4; Sanhedrin 93-a.
23. Herodotus; Clio 1; Trans. by Cary, H.: American Book Co., New York, p. 86.
24. Midrash; Samuel 103:15. Cited by Preuss.
25. Acts 5:15.
26. Geschichte der medizin. Unterrichts, Berlin, 1889, p. 26.
27. Mid. Deuteronomy 6:13; Halacha 11.
28. Talmud; Sanhedrin 5-b.
29. Bechoroth 45-a.
30. De Ossium Natura. Geneva, 1657, p. 274.
31. Ibid.
32. Hyrtle: Das arabische Med. Pp. 166–167.
33. Mid. Tanhuma; Genesis.
34. Mishna Oholoth 1:8; Hulin 128-b.
35. Hulin 128-b.
36. Ibid. 93-a.
37. Ibid. 45-a.
38. Ibid. 45-a, b.
39. Zohar 3:128; Hulin 45-a.
40. Menohoth 37-a.
41. Cited by Perlman: Mid. Rephuah 13.
42. Yebomoth 9-a.
43. Mid. Proverbs 1.
44. Hulin 45-b.
45. Menohoth 37-b.
46. Hulin 45-b.

47. Ibid.
48. Zohar 3: 227–234.
49. Ibid. 3: 221–225.
50. Hulin 47-a.
51. Ibid. 46-a.
52. Brochoth 61-b.
53. Yoma 85-a.
54. Reziel 19.
55. Sanhedrin 77-a.
56. Sukkah 3-a.
57. Pesachim 114-a.
58. Hulin 19-b; 21.
59. Zohar 3:235. See also Hulin 18-a.
60. Hulin 18-a.
61. Zohar 3:235.
62. Mid. Exodus 28.
63. Mid. Genesis 17:8.
64. Sanhedrin 49-a.
65. II Samuel 2:23.
66. Zohar 3:277. Cited by "Midrash Rephua" 1:6.
67. Zohar 3:2.
68. Hulin 46.
69. Ibid. 49-a.
70. Talmud; Bechoroth 55-a.
71. Ezekiel 21:26.
72. Brochoth 61-b.
73. Mid Exodus 24. Cited by "Midrash Rephua."
74. Mid. Numbers 15.
75. Job 6:6.
76. Mid. Numbers 15.
77. Mid. Leviticus 16.
78. Hulin 43-a.
79. Taanith 5-b.
80. Hulin 50-b.
81. Ibid. 19-b, 50-b. See Rashi.
82. Brochoth 61-b.
83. Shabbath 152-a.
84. Brochoth 53-b.
85. Ibid.
86. Talmud; Shabbath 82-a.
87. Ibid.
88. Reziel 13.
89. Mid. Genesis 4:7.
90. Shabbath 82-a; 155-b.
91. Oholoth 11:7; Shabbath, 155-b.
92. Shabbath 155-b.
93. Brochoth 61-b.
94. Proverbs 21:2.
95. Niddah 23-b.

96. Sanhedrin 108-a.
97. Sotha 3-b; Sanhedrin 108.
98. Mid. Sheichel; Tobit. Genesis 16:7.
99. The Semitic race had a propensity to pour out floods of tears; Samuel 3:32; Psalms 6:7; Luke 19:41; Lamentations 3:48.
100. Mid. Sheichel; Tobit 16:24.
101. Lamentations 11:12.
102. Celsus: Rapef. 7 (Galen Admin. Anatomy. Vol. 3:5).
103. Zohar 3:272.
104. Tekunei Hazohar 70.
105. That was a general tradition among medieval scholars, such as the celebrated physicians, Avicenna (980–1037 A.D.) and Abul-Casam (996–1050 A.D.). The seventh tunic, according to the Arabic conception, is anterior to the capsule of the lens.
106. Bechoroth 38-b. This is evidently an Aristotelian teaching (De Anima 3:17, 89).
107. Niddah 23-a.
108. Ibid. 24-b; Bechoroth 40-a.
109. Derech Erez Zuta 9.
110. The term "pupil" has the same significance; it is derived from the Latin pupa, a doll or little person (Pliny: Historia Naturalis 10:37).
111. Bechoroth 3-b.
112. Shabbath 33-b.
113. Ibid. 109-a.
114. Ecc. R. 12:2; Shabbath 151-b; 152-a.
115. Shabbath 151-b; Sanhedrin 104-b.
116. Yalkut Shimoni; Job 12.
117. Sorsby, A.: A Short History of Ophthalmology; John Ball, Sons and Danielson, Ltd., London, 1933, p. 34.
118. Sotha 3:2; Sanhedrin. Cited in Midrash Horephuoth 13; Mid. Tob. Genesis 16:7.
119. Leviticus 8:23.
120. Kedushin 21-b.
121. Mid. Leviticus 8:23.
122. Kethuboth 5-b.
123. Hulin 57-b.
124. Leviticus 14:14.
125. Nedarim 66-b.
126. Hulin 38-a.
127. Hagigah 2-a.
128. Talmud; Trimah 2-a.
129. Targum Isaiah 56:10.
130. Baba Kama 86-a.
131. Hagigah 2-b.
132. Ibid.
133. Ibid.
134. Mag 74-a.
135. Genesis, Rab. 76:3.
136. Baba Kama 91-a.

137. J. Shabbath 6:5; folio 75-b.
138. Abodah Zara 28-b.
139. Shabbath 11-b.
140. T. Shabbath 1:8.
141. J. Shabbath 13-b.
142. Proverbs 14:17.
143. Yebomoth 16:3; Job 39: 19–20.
144. Ibid. 15-a.
145. Talmud; Yebomoth 16:3.
146. Ibid.
147. Taanith 29-a.
148. Kethuboth 7-a.
149. Ibid. 77-a.
150. Odyssey 17:54–55.
151. Problem Sect. 33:7.
152. Brochoth 57-b.
153. Ibid. 24-b.
154. Hulin 42-a.
155. Ibid. 3:1, 47-b.
156. Ibid.
157. Ibid. 3:1, 42-a.
158. Ibid. 48-a.
159. Ibid. 3:1.
160. Ibid. 51-a.
161. Bechoroth 28-b.
162. Hulin 57-b.
163. Ibid.
164. Gittin 70-a
165. Baba Mezia 107-b; Baba Kama 92-b.
166. Shabbath 41-a.
167. Sukah 3.
168. Mid. Samuel 14.
169. Mid. Genesis R. 20.
170. Psalm 91:7; Talmud Brochoth 6-a
171. Brochoth 6-a; Tanhuma Aikab Mishpatim.
172. Brochoth 6-a.
173. Baba Kama 60-b.
174. Brochoth 3-a; Shabbath 151.
175. Mid. Shocher; Tobit. 19.
176. Baba Bathra 73-b. Also Montgomery, J. A.: Aramaic Incantation Texts from
     Nippur. University of Pennsylvania, 1933.
177. Pesachim 112-a.
178. Brochoth 51-a; Hulin 105-a.
179. Gittin 87; Yebomoth 17; Shabbath 69-b.
180. J. Brochoth 54-b.
181. Mid. Ruth 2.
182. Mid. Temurah.
183. Sotah 5-a. Mid. Temurah 3.
184. Baba Kama 92-b; Baba Mezia 107-b.
185. Reziel 12.

187. Baba Bathra 58-a. A change in the condition of the blood; the blood becoming watery is another cause; Mid. Leviticus 15:2.
188. Isaiah 13:24.
189. Job 7:14; 14:11.
190. Aboda Zara 26-b; Hulin 49-a.
191. Hulin 49-b.
192. Gittin 69-b.
193. Aboda Zara 26-b.
194. According to Herodotus and Diodorus the Egyptians attributed most diseases to overeating. They employed laxatives, emetics, and enemas as a routine prophylactic.
195. Gittin 70-a; Bechoroth 52-b.
196. Talmud; Baba Mezia 107-a.
197. Brochoth 62-b.
198. Ibid. 53-b.
199. Shabbath 41-a.
200. Hulin 85-b.
201. Shabbath 41; Numbers Rabba 15.
202. Ibid.
203. Shabbath 41-a.
204. Ecclesiasticus 37.
205. Genesis Rabba 48.
206. Sanhedrin 59-b; Hulin 84-a; Kethuboth 67-b.
207. Yoma 75-b.
208. Hulin 84-a.
209. Pesachim 112-a.
210. Ibid.
211. Gittin 69-b.
212. Callah Rabathi 100-d.
213. Shabbath 10-a.
214. Gittin 70-a.
215. Hupath Eliyahu Rabba.
216. Gittin 70-a.
217. Mid. Mishle 23:17.
218. Niddah 24-b.
219. Gittin 70-a; Callah Rabathi 1.
220. J. Talmud; Shabbath 85-b.

31

Talmudic Diagnosis and Treatment

DIAGNOSIS

THE Talmudists, like other ancients, had but few artificial devices to help them in their diagnosis of disease. In fact, before the middle of the eighteenth century, there were no precision diagnostic instruments and no precise methods with which to identify the location of disease. Auenbruger (1729–1802), the discoveror of percussion, was really the first to render available a means by which the clinician could estimate the advance or regression of lung diseases. He was followed eleven years after by Laennec (1781–1826), the discoveror of indirect auscultation by the use of the stethoscope. Direct auscultation had been employed as early as 2000 B.C. by the Egyptians. The Ebers Papyrus refers to this method of diagnosis. Ancient physicians resorted to their five senses to establish a diagnosis. By inspection, they determined the general appearance of the patient. Changes in the color of the skin, tongue, urine, and feces, growths, tumors, abscesses, dislocations, painful areas, and the existence of dropsy and ascites were noted by direct observation. Direct auscultation enabled the early physician to determine the existence of irregular breathing, pulmonary resonance, and certain pronounced evidences of cardiac disease.

The diagnosis of disease, as today, was based largely on subjective symptoms and objective investigation. Attention was paid to the pulse, the body temperature, the teeth, the condition of the skin, the condition of the eyes, the respiratory sounds, the strength of the voice of the patient, and the functions of the bladder and rectum. The "Hippocratic facies" (indicating the seriousness of a disease and consisting of the following symptoms: sunken eyes, livid skin, cold and leaden ears, pinched nose, hollow temples, and relaxed lips) was probably known to the Talmudic doctors.

The taking of the pulse was one of the few measures known to antiquity in the diagnosis of disease. "A physician that visits a patient takes his pulse."[1] R. Hiyah is reported to have taken the pulse of R. Yochanan. Of course, the clinical thermometer was a late invention. A temperature below 100 or 101 was probably not detected. However, from the several expressions in Talmudic literature with reference to fever, it is evident that different words were used for moderate and very high fevers. *Hamma* and *shimsha* were both etymologically derived from a root designating the sun and were used to indicate a moderate fever; high fever was expressed by the words *eshshatha zemertha*. If one was inflicted with *eshshatha zemertha*, his case was considered sufficiently severe to violate the Sabbath laws.[2] Raba, a third century scholar, entertained an advanced view with reference to fever, "Fever if not the messenger of the Angel of Death, serves as a protection of the body against diseases."[3] It appears that the febrile diseases discussed in the Talmud were mostly malarial in nature and, because of the belief that affliction was a punishment by God for religious violations, the treatment consisted frequently of religious and mystical devices.

Fever was perhaps the first diagnostic sign of disease observed by early man. It usually did not require much diagnostic acumen to perceive a high fever. A mere touch of a neighbor's body could detect a marked febrile condition. Fever was viewed by ancients not as a symptom of some internal disease but as a disease itself. It was dreaded because it was frequently followed by death, particularly when of the pernicious malarial type.

R. Josef, to forestall fever after a chill, engaged in working a hand mill, and R. Shesheth carried lumber in order to induce perspiration.[4] Rabina, when his daughter took sick with fever, violated the law against using the first fruits of tree and administered the juice of figs, a remedy which is often used at the present time.

In addition to pulse and temperature, rapid and particularly labored respiration was undoubtedly noted. The death of a person was established by the absence of breathing or by the stoppage of the pulse beat. R. Pappe thought that the breathing test was more suitable, since it did not necessitate examination of the heart or pulse.[5] The immediate cause of death was generally ascribed to failure of respiration.

R. Ishmael said:

The body is like a leather bottle full of air; as long as the bottle is in good condition, the air remains intact. But as soon as an opening or a crack shows itself, the air escapes. As long as the body is ruled in equal proportions of the four elements, the spirit or pneuma fills the body. But when one of these varies, a change in the person's health is experienced. When the change becomes more marked, the spirit or the air escapes from the body and the body decays.

To the query of R. Akiba as to how children die, he replied, "When one of these forces becomes defective."[6]

Mar Samuel employed a device known as *Beza-Tormita*.[7] This was a method by which an egg was passed many times from hot to cold water until it shrank in size so that a person could swallow it. Somehow, by swallowing the egg completely without breaking it up in the mouth, the healer was informed as to what medicine should be administered. Perhaps this was a kind of test meal administered to patients troubled with gastric disturbances. Another diagnostic device credited to Mar Samuel, mentioned in the Talmud, was called *Kuchla*.[8] This seems to have been a painful procedure, but it is difficult to conjecture just what it was. Perhaps it was a rude kind of a stomach tube.

To identify the origin of blood from the mouth, a straw was dipped into the blood; if the blood stuck to the walls of the straw, it was taken as evidence that the bleeding was pulmonary in character and was curable; if not, it was considered hepatic in origin.[9] Liver defects were considered less than those of the lungs, although hepatic bleeding was thought to be a sign of advanced systemic destruction.

DISEASES AND TREATMENT

In addition to the diseases mentioned in the Old Testament, the Talmud enumerated a number of ailments; not all of these have been identified. The terms *maggepha* and *deber* included many widespread contagious diseases of great mortality, which are presently known as epidemics. They might have included bubonic plague, black death, typhus, cholera, and smallpox. The Mishna,[10] which is a legal work and is precise in its definitions, defined an epidemic disease as one whereby, in a small city like Amiko, out of 500 adult persons, 3 died every day for a period of three days, and in a larger city like Akko, out of 1500 adult persons, 9 died each day for a period of three days. It may be noted that Galen,[11] who was until the sixteenth century accepted as the preeminent medical authority, defined an epidemic as a disease from which many people died in a short time.

Diphtheria: Among the diseases mentioned as highly contagious was *ascara* (croup, or diphtheria). It was said to attack a person during the night. In the case of infants *(tinokoth)*, this disease was considered fatal.[12] Death from *ascara* was caused by suffocation. "The rabbis learned that of the 903 diseases prevailing in the world, *ascara* was the most severe. . . . It is like a thorn in a ball of wool which gets more twisted when one tries to loosen it."[13] *Ascara* was not merely a local disease. It also attacked the gastrointestinal tract. R. Eliezar bar Josse stated that one time he was on board a vessel, and he was stricken with *ascara;* a sailor promptly crossed his throat, causing the *ascara* to pass from his mouth to that of the sailor[14] (indicating that the disease could be communicated from person to person). The statement that the disease passed from the mouth of the rabbi to that of the sailor may be ascribed to the old belief that a disease was taken over completely by the second party, the first party becoming entirely cured ("scapegoat").

"The rabbis taught that there are four kinds of retribution for sin: dropsy *(hadrokan)* is a punishment for sins committed against God; jaundice *(yerokon)* is a chastisement for gratuitous hatred; poverty, a punitive measure against pride; and *ascara*, a punishment for committing slander." R. Nachman stated that the plague *(maggepha)*, brought upon Israel following the return of the twelve men who searched the land, was *ascara* and that it was brought upon them as punishment for their slanderous report about the land.[15] The same rabbi also taught that the 12,000 disciples of R. Akiba, who died in seven weeks between Passover and Pentecost, perished from *ascara*.[16]

Ascara, like other epidemic diseases of a deadly nature, was looked upon as caused by demonic possession and accordingly was treated by magical means. The Talmud, however, mentioned a number of remedies in addition to the magical cures. One of these was blood letting, and such treatment was permitted even on the Sabbath day. R. Mari, citing R. Yohanan, stated that lentils were a good prophylactic against *ascara;* even if only used as a food once in thirty days, lentils would keep *ascara* out of the house.[17] Lentils also formed one of the ingredients in the gargle recommended by Arataeus for croup. Hippocrates and Pliny recommended lentils in ulcerative stomatitis. Other remedies mentioned were salt (perhaps as a gargle) and oil to be brushed in the throat.

Dysentery: *Burdam* has been identified with dysentery. Etymologically, the word *burdam* signified a "cistern of blood" because of the bloody flux accompanying this disease. The symptoms of *burdam*, aside from bloody stools, were swelling of the abdomen and severe pain. Diarrhea was the first sign of the disease, and at that time it behooved one to look for a remedy. *Burdam* was said to cause sudden death. Patients could die while talking. Visiting such a patient was prohibited; even mentioning his name was forbidden, perhaps for psychological reasons.[18]

Eruptive Diseases: Few eruptive diseases were differentiated. They were included under the name *mukei shchin*[19] ("eruption of the skin"); but judging from the strict precaution taken against *mukei shchin*, it would seem that it referred to a particular epidemic ailment, perhaps smallpox, which was known to have raged in the Near East since early times.

Trachoma: Another disease of highly communicative character was *reathan*,[20] which was characterized by lacrimation, discharge from the nose, flow of sputum from the mouth, and a thick mucous discharge from the eyes. I. M. Rabinowitz (1818–1897), in his French translation of the Talmud, opined that *reathan* was an ocular affection. Dr. A. M. Mazia, who practiced medicine in Jerusalem for many years, identified it with trachoma, which, according to his observation, was often marked in the Near East by lacrimation, heavy mucous discharge from the eyes, running nose, and a flow of sputum from the mouth.[21]

R. Jonathan warned against the flies which fed on the eye discharge of people suffering from *reathan (baalei reathan)*. R. Zeira prohibited sitting in front of such a patient for the wind might blow the disease over. R. Eliezer warned against entering the tent of such a patient.[22] From the description of the disease and the strict regulations against contact with such a patient, it is evident that the Talmudic teachers understood its contagious nature. The observation to beware of flies that fed on the discharge shows that it was suspected that flies were carriers of contagion.

Prophylaxis: Epidemic diseases, because of their rapid spread and high mortality, were ascribed to supernatural forces—ruthless fiends or demons sent to possess the person and punish him for his sins.

Mar Samuel ordered a day of fasting in Machoza when he was told that an epidemic was raging in a distant place. When asked why this was necessary when the epidemic was so far away, he replied, "The bridge is not removed for the caravans to pass," implying that disease could be carried from distant places by caravans.[23] R. Judah, when told there was an epidemic among swine, ordered a fast day. When asked whether disease could be carried by animals to man, he answered as a rule not, but swine were an exception because the anatomical structure of their viscera resembled that of man.[24] Prayers, fasting, and charity were the principal measures adopted to prevent and cure epidemic diseases. All these methods are still widely employed.

Pleuritis: *Barsam*, according to the commentator Rashi, applied to sneezing. The word, however, in cognate languages such as Arabic, means "pleuritis." It is to be distinguished from *sarsam*, which signifies "phrenitis." Abayye said that foam or froth was not to be drunk, not because it was unpalatable, but because it might cause *barsam*. The foam of wine was prescribed to counteract the effect of *barsam*; the foam of beer, to counteract the effect of wine; and the foam of water, to neutralize the ill effect of wine *(similia similibus curantur)*; but for the foam of water (evidently polluted), there was no remedy. The following recipe was against *barsam*: Gum ammoniac the size of a pistachio nut; honey galbanum, the size of an almond; white honey, a spoonful; clear wine, the size of a *machuza matia*. Directions: boil (when ammoniac was boiled it was a sign that the remedy was ready for use).[25]

Dropsy: Another important disease mentioned in the Talmud was dropsy *(hadrokan)*. The Talmudists recognized three kinds of *hadrokan:* (1) Anascara *(abah)* where the entire body became dropsical and was usually observed in cases due to chronic heart disease, but also occurred with cirrhosis of the liver or defective metabolism (hypothyroidism) where the water of the body was not extracted normally. This also could be produced by nephritis or severe anemia when the quality of the blood was greatly impoverished. (2) *Hadrokan* where the body appeared large and blown-up perhaps by intestinal gases that were not eliminated. This pseudodropsy was a condition which ancient writers classed under the term "dropsy." (3) *Dak* (leukophlegmasia), a dropsical tendency with general anemia and flabby skin, which was ascribed to sexual sin.[26] R. Osia said, "Those that are given to sin are punished by *hadrokan*."[27] R. Nachman bar Yitzhak said, "*Hadrokan* is a sign of sinfulness." The second kind of dropsy was attributed to witchcraft.[28] R. Gamliel thought that *hadrokan* was due to habitual neglect of defecation.[29] Another Talmudic statement was that three types of disease could cause death while talking—*hadrokan*, *burdam*, and difficult labor.[30] Rabbah bar R. Huna, in the name of R. Ketina, said, "The more one restrains himself from defecation, the more he is likely to be affected with *hadrokan*, and the more one keeps himself back from urination the more he is likely to suffer from *hadrokan*."[31] The term *adripikos* was derived from the Greek *hydropicos* and was another term of *hadrokan*. The Talmud does not suggest any natural remedy for *hadrokan*. The New Testament relates of a sufferer of dropsy who was healed by the touch of Jesus.[32]

Anemia: *Yerokon* (chlorosis or green sickness), so-named on account of the peculiar green or yellowish-green complexion which the patient often presented, was a form of primary anemia resulting from a diminution of the red corpuscles and hemoglobin. The fact that the word *achezu* ("seizure") was used in connection with the attack of *yerokon* shows the popular belief of the day that it was caused by an evil spirit. The cause of *yerokon*, according to the Talmud, was punishment for groundless hating.[33] The immediate cause was given as restraint of the bladder.

As medical treatment, the urine of an ass[34] was recommended. It is interesting to note that Dioscorides suggested the same treatment for renal diseases. The flesh of an ass, although prohibited as a diet, was permitted in the case of *yerokon*.[35] The head of a salted *shibbuta* (fish) boiled in beer, or three measures each of Persian dates, wax, and red aloe boiled in beer were considered efficacious. Date juice was considered an efficient remedy.

Gastrointestinal Diseases: Under the term *holi meayim* were included all gastrointestinal diseases. Owing to the warm climate of the Near East, food easily became decomposed, resulting in various types of gastrointestinal intoxications. Other causes of *holi meayim* were set forth, such as sudden changes in dietary habits,[36] lack of walking exercise after meals,[37] improper food or too much meat,[38] and exposure to cold, night air, and moisture. R. Hiyah recommended the following prophylaxis, "One who does not wish to contract *holi meayim*, shall make a habit of taking regular baths summer and winter, of not indulging in food that he relishes, and of not restraining when the bowels need evacuation."[39] One who felt that a certain food he had eaten was injurious to him, should try to get it out of his system. For this purpose, emetics could be used or the hand could be used in the mouth to induce vomiting.

The treatment of *holi meayim* consisted of massage, with oil and wine[40] internally, and compresses to relieve the pain. *Holi meayim* appeared to have caused excruciating pain. Rab said he would rather suffer any pain than that of *holi meayim*.[41] A folk remedy was to place hot cups on the umbilical region.[42]

For the relief of abdominal pain *(ke'eb-meayim)*, long peppers in wine were used daily. As many as 100 pepper kernels in wine a day were recommended.[43] Rabbin of Naresh cured the daughter of R. Ashi with 150 kernels of pepper.[44] Old apple wine (seventy years old)

was secured for Rabbi Judah when he was troubled with *holi meayim.*[45]
Other remedies were fresh camomile leaves boiled in water[46] and
asparagus wine taken on an empty stomach.[47] Mental occupation was
suggested for pain. The study of Torah was thought to be particularly
effective.[48]

Patients sick with *holi meayim* would not be punished for their sins
in the world to come.[49] The severe punishment they received during
the disease atoned for their sins. Death from *holi meayim* was explained as being due to draining the fluid from the system.

Rabbi, the author of the Mishna, died of *holi meayim.* That day a
faithful female servant of the house, who could not bear to see him
suffer, went on the roof and prayed that the angels above would remove the Rabbi from this troubled world. Persons who died from
holi meayim were deodorized with aromatic substances.[50]

Kolos, according to Jastrow and others, applied to colic. R. Yeho-
shua ben Levi[51] was sick with *kolos* and was advised by R. Haninah
and R. Jonathan to grind cress, mix it with old wine, and drink it. The
meaning of *kolos,* however, is doubtful, since colic prevailed mostly
among children. Musaphia reads it *colum,* a disease known to have
been prevalent in the early part of the present era. It is said that
Emperor Tiberias (14–37 A.D.) died from this disease.[52]

Under the name of *tachtoniyoth,* the Talmud referred to a number
of diseases confined to the rectal passage. These included hemorrhoids,
fistula of the anus, abscess, and pruritus ani. Most frequently it referred
to hemorrhoids.[53] Among the causes of *tachtoniyoth* mentioned by
the Talmud were the use of hard substances to wipe the anus after
defecation, indigestible food, and straining during defecation. Among
the symptoms mentioned were a trembling heart, failing eyes, and
languishing of the soul.[54] The only treatment recommended was dates.

Pica (signifying a depression), referred to any disease situated in
the depression between the two gluteus muscles. The treatment was
application of watercress to the parts, bathing in the hot mineral springs
of Tiberias, and drinking the sap of a cedar tree *(zabliga)*[55] or palm
leaves boiled in water.[56]

Bulimus *(bulimia)* was a disease characterized by excessive appetite
and a morbid hunger excited by the sight or smell of food. The Talmud
used the word *achezu* ("seizure") with reference to this disease. Because of the suddenness of the attack, folk medicine attached a supernatural significance to this disease: possession by a hunger-demon. This
was considered a dangerous disease for it was even permitted to give
a patient suffering with it nonkosher food.[57] The remedy for this ex-

cessive appetite was honey and sweet things, and such other products that would give quick satiety. R. Yochanan once said, "I was seized by *bulimia* and had the presence of mind to run towards the east to a fig tree."[58] While R. Judah and R. Josse were travelling, the former was seized with *bulimia* and obtained food from a shepherd. The following tale illustrates how the very sight of food precipitated an attack: Ameimar, Mar Zutra, and R. Ashi were at the threshold of a certain King Azgur when the cook passed by with food intended for the king. Mar Zutra noticed that R. Ashi was pale. He quickly touched with his finger the food being carried to the king and brought it to the mouth of R. Ashi. Said the latter to Mar Zutra, "You risked your life to save me; you have spoiled the king's meal."[59]

Podagra: *Podagra* appears to have prevailed in Talmudic times. Rab was of the opinion that the disease of the legs which afflicted King Asa in his old age was *podagra*.[60] Mar Zutra described the pain of *podagra* as a "needle" sensation.[61] The Mishna stated that *podagra* was a swelling of the soles of the feet; Aretaeus remarked that *podagra* was marked by pain all over the body, which could indicate arthritis. The causes of *podagra* were narrow shoes, short beds, and excessive sexual intercourse.

Skin Disease: In addition to leprosy which has been discussed in the chapter of Ancient Hebrew Medicine, there have been many other diseases in the ancient East characterized by skin eruption. The term *muchei shchin* included a large number of skin affections that were not identified individually. All of them received similar treatment; many of them perhaps may have been syphilitic in character, as may be seen from the following comment in the Midrash.[62] Commenting on the passage of Leviticus 13:20, the Midrash explained that skin eruptions resulted from lechery. Rabo stated, "One shall not wed a woman from a family addicted to skin disease."[63]

Heart Disease: The Talmud gave few details with respect to heart disease. It mentioned only heart symptoms. Rab said, "I can bear any pain except *ke'eb leb*[64] (anginal syndrome)." Another heart condition *khulsha d'libba* (heart weakness), generally affecting the hungry, was described. The Talmud related that R. Hisda and R. Abba bar Huna, while serving for a long period as judges, were stricken with *khulsha d'libba*.[65] R. Zeira was prevented from delivering his discourse because he was attacked by *khulsha d'libba*.[66] R. Ayva feared an attack of *khulsha d'libba* when he went on an empty stomach to listen to the lengthy discourse of R. Joseph;[67] this was perhaps a fainting spell. The disease could be brought on by using *khardal* (mustard) daily. "*Khar-*

dal taken monthly is valuable for many diseases but taken daily is injurious to the heart."[68]

Purcha d'libba (flying of the heart) probably referred to tachycardia; no details of the condition were given.[69]

It is not certain whether "heaviness of the heart" *(yukra d'libba)* referred to a heart that was physically heavy (that is hypertrophied) or whether is connoted a spiritually heavy heart or a sense of precardial constriction. To treat *yukra d'libba,* three shekels of assat *(chilthith)* in cold or warm water were advocated to be drunk daily. One should be careful to be certain that the patient did not vomit, for vomiting was considered dangerous to the heart.[70]

Groaning from the heart *(gonach millibba)* referred to asthmatic bronchitis rather than to heart trouble. Loud asthmatic wheezes and rales are still frequently mistaken by the laity for heart disease; of course, at times they may be symptomatic of "cardiac" asthma. It would appear from a statement by R. Mrimus[71] that the term was even used to refer to a person that groaned. It is related that R. Judah ben Baba suffered from a groaning heart and was advised to suck milk directly from the udder of a goat every morning and evening.[72]

Tzirca d'libba, according to Rashi,[73] meant severe pain in the heart. Jastrow thought this to be angina pectoris,[74] and it could refer to an anginal syndrome, with or without coronary occlusion. The Talmudic therapeutics against heart disease was largely folkloristic. Drugs mentioned were black cumin *(ketzah).* "He that is in the habit of using black cumin will never have pain in the heart."[75] The mother of R. Yirmeyahu was against using *ketzah* because of the smell it produced. She scraped the *ketzah* off the bread before she disposed of it.[76] The mother of Abayye, who knew a large number of folk remedies, advised the patient to eat roast meat, taken from the right hip joint of a male animal, followed by wine.[77]

Diseases of the Mouth and Teeth: Among diseases of the mouth mentioned *fetor ex ore,* stomatitis, ranula, and abscess. R. Muna, citing R. Judah said, "One that touches his hand to his mouth deserves to have his hand cut off." The hand was responsible for polypus.[78] Abayye said polyps caused *fetor oris.*

One who ate foods without salt and drank all drinks, but no water, could get a fetid breath.[79] Indigestion was given as the cause of offensive breath. To aid digestion, one was advised to take short walks after meals.[80] Lentils, which were a favorite dish in Palestine, were thought to corrupt a person's breath if eaten daily.[81] A certain fish *(benito)* produced a heavy breath.[82] One who ate raw cabbage should not speak to people that day as cabbage emitted a foul odor. Long fast days tended to produce an offensive odor from the mouth.[83]

Zapidna (gingivitis) could be mentioned among dental diseases. "It begins in the mouth and travels quickly through the stomach and intestines."[84] One of the symptoms was bleeding of the gums, for "as soon as food touches a molar tooth the gums around that tooth begin to bleed." R. Yohanan[85] and Rabbi were said to have been troubled with *zapidna*. The disease was ascribed to the practice of eating very cold or very hot food. R. Yohanan was cured of it by a Roman lady, the daughter of a certain Domitian, who kept her formula secret. He visited her home on a Thursday and Friday and she herself administered the remedy. Not being able to visit her on Saturday because her home was too far away to walk on the Sabbath day, she consented to give him the formula, which consisted of fermented dough, olive oil, and salt. It was applied with a goose feather to the mouth.[86] Abayye recommended young olives roasted on a new iron plate and applied to the bleeding gums.

That the teeth were the source of human strength[87] (and should be taken care of) was a Talmudic statement. R. Meir was in the habit of saying, "Grind with your teeth and you will find it in your step."[88]

As a toothache sedative, a grain of salt was applied to the cavity.[89] Fruit-vinegar was another remedy for toothache.[90] The use of spleen as a food was recommended as a preservative of teeth. The spleen was to be well chewed but not swallowed.[91] Hygiene of the mouth was insisted upon. *Fetor ex ore* was referred to in the Talmud, "One that omits salt from a meal will be troubled with a fetid odor from his mouth."[92] The steam of a bath was perilous to teeth.[93]

As a prophylaxis against foul breath, the use of peppers or mastic was recommended.[94] Peppers were a favorite drug of Dioscorides and are still used in certain countries for fetid breath. *Hinchi,* perhaps ulcerative stomatitis, was only mentioned by name. The treatment was *chumithi ki mamru,* the meaning of which is not clear. This remedy was to be kept in the mouth.[95] Another recipe was a mixture of coarse bran, green lentils, carub, beans, and hop-buds, made in the size of a nut and kept in the mouth. The juice of white cress drawn into the mouth through a straw was also suggested. A fetid breath was considered a physical deformity; and if one married a woman with the understanding that she was physically sound and it turned out that she had a fetid breath, the marriage could be dissolved.[96]

Diseases of the Ear: Very little was known of the interior machinery of the ear, and consequently the deviation from the normal was not recognized. Common observation, of course, dictated that abnormal secretion of the ear was pathologic.[97] The treatment of catarrh of the ear (in addition to the remedies mentioned in the first chapter) was a plug of (cotton) saturated in oil and inserted into the aural cavity. Two affections of the nose were identified: catarrhal rhinitis and polyps; the treatment was folklorish.

Mental Diseases: Mental diseases have always been regarded by ancient peoples as of supernatural origin. The insane person was supposed to be possessed by a frenzied, avenging demon. The appearance and behavior of the insane, who no longer expressed the customary thoughts and no longer spoke with the familiar voice, suggested that some strange being had entered that person. The remedies administered to the insane were not intended for the patient but for the expulsion of the possessing demon; and consequently, the fouler the remedy, the quicker the demon would be forced to leave the body of the sick. Indeed before Phillippe Pinel (1745–1826), insane persons were treated savagely. The cruel treatment was directed, not so much against the patient, since it was believed that the insane had no sense of feeling, but as a means of expelling the evil spirit that took possession of him. "The insane," stated the Talmud, "have no sensation and no judgment." One of the treatments to get rid of the evil spirit was the burning of a certain root; the unpleasant smoke was supposed to induce the demon to leave the body of the insane.

The worst form of mental disorder was considered to be epilepsy *(nikhpe)*. Throughout antiquity, it was looked upon as a sacred disease. According to the Old Testament, Balaam prophesied while he was under the influence of an epileptic spell. Ancient Greeks viewed epileptic seizures as a manifestation of the activities of the gods. The Talmud recognized epilepsy as of hereditary nature, "One is prohibited to marry from a family of epileptics. . . . There are two kinds of epileptics, those that have periodic seizures and those whose spells come on irregularly."[98]

Ocular Diseases: The Talmudists identified a number of external ocular affections, including lagophthalmos, blepharitis ciliaris, conjunctivitis, hyperemia of the conjunctiva, hemorrhage, subconjunctival hemorrhage, trachoma (or ophthalmia granulosa), gonorrheal ophthalmia, ophthalmia neonatorum, ankyloblepharon, nystagmus, strabismus, pterygium, macula, leukoma, interstitial keratitis, hypopyon, keratitis, coloboma, cataract, ophthalmomycosis, parasitic ophthalmia, exophthalmos, and phthisis bulbi.[99]

Spittle was among popular therapeutic agents used in ocular practice by ancient physicians. It was taken from a healthy persons before breakfast.[100] One reads in Mark, "And he took the blind man by the hand and led him out of the town, and when he had spit on his eye and put his hand upon him, he asked him if he saw aught, and he saw things clearly."[101] The cure of inflammatory diseases of the eye with spittle was also popular among the Romans and Egyptians. Tacitus stated that "the eyes of Emperor Vespasian were cured with spittle."[102] In Egypt, spittle was used as a solvent for disturbing films in the eye.

The spittle of the seventh son of the same wife was particularly effective; and the father of seven sons was in an enviable position, demanding a high price for this much-sought remedy. The Talmud preferred the spittle of the first-born son.[103] Next to spittle was mothers' milk, a still popular remedy.

Ancient writers mentioned a popular remedy called "collyrium." Unlike modern eye lotions, collyrium was made in three different forms (that is liquid, semisolid, and powder). The Greek collyrium contained oxide of antimony as one of its ingredients. In Palestine, collyria were sold in public market places with other merchandise; the ingredients were not disclosed. It was often made in paste form. Pliny stated that a cataplasm collyrium consisted of soaked bread, wine, water, milk or white of an egg, in addition to the regular ingredients. It was made up in the form of small bars. In Rome, the ingredients were stamped on the bars. In Palestine, the bars were sold under the name *kilirith*.[104] Celsus named ten different collyria and gave the ingredients of each. They seem to have been well known, for, in prescribing, physicians identified the different collyria by numbers.[105]

Dry collyrium (xerocollyrium) was used in powdered form, intended to be dusted in the conjunctival sac. The use of the powder appears to have been a painful procedure. Once the famous patriarch Rabbi was suffering from some ocular disease, and he was advised by his physician to use the powdered collyrium. Rabbi refused to be treated with this irritant.[106] Mar Samuel, a prominent physician of the third century, had no faith in any of the collyria. He said, "A few drops of cold water in the morning and a general bath in the evening is better than all the collyria in the world."[107] Another popular drug, often spoken of in Talmudic writings, was *cohol*. According to Kohut, it was an herb that colored the tissue of the eye, somewhat like mild silver protein, and was supposed to strengthen the muscles of the eye.[108] It was applied on the lids and within the conjunctiva. Until forty years of age, *cohol* was supposed to have a beneficial effect on the eyesight, but after forty it had no effect.[109] Another collyrium known as *puch*, rendered *stibium*, was recommended for the growth of falling eye-lashes.[110]

The gall of reptiles, animals, and fish was used for various diseases of the eye, particularly to absorb films on the cornea as in the case of Tobit.[111] In ancient Babylon, the gall of frogs was used in certain diseases of the eye. Diluted reptile gall was used by the Egyptians for absorbing obscuring films.

Blood, particularly that of a bat, was used frequently by ancient oculists. According to the Ebers Papyrus, it was a specific in trichiasis. Galen also recommended it in certain ocular diseases. The Talmud found it efficient in leukoma and proptosis.[112] Bat's blood is a popular remedy in some countries to this day. It is believed that, when one paints his eyes with this blood, he will see at night as well as during the day.[113] Hippocrates' treatment for nyctalopia was the administration of ox liver in honey, purgatives to drive the humors away. Counter-irritants were used, such as strong gargles and sharp masticatories, to drive away the injurious humors or fluxors from the eyes. Local applications were seldom employed in acute cases for fear they would increase the fluxors.

The Talmudic writers recommended heat for inflamed parts,[114] an old theory being that disease might be cured by remedies which, if given to healthy persons, would produce diseases;[115] this antedated Hahnemann's theory: *similia similibus curantur*.

Among the favorite drugs the leaves of coriander, *kusbarta*, were considered effective on inflamed lids,[116] and *gargira*, the leaves of white mustard, were recommended by R. Huna for the same condition.[117]

The therapeutic measures taken against trachoma, reathan, or *enei dolphos* by ancient Hebrew physicians were of an empiric nature (most of the remedies cannot be identified). The bark of nut and fig trees was mentioned,[118] and shavings of hides[119] appear to have been a favorite local remedy. Evidently these therapeutic agents were intended for the purpose of rubbing the conjunctival surfaces. The old Egyptian treatment, according to the Ebers Papyrus, was to apply ver-digris with onion on the lids.[120] Hippocrates advised rubbing the inner surface of the lids with Milesian wool wrapped around an applicator until the blood ceased flowing and a thin fluid took its place.

The medical treatment for cataract, which was known as "the mounting of water in the eye" *(efuso ocularium)*, was to abstain from drinking water and eating food that would make one thirsty, such as fish, in order to keep away the fluid of the body. In the Talmud, it was known as *mayim-hakbuim*.[121]

The question of whether or not the loss of sight had a compensatory effect on other sensory organs, such as hearing, touch, taste, and smell (a subject much discussed by ancient as well as by modern observers), was decided in the affirmative by Talmudic authorities. In the blind, all the special senses were more developed than in the seeing persons. "A blind child can recognize the mother by the odor of her breasts and the taste of the nipples."[122]

Another interesting observation made by the Gemara was that the blind had excessive appetites, "They eat, but they do not fill up." The "filling up" was influenced by the visual organs.[123] This Talmudic statement was corroborated by the observations of superintendents of institutions for the blind, who also noticed this strange phenomenon in the blind.

Hydrophobia: Hydrophobia was a well known disease in Talmudic times. It was considered fatal. "No man has appeared who could say that he has seen a man live who was bitten by a mad dog." The treatment of hydrophobia, according to Mathiah ben-Heresh, consisted of killing the dog and using its liver as a remedy against the disease. In order that the man stricken with hydrophobia might dismiss his mind from water, he was made to drink through a tube from a vessel in which the water was not exposed.[124]

MATERIA MEDICA

Medicaments were chiefly vegetables; less frequently, animal products. The therapeutic efficacy of fresh air, sunlight, and baths was well understood. Aside from herbs and animal substances, the Talmudic pharmacopeia contained metal and mineral ingredients, such as mercury, iron, lead, antimony, and copper. The term *sam* (Aramaic *sama*) designated all kinds of materials used in medicine, including poisonous and narcotic substances. Where the physiological action of the drug was known, a description of its action was added to the word *sama*. For example, *sama deshanta*[125] signified a hypnotic drug; and *sama di naphiza*,[126] an abortifacient. Poisonous drugs of any origin were known as *sama demotha*, or *sam hamaveth*.[127] Drugs were often administered in powder form. A story is told of a wet nurse who sprayed poisonous powder *(sama mitha)* on her nipples to kill a nursing baby.[128] A restorative was known as *sam hayim*,[129] or *sama dechaye. Samthar* was used as an analgesic in sciatica and stab wounds.[130] Pungent or strong medicines were known as *sama harifta*.[131] Some drugs, such as *aphikte phisin*, an emetic, retained their Greek names.[132]

Olive oil was used as a base for ointments, to soak dressings on wounds, and as a gargle for sore throat.[133] Vinegar was used as a hemostatic. Wine, mixed with peppers, was prescribed for a disordered stomach. Goat milk was employed for dyspnea; and if fresh from the udder,[134] for acute and chronic coughs. A mixture of oil and turpentine was a favorite remedy for *cholelithiasis*. This drug was instilled rectally. Onions were a remedy for intestinal parasites.[135] Hydrophobia was treated with the liver of the dog that caused it. Cold water in the morning and a warm foot bath in the evening were recommended for sore eyes,[136] and emetics were prescribed for nausea.

Honey was extensively used by all ancient peoples. The old dictum, "with sweet, man heals bitterness,"[137] was adhered to in the Talmud. It was administered to persons troubled with *bulimia*[138] and in many diseases of the eye. The hot sulfur baths of Tiberias were recommended for bodily pain, colds, before venesection, and for plethora. Exposure to the sun was ordered for many abnormal conditions.[139] Wine was frequently used for the treatment of wounds, possibly because of its alcoholic content which acted as an antiseptic.[140] As an antipyretic measure, fresh watermelon was applied to the head.[141]

Plasters and poultices were used for external inflammatory conditions. A *retiyah* (plaster) had wax or tallow for its base. "One whose skin was stabbed with an *izmel* (a scalpel) should place a *retiyah* on the wound."[142] The fact that it was forbidden to keep a *retiyah* in the house during Passover indicates that it probably contained flour as a base. *Espelanish*[143] and *neshiftha* were names of various plasters. The first was perhaps a corruption of the Greek *emplastron*. It was made of fat with a small quantity of wax. This local application was considered to be a pain reliever. The fact that the contents of *espelanish* were placed in a leather or cloth bag would indicate that it was a poultice rather than a plaster. It was administered while warm to the affected parts.

Melugma[144] was probably an ointment; it was composed of a variety of foodstuffs, including wheat products mixed with figs.[145]

A folklore remedy was a plaster composed of the fat of an ox that had killed a person and was afterwards stoned to death. It was believed that such a plaster would kill pain as the ox had killed the human being.

Drugs were to be taken on an empty stomach. An important factor in the therapy was the day of the week and the time of the year that the drugs were administered. Vermifuges, for example, were administered on the first day of the lunar month for astrologic reasons. The first seven days of the lunar month were considered most propitious for the taking of medicine.

As early as 1600 B.C., drugs were ordered in the form of written prescriptions. According to the Ebers Papyrus, the Egyptian physicians wrote down the ingredients on reed leaves. The name of each ingredient was specified and the amount to be used expressed in units to be weighted out on scales. About 100 such prescriptions were published by George Ebers in Leipzig in the year 1875. The Jewish physicians appear to have adopted a similar practice when ordering medicine for the sick. The prescription was known as *leitha*, and this word formed the superscription of the medical substances ordered. The following was an example of a prescription for sterility ordered by R. Yochanan,[146] a well-known physician of the third century:

Leitha:

Gum Arabic (Alexandrian) . . . . .zuz i
Alum . . . . z i
Crocus (saffron) . . . . z i

The following is an ointment for external use, the formula of which was credited to R. Abayye:[147]

Leitha:

Adepis . . . . .part vii
Cera (wax) . . . . .part i

Frequently, when the exact weight was not important, the amount of the drug was measured by the fistful. The following was given for hemorrhages:[148]

Leitha:

Karum (caroway seed)
Crocus (saffron)
Mix in wine, boil, and drink, and say, "Arouse yourself from the hemorrhage."

Celsus mentioned a Jewish plaster *(Judaei emplastrum fracto capiti accommodatum)* which contained as many as twelve ingredients.[149] It seemed that this plaster was very popular for many centuries, for it was mentioned again by the famous fifth century Byzantine physician Aetius. Another popular Hebrew preparation for diseases of the spleen was the *"ad Splenum remedum singulara,"* which was associated with the name of Gamliel Bathrai, and was mentioned by the Roman physician Marcellus Empicurus in his book "De Medicamentis."[150]

RULES FOR CARE OF THE SICK

The physician's behavior toward the patient and his bedside manner were regulated. When entering the sick room, the physician was instructed first to grasp the patient's hand[151] and then inquire about his condition. Next he had to investigate whether the dietary regulations had been carried out by the attendant. He had to ascertain that the patient's bed was comfortable and particularly that the linen was not damp. Following these preliminaries, the doctor proceeded with the examination. If the physician found that his patient's condition was hopeless, he was not to disclose this fact to the patient, although he could reveal it to the family. In such a case, he instructed the attendants not to limit the patient's diet in any way but to give him anything he desired. The physician himself, however, should never give up hope.[152]

Like all ancient peoples, the Hebrews believed in omens for prognosis. An unfavorable omen was when the patient was apathetic, preferring to keep his face towards the wall. Among the favorable omens were perspiration, free defecation and urination, restful sleep, dreams, seminal emission, and sneezing.[153] If the case were hopeless, the doctor warned the attendants not to move the patient. R. Meir compared a dying patient to a flickering candle. When the candle was moved, the light was extinguished.

The visiting hours for the patient were regulated. R. Eliezer instructed his son, when visiting the sick, to make an effort to be pleasant and cheerful and not stay too long because such might fatigue the patient.[154] Visiting hours should be early in the morning because during the morning hours the condition of the sick was better. During late hours, the sickness was generally worse, and the visitor might carry away a wrong impression. Only relatives could see the sick during the first three days of the illness. After three days (presumably when the patient's condition was better), strangers could visit him.

EQUIPMENT OF THE PHYSICIAN

The outfit of the Talmudic physician consisted of a bag (nartik),[155] a scalpel (izmel),[156] a trephine ("the nail") for blood letting, a sharp-pointed probe (makdeiach,[157] which might have been used for puncturing abscesses and exploring places not easily reached with the fingers), a pair of scissors (misporayim),[158] a speculum (tarvad), a spoon (pointed at the top and curved at the end), a tube which contained a stem with a tip,[159] a forceps (kalbo),[160] cupping glasses, and a stomach tube (kulcha).[161] The last was designed by the famous physician Mar Samuel, who used it on himself. There was also the *gubtha,* perhaps a catheter. The professional office apparel consisted of a leather apron, or *shel harophe.*[162] *Migdal,*[163] a chest or desk, probably constituted the main piece of office furniture. The *kisei tani,*[164] an iron box, or basket, was perhaps for the instruments, medicine, and appliances used by the physician when making the rounds of his patients.[165]

SURGERY

Ancient surgery dealt mostly with setting broken bones, reducing dislocations, stopping hemorrhages, removing arrows, and healing wounds.

Hemorrhage was stopped with styptics, such as rabbit's hair, mill dust, and moss (from skulls found in the graveyard). Wounds were irrigated with boiling oil or wine to neutralize poisonous substances. Fractures were common among early man, who did his best to set them. To relieve pain by immobilization, he placed his fractured limb in loam, mud, or clay. He also used splints of wood to immobilize the fractured parts.

Judging from the description of the wounds in the Old Testament period, wound surgery was fairly well developed. Wounds in different parts of the body caused by weapons were mentioned in the Old Testament;[166] for example: a perforating wound inflicted by a *romach* (javelin or dagger);[167] a penetrating wound of the abdomen, by a sword;[168] a piercing wound into the chest cavity at the region of the fifth rib, by a spear; a perforating wound through the heart, with three darts;[169] a wound in the area of the fifth rib, caused by a sword; a fractured skull effected with a nail and workman's hammer;[170] and a mortal wound inflicted on King Gesah by an arrow.

During the Talmudic period, surgery obtained a comparatively high degree of development. Many physicians devoted themselves to surgery, and many surgical instruments were devised.

In severe operations, the patient was given a sleeping potion *(sama de shinta)*[171] which might have opium *(oufion)* as one of its ingredients.[172] Hot compresses before the operation were used for local anesthesia.

A large variety of wounds were mentioned in Talmudic literature. Not all of them, however, can be identified. Judging from the various designations applying to wounds, wound surgery was already well advanced. The term *petza*[173] was applied to a stab wound.[174] *Habbura,* according to the Tosephta, was a blow resulting in the extravasation of blood in the parts; it was either an open wound or one in which the blood gathered under the skin[175] as in simple or infected hematomata.

Mazor[176] was a boil, or abscess, containing septic matter; it was also known in the Talmud as *mursa*. It could open spontaneously or might have to be opened surgically to permit the pus to escape.[177] The general term for a wound was *makka*. *Retiyyah* was a wound resulting from a burn; *tzarebeth*[178] had the same meaning. Three kinds of *makkoth* were described: *makka teriyyah*, a festering wound;[179] *makka nachlah*,[180] a grievous wound; and *makka anusha*,[181] a wound that did not heal. The treatment for wounds was oil and wine, dressings, and bandaging.[182]

The healing of an abscess *(mursa)* was brought about by getting rid of the pus.[183] *Enabatha*, a swelling resembling a large white grape (cognate to the Hebrew *einab*) was perhaps a carbuncle. The treatment for this consisted of a poultice made of a certain vegetable *(tigna)*, mixed with honey or *karpaso*, and mixed with strong wine.[184] The meaning of *nimo* is not clear. According to Jastrow, it was a corroding ulcer, but it was more likely a cancer, for the Talmud posed the following question, "If one has a *nimo* on his foot or on his hand shall he have it cut out and live or let it go and die?"[185] The Midrash related that the son of King Izates developed a *nimo* on his prepuce; thereupon King Izates followed the advice of a court physician and had the boy circumcised.[186] *Simta*,[187] the meaning of which is also not clear, was perhaps a furuncle. *Katith* was a superficial wound or a scab due to a brush burn. Honey was recommended for the treatment of *katith*.[188] *Silu* was a sore effected by injuring the skin by a thorn.[189] *Pedatha* was a lacerated wound produced by a metal weapon, such as a sabre. Mar Samuel said that a wound caused by a metal weapon was always dangerous. He also said that the wound effected by a Persian lance was always fatal.[190]

There was a tradition among the sages of Caesarea that the bite of a spider *(achshemonitha)* was dangerous.[191] R. Samuel bar R. Yitzhak said that a *gumartha* (carbuncle) was a dangerous growth.[192] First-aid treatment for dislocation and contusions was the application of cold compresses to prevent swelling.[193]

There were persons whose wounds healed readily, and there were those whose wounds did not heal.[194] An older person did not respond to treatment as well as a child.[195]

The treatment of wounds consisted first, in cleansing the wound with warm water, then applying dry sponges, dry layers of wool, and lawn or reed grass.[196] R. Ishmael said sponges were used, not because of their absorbent qualities, but because of the protection they gave to the wound.[197] This was disputed by another teacher who said they were placed on the wound to absorb the moisture.[198] Warm water and oil were the two substances with which wounds were cleansed and the dressings saturated.[199] For softening an abscess, a poultice made of fat and wax or a plaster made of certain drugs mixed with herbs was applied either on the skin or on the top of the shirt over the abscess. Fine ashes removed from the top of burned coals were recommended as a dusting powder.[200] The skins of onions and garlic were applied to the wounds as a healing or protective[201] agent. Grape leaves were thought to possess healing virtues.[202] Dyer's madder was considered to have healing virtues,[203] particularly when made from a plant that had five, seven, or nine garlands.[204] A hot towel applied to a wound was thought to be of therapeutic value.[205] Abaye quoted his mother to the effect that the ingredients of an *ispalonith* were wax, resin, or tar.[206]

External wounds were closed by sutures. The edges of open wounds that would not heal were trimmed in order that union might be effected.[207]

The first surgery mentioned in the Old Testament was that of circumcision. The Egyptians performed this operation from time immemorial. This operation among Jews was, and still is, largely performed by circumcision specialists *(mohel, or rophe mumhe, a practical surgeon)*,[208] although an authorized physician *(rophe uman)* was considered preferable.[209] This operation frequently was associated with prolonged and serious symptoms. Owing to the frequent deaths resulting from the operation, it was decided that, if more than two children from the same mother died as a result of circumcision, the third child did not have to be circumcised.[210]

Trephining of the skull was another operation referred to in the Talmud. The closure of the opening, when there was a loss of bone substance, was made by a plate *(kidduk shel kruyah)*,[211] Trephining was performed to relieve pressure from a growth within the head.[212]

Abdominal operations were performed for the removal of excessive fat.[213] An operation for making an artificial anus in the newborn (congenital imperforate anus) was described.[214] Extirpation of the spleen was performed[215] as was Cesarean section when the mother died during labor, and it was thought that the fetus still survived.[216] It is not clear whether the Cesarean operation was also performed on living mothers. Embryotomy was performed to save the mother.

Intubation of the larynx *(kerumith kaneh)* was practiced on animals. The couching operation for cataract *(depressio cataractae)* was a favorite one. There was a cataract specialist *(ikutta)* in every sizable town of

Palestine. Thus said the Midrash, "Woe to the community whose *ik-kuta* himself is blind."[217] Umbilical hernia in the newborn was prevented by applying a round object over the umbilicus, which was kept in position by a bandage.[218] This form of treatment still prevails. Plastic surgery of the head was referred to.[219] Orthopedic appliances, such as crutches and braces, were used.[220]

PHLEBOTOMY

Phlebotomy was largely practiced as a prophylaxis. It was believed that too much blood was the cause of skin eruptions and many other diseases. According to Samuel, blood letting should be performed not more than once in thirty days to keep the body in normal health, and its practice should be gradually lessened with the age of the person.

The Talmud did not specify at what age blood letting should begin and at what age it should be stopped. It should be borne in mind that Galen established the age of blood letting as between fourteen and sixty years, barring exceptional cases. "It should not be performed when the individual runs a high temperature. . . . In febrile diseases, it may be done on the second day."[221] This recalls the teaching of Celsus, who thought it was dangerous to draw off blood during high fever. "Venesection should not be performed on a full stomach."[222] Food and a moderate quantity of wine should be administered to the patient soon after the operation."[223] "The back of the shoulders and the head were the favorite positions for venesection."

R. Muna warned not to touch the wound caused by drawing off the blood. As late as the sixteenth century, venesection was performed on young children in the cities of Venice and Padua, Italy. One hundred years later, Sanden collected twenty-three cases of blood letting in children of tender age. Chemnitz reported cases of blood letting in the newborn. The blood was drawn off from the navel before the cord was tied. In the Middle Ages, well-organized churches had phlebotomists in an adjoining room to the church. Bleeding was also suggested by means of leeches[224] and cupping.[225] Pure wine and fat meat roasted on coals were recommended as a restorative diet.

OBSTETRICS AND GYNECOLOGY

The anatomy of the female genital organs was not described in detail. Vaginal examination was conducted by female assistants, and the findings were reported to the physician.

The menstrual period, which was stated normally to last seven days, was said to be marked by pain around the navel, and by yawning, sneezing and chills. Cohabitation with women, bleeding from the vagina, regardless of the cause, was forbidden.

R. Simon said that the female genital organs were constructed in chambers and well-defined passages. If it were not for this, delivery of the child would come on abruptly without any warning.[226] Cephalic presentation was considered the only normal position for the fetus to assume before delivery. The delivery was made on a birth stool. Post-mortem Cesarean section was performed to save the life of the child.[227] In extreme cases, embryotomy was resorted to, to save the life of the mother.[228] Soon after delivery, the newly born was bathed and oiled;[229] it was put to the breast after twenty-four hours. Nursing the child was considered the sacred duty of the mother. When this was impossible, a wet nurse was employed. Special care was exercised before the wet nurse was permitted to attend to the child. Her physical and moral standards were carefully examined.

It was of paramount importance, for ritual reasons, to ascertain the source of vaginal bleeding to eliminate menstrual blood that would necessitate a seven-day period of purification from the time the hemorrhage stopped. Arrest of menstruation was not considered the only symptom of pregnancy. The Talmudists were aware that pregnancy, in rare cases, could occur in the presence of menstruation and that amenorrhea did not positively signify pregnancy.[230] Other symptoms of pregnancy were facial pallor or greenish appearance and "heaviness of heart and body." The origin of milk in female breasts was regarded as a conversion from the menstrual blood,[231] which ceased to flow. The duration of pregnancy was calculated to be 271, 272, or 273 days.[232]

For a period of fifteen centuries, there was a gross ignorance of embryology. This was particularly anomalous, since the preservation of the species was the natural urge of all races. The very discussion of procreation was considered taboo and sacrilegious. Philosophers and theologians confined themselves to discussing how the soul or the spiritual part of man came into being but were reluctant to speak on how the physical man came into existence.

In view of the general attitude towards the enigma of birth, it will be of interest to learn that the Talmudic teachers freely discussed embryologic problems. A few references will show how the subject of embryology was understood by Talmudic teachers during the first five centuries A.D., "At the end of forty-one days from the time of conception, the embryo assumes human form and may be recognized as such." This statement was based on observation of a case: An autopsy was made on a servant of the Egyptian Queen Cleopatra, who was sentenced to death for adultery. Her womb was examined forty-one days after intercourse, and it showed a fully formed embryo.[233] Abba Saul described the appearance of an embryo at its first formation (about six weeks), "Its size is that of a locust; its eyes are like two specks of a fly at some distance from each other; so are the nostrils and ears; its feet like two silken cords, the mouth like a hair . . ."[234]

Mar Samuel Yarchanai thought it impossible to recognize the sex before the end of the fourth month. "Both parents contribute equally to the physical part of the body."[235] "The human embryo is formed by the male element and is hatched in the coagulated blood of the female uterus"[236]—an old Aristotelian teaching.

"The male seminal fluid originates in the head and follows along the spinal column to the productive organs"[237]—a Galenic doctrine. "Only the essence of the seminal fluid is necessary for fecundation, not the fluid as a whole"[238]—an observation which anticipated the discovery of Von Baer and Newport that only one spermatozoon was engaged in fertilization.

"The seminal fluid possesses the elements of all organs."[239] "A woman can only conceive when close to her menstrual period."[240] R. Hiyah recalled a tradition that a woman who had more menstrual blood was more productive than one who had little blood. "Seminal discharge, after three days, becomes impotent."[241] "The whole structure is developed simultaneously and not organ by organ. . . . Physical deformities in the newborn were not caused by hereditary influence through the seminal fluid, for if this would be the case, blind and lame parents would transmit their abnormalities to their children."[242] "The birth of male or female depends upon the one who plants the seeds first. If the female plants first,[243] the offspring will be a male; if the male has the priority, it will be a female. If both plant at the same time, a twin conception will result."[244] Another opinion was that twin pregnancies were caused by the division of the "drop."[245] The umbilical cord supplied nourishment to the fetus and connected the fetus with the mother. R. Shimlai gave a characteristic description of the fetus as it lay crouched in the uterus; its hands were on its temples; its elbows touched its thighs; its heels touched its buttocks; its mouth was closed. It was nourished from the mother's food. It did not defecate, since this would kill the mother.[246]

Certain diseases have long been known to follow the laws of heredity. In choosing a wife, the Talmud advised to investigate her family history.[247] The bride had to subject herself to an examination in the town bathhouse by female relatives of the bridegroom.[248] Bodily defects and skin diseases could easily be detected by such methods. Physical stature and complexion were considered by the Talmudists to be controlled by hereditary influence. Thus said Reish Lakish, "A tall man shall not marry a tall woman lest they will give birth to a giant . . . a dwarf shall not marry a dwarf lest they will give birth to a pigmy . . . a blonde shall not marry a blonde lest they may give birth to an albino (boheik)."[249] "A man of dark complexion shall not marry a dark woman lest the child be black."[250]

R. Hiyah cited a case, which came before R. Simeon ben Gamliel, of four sisters who lost three children each, through hemorrhage following circumcision. The rabbi gave his opinion that the sisters possessed an inherited blood disease and that they did not need to resort to the operation again, adding that there were families having thin blood whose hemorrhages were hard to control.[251] Incidentally, the Talmud hinted that hemophilia was a sex-linked disease passed on only to males and only through females.

Talmudic views with regard to heredity were illustrated by the fact that two mentally deficient persons were not permitted to marry, whereas two deaf-mutes were given such permission. The explanation of this may be that deafness could be acquired as a result of upper respiratory infection and thus might not necessarily be transmissable, whereas mental deficiency was more apt to be hereditary.

Talmudic medical discussions were not confined to the closed doors of the academies. There were occasional discussions with nonJewish scholars. R. Judah (the Prince) frequently held discussions with the Roman Emperor Antoninus; both were contemporaries of Galen. On one occasion, Antoninus expressed himself that the vital principle of a person joined the embryo at the time of conception. On the other hand, R. Judah was of the opinion that it entered the body at the time of birth. "Would the embryo not perish within the womb if it did not possess a vital principle?" questioned Antoninus. This argument seems to have convinced the rabbi that the vital principle entered the embryo at the time of conception.[252] He held, however, that the germ of mentality and concomitant inclinations for good or evil entered the body at the time of birth.

TALMUDIC PHYSICIANS

One of the most prominent Talmudic physicians of the Rabbinic class was Mar Samuel ben Abba ha Cohen (160–257), popularly known as Samuel (Yarchanai), the Astronomer. His biography is of more than passing interest and may prove interesting reading. Samuel was born in Nehardea (Babylonia) in the year 165 of the present era. His father Abba bar Abba, although a prominent teacher of the law, did not use his learning as a "pickaxe to dig with."[253] He was a silk merchant. On frequent occasions, his commercial ventures took him to Palestine. Samuel had shown unusual mental faculties from early childhood. His local teachers, after instructing him for a brief period, proved to be unequal to the task of instructing this young genius. His father, who was also a learned man, soon realized that Samuel was getting ahead of him. He therefore sent him to the neighboring town of Nisibis to the academy of R. Judah. It is not stated how long young Samuel studied at Nisibis; but when he returned to Nehardea, he was qualified to become the disciple of the celebrated sage Levi ben Sisi. His progress was so great that in a short time he became an associate instead of a disciple of his teacher.

Aside from his eminence as a student of law, ethics, and astronomy, he excelled in the art of medicine, as may be seen from his medical aphorisms and dietetic rules scattered through all the Talmud. He emphatically opposed the views that disease was caused by evil spirits, insisting that all sickness was brought on by the noxious influences in the air and the effects of climatic conditions upon the human organism. Cleanliness, he maintained, was the most important factor to normal health.

He did not call himself "physician," perhaps because it was considered sacrilegious for a human to call himself *rophe* ("healer"), which was a divine attribute, and it was certainly not becoming for the head of a Talmudic academy and a judge. Perhaps he only attended to exceptional cases, such as that of R. Judah (the Prince). The science of medicine in antiquity was largely a part of general culture, which included also the sciences of mathematics, astronomy, philosophy, and metaphysics. Not all who theorized and wrote on medical subjects were practical physicians.

His wide reputation as astronomer and physician perhaps hindered him from being ordained as a rabbi. It is related that when Samuel saw that R. Judah was sorry that he couldn't confer on him the degree of Rabbi, he humorously remarked to R. Judah not to be sorry for him, "I have seen in the Book of Adam that it is written, Samuel the Astronomer, shall be called Hakim (wise) not Rabbi."[254]

Because of his liberal views, his opinions were followed in matters pertaining to civil law. On questions pertaining to religious law, the decisions of Rab, his colleague, were preferred.

Mar Samuel was one of the few Talmudic sages who devoted his time to medicine as a science. It is not stated definitely whether he was a practicing physician. He probably attended to exceptional cases, such as that of R. Judah. His time was occupied as a teacher and a judge. The science of medicine in antiquity was a part of general culture, such as the sciences of mathematics, astronomy, philosophy, and metaphysics. Not all who theorized and wrote on medical subjects were practical physicians. It is doubtful whether Aristotle, Plato, and later the Roman Celsus adopted medicine as their profession.

It is not stated what made him leave Palestine abruptly. He returned to his native town of Nehardea, where his reputation as a teacher of law soon attracted many students around him. Among them was the Exilarch Mar Ukba who appointed him to the exalted position of judge of the Diaspora.[255] He succeeded as head of the academy of Nehardea upon the death of R. Shilah. This appointment was the beginning of the brilliant phase in his life's history.

Mar Samuel was very unfortunate in his family life; he had no sons. His two daughters were captured by Roman soldiers during the war and were taken to Sepphoris (Palestine). They were eventually ransomed by the Jewish community of that city. They died in early life after having been married successfully.[256]

Among the last of the Talmudic physicians R. Gamliel Bathrai should be mentioned, the last prince of the house of Hillel to occupy the position of Nasi (Exilarch) from 400 to 425 A.D. under the reign of Theodosius II. Marcellus Empericus from Bordeaux, the court physician of Emperor Theodosius, in his work "de Medicamentis Empericis Physicis,"[257] cited Gamliel's formula for diseases of the spleen.

SCOPE OF TALMUDIC MEDICINE

It is often questioned, if Talmudic medicine was in such a high state of development, why did it not become more known to the outside world and why did the Talmudic doctors leave no written records. The answer is that Talmudic medicine had not been transmitted as works of medicine, pure and simple, and were not set down as medical facts, but were to illustrate certain points of law. Furthermore, the Talmudic style had been very difficult for the student of medicine to understand. The subject was not systematically arranged. In many instances, it was hard to identify Aramaic and other terms for diseases. Many mistakes have also crept in while copying from one manuscript to another. Some medical terms lost their original significance during their centuries of wandering through countries where the Talmudic dialects were no longer spoken. The true meaning of the sickness and symptoms in some cases could only be identified by the account of the case. When no description was given, one was compelled to search for corresponding words in cognate languages, such as Hebrew, Arabic, Syriac, Assyrian, Ethiopic, and Coptic. Frequently Latin and Greek dialects also had to be resorted to. The nomenclature of remedies was also dependent on the studies of the philologist.

Attention should also be called to the fact that the Talmud was not the work of one man; it was a collection of opinions and decisions of more than 3000 scholars, covering a period of about 650 years. In other words, it was an encyclopedic work embracing all matters known to antiquity. In a work of this kind, one should expect to find contradictory statements and divergent views. One scholar displayed essential knowledge, while another showed no attempt to reach higher standards than the period in which he lived. In one place, originality and initiative were revealed, while in another place dependence and subservience to tradition were manifested. On one point, foreign influence was dominant, and in another foreign ideas were barred. To speak, therefore, of the Talmud as the opinion of one person, as often expressed by writers, and to hold up the opinion of one as that of the Talmud at large is unsound.

In concluding this chapter, it might be well to cite Dr. Fielding H. Garrison in his "History of Medicine" on Hebrew physicians:

Through their peculiarly analytical cast of mind, their intensive mode of thought, and their appreciation of the value of theoretical experimentation, they acquired a correct materialistic way of looking at concrete things. While medical men under Christianity were still trifling with charms, amulets, saintly relics, and other superstitions, the Jewish physician looked upon these things with a secret contempt.

References and Notes

1. Yalkut Shimoni; Psalm 73; Mid Shocher Tob 73.
2. Abodah Zarah 28-a.
3. Ibid.
4. Gittin 67-b.
5. Yoma 85-a.
6. Trumah 1.
7. Nedarim 50-b.
8. Ibid.
9. Gittin 69-a.
10. Taanith 3:4; 21-b.
11. Galen: De Acut. Morb. Victu 1, 8.
12. Brochoth 8-a; Sofrim 17:5.
13. Taanith 27-b; Brochoth 8-a.
14. Cited by Perlman, M.: Vol. 2, p. 27.

15. Sotah 35-a.
16. Yebomoth 62-b.
17. Brochoth 40-a.
18. Nedarim 41-b.
19. Kethuboth 77-b.
20. Ibid.
21. See Gordon, B. L.: Ophthalmology in the Bible and the Talmud. Arch. Ophth., May, 1933.
22. Kethuboth 77-b.
23. Taanith 21-b.
24. Ibid.
25. Gittin 69.
26. Erubin 41-b; Shabbath 33-a.
27. Shabbath 33-a.
28. Ibid.
29. Bechoroth 44-b.
30. Brochoth 62.
31. Y. Shabbath 14-d.
32. Luke 14:2.
33. Shabbath 33-a.
34. Bechoroth 7-b.
35. Yoma 84-a.
36. Kethuboth 110-b.
37. Shabbath 41; Baba Meziah 113.
38. J. Shekalim 5:2.
39. Gittin 70-a.
40. Shabbath 147-b.
41. Ibid. 11-a.
42. Shabbath 66-b.
43. Gittin 69-a.
44. Ibid.
45. Abodah Zarah 40-b.
46. Gittin 69.
47. Ibid. 51-a.
48. Erubin 54-a.
49. Shabbath 118-b.
50. Moed Katan 27.
51. J. Shabbath 14:4.
52. Pliny 26:6.
53. Shabbath 81-a; Brochoth 55-a.
54. Nedarim 22-a.
55. Abodah Zarah 28.
56. Ibid.
57. Yoma 83.
58. Ibid.
59. Kethuboth 61-a.
60. I Kings 15–23.
61. Sotah 10.
62. Tanchuma Tazria.
63. Yebomoth 64.

64. Shabbath 11-a.
65. Ibid. 10-a.
66. Erubin 29.
67. Brochoth 40-a; 28-b.
68. Ibid. 40, 48-a.
69. Gittin 69.
70. Ibid.
71. Kethuboth 60.
72. Baba Kama 80-a.
73. Gittin 69-b.
74. Jastrow: Talmudic and Aramaic Dictionary.
75. Brochoth 40-a.
76. Ibid.
77. Erubin 29-d.
78. Shabbath 108.
79. Brochoth 41-a.
80. Shabbath 40-a.
81. Brochoth 40-a.
82. Ibid.
83. Ibid.
84. Abodah Zarah 28-a.
85. Yoma 84.
86. Abodah Zarah 28-a.
87. Yalkut Shimoni; Song of Songs 988.
88. Shabbath 152-a.
89. Ibid. 65.
90. Ibid 111-a.
91. Brochoth 44-b.
92. Ibid. 40-a.
93. J. Abodah Zarah 3.
94. Shabbath 90-a.
95. Gittin 69-a.
96. Kethuboth 75-a.
97. Baba Meziah 107.
98. Kethuboth 77-a; Num. R. 19.
99. Gordon, B. L.: Ophthalmology in the Bible and the Talmud. Arch. Ophth. 9:751–788, May, 1933.
100. Shabbath 108-b.
101. Mark 8:23; John 9:6, 7.
102. Tacitus 4, 81.
103. Baba Bathra 126-b.
104. Shabbath 107-b.
105. Wood, C. A.: American Encyclopedia and Dictionary of Ophthalmology. Cleveland Press, Chicago, 1913–1917, Vol. 3.
106. Baba Meziah 85-b.
107. Shabbath 108-b.
108. Aicho Rabba 2.
109. *Cohol* must have been a popular drug. According to Stein, an oculist in Persia and Turkey, it is still called *cohol* (Turkai 1-66). In Arabia, oculists are called *Cahalin*.

110. Shabbath 109-a.
111. Tobit 6:6.
112. Shabbath 78-a.
113. Buck: Medizinische Volksglauben aus Schwaben. Berlin, 1898, p. 44.
114. "Heat withdraws heat" is an old Talmudic aphorism. Shabbath 41-a.
115. Numbers Rabba 18:22; Leviticus Rabba 22.
116. Shabbath 109-a.
117. Ibid.
118. Kethuboth 77-b.
119. Ibid.
120. "American Encyclopedia and Dictionary of Ophthalmology." Chicago.
121. Bechoroth 38-b.
122. Kethuboth 60-a.
123. Yoma 74-b.
124. Yoma 84-a.
125. Baba Meziah 83.
126. Niddah 30-b.
127. Shabbath 88-b.
128. Abodah Zarah 26-a.
129. Yoma 72-b; Shabbath 88-b.
130. Baba Bathra 47-b.
131. Baba Kama 85-b.
132. Shabbath 147-b.
133. Brochoth 36-a; Shabbath 134-b.
134. Baba Kama 80.
135. Ibid. 82-a.
136. Shabbath 108-b.
137. Mid. Tanchuma B'Shalach.
138. Yoma 83.
139. Niddah 8-b.
140. Shabbath 134.
141. Yoma 78-b.
142. Kedushin 30-b.
143. Kelim 28:3.
144. Ibid.
145. Ibid.
146. Shabbath 110-a.
147. Cited by Epstein, W.: Medizin im Neuen Testament und im Talmud. Stuttgart, 1903, p. 288.
148. Shabbath 110-b.
149. Libra 5:19–22.
150. Libra 23–27.
151. Mid. Psalms 73.
152. Exodus Rabba 30.
153. Brochoth 57-b; Kethuboth 103-b.
154. The will of R. Eliezer.
155. J. Brochoth 5–6.
156. Bechoroth 38.
157. Ibid.
158. Keilim 16:8.

159. Kelim 17:12.
160. Ibid.
161. Nedarim 50-b
162. Kelim 27:5.
163. Ibid. 2:4.
164. Ibid. 12:3.
165. Ibid.
166. Isaiah 1:6.
167. Judges 5:8.
168. II Samuel 20:10.
169. Ibid. 18:14.
170. Judges 5:26.
171. Baba Meziah 83-a.
172. J. Abodah Zarah II 40-d.
173. Isaiah 1:6.
174. Ibid.
175. T. Shabbath 8:23.
176. Hosea 5:13.
177. Eduyoth 2:5.
178. Leviticus 13:28.
179. Isaiah 1:6.
180. Jeremiah 10:19.
181. Ibid. 15:18.
182. Isaiah 1:6.
183. Eduyoth 2:5.
184. Abodah Zarah 28-a.
185. Abodah Zarah 10-b.
186. Mid. Genesis 46:10.
187. Abodah Zarah 28-a.
188. Shabbath 77.
189. Abodah Zarah 28.
190. Gittin 70-a.
191. J. Shabbath 14:4.
192. Ibid.
193. Shabbath 148-a.
194. Baba Kama 84.
195. Baba Meziah 107-b.
196. Shabbath 134.
197. Mid. Leviticus 15.
198. Kelim 28:3.
199. Shabbath 134-b.
200. Pesachim 39; Kelim 28:3.
201. Tosephta Shabbath 6:3.
202. Ibid. 6:2.
203. Ibid.
204. Ibid.
205. J. Shabbath 9:3.
206. Shabbath 133.
207. Hulin 77-a.
208. Abodah Zarah 27-a.

209. Sanhedrin 91-a.
210. Shabbath 134; Hulin 47.
211. Hulin 57; Kethuboth 57-b; Oholoth 2:3.
212. Abodah Zarah 5:2.
213. Baba Meziah 83-b.
214. Shabbath 134-b; Niddah 41.
215. Abodah Zarah 44-a; Sanhedrin 21.
216. Arechin 7-b; Aboth di R. Nathan 40-b.
217. Mid. Leviticus 5:6.
218. Shabbath 66-b.
219. Hulin 77-b; T. Oholoth 2.
220. Shabbath 65-a.
221. Nedarim 54.
222. Shabbath 129-a.
223. Gittin 70-a; Shabbath 129-a.
224. Abodah Zarah 12-b.
225. Shabbath 145-b.
226. Mid. Leviticus 18.
227. Arechin 7-a.
228. Oholoth 7:6.
229. Shabbath 129.
230. Hagigah 14-15; Niddah 31-a.
231. Niddah 9.
232. Ibid. 38.
233. Ibid. 30.
234. Ibid. 25-a.
235. Ibid. 31-a.
236. Mid. Leviticus Rabba 14.
237. Cited by Mid. Rephuah 3:3.
238. Niddah 31-a.
239. Mid. Trumah 3.
240. Niddah 31.
241. J. Shabbath 9:3.
242. Hulin 69.
243. Niddah 31-a.
244. Ibid. 25-b.
245. Ibid. 27; Yebomoth 98.
246. Niddah 30-b; 51-a.
247. Yebomoth 64-b.
248. Kethuboth 5-b.
249. Bechoroth 45-b.
250. Ibid. 45-b.
251. Yebomoth 64.
252. Sanhedrin 91.
253. Abboth 4:7.
254. Baba Meziah 85-b; 86-a.
255. Sanhedrin 17-b.
256. Kethuboth 23-a.
257. Libra 21

INDEX

INDEX

Note: Page numbers in *italics* refer to illustrations.

797